Thoracic Radiology THE REQUISITES

SERIES EDITOR   **James H. Thrall,** M.D.
Radiologist-in-Chief
Department of Radiology
Massachusetts General Hospital
Juan M. Taveras Professor of Radiology
Harvard Medical School
Boston, Massachusetts

OTHER VOLUMES IN THE REQUISITES™ SERIES   Gastrointestinal Radiology

Pediatric Radiology

Neuroradiology

Nuclear Medicine

Ultrasound

Musculoskeletal Imaging

Cardiac Radiology

Genitourinary Radiology

Mammography

Vascular and Interventional Radiology

Thoracic Radiology

THE REQUISITES

THERESA C. McLOUD, M.D.

Director of Thoracic and Cardiac Radiology
Associate Radiologist-in-Chief
Director of Education
Massachusetts General Hospital
Professor of Radiology
Harvard Medical School
Boston, Massachusetts

with 822 illustrations

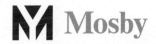 Mosby

St. Louis Baltimore Boston Carlsbad Chicago Minneapolis New York Philadelphia Portland
London Milan Sydney Tokyo Toronto

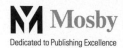

Dedicated to Publishing Excellence

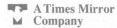
A Times Mirror
Company

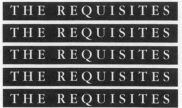

THE REQUISITES is a proprietary trademark
of Mosby, Inc.

Publisher: Geoff Greenwood
Editor: Elizabeth Corra
Development Editor: Mia Cariño
Project Manager: Linda Clarke
Senior Production Editor: Veda King
Senior Composition Specialist: Pamela Merritt
Design Manager: Carolyn O'Brien
Manufacturing Manager: Willam A. Winneberger, Jr.

Printed in the United States of America
Composition by Mosby Electronic Production, Philadelphia
Printing/binding by R.R. Donnelley & Sons Co.

Mosby, Inc.
11830 Westline Industrial Drive
St. Louis, MO 63146

Library of Congress Cataloging-in-Publication Data

McLoud, Theresa C.
    Thoracic radiology : the requisites / Theresa C. McLoud.
        p.   cm. — (Requisites series)
    Includes bibliographical references and index.
    ISBN 0-8016-6354-7
    1. Chest—Imaging.   I. Title.   II. Series.
    [DNLM: 1. Thoracic Diseases—radiography.   2. Lung Diseases—
radiography.   3. Radiography, Thoracic—methods.   WF 975 M478t
1998]
    RC941.M356   1998
    617.5'407572—dc21
    DNLM/DLC
    for Library of Congress   98-18593
                                                                   CIP

98 99 00 01 02 03 / 9 8 7 6 5 4 3 2 1

Contributors

Meenakshi Bhalla, M.D.
Former Assistant Professor of Radiology
New York University Medical Center
New York, New York

Phillip M. Boiselle, M.D.
Director of Thoracic CT
Assistant Professor of Radiology
Temple University School of Medicine
Philadelphia, Pennsylvania

Jo-Anne O. Shepard, M.D.
Associate Professor of Radiology
Harvard Medical School
Associate Radiologist
Massachusetts General Hospital
Boston, Massachusetts

Beatrice Trotman-Dickenson, M.D., M.R.C.P.,
    F.R.C.R.
Clinical Assistant in Thoracic Radiology
Massachusetts General Hospital
Boston, Massachusetts

To my nephews,
Malcolm and Paul

Foreword

Thoracic Radiology: THE REQUISITES is the ninth book in a series designed to provide core material in major subspecialty areas of radiology for use by residents during their training and by practicing radiologists seeking to review or expand their knowledge.

Thoracic radiology presents a special challenge to the development of a book for THE REQUISITES™ series, because imaging studies of the chest continue to represent the largest aggregate number of procedures performed in contemporary radiology. How beguiling is the simple "chest x-ray" and yet how infinite are the diagnostic possibilities! Dr. Theresa McLoud and her contributors have done a magnificent job of distilling the essential facts and concepts of thoracic radiology into a text that will serve the resident and practicing radiologist equally well.

Each volume of THE REQUISITES™ series lends itself to a unique organization. In *Thoracic Radiology: THE REQUISITES,* Dr. McLoud has structured the text in a logical fashion, which first examines technical and anatomic considerations in imaging the chest and investigates the important radiographic signs used in the diagnosis of chest disease. The book then explores the lung, airways, pulmonary vasculature, mediastinum and pleura. These discussions are further subdivided by anatomy and disease category. By organizing the text in this way, Dr. McLoud allows the reader to access desired information quickly and to use the book efficiently for both initial introduction to and regular review of this complex subspecialty.

A major strength of THE REQUISITES™ series is that each author prepares a truly new book. The latest information on all imaging modalities is placed in the context of radiology practice today rather than grafted onto a preexisting text of historic approaches. Dr. McLoud and her contributors have used their fresh canvas to excel-

lent advantage. They depict thoracic radiology in a modern clinical and methodological context. In particular, the continued emergence of computed tomography for studying the thorax is strongly addressed.

In some sense, those entering training in radiology are forced to "start over" in developing their medical knowledge base. The fundamental principles of basic science and clinical medicine that are learned in medical school provide the necessary background for training in radiology. However, the task of acquiring the specific knowledge and skills required to interpret radiologic examinations is left almost entirely to residency training. Therefore, a resident entering a subspecialty rotation in a radiology training program faces the formidable challenge of obtaining a working knowledge of subspecialty specifics in a very short period of time.

This observation was the basis for creating THE REQUISITES™ in Radiology series. One volume in the series is devoted to each of the major subspecialty areas. The length and format of each volume is dictated by the material being covered, but the principal goal is to equip the resident with a text that provides the basic factual, conceptual, and interpretive material required for clinical practice.

I believe residents in radiology will find *Thoracic Radiology: THE REQUISITES* to be an excellent tool for learning the subject. The book provides both basic and state-of-the-art information in all chapters. In keeping with the philosophy of the series, the book can be reasonably read and reread during successive thoracic radiology rotations in a residency program. Physicians in practice and those participating in fellowship programs should find *Thoracic Radiology: THE REQUISITES* attractive for the same reason—it serves as a concise and useful way to build and refresh their knowledge in the area. Furthermore, I hope that chest physicians, cardiologists, pulmonary specialists, thoracic surgeons, and emergency medicine physicians, as well as their residency and fellowship trainees, will consider this a user-friendly vehicle for exploring imaging of the chest.

I congratulate Dr. Theresa McLoud and her contributors for an outstanding contribution to THE REQUISITES™ in Radiology.

James H. Thrall, M.D.

Radiologist-in-Chief
Department of Radiology
Massachusetts General Hospital
Juan M. Taveras Professor of Radiology
Harvard Medical School
Boston, Massachusetts

Preface

THE REQUISITES™ in Radiology series is designed to provide standard textbooks in each of the subspecialties of radiology, primarily for use by radiology residents throughout their years of training. This particular book in thoracic radiology is also designed to meet the educational needs of those training in pulmonary medicine, thoracic surgery, and critical care. This book defines the basic knowledge that radiology students need to master. It attempts to integrate a number of imaging modalities that are essential in the diagnostic imaging approach to clinical problems. These include standard chest radiography, computed tomography (CT), and magnetic resonance imaging (MRI).

The book begins with chapters dealing with technical factors and the anatomy of the thorax. This is followed by an extensive review of important readiographic signs used in the diagnosis of chest disease. The approach is integrated, emphasizing signs on standard radiographs as well as cross-sectional imaging including CT and MRI. The remainder of the text is devoted to specific disease processes with particular emphasis on anatomic areas such as the lung, the airways, the mediastinum, and pulmonary vasculature. The final chapter provides a brief summary of the important interventional techniques used by the radiologist in the diagnosis of thoracic disease.

Each of the chapters is extensively supplemented with tables and boxes that provide summaries of information presented in the text, including clinical features of disease processes, pathology, and radiographic signs. The intent of such a format is to allow the radiology resident to correlate clinical findings, pathophysiology, and radiographic observations in important disease processes.

Emphasis is placed on fairly common thoracic diseases, although uncommon diseases are addressed briefly, particularly if the imaging features are diagnostic. Tables of differential diagnosis are provided as appropriate.

The standard chest radiograph still remains the most frequently ordered imaging study. The number of disease processes affecting the thorax is legion, and it has been challenging to encompass all the necessary material in simple and direct form. However, the aim of this book is to provide a curriculum of the most important requisites in thoracic radiology, which will be beneficial to residents at any level of training, to fellows in allied clinical fields, and to physicians in practice. Hopefully it will serve as a valuable learning tool for all of its readers.

Theresa C. McLoud, M.D.

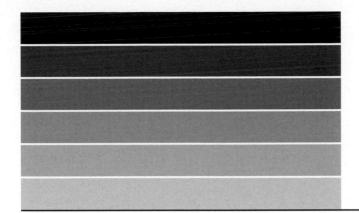

Acknowledgments

I am indebted to several individuals who have contributed directly or indirectly to *Thoracic Radiology: THE REQUISITES*.

First of all, Dr. James H. Thrall, Radiologist-in-Chief at Massachusetts General Hospital (MGH), Series Editor for THE REQUISITES™, provided me with the encouragement to see the project through to completion.

A number of my colleagues at the Department of Radiology at MGH have contributed chapters. I am indebted to Dr. Jo-Anne O. Shepard, Dr. Beatrice Trotman-Dickenson, Dr. Meenakshi Bhalla, and Dr. Phillip Boiselle (a former fellow at MGH) for their unique contributions to this book. Together we have attempted to craft a textbook that reflects not only a large body of factual material about thoracic diseases, but that also offers our own approach to radiographic interpretation and diagnostic investigation.

I also wish to acknowledge all of my clinical colleagues in pulmonary medicine, critical care, and thoracic surgery who over the years have provided both the inspiration and the education in clinical decision-making that have helped to make this book possible. It is only appropriate to recognize the outstanding mentors who have helped to foster and support my career as a thoracic radiologist. Foremost is Dr. Robert Fraser under whose tutelage I trained and with whose textbook mine, of course, will never be able to compete. Dr. Juan Taveras provided me with the opportunity to flourish as a junior staff member and eventually as a division head at MGH. Finally, I wish to acknowledge Dr. Edward Gaensler, a thoracic surgeon, pulmonologist, and clinical researcher extraordinaire, who helped to develop my interest in infiltrative and occupational lung disease.

Finally, this book would not have been possible without the dedication of many people involved in all stages of book preparation. Virginia Raulinaitis typed the manuscript and was never deterred by my many revisions and additions. Gail Abbass, a professional medical writer, edited portions of the manuscript and helped to maintain a consistent style and format throughout the book. Nancy J. Speroni, M.Ed., illustrated the graphic drawings and supervised the photography. I also wish to thank and recognize all the professionals with whom I have worked at Mosby, Inc., especially Anne Patterson, Elizabeth Corra, Mia Cariño, and Veda King. Their support and encouragement over the past few years have made this publication possible.

T.C.M.

Contents

Thoracic Radiology   THE REQUISITES

CHAPTER 1

Thoracic Radiology: Imaging Methods, Radiographic Signs, and Diagnosis of Chest Disease

EXAMINATION TECHNIQUES AND INDICATIONS

Chest Radiography

The plain chest radiograph is the most commonly performed imaging procedure in most radiology practices, generally constituting between 30% and 50% of studies. The standard routine chest roentgenogram consists of an erect radiograph made in the posterior-anterior (PA) projection and a left lateral radiograph, both obtained at full inspiration. The target film distance is six feet. Chest radiographs should be exposed using a high kvp (kilovoltage peak) technique in the range of 100 to 140 kvp (Fig. 1-1). With this technique a grid or air gap is required to reduce scatter radiation. The main advantage of this technique is that the bony structures appear less dense, permitting better visualization of the underlying parenchyma as well as better visualization of the mediastinum. The only drawback is the decreased detectability of calcified lesions and loss of bony detail. Additional views of the chest may be required in special instances (Table 1-1). Shallow oblique radiographs (15°) may be useful in confirming the presence of a suspect-ed nodule. Forty-five degree oblique radiographs are recommended for the detection of asbestos-related pleural plaques. Apical lordotic views (Fig. 1-2) project the clavicles above the chest, improving visualization of the apices and also the middle lobe, particularly in cases of middle-lobe atelectasis. You can use expiration chest radiographs either to detect air trapping or to confirm small pneumothoraces. Lateral decubitus radiographs are commonly used to determine the presence or mobility of pleural effusion. These views can also be

Table 1-1   Indications for nonstandard chest radiography

Projection	Indications
Obliques	Suspected nodule
	Plaques
Lordotic	Apical and middle-lobe disease
Expiration	Air trapping
	Pneumothorax
Lateral decubitus	Pleural effusion
	Pneumothorax

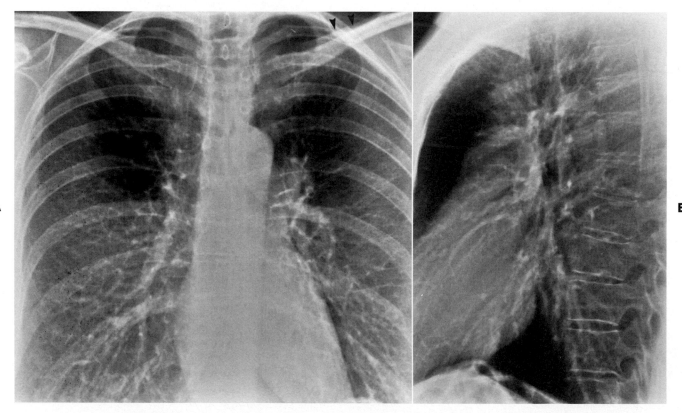

A   B

Fig. 1-1.   Standard PA and lateral chest radiographs obtained at 140 kvp, 12 to 1 grid, and automated phototimed exposure. Note the visibility of retrocardiac vessels and mediastinal structures. Companion shadow of left clavicle (*arrow*).

obtained to detect small pneumothoraces, particularly in patients who are confined to bed and unable to sit or stand erect. Bedside portable examinations may account for as much as 50% of chest radiographs obtained on in-patients. The diagnostic quality of such images is usually limited because of the increased exposure time needed, which results in respiratory motion. Because the target film distance is considerably less than six feet, magnification occurs, particularly of the heart and anterior structures. Many very ill patients, including patients in the intensive care units, must be radiographed at the bedside, resulting in radiographs with limited diagnostic information.

Conventional Chest Tomography and Fluoroscopy

Both of these techniques have become rather obsolete with the widespread application and utilization of computed tomography (CT) (Table 1-2). Fluoroscopy is mainly restricted to the evaluation of diaphragmatic motion. The patient is placed in an oblique position so that both hemidiaphragms can be visualized simultaneously. If diaphragmatic paralysis is present the affected hemidiaphragm will move up during a rapid inspiratory maneuver (such as a sniff).

Conventional tomography has largely been replaced by computed tomography. Occasionally focal lung tomography is still used in the evaluation of the solitary pulmonary nodule, particularly for the detection of calcification. In such cases low kilovoltage technique (65 kvp to 85 kvp) with four to six tomograms at 5 mm intervals and a 20° arc is preferred. However, the more universally utilized procedure for this purpose is CT.

At our institution, conventional tomography is limited to the evaluation of the trachea and major bronchi (Fig. 1-3). Such a study is usually performed as a preliminary to tracheal or carinal resection for central tumors. The

Table 1-2	Indications for chest fluoroscopy and tomography	

Technique	Indications
Fluoroscopy	Diaphragmatic movement
Tomography	Detection of calcification in solitary nodule
	Major airways—trachea

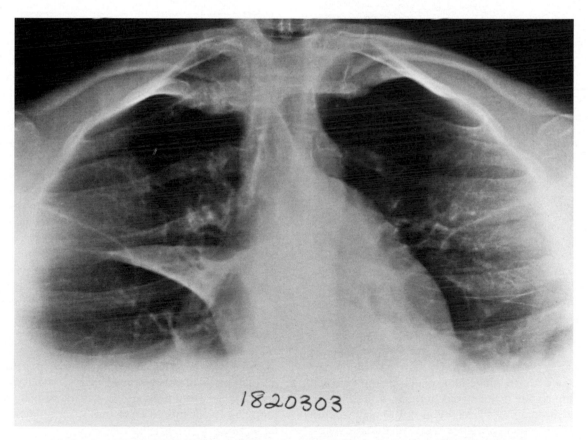

Fig. 1-2. Apical lordotic view. The clavicles are projected above the apices of the lungs. There is an excellent demonstration of right middle-lobe collapse.

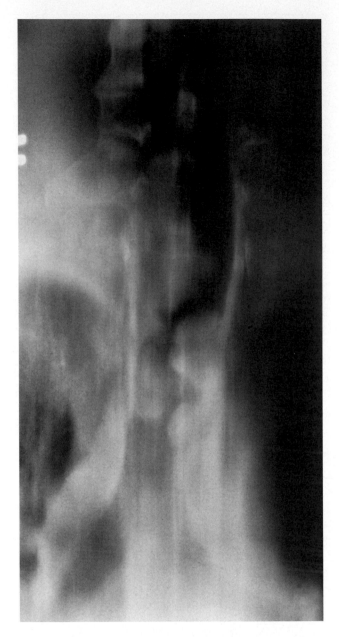

Fig. 1-3.   Tomogram of the trachea. AP view demonstrating multiple tracheal tumors (papillomatosis).

study is done in the range of 90 to 100 kvp using an aluminum filter, a 20° arc, and a high speed screen. Conventional tomography of the airways allows for direct imaging in the coronal and sagittal planes without the need for reconstruction as occurs with conventional CT and results in image degradation. Helical CT will soon supplant conventional tomography for this purpose. Chest tomography may be done with a unit that uses pleuridirectional movements, such as the tri-spiral variety, although the majority of tomography is still done with conventional linear technique. Although pleuridirectional movement provides truer sectional images, it does not provide significantly incremental information.

Box 1-1 Computed Tomography— Common Indications

ABNORMAL CHEST RADIOGRAPH

Staging bronchogenic carcinoma
Solitary nodule, mass, opacity
Infiltrative lung disease
Mediastinum
   Widening
   Mass
   Other abnormality
Pleural abnormalities
Chest-wall lesions

OCCULT DISEASE—NORMAL CHEST RADIOGRAPH

Metastases
Hemoptysis
Suspected bronchiectasis
Myasthenia gravis (thymus)
Endocrine abnormalities (suspect lung tumor or mediastinal parathyroid adenoma)
Unknown source of infection (immunocompromised)
Suspected infiltrative lung disease
Suspected aortic dissection

Computed Tomography

Computed tomography is generally used as a diagnostic study, usually following a standard chest radiograph or when the chest radiograph is considered to be abnormal (Box 1-1). Indications for CT include (1) the staging of bronchogenic carcinoma; (2) a solitary pulmonary nodule, mass, or opacity; (3) diffuse infiltrative lung disease; (4) widened mediastinum, a mediastinal mass, or other abnormality of the mediastinum; (5) an abnormal hilum; (6) pleural abnormalities or the need to differentiate pleural from parenchymal abnormalities; and (7) chest-wall lesions. CT may also be used for the detection of occult disease. Indications include the following: (1) detection of metastatic disease in tumors with a propensity for metastases to the lungs; (2) hemoptysis and/or suspected bronchiectasis; (3) evaluation of the thymus in patients who have myasthenia gravis; (4) evaluation of patients with endocrine abnormalities that are associated either with a suspected lung tumor or parathyroid adenoma; (5) search for an unknown source of infection, especially in the immunocompromised population; (6) evaluation of the pulmonary parenchyma in patients with normal chest films and suspected diffuse infiltrative lung disease or emphysema; and (7) suspicion of aortic dissection.

CT scans should be performed in deep inspiration at total lung capacity. For routine CT of the chest, 8- to 10-

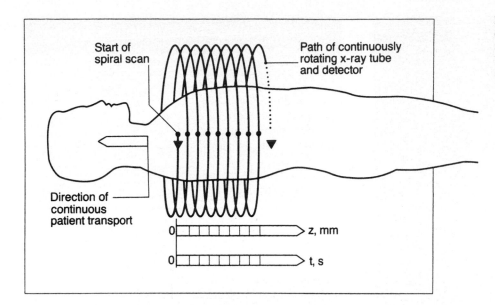

Fig. 1-4. Helical CT scan principle. (From Kalender WA, Seissler W, Vock P: Single breath hold spiral volumetric CT by continuous patient translation and scanner rotation, *Radiology* 173(P):414, 1989.)

Box 1-2 Helical CT—Indications

Routine
Solitary pulmonary nodule
Metastatic disease
Airways
Vascular lesions
Peridiaphragmatic lesions
Pulmonary embolism

---

mm sections are recommended at 1-cm intervals. Thinner 1- to 2-mm sections can be used to study fine details of the pulmonary parenchyma (high-resolution CT [HRCT]). Generally, contiguous spacing throughout the chest is recommended. A short scan time of 1 to 2 seconds is necessary to reduce the effect of respiratory motion. On routine studies the field of view should be adjusted to the size of the thorax, but smaller fields of view may be selected for smaller anatomic parts that require study. A smaller field of view will improve spatial resolution.

In regard to window settings, the routine is to obtain at least two sets of window settings, one for the lung parenchyma and the other for the mediastinum. Suggested settings for the mediastinum are window level of +30 to +50 and window width of +350, and for the lung windows, a width of +1500 and a window level of −500 to −700. The algorithm of reconstruction may be modified either for the mediastinum or lung. In the mediastinum a smoothing or standard algorithm is recommended. This is also sufficient for routine studies of the lung. However, high-rcs-

olution CT requires an algorithm with high spatial resolution that, on most scanners, corresponds to the bone algorithm.

With a proper knowledge of mediastinal and hilar anatomy, contrast material is not required for routine CT of the thorax. However, contrast enhancement may be necessary for the evaluation of known or suspected vascular abnormalities (e.g., aortic aneurysm or dissection), for evaluation of the abnormal hilum, or for certain abnormalities of the pleura. Approximately 100 to 150 ml at an injection rate of 2 ml/sec using an agent with 30% to 40% concentration of iodine is recommended. In hemodynamically normal individuals, the transit time of contrast from an antecubital vein to the right heart is about 3 seconds, 6 seconds to the pulmonary arteries, 9 seconds to the left heart, and 12 to 15 seconds to the major arteries. Although transit times will vary among patients, we recommend as a routine a delay of at least 15 seconds between the onset of the injection and the first image. A power contrast injector should be used.

Recent improvement in scanner technology has led to the introduction of spiral or helical volumetric CT (Box 1-2). Such a CT scanner acquires data continuously and as the patient is transported through the scanner during a single breathhold (Fig. 1-4). Reconstruction of planar slices is produced from the volume scanned. The main advantage of this method is that it permits imaging of a volume of the chest without misregistration due to respiratory motion. Studies indicate that spiral CT is useful in the evaluation of the solitary pulmonary nodule for densitometry as well as for the detection of metastatic disease. Contrast media studies may be used for the detection of pulmonary thromboembolism. High-quality three-dimensional reconstructions as well as two-dimen-

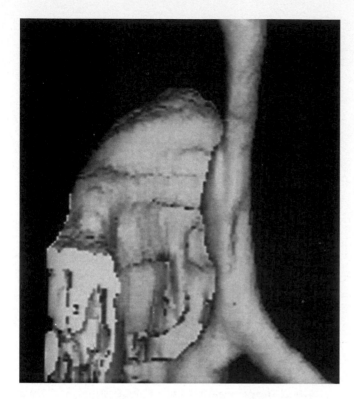

Fig. 1-5. Three-dimensional shaded surface display of the trachea.

sional reformatting in coronal and sagittal planes are possible (Fig. 1-5).

Magnetic Resonance Imaging

Magnetic resonance imaging (MRI) has not had extensive application in the thorax mainly because of problems due to motion artifacts secondary to cardiac and respiratory movements. In addition, the normal lung does not produce an MR signal because of magnetic susceptibility effects. However, MR does provide excellent images of both the mediastinum and the chest wall and does permit direct imaging in the coronal and sagittal as well as the axial planes. General indications for MR in the chest include the following: (1) evaluation of the mediastinum or vascular structures in patients in whom contrast media is contraindicated; (2) diagnosis of aortic dissection and congenital abnormalities of the aorta; (3) evaluation of superior sulcus tumors; (4) imaging of chest-wall lesions and brachial plexus abnormalities; (5) staging of bronchogenic carcinoma with particular reference to direct chest wall and mediastinal invasion; (6) evaluation of posterior mediastinal masses; and (7) follow-up of patients with lymphoma (Box 1-3).

Some general recommendations can be made in regard to technique. Techniques can be varied depending on the clinical indication. In general a body coil is used, and images are obtained in the axial plane using

Box 1-3 Magnetic Resonance—Indications

Contraindication to contrast medium; mediastinal or vascular abnormality
Aortic dissection
Superior sulcus carcinoma
Chest-wall and brachial plexus lesions
Suspected chest-wall and mediastinal invasion by lung cancer
Posterior mediastinal masses
Follow-up lymphoma

two different spin-echo sequences. With high field-strength magnets, ECG gating should be employed. T1-weighted multislice single-echo (echo-time [TE] values of 15 to 30 msec) sequences are always obtained and a T2-weighted sequence with two echoes (TE 60 to 100 msec) is obtained in most instances. T1-weighted images give information concerning diagnosis of masses and the best information on vascular anatomy. The T2-weighted images may render fluid collections distinguishable from solid masses and may also help separate tumor from fibrosis (Fig. 1-6).

In addition to ECG gating, there are several other techniques that can be used to limit or correct motion artifacts. Respiratory compensation and presaturation (destroying the magnetization of incoming blood by repeatedly imposing radiofrequency pulses to the areas adjacent to the image volume) in order to eliminate the artifacts related to blood motion are frequently used. Rapid scanning techniques that allow for acquisition of single or multiple images during a single breathhold (GRASS or FLASH) have been developed. These techniques use decreased flip angles, gradient refocused echoes, and short TR and TE values.

Because MR is often used as a problem-solving procedure, it needs to be correlated carefully with CT scans. For this reason images are usually obtained in the transaxial plane. However it is possible with MR to have direct imaging in the sagittal and coronal planes. The benefits of imaging in the sagittal and coronal planes are that they better elucidate structures oriented longitudinally, and they also reduce the chance of misinterpretation of findings due to volume averaging.

Fast imaging techniques sometimes referred to as "cine-MR" are available for imaging vascular structures and diagnosing vascular abnormalities. These are discussed in more detail in the series dealing with vascular diseases and cardiac imaging. *

---

*Miller SW: *Cardiac Radiology: THE REQUISITES*, 1996.

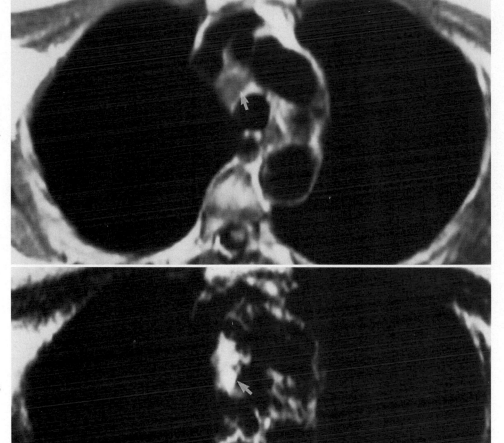

Fig. 1-6. MR of bronchogenic cyst. **A,** T1-weighted image shows low signal intensity of the right paratracheal mass. The low signal intensity is due to the water content of the cyst. **B,** On the T2-weighted image the cyst has greater signal intensity than fat or muscle because of the long T2 value of water.

ANATOMY

Airways

Trachea and main bronchi

The trachea is a midline structure that generally ranges in length from 6 to 9 cm. The wall contains horseshoe-shaped cartilage rings at regular intervals, but the posterior wall is membranous. The upper limits for coronal and sagittal diameters are 25 and 27 millimeters for men and 21 and 23 millimeters for women. The lower limit of normal in both dimensions is 13 mm in men and 10 mm in women. The trachea divides into two major bronchi at the carina. The carinal angle usually measures around 60°, but a wide range of 40° to 75° can be seen in normal adults. The right main bronchus has a more vertical course than the left and its length is considerably shorter. The air column of the trachea, both major bronchi, and the intermediate bronchus are usually visible on well-exposed standard radiographs of the chest in the frontal projection (Figs. 1-7 and 1-8). The right lateral and posterior walls of the trachea are identifiable on PA and lateral chest radiographs as vertically oriented linear opacities called the right paratracheal and posterior tracheal stripes. These are described in more detail in the section on the mediastinum.

Lobar bronchi and bronchopulmonary segments

Table 1-3 summarizes the bronchopulmonary segments of the right and left lung.

Right side The bronchus to the right upper lobe (Fig. 1-9) arises from the lateral aspect of the mainstem bronchus, approximately 2.5 cm from the carina. It then divides into three branches—the anterior, posterior, and apical—each supplying a segment of the right upper lobe. The intermediate bronchus continues distally for 3 to 4 cm from the takeoff of the right upper-lobe bronchus and bifurcates to become the bronchi to the middle and lower lobes. The middle-lobe bronchus arises from the anterolateral wall of the intermediate bronchus almost opposite the origin of the superior segmental bronchus of the lower lobe. It then bifurcates into lateral and medial segments.

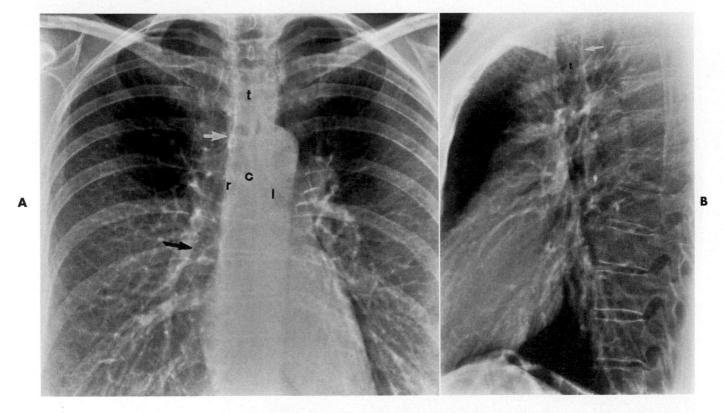

Fig. 1-7.   Tracheal and bronchial anatomy on standard PA and lateral views. *t*, trachea; *c*, carina; *r*, right main bronchus; *l*, left main bronchus; *white arrow*, right paratracheal stripe; *large black arrow*, right intermediate bronchus; *white arrow*, posterior paratracheal stripe.

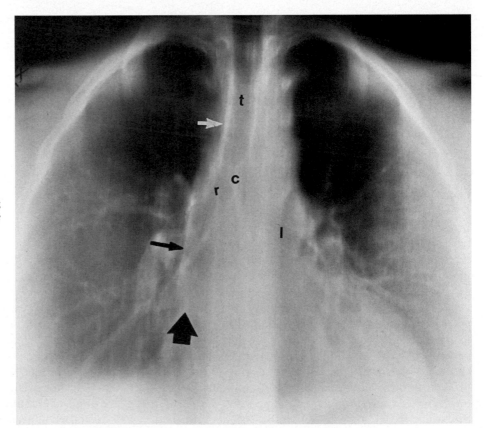

Fig. 1-8.   AP tomogram illustrating anatomy of tracheobronchial tree. *Black arrowhead*, venous confluence.

RIGHT BRONCHIAL SEGMENTS

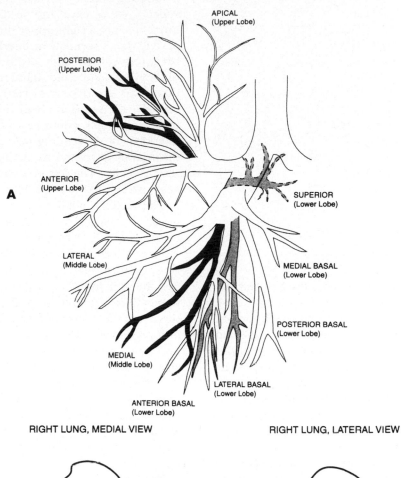

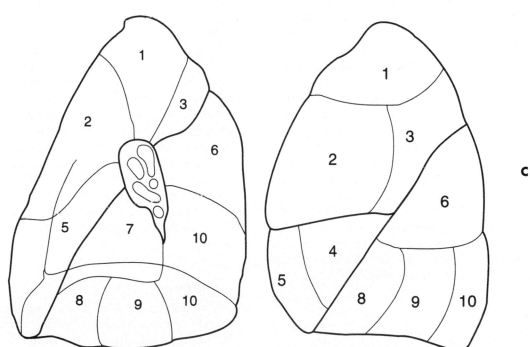

Fig. 1-9.   A, Anatomy of right bronchial tree including bronchial segments. **B** and **C,** Segmental anatomy viewed from the medial and lateral surfaces of the right lung.

Table 1-3 Bronchopulmonary segments

Right Lung	Left Lung
UPPER LOBE	**UPPER LOBE**
1—Apical	1 & 2—Apical posterior
2—Anterior	3—Anterior
3—Posterior	4—Superior lingula
	5—Inferior lingula
MIDDLE LOBE	
4—Lateral	**LOWER LOBE**
5—Medial	6—Superior
	7 & 8—Anteromedial basal
LOWER LOBE	9—Lateral basal
6—Superior	10—Posterior basal
7—Medial basal	
8—Anterior basal	
9—Lateral basal	
10—Posterior basal	

The superior segmental bronchus is the first segment originating in the lower lobe. It arises from the posterior aspect of the lower-lobe bronchus immediately beyond its origin and directly posterior to the takeoff of the middle-lobe bronchus. There are four basal segments that subsequently arise from the root bronchus of the right lower lobe. These are the anterior, lateral, posterior, and medial. This is the order of the basal bronchi from the lateral to the medial aspect of the hemithorax on a standard PA radiograph.

Left side The left upper-lobe bronchus (Fig. 1-10) arises from the left main bronchus and then either bifurcates or trifurcates. The upper division is the main left upper-lobe bronchus and the lower division is the lingular bronchus. The upper division almost immediately divides into two segmental branches, the apical posterior and anterior. The lingular bronchus is analogous to the middle lobe bronchus of the right lung. The lingular bronchus then bifurcates into superior and inferior divisions or segments.

The divisions of the left lower lobe bronchus are in name and anatomic distribution identical to the right lower lobe bronchus except that there are usually three basal bronchi—the anteromedial, lateral, and posterior. The distribution from lateral to medial on the frontal radiograph is ALP. The lingular bronchus like its corollary on the other side, the middle lobe bronchus, usually comes off directly anterior to the takeoff of the superior segmental bronchus of the lower lobe.

Pulmonary Vessels

See Figs. 1-11 and 1-12.

The main pulmonary artery originates in the mediastinum at the pulmonic valve and passes upward, backward, and to the left before bifurcating within the peri-cardium into the short left and long right pulmonary arteries. The right pulmonary artery courses to the right behind the ascending aorta before dividing behind the superior vena cava and in front of the right main bronchus into a right upper branch (the truncus anterior) and the descending or interlobar branch. The interlobar artery subsequently divides into segmental arteries to the right middle and right lower lobes. The higher left pulmonary artery passes over the left main bronchus. It may give off a separate branch to the left upper lobe or, more commonly, continues directly into a vertical left interlobar or descending pulmonary artery from which the segmental arteries to the left upper and lower lobes arise directly. The left descending or interlobar artery lies posterior to the lower lobe bronchus.

The upper limit of normal diameters for the pulmonary arteries have been determined in normals on the basis of CT scans. They are the following: main pulmonary artery 28.6 mm, left pulmonary artery 28 mm, and proximal right pulmonary artery 24.3 mm. In addition the right interlobar artery can often be measured on standard radiographs with the intermediate bronchus serving as the medial border. The mean diameter for men is approximately 13 mm and for women approximately 12.5 mm. Another method for estimating changes in arterial caliber is the artery-to-bronchus index. Normally the ratio of pulmonary artery to bronchus size at any point distal to the takeoff of the upper-lobe bronchi is approximately 1.3-1.4:1. On CT scans the more peripheral arteries can be visualized in the bronchovascular bundles, and the arterial bronchial index is approximately 1:1.

The right superior pulmonary vein drains the segmental veins of the right upper lobe and descends medially into the mediastinum to the upper and posterior aspect of the left atrium. The middle-lobe vein after passing under the middle-lobe bronchus usually joins the left atrium at the base of the superior pulmonary venous confluence. The left superior pulmonary vein drains the left upper lobe and lingula and also courses in an oblique fashion medially into the mediastinum to join the superior part of the left atrium. In the lower lobes the right and left inferior pulmonary veins have a horizontal rather than an oblique course and drain into the left atrium medially. They form inferior pulmonary venous confluences.

Pulmonary Hila

The pulmonary hila or root of the lungs contain bronchi, pulmonary and systemic arteries and veins, autonomic nerves, lymph vessels, and lymph nodes.

Standard PA and lateral chest radiograph
See Fig 1-12.

LEFT BRONCHIAL SEGMENTS

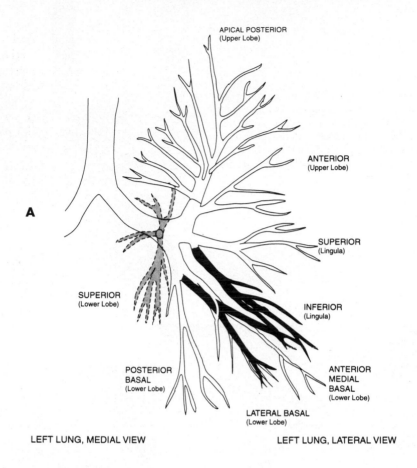

Fig. 1-10. **A,** Anatomy of the left bronchial tree including bronchial segments. **B** and **C,** Segmental anatomy viewed from the medial and lateral surfaces of the left lung.

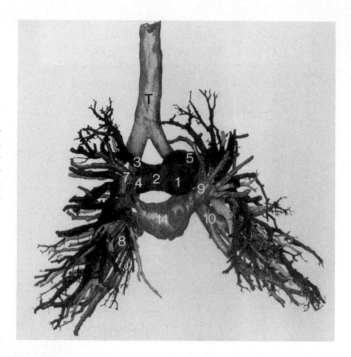

Fig. 1-11. Central pulmonary vasculature. (*1*) main pulmonary artery, (*2*) right pulmonary artery, (*3*) truncus anterior, (*4*) right interlobar artery, (*5*) left pulmonary artery, (*7*) right superior pulmonary vein, (*8*) right inferior pulmonary vein, (*9*) left superior pulmonary vein, (*10*) inferior pulmonary veins, (*14*) left atrium. (From Genereux GP: Conventional tomographic hilar anatomy emphasizing the pulmonary veins, *AJR* 141:1241-1257, 1983.)

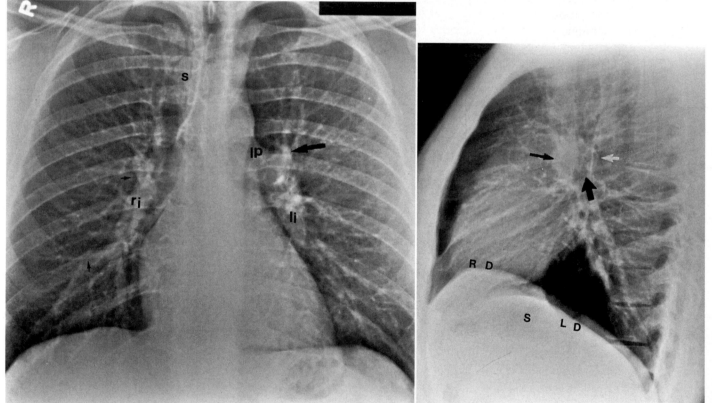

Fig. 1-12. Central pulmonary vasculature. **A,** *lp,* left pulmonary artery; *li,* left interlobar artery; *ri,* right interlobar artery; *s,* sternum. *Small black arrows* on right indicate the right superior pulmonary vein that forms the upper border of the right hilum and a V configuration with the right interlobar artery. *Lower black arrow* on the right points to the horizontal course of the inferior pulmonary vein. *Large black arrow on left,* left superior pulmonary vein. **B,** Lateral view. Anterior portion of the hilar structures is made up mostly by the right pulmonary artery (*black arrow*). The left pulmonary artery (*white arrow*) is seen as a longitudinal structure arching over and passing posterior to the left upper-lobe bronchus (*large black arrow*). *RD,* right hemidiaphragm; *LD,* left hemidiaphragm; *S,* stomach bubble.

The hila can be conveniently divided into upper and lower zones and specific anatomic structures can be identified in each area. The upper part of the right hilum consists of the right superior pulmonary vein and the truncus anterior branch of the right pulmonary artery. A short segment of the upper-lobe bronchus and the end-on anterior segmental artery and bronchus can often be identified. The lower portion of the right hilum is formed by the interlobar artery, which descends in a vertical manner and lies lateral to the intermediate bronchus. The horizontally oriented inferior pulmonary vein lies posteroinferior to the hilum. On the left side the upper part of the left hilum is formed by the distal left pulmonary artery and the left superior pulmonary vein. The proximal left pulmonary artery is almost always higher than the highest point of the right interlobar artery, the left hilum therefore being higher than the right. The lower portion of the left hilum is formed by the distal interlobar or descending artery and more caudally by the left inferior pulmonary vein. The air columns of the lingular and left lower-lobe bronchus may be identified.

Occasionally the venous confluences may be extremely prominent and produce vascular pseudotumors. This is particularly common in the right retrocardiac area when the inferior right venous confluence is prominent (Fig. 1-8).

Understanding hilar anatomy on the lateral projection is critical (Fig. 1-13). The tracheal air column is always clearly visible and ends caudally in a rounded radiolucency that represents the distal mainstem or proximal left upper-lobe bronchus seen end on. The right pulmonary artery is projected as a circular opacity anterior to this bronchus. The left pulmonary artery is tubular in configuration and arches over the left mainstem or left upper-lobe bronchus. The right upper-lobe bronchus can be identified approximately a centimeter above the left upper-lobe bronchus. Between the right and left upper-lobe bronchi, which are seen end on, is a thin vertical white line representing the posterior wall of the bronchus intermedius that courses inferiorly. It separates the lumen of the bronchus intermedius from the aerated right lung and the azygoesophageal recess posteriorly. The area beneath the left mainstem bronchus is sometimes referred to as the "inferior hilar window." It should be clear and radiolucent. If you see an opacity, particularly a rounded opacity, in this area, it suggests the presence of hilar or subcarinal adenopathy. Abnormalities of the hilum on standard radiographs may be increased opacity or changes in size, shape, or lobulation.

Computed tomography

The pulmonary hila are probably best evaluated with CT. They can be well visualized either with or without the use of intravenous contrast medium. However, dense opacification of the pulmonary or the hilar vessels sim-

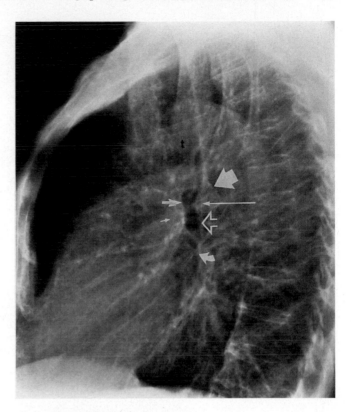

Fig. 1-13. Hilar anatomy on the lateral view. *t,* trachea; *large white arrow,* right upper-lobe bronchus; *white open arrowhead,* left upper-lobe bronchus; *small white arrow,* right pulmonary artery; *large white arrowhead,* left pulmonary artery; *long white arrow,* posterior-wall right intermediate bronchus; *curved white arrow,* "inferior hilar window."

plifies interpretation. The bronchial tree is best assessed at wide windows, that is, 1500 to 2000 Hounsfield units (HU). Visualization of hilar structures is also improved by thin, that is, 5-mm, sections.

The anatomy of the hila is illustrated in the accompanying figure (Fig. 1-14) and the figures of mediastinal anatomy (see Figs. 1-23 & 1-24).

Magnetic resonance

There are several advantages to the use of MR in imaging the hila. Contrast is not required because flowing blood within hilar vessels generates no signal and can be easily differentiated from the lymph nodes and masses in the hila. The anatomy is identical, of course, to that described on CT in the axial plane. MR also has the advantage of direct imaging in the coronal and sagittal planes.

However, the spatial resolution of MR is less than CT and occasionally on T1-weighted spin-echo images signal may be generated from soft tissues in the normal hilum that can be confused with enlarged nodes or masses. This is most likely due to focal hilar fat and normal sized lymph nodes. For these reasons, CT with contrast is the preferred method for evaluating the hila. However, MR

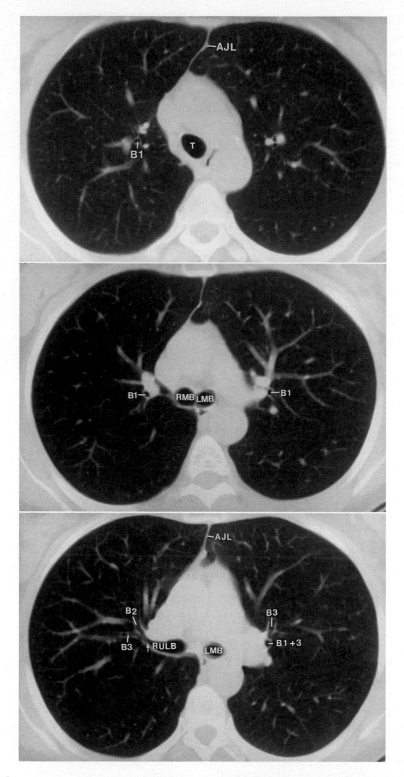

Fig. 1-14. CT hilar anatomy. Sequential CT sections demonstrate anatomy of the major airways and central pulmonary vessels. *AJL,* anterior junction line; *B1,* apical segmental bronchus upper lobe; *B2,* anterior segmental bronchus upper lobe; *B3,* posterior segmental bronchus upper lobe; *B6,* superior segmental bronchus-right lower lobe and left lower lobe; *BI,* bronchus intermedius; *LB,* lingular bronchus; *LDPA,* left descending (interlobar) pulmonary artery; *LLB,* left lower-lobe bronchus; *LLLB,* left lower-lobe bronchus; *LMB,* left main bronchus; *LULB,* left upper-lobe bronchus; *RIA,* right interlobar artery; *RLLB,* right lower-lobe bronchus; *RMB,* right main bronchus; *RMLB,* right middle-lobe bronchus; *RULB,* right upper-lobe bronchus; *T,* trachea.

Continued

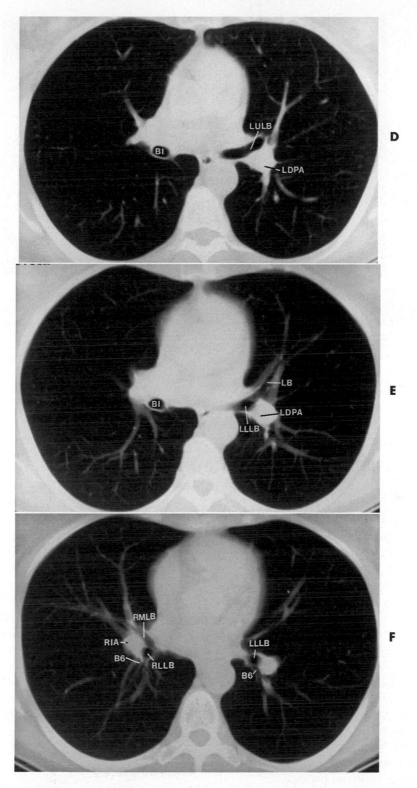

Fig. 1-14, cont'd.   For legend, see opposite page.   *Continued*

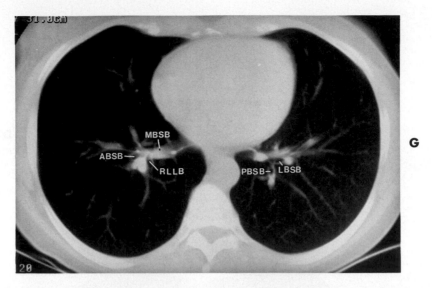

Fig. 1-14, cont'd.   CT hilar anatomy. Sequential CT sections demonstrate anatomy of the major airways and central pulmonary vessels. *ABSB,* anterior basal segmental bronchus; *LBSB,* lateral basal segmental bronchus; *MBSB,* medial basal segmental bronchus; *PBSB,* posterior basal segmental bronchus; *RLLB,* right lower-lobe bronchus.

may be useful particularly in patients who cannot tolerate intravenous contrast.

Pulmonary Parenchyma

The pulmonary acinus

The pulmonary acinus is often considered an anatomic as well as functional unit of the lung parenchyma (Fig. 1-15). It refers to the gas-exchanging unit of the lung and is defined as that portion of the lung distal to the terminal bronchiole (the last purely conducting airway) comprised of the respiratory bronchioles, alveolar ducts, alveolar sacs, and alveoli. There has been considerable debate about whether the acinus is radiologically visible. Experimentally, the acinus can be filled with bronchographic contrast medium and the radiographic opacities that are produced are nodular opacities with a rosette appearance and a diameter of approximately 6 to 10 mm. However, it is debatable whether such "acinar shadows" can be identified with confidence in disease processes creating opacification in the lungs in living patients.

Secondary lobule

The secondary lobule is defined as the smallest discrete portion of the lung that is surrounded by connective tissue septa (Fig. 1-16). It is composed of 3 to 5 terminal bronchioles with their accompanying airways and parenchyma. It is usually polyhedral in shape and generally ranges from 1 to 2.5 cm in diameter. The secondary lobule has been recognized by some authors as the radiographically visible basic structural unit of the lung. It is certainly the unit of the lung that is readily identified on high-resolution CT. However, the distribution of lobules is not uniform throughout the lung and the septa are better developed and more numerous in the lateral and anterior surfaces of the lower lobes. The secondary pulmonary lobule consists of core structures, which are the bronchus and accompanying pulmonary artery, and peripheral structures within the interlobular septa, which are the pulmonary veins and lymphatics.

In diffuse infiltrative lung diseases (see Chapter 7), the lobular architecture can often be readily identified on high-resolution CT, and the relationship of the disease process to either the center or the periphery of the lobule may be helpful in diagnosis. However, lobular architecture is impossible to appreciate on standard chest radiographs.

The Pleura

The pleura consists of two layers, the parietal and visceral. It is not of sufficient thickness to be visible on standard chest radiography. The pleura becomes visible when it is thickened, particularly over the lateral surfaces of the lungs and over the convexity, but such thickening cannot be appreciated along the mediastinal or diaphragmatic surfaces.

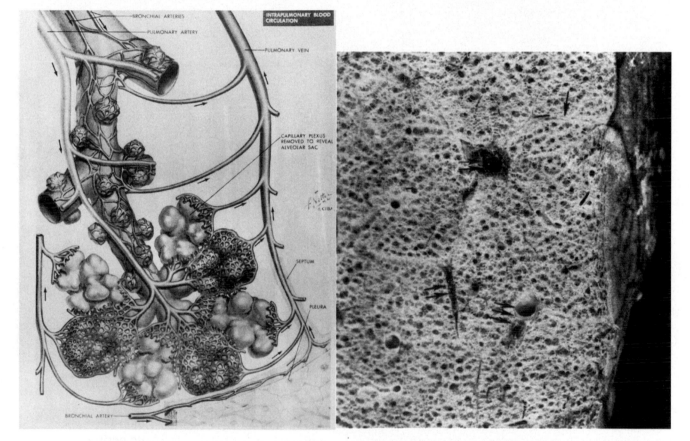

Fig. 1-15. The pulmonary acinus. *TB,* terminal bronchiole; *RB,* respiratory bronchiole; *AD,* alveolar duct; *AS,* alveolar sac. (From Thurlbeck WM: In Sommers SC, editor: *Pathology annual,* New York, 1968, Appleton Communications.)

Fig. 1-16. **A,** Secondary pulmonary lobule. Schematic drawing demonstrating the pulmonary arteriole and airway in the center of the lobule. Pulmonary veins lie in the interlobular septum. (Copyright © 1989, Novartis. Reprinted with permission from *Atlas of Human Anatomy,* illustrated by Frank H. Netter, M.D. All rights reserved.) **B,** Photograph of cut surface of inflated fixed lung. The margin of the secondary pulmonary lobule is formed by the interlobular septum, which is continuous with the pleural surface (*single arrow*). The pulmonary arteriole and airway are seen in the center of the lobule (*three arrows*), the pulmonary veins in the septa (*two arrows*). (From Groskin SA: *Heitzman's the lung: radiologic pathologic correlations,* ed 3, St. Louis, 1993, Mosby, Inc.)

Interlobar fissures

Between the lobes, contiguous layers of visceral pleura called the interlobar fissures separate individual lobes and can be visualized on standard chest radiographs (Fig. 1-17) as well as on CT. The fissures may or may not be complete, and incomplete fissures allow collateral air drift or spread of disease from one lobe to the other. The major or oblique fissures separate the upper, and on the right, the middle lobe from the lower lobes. They extend

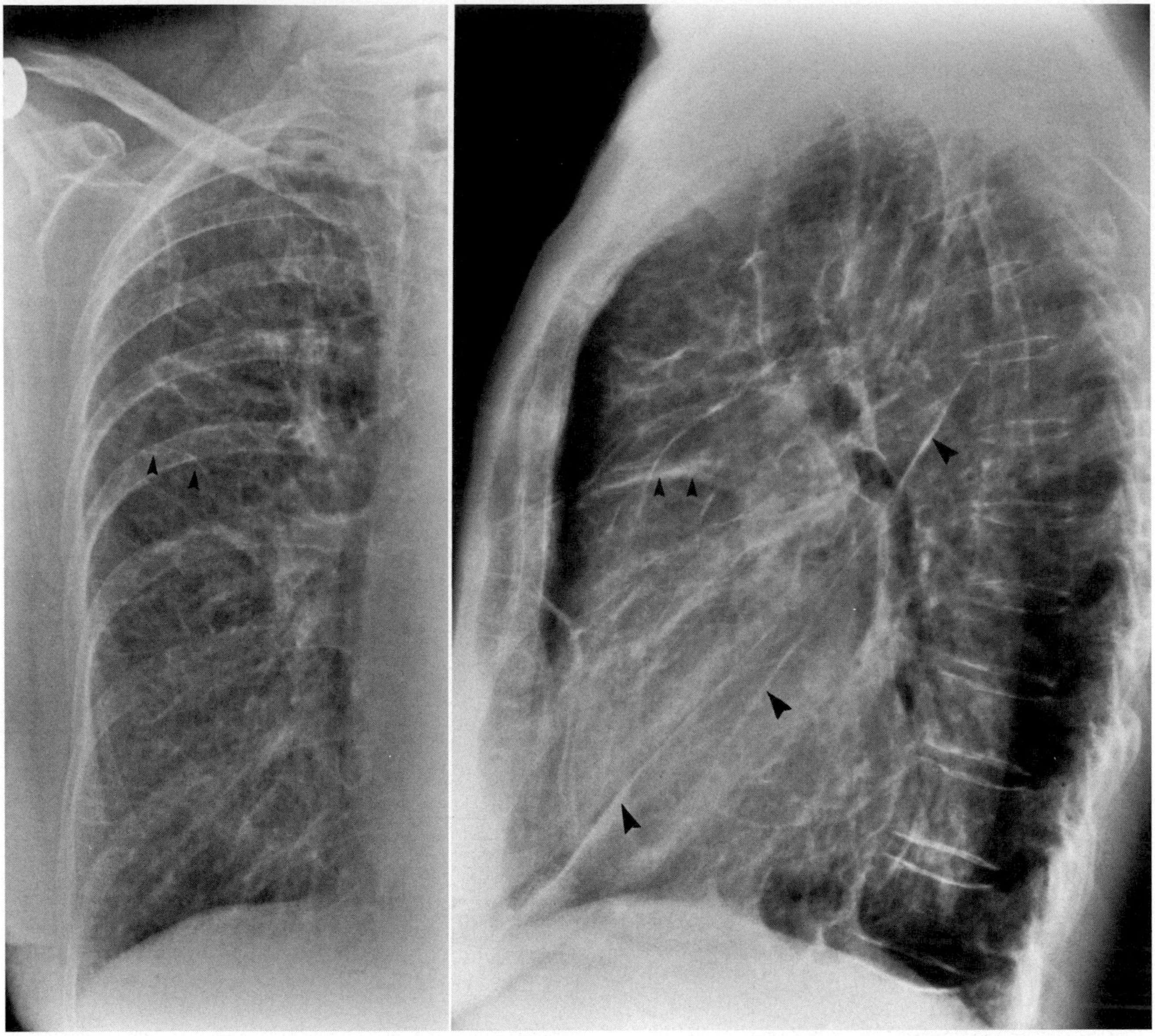

A

B

Fig. 1-17.   Interlobar fissures. PA and lateral chest radiographs in a patient with congestive heart
failure. Minor fissure *(small arrowheads),* major fissures *(large arrowheads).*

from about the level of the fifth thoracic vertebra
obliquely downward and forward roughly paralleling the
sixth rib to the diaphragm a few centimeters behind the
anterior costophrenic angle. The minor or horizontal fissure separates the anterior segment of the right upper
lobe from the middle lobe and lies in a horizontal plane
at about the level of the fourth rib anteriorly. On the lateral chest radiograph the posterior extent of the minor
fissure is sometimes projected behind the hilum and the
right major fissure due to the undulating course of the
fissures. The position of the interlobar fissures is critical
in the diagnosis of pulmonary volume changes such as
lobar collapse. It is uncommon to see the normal major
fissure on a frontal projection, and if it is visualized it usually indicates thickening or fluid within the fissure or an

abnormal position of the fissure due to volume loss and
atelectasis.

The pleural fissures can usually be identified on CT
scans (Figs. 1-18 and 1-19) On thick section scans they
usually appear as lucent bands that are devoid of vessels
and only occasionally as thin lines. However, on thinner
section CT the fissures will usually appear as thin lines or
dense bands. On conventional thick-section CT the
minor fissure, because it is tangential to the CT scan,
appears as a lucent area relatively devoid of vessels (Fig.
1-20).

Accessory fissures

Accessory pleural fissures may occur between segments. Such fissures are more frequently incomplete and

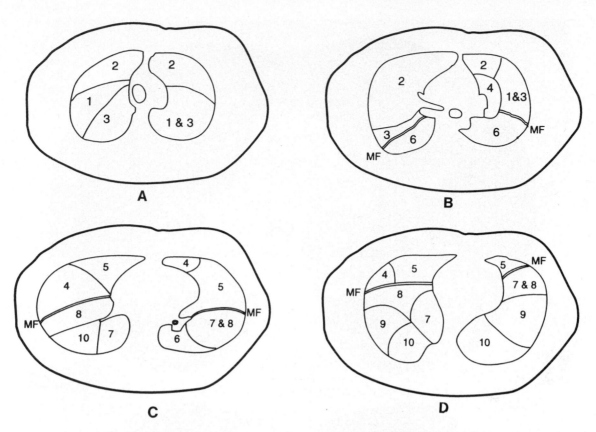

Fig. 1-18.   CT line drawings of four levels **A-D** from cephalad to caudad illustrating the course of the major fissures *(MF)*. The bronchopulmonary segments are numbered. (Modified from Freundlich IM: Anatomy. In Freundlich IM, Bragg DG: *A radiologic approach to diseases of the chest,* ed 2, Baltimore, 1992, Williams & Wilkins).

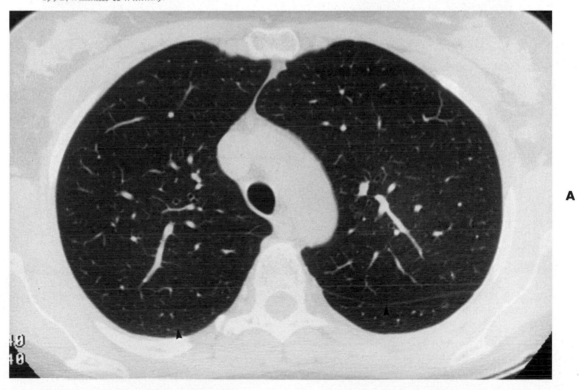

Fig. 1-19.   Comparable CT sections demonstrating the major fissures bilaterally. They appear as lines because of the thinness of the slices (1.5 mm) *(arrowheads).*

Continued

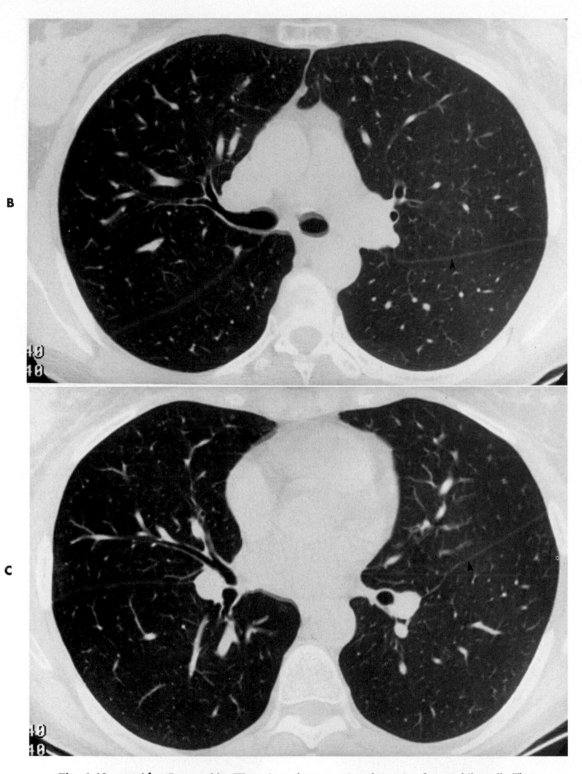

Fig. 1-19, cont'd.   Comparable CT sections demonstrating the major fissures bilaterally. They appear as lines because of the thinness of the slices (1.5 mm) *(arrowheads).*

Continued

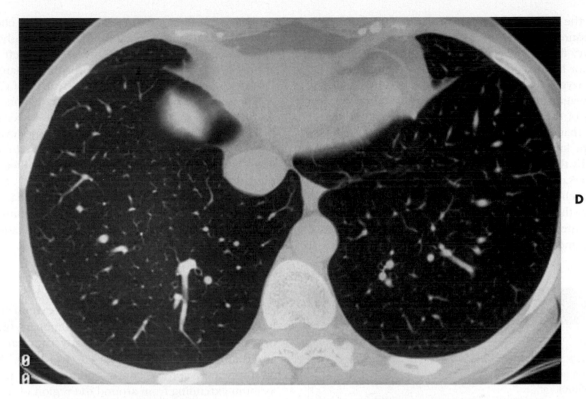

D

Fig. 1-19, cont'd. Comparable CT sections demonstrating the major fissures bilaterally. They appear as lines because of the thinness of the slices (1.5 mm) *(arrowheads)*.

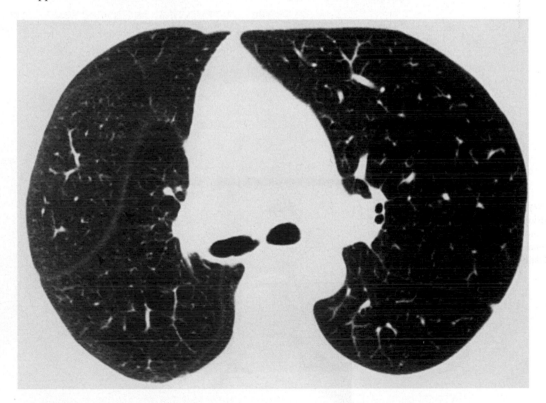

Fig. 1-20. Minor fissure. Thin section CT at the carina demonstrates the minor fissure as a band-like structure *(arrowhead)*.

vary in the degree of development. The common accessory fissures include the azygos fissure, the inferior accessory fissure, the superior accessory fissure, and the left minor fissure (Box 1-4).

The azygos fissure (Fig. 1-21) is created by the downward invagination of the azygos vein through the apical portion of the right upper lobe. It creates a curvilinear opacity that extends obliquely from the upper portion of the right lung, and it terminates in a teardrop shadow caused by the vein itself above the right hilum. It contains four layers of pleura. This fissure is visible in approximately .4% of chest radiographs. The portion of the lung lying medial to the fissure is often referred to as the azygos lobe.

The inferior accessory fissure separates the medial basal segment from the remainder of the lower lobe. It

can often be identified on conventional PA chest radiographs. The fissure extends superiorly and slightly medially from the inner third of the right or left hemidiaphragm. It is seen on either side in approximately 8% of PA chest radiographs, but up to 15% to 16% of CT scans.

The superior accessory fissure separates the superior segment from the basal segments of the lower lobes. It lies in a horizontal plane at about the same level as the minor fissure with which it may be confused on the PA chest radiograph, although it can be clearly identified on the lateral view.

The left minor fissure separates the lingula from the rest of the left upper lobe. It is usually incomplete and may be identified in 1% to 2% of PA chest radiographs and more frequently on CT.

Inferior pulmonary ligament

The inferior pulmonary ligaments bilaterally are reflections of the parietal pleura that extend from just below the inferior margins of the pulmonary hila inferiorly and to the diaphragm posteriorly. They can be visualized in normal individuals on CT (Fig. 1-22). They usually appear as broad bands connected to the mediastinum extending from around the region of the esophagus to the diaphragm. The right inferior pulmonary liga-

---

Box 1-4 Accessory Fissures

Azygos
Superior accessory
Inferior accessory
Left minor

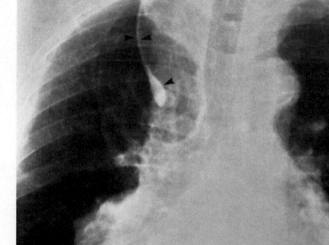

Fig. 1-21. Azygos fissure. **A,** PA view demonstrates the curvilinear opacity produced by the azygos fissure and the teardrop opacity of the azygos vein *(arrowheads)*. The fissure is prominent because it contains fluid.

Continued

A

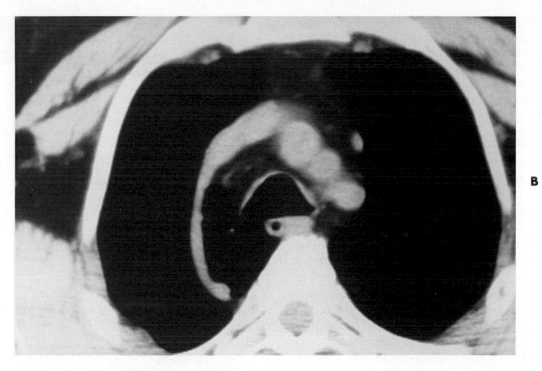

B

Fig. 1-21, cont'd.   B, CT appearance of azygos fissure.

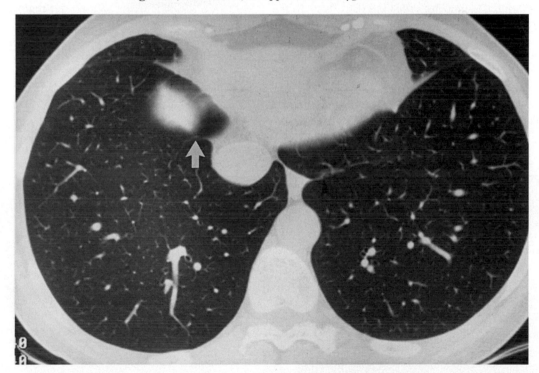

Fig. 1-22.   Inferior pulmonary ligament. Left inferior pulmonary ligament can be seen as a band extending from and connected to the mediastinum just to the left of the esophagus *(black arrowhead).* Right phrenic nerve is seen adjacent to the inferior vena cava *(white arrow).*

ment generally lies adjacent to the esophagus and posterior to the inferior vena cava. The ligaments should be distinguished from the phrenic nerves, which are nearby. The left phrenic nerve is generally identified lying adjacent to the pericardium, whereas the right phrenic nerve is only occasionally visualized.

Mediastinum

The anatomy of the mediastinum on CT and MR is illustrated in Figures 1-23 and 1-24.

Lymph nodes

A number of lymph-node classifications exist, the most important being that of Rouvière (Table 1-4). The American Thoracic Society has developed a numbered map of mediastinal lymph nodes that is used in the staging of bronchogenic carcinoma (Fig. 1-25).

Normal-sized lymph nodes can be identified on CT, and there is a range in size of normal lymph nodes. Most normal nodes are 7 mm or less in diameter, but normal nodes up to 11 mm and occasionally 15 mm in diameter may be observed. For practical analysis lymph nodes up to 1 cm in diameter should be considered to be within normal limits for size (Fig. 1-23, *F*). Normal lymph nodes on CT may occasionally have low attenuation or fatty centers, a reliable indication that they are not involved with malignancy.

Anterior mediastinal lymph nodes

INTERNAL MAMMARY NODES   The internal mammary nodes are parietal lymph nodes that drain the chest wall.

Text continued on page 30.

Table 1-4 Lien and Lund's modification of Rouvière's classification system	
Lymph Node Group	**Drainage Area**
ANTERIOR MEDIASTINAL NODES	
Parietal group	Breasts, liver, anterior chest and
Internal mammary nodes	abdominal wall diaphragm,
Superior diaphragmatic nodes	pleura, pericardium
Prevascular group	
Right anterior nodes (prevenous)	Thymus
Intermediate anterior nodes	Heart
Left anterior nodes (prearterial)	Pericardium
	Lungs, especially left
	upper lobe
MIDDLE MEDIASTINAL NODES	
Paratracheal group	
Right lateral nodes	Lungs
Left lateral nodes	Trachea
Pretracheal nodes	Bronchi
Retrotracheal nodes	Esophagus
Intertracheobronchial	Pericardium
(subcarinal group)	
Tracheobronchial	
(pulmonary root) group	
POSTERIOR MEDIASTINAL NODES	
Paraesophageal nodes	Esophagus, pericardium
Paraaortic nodes	diaphragm, lower-lung lobes
Paravertebral group	
Prevertebral nodes	Posterior chest wall
Laterovertebral nodes	Vertebrae

From Lien HH, Lund G: Computed tomography of mediastinal nodes: anatomic review based on contrast enhanced nodes following foot lymphography, *Acta Radiol Diagn* 26:641-647, 1985.

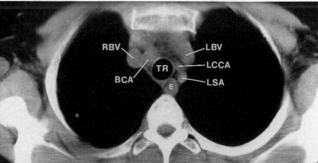

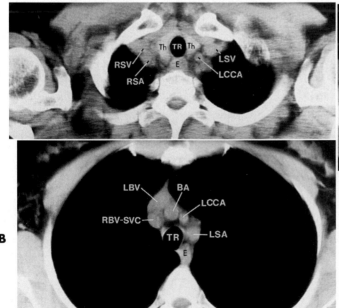

Fig. 1-23. Sequential CT slices from the thoracic inlet to the diaphragm illustrating normal mediastinal and hilar anatomy. **A,** *TR,* trachea; *Th,* thyroid gland; *RSV,* right subclavian vein; *RSA,* right subclavian artery; *E,* esophagus; *LSV,* left subclavian vein; *LCCA,* left common carotid artery. **B,** *RBV,* right brachiocephalic vein; *BCA,* brachiocephalic artery; *LBV,* left brachiocephalic vein; *LSA,* left subclavian artery. **C,** *RBV-SVC,* right brachiocephalic vein–superior vena cava junction.

Continued

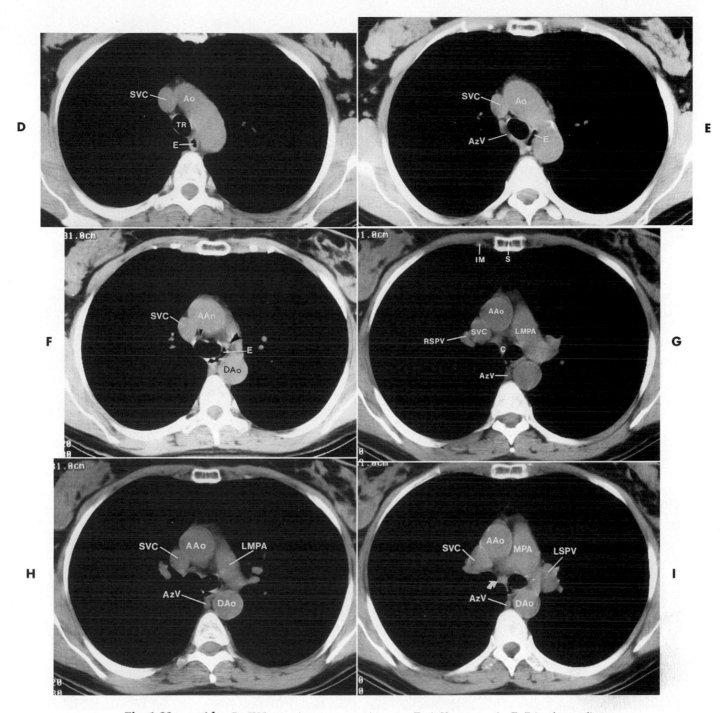

Fig. 1-23, cont'd.   D, *SVC,* superior vena cava; *Ao,* aorta. **E,** *AzV,* azygos vein. **F,** *DAo,* descending aorta. **G,** *RSPV,* right superior pulmonary vein; *LMPA,* left main pulmonary artery; *IM,* internal mammary vessels; *S,* sternum; *C,* tracheal carina; *MPA,* main pulmonary artery. **I,** *LSPV,* left superior pulmonary vein.   *Continued*

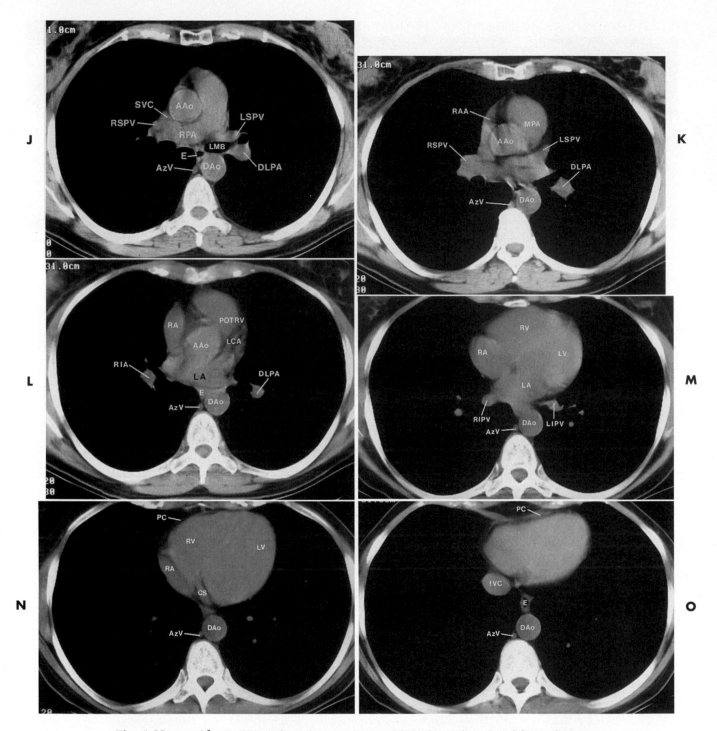

Fig. 1-23, cont'd.   J, *RPA,* right pulmonary artery; *DLPA,* descending (interlobar pulmonary artery); *LMB,* left main bronchus. **K,** *RAA,* right atrial appendage. **L,** *RIA,* right interlobar artery; *RA,* right atrium; *POTRV,* pulmonary outflow tract of the right ventricle; *LCA,* left coronary artery. **M,** *LA,* left atrium; *RIPV,* right inferior pulmonary vein; *RV,* right ventricle; *LV,* left ventricle; *LIPV,* left inferior pulmonary vein. **N,** *PC,* pericardium; *CS,* coronary sinus. **O,** *IVC,* inferior vena cava.

Continued

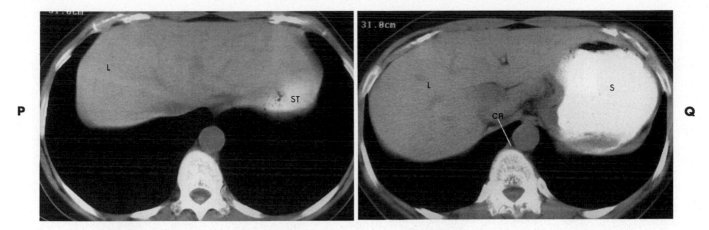

Fig. 1-23, cont'd. **P,** *L,* liver; *ST,* stomach. **Q,** *CR,* crus of diaphragm. Normal sized right paratracheal lymph node *(small black arrowhead);* aorticopulmonary *(A-P window)* lymph node *(large black arrowhead);* subcarinal lymph node *(curved white arrow).*

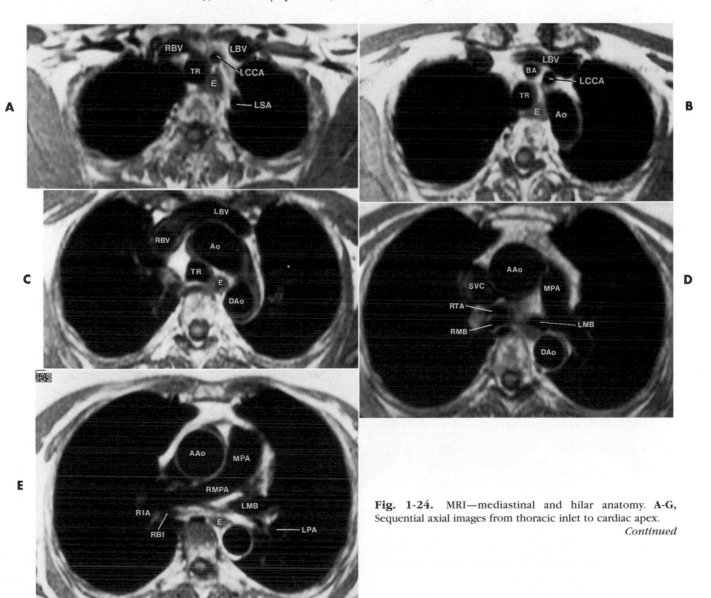

Fig. 1-24. MRI—mediastinal and hilar anatomy. **A-G,** Sequential axial images from thoracic inlet to cardiac apex.

Continued

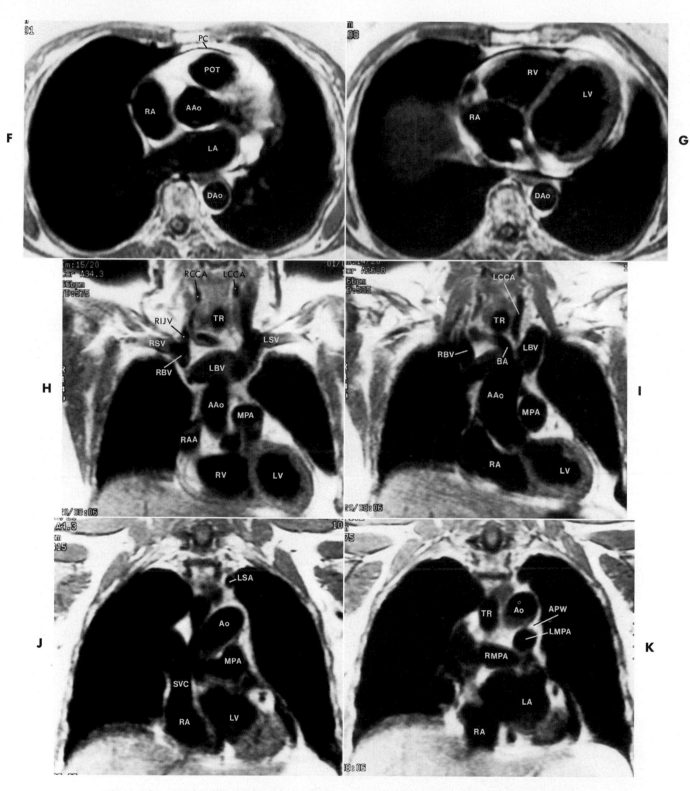

Fig. 1-24, cont'd.   MRI—mediastinal and hilar anatomy. **A-G,** Sequential axial images from thoracic inlet to cardiac apex. **H-M,** Coronal images proceeding from anterior to posterior. **N-Q,** Sagittal images from right to left. *RTA,* right truncus anterior artery (right upper-lobe branch); *RMB,* right main bronchus; *RBI,* right bronchus intermedius; *RCCA,* right common carotid artery; *APW,* aorticopulmonary window; *RIB,* right intermediate bronchus.

Continued

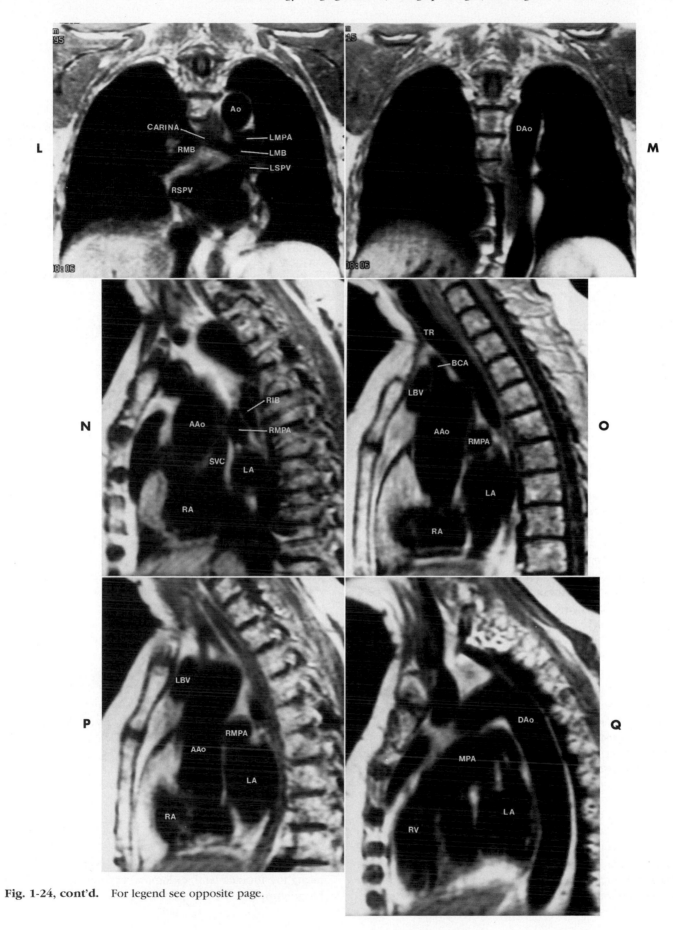

Fig. 1-24, cont'd. For legend see opposite page.

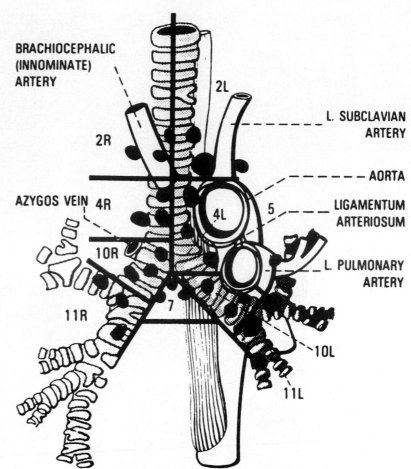

Fig. 1-25. American Thoracic Society lymph node classification. *2R & 2L*, high paratracheal; *4R & 4L*, lower paratracheal; *5*, aorticopulmonary; *7*, subcarinal; *10R & 10L*, tracheobronchial; *11R & 11L*, bronchopulmonary (hilar).

They are located close to the anterior chest wall on either side of the sternum. They are usually not identified on standard radiograph unless they are markedly enlarged, but they are easy to identify on CT adjacent to the internal mammary vessels (Fig. 1-23, *G*).

Prevascular nodes Prevascular nodes are defined as those nodes located anterior to the great vessels. They usually occur on the left side. The lowest node of this group is often referred to as the "aorticopulmonary window" or "ductus node" and is situated just above the left pulmonary artery near the ligamentum arteriosum (Fig. 1-23, *F*).

Anterior diaphragmatic lymph nodes These lymph nodes are also parietal lymph nodes that occur on the anterior surface of the diaphragm. They are identified on CT. The most medial node is referred to as the pericardiac node.

Middle mediastinal lymph nodes

PARATRACHEAL NODES There are right and left paratracheal chains along the anterolateral walls of the trachea (Fig. 1-23, *F*). On the right side these drain mainly the right upper lobe, but they may drain the right middle and lower lobes indirectly. The lowest node of this chain is called the azygos node. It is usually the largest and is located in the tracheobronchial angle. The left paratracheal nodes are fewer in number and smaller than on the right side.

SUBCARINAL LYMPH NODES The subcarinal lymph nodes are visceral lymph nodes that lie below the tracheal bifurcation anteriorly or posteriorly, and they extend along the inferior margins of the main bronchi (Fig. 1-23, *I*).

Posterior mediastinal lymph nodes These nodes occur in the paraesophageal, paraaortic, and prevertebral nodal groups. Even when enlarged they are difficult to see on the standard chest radiograph. These nodes may drain to the thoracic duct, subcarinal nodes, and intraabdominal nodes. On CT they are usually not identified unless enlarged.

Hilar nodes (tracheobronchial lymph nodes) These are the nodes of the lung hila. They occur most frequently at the bifurcations of the bronchi and vessels. Illustrations of nodal enlargement in each of these locations can be found in Chapter 17.

Other mediastinal anatomy

Other features of known mediastinal anatomy are discussed in the chapters dealing with the mediastinum.

The Diaphragm

The diaphragm is a muscular tendinous sheath separating the thoracic and abdominal cavities. It receives its blood supply from the phrenic and intercostal arteries and from branches of the internal mammary artery. Its nerve supply comes from the phrenic nerve. In most individuals, on standard PA radiographs the right hemidiaphragm is approximately half an interspace above the left (Fig. 1-12). The anterior portion of the left hemidiaphragm is obscured by the heart and lies above the stomach bubble. The diaphragm usually has a smooth contour, but scalloping may occur—that is, smooth arcuate elevations may be observed in about 5% of normal individuals.

Chest Wall

Certain soft-tissue structures in the chest wall can be identified on standard roentgenograms. The pectoralis muscles form the anterior axillary fold. Calcification of the rib cartilages is a common and normal finding and increases with age. There is a difference in the pattern of calcification between men and women. Among men the upper and lower borders of the cartilage become calcified first whereas in women the cartilage tends to calcify initially in a central location. Companion shadows can be seen outlining the clavicles and ribs (Figs. 1-1, *A* and 1-26). They are smooth soft-tissue opacities that parallel these bones and measure 1 to 2 mm in diameter, particularly along the axillary portions of the lower ribs. They are caused by visualization in tangential projection of the parietal pleura and soft tissues immediately external to the pleura. You should not confuse these with pleural thickening. Congenital anomalies of the ribs include supernumerary ribs, that is, cervical ribs that arise from the seventh cervical vertebra. Intrathoracic ribs are rare congenital anomalies. These usually arise from a vertebral body and extend downward and laterally to end at or near the diaphragm. The normal thoracic spine is straight in frontal projection and concave anteriorly in the lateral projection (Fig. 1-1). The lateral and superior borders of the manubrium may be visible on standard PA chest radiographs (Fig. 1-12, *A*).

SIGNS OF DISEASE AND PATTERN RECOGNITION

In this section the important radiographic signs of lung disease that must be recognized in interpreting standard chest radiographs are discussed. Abnormalities on CT scanning often parallel the changes observed on standard radiographs. However, the axial imaging of CT often provides more detailed information because it eliminates superimposition of abnormalities and provides more detailed and accurate anatomic localization even to the level of the secondary pulmonary lobule. CT signs of disease are dealt with more specifically in each of the chapters dealing with disease entities. Radiographic signs of

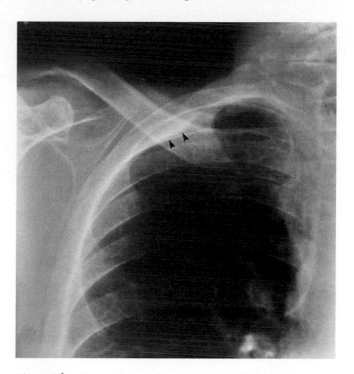

Fig. 1-26. Companion shadow of second rib on right *(arrowheads).*

pleural and mediastinal disease are also dealt with in their own respective chapters.

Alveolar Consolidation

It has been traditional to divide disease processes involving the pulmonary parenchyma into those that primarily involve the air spaces (i.e., the alveoli or distal acinus) and those that involve the interstitium. However, this approach to pattern recognition has many limitations, particularly poor correlation with histology. Also many diffuse disease processes in the lung involve both the alveoli and the interstitium, and additionally it is almost impossible radiologically to differentiate nodules that are produced by disease in the interstitium from nodules that are due to acinar or airspace filling. However, it is useful to consider homogeneous amorphous opacification often with air bronchograms and ill-defined margins as representing alveolar consolidation with airspace filling (Box 1-5). The term "alveolar consolidation" or "alveolar disease" will be used in this textbook to describe such processes. The appearance may be caused by accumulation of edema, hemorrhage, or neoplastic elements within the alveolar spaces, and of course the interstitium may be involved as well. Parenchymal consolidation is usually characterized radiographically by coalescent opacities that usually do not respect segmental boundaries (Fig. 1-27). The edge characteristics are ill defined and show poor margination. An example of this is the "butterfly" or "bat's wing" appear-

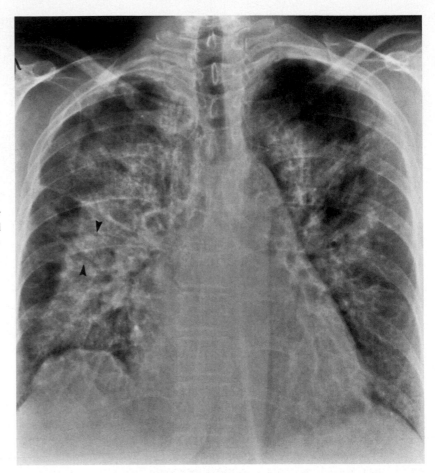

Fig. 1-27. "Alveolar disease"—pulmonary edema. There are diffuse poorly marginated central opacities with air bronchograms *(arrowhead)*. "Butterfly" or "bat's wings" appearance.

Box 1-5 Signs of Alveolar Consolidation
Homogeneous amorphous opacification
Ill-defined margins
Air bronchograms
Coalescence
Absence of volume loss
Ground glass (on CT)

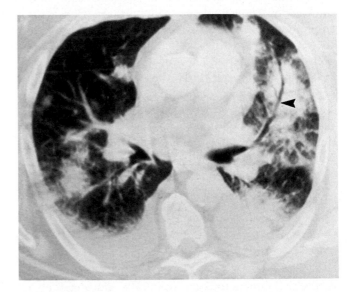

Fig. 1-28. Bilateral pneumonia. There are prominent air bronchograms in the left upper lobe *(arrowhead)*.

ance of acute pulmonary edema in left-sided congestive heart failure. Consolidation of the lung parenchyma often produces an air bronchogram (Fig. 1-28). The normally invisible air within the bronchial tree becomes apparent because of the surrounding consolidation. On standard films this sign is seen for the most part when the bronchus is not occluded, for example, by a lung carcinoma, although on CT air bronchograms can definitely be observed even distal to a bronchial obstruction. Occasionally rather minute radiolucencies may be seen within parenchymal consolidation. These may represent incompletely filled bronchioles and alveoli. This occurrence is sometimes called the "air alveologram" or sometimes it is referred to as "pseudocavitation". One of the important features of airspace consolidation is the absence of volume loss or atelectasis.

There are many etiologies of parenchymal consolidation. The process may be either localized or diffuse. You may find it helpful to consider that the parenchyma of

Box 1-6 Causes of Alveolar Consolidation

EDEMA

Hydrostatic
   Congestive heart failure
   Volume overload
   Renal failure
Capillary leak
   Acute respiratory distress syndrome

INFECTION

HEMORRHAGE AND VASCULITIS

Trauma—contusion
Overanticoagulation—hemorrhagic diathesis
Goodpasture's stain syndrome
Pulmonary—renal syndromes
Vasculitis
   Wegener's granulomatosis
Idiopathic pulmonary hemorrhage (hemosiderosis)

CHRONIC INFILTRATIVE LUNG DISEASE

Bronchiolitis obliterans-organizing pneumonia
Pulmonary alveolar proteinosis
Eosinophilic pneumonias

NEOPLASM

Bronchoalveolar carcinoma
Lymphoma

ASPIRATION

Lipid pneumonia
Near drowning
Gastric contents
Oropharyngeal material

Box 1-7 Interstitial (Infiltrative) Lung Disease

INTERSTITIUM
Compartments

Axial
Parenchymal

SIGNS OF INTERSTITIAL DISEASE
Patterns

Linear or reticular
Fine
Coarse
Nodular (less than 1 cm)
Reticulonodular
Ground glass (on CT)

Other features

Septal lines
Honeycombing (fibrosis)

the lung and the alveoli may be filled with water, pus, blood, cells, or protein. Box 1-6 lists some of the more common causes of alveolar consolidation.

Infiltrative (Interstitial) Lung Disease

Many of the diffuse diseases involving the lungs arise primarily in the interstitium, although they may eventually involve the alveoli. This group of diseases is now referred to as "infiltrative lung disease" rather than purely "interstitial" because both compartments are often involved. However, from the radiologist's point of view, you will find it useful to identify certain patterns that may occur in these diffuse diseases (Box 1-7). These patterns may be related to primary histologic involvement of the interstitium. Examples of such diseases include sarcoidosis, lymphangitic carcinomatosis, and idiopathic pulmonary fibrosis. A few of these infiltrative lung diseases primarily produce alveolar consolidation. They include such entities as chronic eosinophilic pneumonia and pulmonary alveolar proteinosis.

The interstitial space consists of two major anatomic compartments: the axial interstitial space and the parenchymal interstitial space. The former surrounds the bronchovascular bundles and occurs primarily in the central portions of the lung. The axial interstitium also extends out to the level of the terminal bronchioles. The parenchymal interstitial space lies between the alveolar and capillary basement membranes in the peripheral portions of the lung, in other words, the alveolar walls. Many interstitial or infiltrative lung diseases will involve both compartments, a classic example being interstitial pulmonary edema (Fig. 1-29). The interlobular septa contain the veins and lymphatics. Thickening of the interlobular septa produces the classic short subpleural lines that lie perpendicular to the pleural space. Such septal lines are also called "B" lines of Kerley.

There are two major patterns of small opacities that can be identified in interstitial lung disease, linear or nodular. The linear pattern may be fine, medium, or coarse. The nodular pattern consists of small rounded opacities that are less than a centimeter in diameter (Fig. 1-30). Nodules 1 to 2 mm in diameter are sometimes to referred to as a "miliary" or "micronodular" pattern as seen in miliary tuberculosis. The two types of small opacities may be combined producing a reticulonodular pattern. A distinctive type of opacification may be identified in infiltrative lung disease on CT. This is referred to as "ground-glass" opacification, an amorphous increase in attenuation in the lung parenchyma through which the normal pulmonary vessels can be visualized (Fig. 1-31). The latter characteristic distinguishes ground-glass

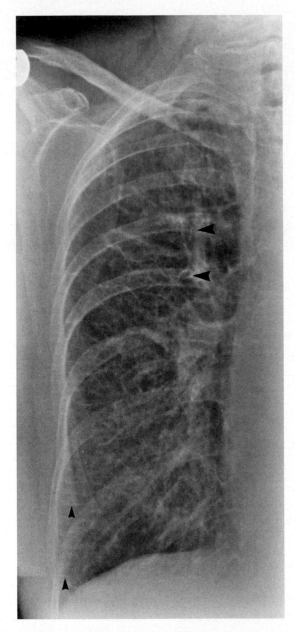

Fig. 1-29.   Interstitial edema. There is thickening of the axial interstitium by edema fluid (manifested by thickened bronchial walls [*larger arrowheads*]). The interlobular septa are also thickened *(Kerley B lines)* by edema fluid. These short subpleural lines are best seen at the lung bases *(smaller arrowheads)*.

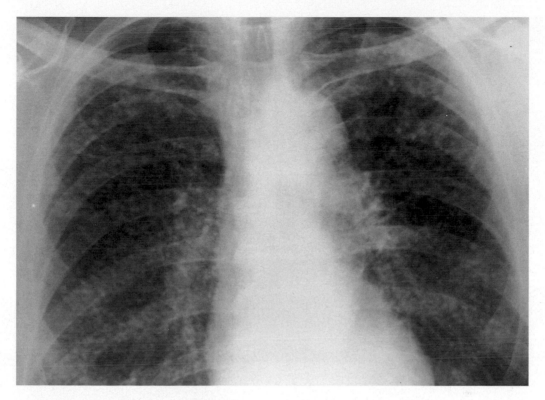

Fig. 1-30. Nodular pattern. Silicosis. There are multiple small, rounded opacities or nodules ranging in size from 2 to 4 mm.

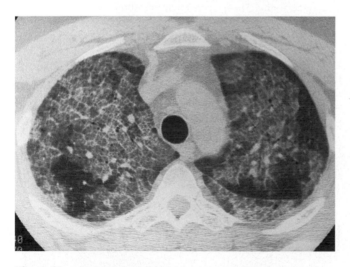

Fig. 1-31. Ground-glass attenuation or pattern. Pulmonary alveolar proteinosis. CT demonstrates diffuse increased opacification in both lungs. Pulmonary vessels in these areas can still be visualized. There are no air bronchograms as are found in true consolidation.

opacification from alveolar consolidation, which produces higher attenuation and usually obliterates the vessels within the lung parenchyma.

Linear or reticular opacities may be fine to coarse in nature, and the more coarse the reticular pattern generally the more severe the underlying disease (Fig. 1-32). The linear or reticular pattern is most frequently seen in diseases that cause diffuse fibrosis in the lung. Severe

fibrosis may result in end-stage lung (Fig. 1-33). This term refers to severe irreversible and chronic pathologic change. Typically the lung consists of cystic spaces that result from the breakdown of alveolar walls or dilatation of terminal and respiratory bronchioles. These cystic spaces are thick walled and lined by fibrosis. Usually the spaces are 1 cm or less in diameter, but they may be larger. Diseases that produce such honeycombing include idiopathic pulmonary fibrosis, fibrosis associated with collagen vascular disease (rheumatoid lung, systemic sclerosis) asbestosis, and occasionally end-stage sarcoidosis.

Examples of diseases causing a diffuse nodular pattern include the pneumoconioses such as silicosis and coal workers' pneumoconiosis, the granulomatous diseases such as sarcoidosis and hematogenous dissemination of granulomatous infection (e.g., "miliary" tuberculosis).

The CT and high-resolution CT (HRCT) findings of small interstitial opacities are discussed in detail in the chapter dealing with infiltrative lung diseases (Chapter 7).

Atelectasis

Atelectasis may be defined as decrease in volume of a lung or a portion of the lung. You may hear atelectasis referred to as "collapse" although this definition is somewhat simplistic. There are a number of types of atelectasis that are related to the mechanism by which the loss

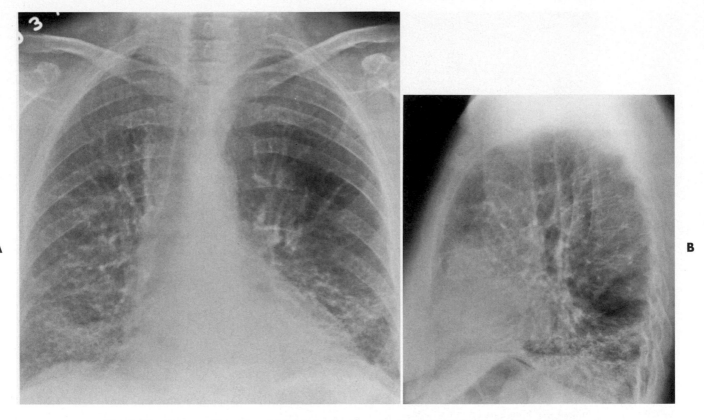

Fig. 1-32.   Linear pattern. PA and lateral chest radiographs demonstrate fine to medium coarse linear opacities at both lung bases. Desquamative interstitial pneumonitis (DIP), a form of chronic interstitial pneumonia.

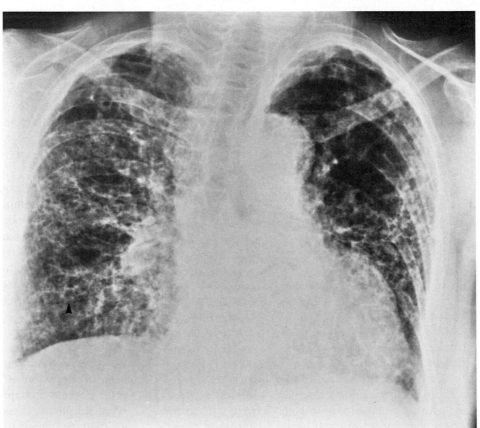

Fig. 1-33.   End-stage lung with honeycombing. Rheumatoid lung with diffuse fibrosis. **A,** PA chest radiograph shows multiple cystic spaces *(arrowhead)* that are thick walled and less than 1 cm in size.

Continued

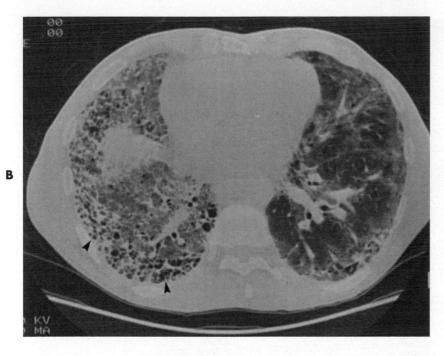

B

Fig. 1-33, cont'd.   **B,** High-resolution CT scan demonstrating subpleural honeycomb spaces more marked on the right side *(arrowheads).*

in lung volume occurs (Box 1-8). The most common type is that due to central bronchial obstruction that usually leads to lobar or less frequently segmental collapse. When such obstruction occurs gas is resorbed from the alveoli. This type of atelectasis is sometimes referred to as *resorption atelectasis.* The second major type is *passive atelectasis,* which is collapse caused by extrinsic pressure on the lung either from air, fluid, or both in the pleural space or at the edge of a local space-occupying lesion such as a mass in the lung. The third type, *cicatrization atelectasis,* occurs in areas of pulmonary fibrosis. Occasionally atelectasis can be patchy and caused by widespread collapse of alveoli. This occurs in the postoperative situation or in the adult respiratory distress syndrome. This has been termed *adhesive atelectasis.*

Lobar collapse

Collapse of a lobe may be complete or incomplete. The most common cause is obstruction of a central bronchus. The major or primary signs are opacification due to airlessness of the affected lobe and displacement of the interlobar fissures. There are multiple secondary signs, which include the following: (1) elevation of the hemidiaphragm; (2) mediastinal displacement (heart, trachea, other mediastinal structures); (3) hilar displacement; (4) crowded vessels in the affected lobe if it is still partially aerated; and (5) compensatory overinflation of the remaining lung (Box 1-9). If the obstruction of the lobar bronchus is caused by a large tumor mass, it may cause a bulge in the contour of the collapsed lobe (Fig. 1-34), and alternatively if the entire lobe is replaced by tumor, the lobe may appear lobular with undulation of

the affected fissure. These signs, of course, also apply to CT features of lobar collapse. However, you should look for the following additional features on CT. Air bronchograms may be present but if there is central endobronchial tumor causing the lobar collapse, the bronchus will be narrowed or occluded. The involved lobe usually becomes pie shaped rather than hemispherical in cross section with the apex of the triangle situated at the origin of the affected bronchus. Loss of volume also produces a reduced zone of contact between the pleural surface of the lobe and the chest wall.

Right upper-lobe atelectasis   The right upper lobe collapses superiorly and medially, creating a wedge-shaped opacity in the right upper hemithorax (Fig. 1-34). When collapsed completely the right upper lobe progressively pancakes against the mediastinum. The minor fissure is displaced upward, and the major fissure is displaced anteriorly. If there is a large central mass causing lobar collapse a convex bulge in the central medial portion of the minor fissure can be observed, which curves around the mass, the so-called "reverse S sign of Golden" (Fig. 1-35). On the lateral projection the collapsed lobe may appear as an indistinctly defined triangular opacity with its apex at the hilum and its base at the parietal pleura at the apex of the hemithorax. On CT the collapsed right upper lobe appears as a wedge of opacification extending along the mediastinum to the anterior chest wall (Fig. 1-35). Hyperaeration of the middle and lower lobes will occur, and the vessels in those lobes will typically be spread apart.

Left upper-lobe atelectasis   The major difference between collapse of the left and right upper lobes is the absence of the minor fissure on the left. With left upper-

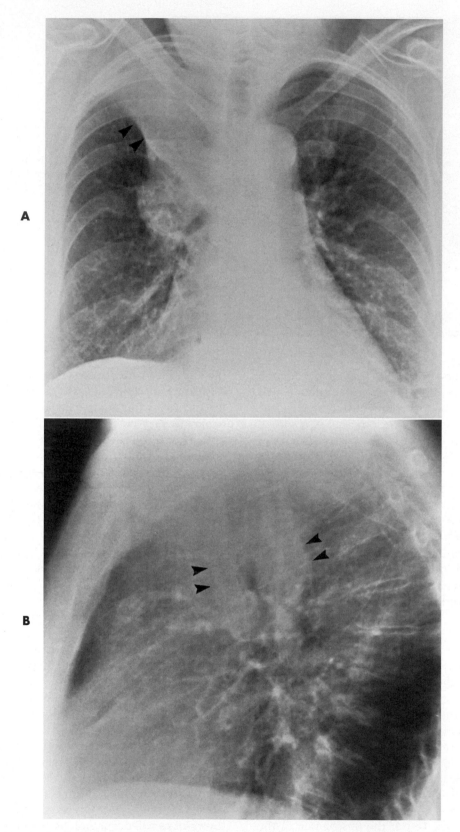

Fig. 1-34.   Right upper-lobe atelectasis. **A,** PA view demonstrates opacification of the right upper lobe and elevation of the minor fissure *(arrowhead).* There is a large mass in the right hilum (lung carcinoma) that is elevated (slightly above the left hilum). **B,** The atelectasis is less visible on the lateral view. It appears as a wedge-shaped opacity in the center of the chest *(arrowheads).*

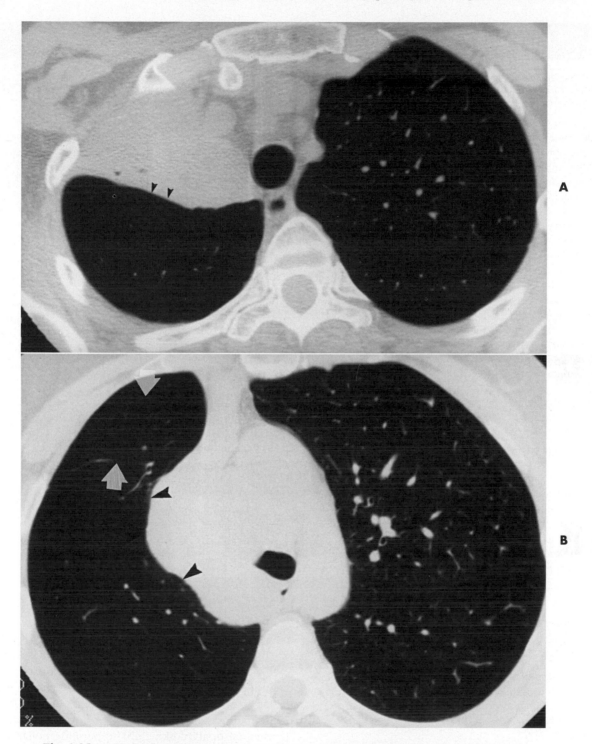

Fig. 1-35.   CT of right upper-lobe atelectasis. The major fissure is displaced forward *(small black arrowheads)* and the minor fissure displaced around a central mass *(larger black arrowheads)*. The remaining right middle lobe *(large white arrowheads)* and right lower lobe *(posteriorly)* are hyper-inflated and their vessels spread apart.

Box 1-8 Etiology and Types of Atelectasis

CENTRAL BRONCHIAL OBSTRUCTION (RESORPTION ATELECTASIS)
Endobronchial

Lung cancer
Other neoplasms
   Carcinoid
   Mucoepidermoid carcinoma
   Hamartoma
   Lipoma
   Metastases
      Breast
      Thyroid
      Melanoma
      Renal-cell carcinoma
   Lymphoma
Foreign body
Mucoid impaction
Sarcoid
Misplaced endotracheal tube
Middle-lobe syndrome—postinflammatory
Stricture
   Tuberculosis
   Trauma

Exobronchial

Lymphadenopathy
   Malignant
      Lung cancer
      Lymphoma
      Metastases
   Benign
      Sarcoid
      Tuberculosis ⎤
      Histoplasmosis ⎦ particularly if nodes are calcified

Enlarged left atrium
Mediastinal or adjacent mass

PASSIVE (COMPRESSION)
Pleura

Pneumothorax
Pleural effusion
Rounded atelectasis

Lung (adjacent space-occupying lesion)

Bulla
Mass
Abdominal disease (e.g., ascites)

CICATRIZATION
Granulomatous

Infection
   Tuberculosis
   Fungal
Sarcoidosis

Pneumoconiosis

Interstitial fibrosis

ADHESIVE
Adult acute respiratory distress syndrome

Postoperative (lower lobes)

OTHER
Subsegmental, plate-like, discoid

Box 1-9 Signs of Lobar Collapse

Opacification of affected lobe
Displacement of fissures
Elevation of hemidiaphragm
Mediastinal displacement
   Heart
   Trachea
   Other mediastinal structures
Hilar displacement
Crowding of vessels
Compensatory overinflation of remaining lung

lobe collapse the major fissure is displaced forward roughly parallel to the anterior chest wall (Fig. 1-36). This fissure is well depicted on the lateral view where it can be seen to parallel the sternum. The opacity of the left upper lobe is anterior to the fissure extending from the apex of the lung to the diaphragm. On the PA view the left upper-lobe collapse does not appear as a wedge-shaped opacity like right upper-lobe collapse. There is often a hazy opacification present that obliterates the left-heart border in the frontal projection ("silhouette" sign). The overinflated superior segment of the lower lobe occupies the far apex of the lung. There may be a paraaortic lucency on PA radiographs due to the hyper-aeration of the left lower lobe. On CT the left upper lobe generally retains more contact with the anterior and left lateral chest wall than the right upper lobe, which collapses against the mediastinum. Superiorly the collapsed

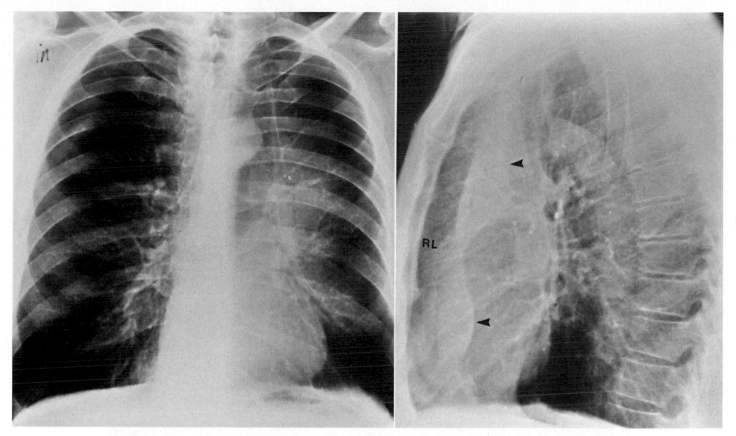

Fig. 1-36.   Left upper-lobe collapse. **A,** PA view shows hazy opacification in the left perihilar area with partial obliteration of the left heart border. The apex is aerated and occupied by the left lower lobe. **B,** The lateral view demonstrates forward displacement of the major fissure *(arrowheads)* parallel to the chest wall. The retrosternal lucency in front of the collapsed lobe is due to herniation of the overinflated right lung *(RL).*

upper lobe has a wedge-shaped triangular configuration (Fig. 1-37). Hyperinflation of the lower lobe is somewhat greater than that seen in right upper-lobe collapse. The left hilum is frequently elevated.

Middle lobe atelectasis   When the right middle lobe collapses it often does not produce a discrete opacity on the PA projection (Fig. 1-38). The right middle lobe collapses medially toward the right heart border obliterating this border, the so-called "silhouette" sign. On the lateral projection the right middle lobe is seen as a linear band or a wedge-shaped triangle with displacement of the minor fissure inferiorly and the major fissure superiorly. Right middle-lobe atelectasis may be seen to better advantage with a lordotic view. The lobe appears as a thin triangular opacity with the apex of the opacity directed away from the hilum and the base abutting the right cardiac border. Compensatory signs of middle-lobe atelectasis are less marked than with other lobes because of the small volume of the middle lobe. On CT the medial margin of the lobe will abut the right heart border and the posterior margin of the lobe is displaced anteromedially (Fig. 1-39).

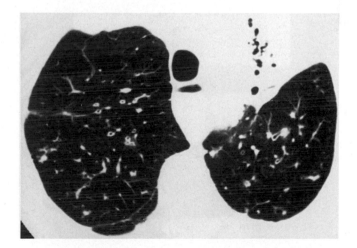

Fig. 1-37.   CT. Left upper collapse with wedge-shaped configuration. There are dilated bronchi in the collapsed lobe indicating bronchiectasis.

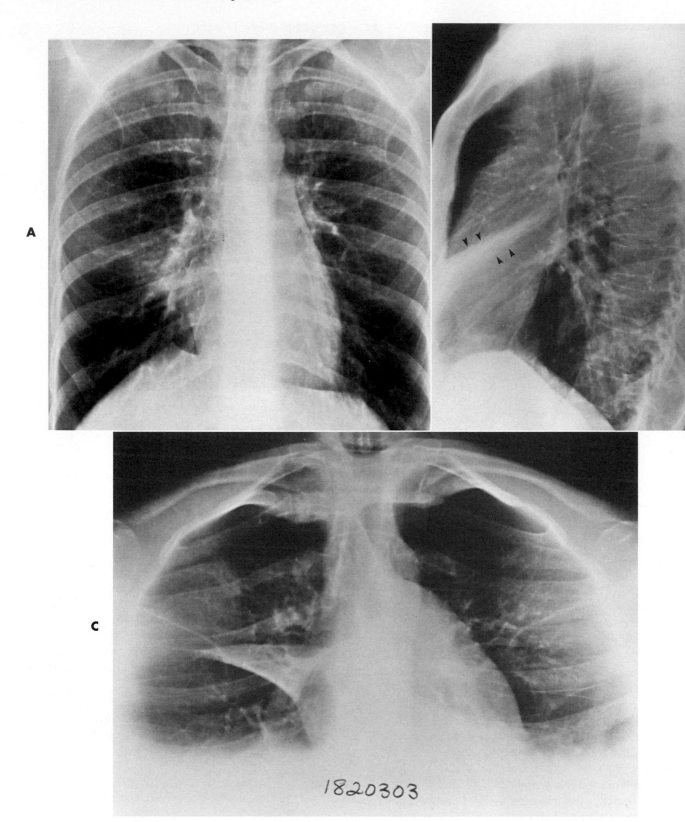

Fig. 1-38.   Right middle-lobe atelectasis. **A,** PA view shows loss of definition of the right heart border ("silhouette" sign). There are no signs of volume loss. **B,** The lateral view demonstrates a wedge-shaped triangle bordered by the minor fissure above and major fissure below (*arrowheads*). **C,** On the lordotic view the middle-lobe collapse is clearly evident.

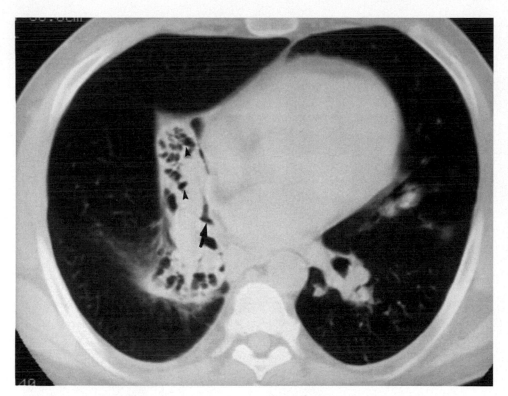

Fig. 1-39. CT—right middle-lobe atelectasis. The lobe is collapsed medially along the right heart border. The lobe was chronically collapsed due to bronchiectasis. Dilated air-filled bronchi are seen in the lobe (*arrowheads*) and the origin of the middle-lobe bronchus is patent (*arrow*).

Although right middle-lobe atelectasis may be caused by a central endobronchial tumor this lobe appears to be susceptible to chronic collapse secondary to prior inflammatory episodes. This is sometimes called "the right middle-lobe syndrome." Typically the middle-lobe bronchus is patent but narrowed in this condition, and bronchiectasis is present peripherally in the collapsed lobe. You can identify the open bronchus and the absence of a mass on CT. Patients may be asymptomatic or occasionally have recurrent pneumonias involving the lobe (Fig. 1-39).

Lower-lobe atelectasis The pattern of lower-lobe collapse is similar on both sides because of the equivalent anatomy bilaterally (Fig. 1-40). Both lower lobes collapse in a posterior medial and inferior direction. The upper part of the major fissure swings downward and the lower half backward. The upper half of the fissure becomes evident on the PA projection and the lower part of the fissure can be seen to be displaced backward on the lateral projection. Eventually as the collapse becomes complete the lobe occupies a position in the posterior costophrenic gutter and medial costovertebral angle. Often no discrete opacity can be seen on the lateral view except for a slight increase in opacification overlying the lower thoracic vertebra (normally the vertebrae become relatively more radiolucent from above downward) with loss of the contour of the posterior part of the hemidiaphragm. On a well-penetrated PA view the collapsed lobe will appear as a triangular-shaped opacity behind the heart and adjacent to the spine. The CT appearance

can be induced from the above description (Fig. 1-41). The right and left lower lobes collapse posteromedially against the posterior mediastinum and spine. The lateral contour of the collapse, though, may be convex if a central tumor is present.

Combined lobar atelectasis Combined right-middle and lower-lobe atelectasis can occur when a tumor obstructs the intermediate bronchus. The major and minor fissures in such an instance are displaced downward and backward creating on the PA view an opacity that obliterates the right dome of the diaphragm. The upper surface of the opacity may be either concave or convex. You should not confuse this with a medially loculated pleural effusion.

Combined right-upper and right-middle lobe atelectasis is unusual because the bronchi to these lobes are remote from each other. However, when this combination occurs the appearance is identical to upper-lobe atelectasis on the left.

Segmental and subsegmental atelectasis

It is unusual for a segment to undergo atelectasis because of channels that produce collateral air drift even when a segmental or subsegmental bronchus within a lobe is occluded. These forces tend to keep the segment aerated and obstructive overinflation and air trapping occurs rather than atelectasis.

Subsegmental, discoid, or plate atelectasis are terms used synonymously for linear opacities that range in thickness from 1 to 3 mm and 4 to 10 cm in length

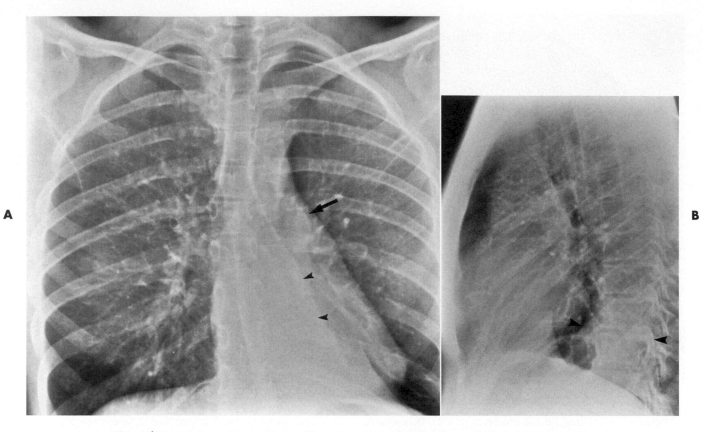

Fig. 1-40. Left lower-lobe atelectasis. There is a triangular opacity seen behind the heart on the PA view (*arrowheads*). The heart is shifted to the left and the left hilum is depressed (*arrow*). On the lateral view there is loss of visualization of the left hemidiaphragm and increased opacity overlying the lower thoracic vertebrae (*arrowheads*) in the posterior costophrenic gutter.

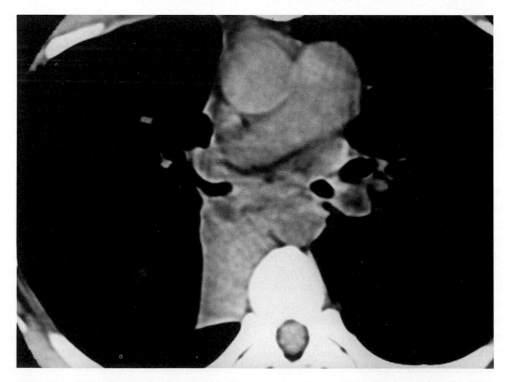

Fig. 1-41. CT of right lower-lobe collapse. The lobe is collapsed posteriorly and medially along the posterior mediastinum and spine.

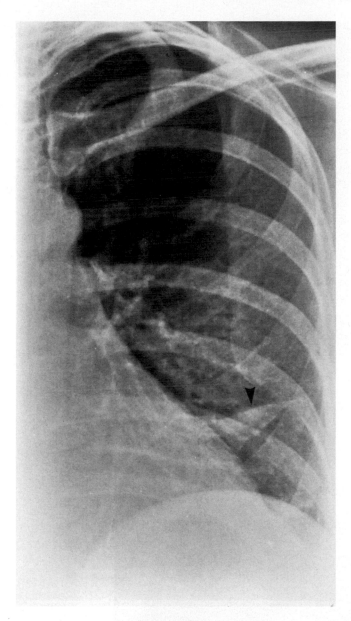

Fig. 1-42. Platelike atelectasis. There is a broad band of increased opacity at the left base paralleling the left hemidiaphragm (*arrowhead*).

(Fig. 1-42). They are usually located in the lower-lung zones and occur in a horizontal plane paralleling the diaphragm, although occasionally they may be oblique. These linear opacities are almost invariably associated with disease processes that diminish diaphragmatic excursion and are commonly seen after thoracic or abdominal surgery or in patients who are bedridden and who are kept in the supine position.

Total collapse of the lung

When an entire lung collapses the hemithorax on that side becomes completely opaque (Fig. 1-43). There is shift of the mediastinum to the affected side. Elevation of the hemidiaphragm can be recognized only indirectly on the left side by the high position of the stomach bubble. The opposite lung will overinflate and move across the midline particularly anteriorly behind the sternum creating a large retrosternal air space on the lateral view. The appearance differs from that of a massive pleural effusion, which will cause similar opacification of a hemithorax. In this condition an increased retrosternal clear space will not be noted, and there will be shift of the mediastinum to the opposite side. In addition on the lateral view a hazy opacification or uniform "filter effect" is observed.

Postobstructive pneumonitis and drowned lung

When a bronchus is obstructed, atelectasis is always accompanied by some fluid exudation or sequestration of blood in the obstructed lobe. Sometimes the amount of fluid can become quite voluminous, resulting in a radiographic appearance in which there is very little volume loss noted within the lobe despite the endobronchial obstruction. This appearance is sometimes referred to as "drowned lung" (Fig. 1-44). Infection may also occur distal to an obstructed bronchus, and the development of inflammatory exudate may also result in little loss of volume of the affected lobe.

Passive atelectasis

This term, also called "relaxation atelectasis," refers to pulmonary collapse that occurs as a result of pneumothorax or hydrothorax (Fig. 1-45). If there are no pleural adhesions, the collapse of any portion of the lung is proportional to the amount of air or fluid in the adjacent pleural space. When a pneumothorax is large, the pulmonary collapse may be total, however the opacity of the lung usually does not increase until it is approximately one-tenth of its normal area at total lung capacity. More specific discussion of pneumothorax and pleural effusion can be found in the chapter on pleural disease (Chapter 18). "Compression atelectasis" is a similar phenomenon and describes focal parenchymal collapse adjacent to a space-occupying mass within the thorax.

Another type of focal atelectasis is rounded atelectasis. This type of atelectasis (which is often an incidental finding on a chest radiograph) is a peripheral rounded type of atelectasis that is always associated with pleural thickening or, less commonly, pleural effusion (Fig. 1-46). It appears as a sharply defined mass abutting the pleura and ranging in size from 2 to 7 cm in diameter usually located posteriorly in the lower lobes. Air bronchograms or focal collections of air ("pseudocavitation") may be present within the atelectasis. The most distinctive finding is that vessels and bronchi located more centrally than the peripheral area of atelectasis are crowded together in a "whorled" pattern coursing like a "comet tail" toward the hilum. On CT the finding is that of a

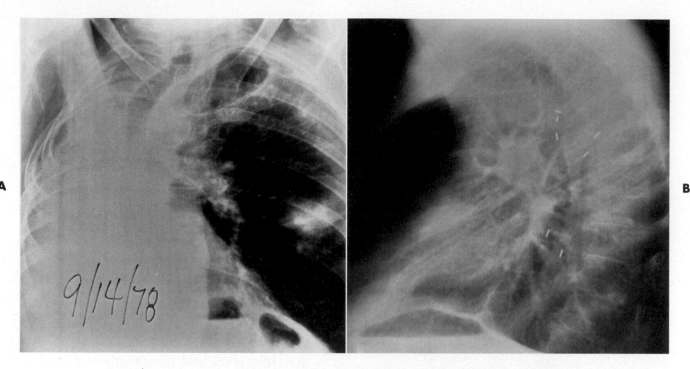

Fig. 1-43. Right pneumonectomy. Appearance is equivalent to complete right-lung collapse. **A,** On the PA view there is a completely opaque right hemithorax with shift of the mediastinum toward that side. **B,** On the lateral view there is large retrosternal clear space and loss of visualization of the right hemidiaphragm (recurrent lung cancer in the left lung).

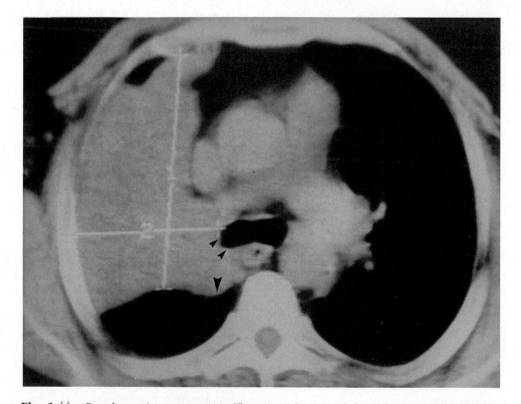

Fig. 1-44. Postobstructive pneumonitis. There is atelectasis of the right upper lobe and the bronchus is obstructed (*small arrowheads*). There is no loss of volume and a lobulated contour of the fissure can be identified due to tumor (*large arrowhead*).

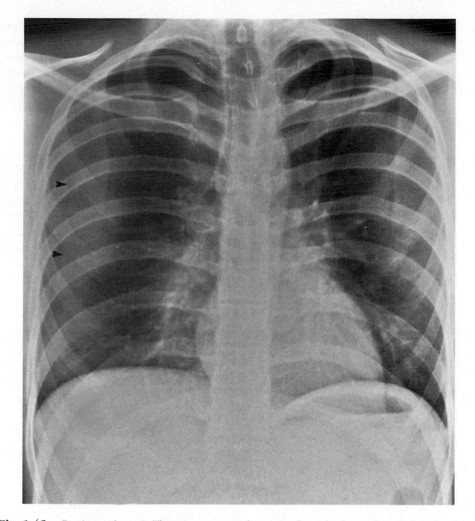

Fig. 1-45.   Passive atelectasis. There is a pneumothorax on the right (*arrowheads*), but the density of the partially collapsed right lung has not changed.

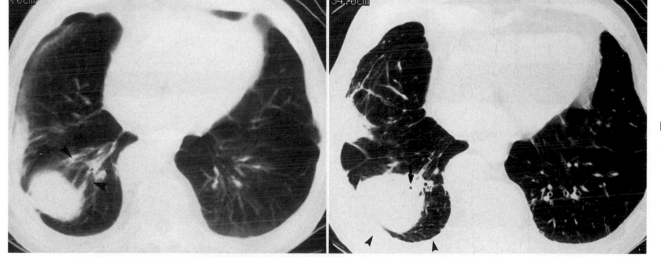

Fig. 1-46.   CT scan of rounded atelectasis. There is a mass abutting the pleura that is thickened (*small arrowheads*). The pulmonary vessels are crowded together medial to the mass (*large arrow heads*) producing a "comet-tail" appearance. Areas of pseudocavitation are present (*arrow*).

rounded peripheral lung mass associated with pleural thickening. The comet-tail appearance is more easily visualized. Rounded atelectasis can be associated with any cause of pleural thickening but particularly with asbestos-related disease.

Cicatrization atelectasis

Cicatrization atelectasis is a form of loss of volume that may be focal or diffuse. It is a form of collapse resulting from scarring and fibrosis. It is most typically associated with old granulomatous infection, particularly tuberculosis. Endobronchial obstruction is absent and bronchiectasis is a frequent feature. When an entire lobe is involved, the degree of volume loss is more marked than with other forms of lobar atelectasis (Fig. 1-47).

More generalized fibrosis in the lungs may be associated with general loss of lung volume.

Adhesive, nonobstructive, or microatelectasis

This form of atelectasis is usually related to a number of forces and with decrease in the amount of surfactant. An example is diffuse microatelectasis associated with the adult respiratory distress syndrome.

Nodules and Masses

The definition of nodules and masses is somewhat arbitrary, but usually both are considered to be lesions that are roughly spherical; a nodule is usually less than 3 cm in diameter and a mass greater than 3 cm in diameter. Nodules that are greater than 3 cm in size are highly likely to represent primary or secondary malignant disease in the lung. A more detailed discussion of nodules and masses is considered in the chapter on neoplasms (Chapter 11), specifically the discussion of the solitary pulmonary nodule. The smoothness of contour and edge

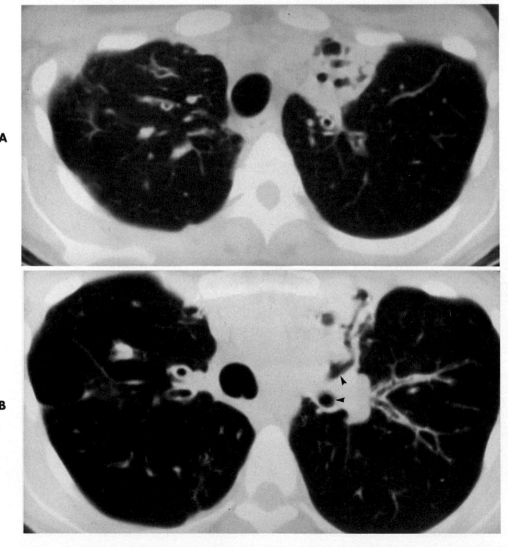

Fig. 1-47. Cicatrization atelectasis—CT. **A,** There is atelectasis of the left upper lobe with bronchiectasis secondary to old tuberculosis. **B,** The upper-lobe segmental bronchi are patent

characteristics of a nodular mass may be important. In general a smooth contour suggests benign disease and nodularity or lobulation indicates malignancy, although these findings are relatively nonspecific and cannot be relied on to distinguish malignant from benign disease (Figs. 1-48 and 1-49). Nodules and masses may be associated with "satellite" lesions. These are usually small, often rounded, opacities that lie in close proximity to the larger nodule or mass. They are more suggestive of an infectious etiology, such as tuberculosis, rather than a lung carcinoma. The relation of a mass or a nodule to the pleura or chest wall is important. A mass or nodule that arises within the extrapleural space in the chest wall will create an obtuse angle with the chest wall whereas an intraparenchymal lesion usually has an acute angle with the contiguous pleura. Extrapleural masses may have better defined margins than lung masses (Fig. 1-50).

Calcification and Ossification

Intrathoracic calcification is an important feature of pulmonary disease (Box 1-10). It is usually dystrophic, that is, it occurs in areas of necrosis. Less commonly it is metastatic, that is, related to hypercalcemia. Calcification may occur in focal lesions such as solitary pulmonary nodules (Fig. 1-51). The distribution and character of the calcification is important. This is discussed in more detail in the chapter on solitary pulmonary nodules (Chapter 11). Occasionally ossification can occur diffusely in the lung.

Diffuse pulmonary calcification can occur in a number of entities (Fig. 1-52). One is pulmonary alveolar microlithiasis, a hereditary disease in which calcified spherules occur within the alveoli. Other conditions with diffuse calcification include: silicosis, end-stage mitral stenosis with hemosiderosis, and certain healed disseminated granulomatous or viral infections. Examples of these include tuberculosis, histoplasmosis, and varicella pneumonitis. The radiographic pattern consists of diffuse round or punctate calcific opacities. Interstitial ossification is rare but has been occasionally reported in idiopathic pulmonary fibrosis and long-term busulfan therapy. The radiographic pattern is one of branching opacities distributed along the bronchovascular bundles.

Metastatic pulmonary calcification may occur with long-standing hypercalcemia. It is most common in patients with chronic renal disease who are maintained on dialysis and have secondary hyperparathyroidism. Metastatic calcification usually occurs in the apical and subapical lung zones, but it may be diffuse.

Cavities and Cysts

Abnormal air-filled spaces in the lung may develop in a variety of lung diseases, which include infection, vas-

cular embolic disorders, bronchiectasis, emphysema, pulmonary fibrosis, adult respiratory-distress syndrome, lymphangioleiomyomatosis, and histiocystosis X (Box 1-11).

General features

A pulmonary cyst is usually defined as a thin-walled (usually less than 3 mm), well-marginated, and circum-

---

Box 1-10 Etiology of Calcification

TYPES

Dystrophic
Metastatic

NODULES

Benign
   Tuberculosis
   Histoplasmosis
   Hamartoma
Malignant
   Lung cancer
   Metastases
      Osteogenic sarcoma (ossification)
      Chondrosarcoma
      Mucin-producing adenocarcinoma

DIFFUSE

Pulmonary alveolar microlithiasis
Silicosis
End-stage mitral stenosis (ossification)
Healed disseminated infections
   Varicella
   Tuberculosis
   Histoplasmosis
Secondary hyperparathyroidism—renal failure
Idiopathic pulmonary fibrosis

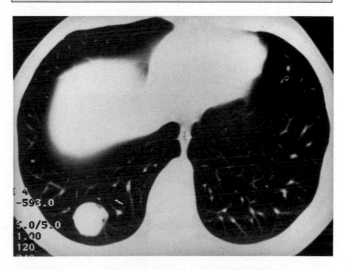

Fig. 1-48. Benign nodule. Hamartoma. CT shows a 2.5 cm nodule with smooth borders in the right lower lobe.

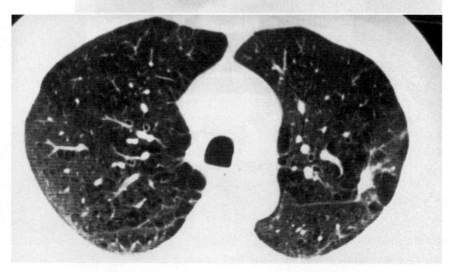

Fig. 1-49. Lung carcinoma. **A,** There is a small irregular nodule (*arrowhead*) in the left upper lobe on the PA view. **B,** CT demonstrates that it has spiculated and irregular margins.

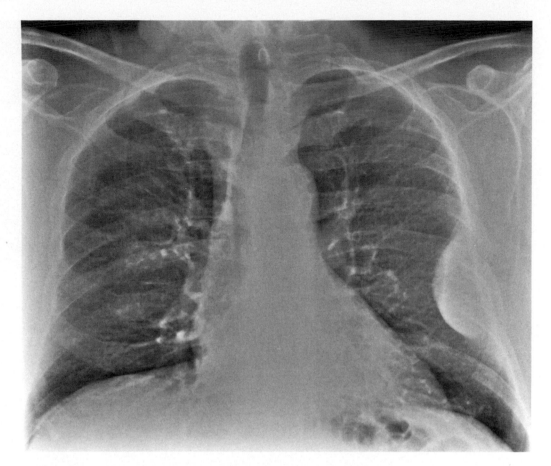

Fig. 1-50.   Extrapleural mass. PA view shows a large well-defined mass having obtuse angles with the chest wall. The sixth anterior rib cannot be visualized due to destruction. Metastatic renal-cell carcinoma.

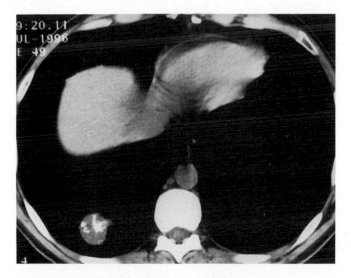

Fig. 1-51.   CT scan of calcified nodule (hamartoma).

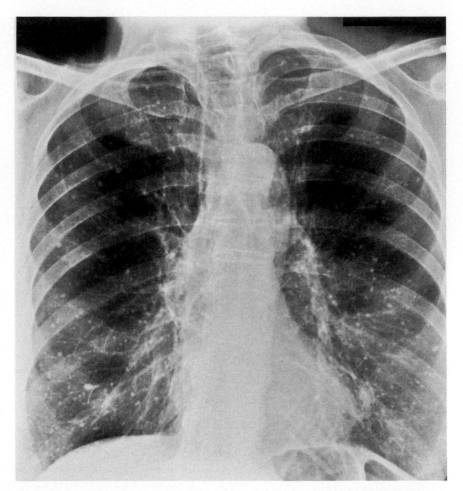

Fig. 1-52. Diffuse pulmonary calcification in healed varicella pneumonia. There are multiple small, dense nodules in both lungs.

Box 1-11 Cysts and Cavities

DEFINITION

Cyst
  Thin wall (<3 mm)
  Fluid- or air-filled
  Air/fluid level (occasional)
Cavity
  Thick wall (>3 mm)
  Always contains air
  Air/fluid level

TYPES

Congenital
  Bronchogenic
  Cystic adenomatoid malformation
Acquired
  Infection
    Postinfectious pneumatocele
    Abscess
    Nonpyogenic
      Tuberculosis
      Fungal
    Septic infarcts
Vasculitis and granulomatosis
  Wegener's
  Lymphatoid granulomatosis
Rheumatoid nodules
Neoplasms
  Primary lung carcinoma (squamous cell)
  Metastatic
    Squamous cell
    Sarcomas
Trauma
  Posttraumatic pneumatocele (laceration)
Emphysema
  Bulla
Bronchiectasis
Diffuse infiltrative lung disease
  Langerhans' histiocytosis
  Lymphangioleiomyomatosis
  Honeycombing

scribed air- and/or fluid-containing lesion that is 1 cm or more in diameter (Fig. 1-53). A cavity on the other hand is a lucency within a zone of pulmonary consolidation, a mass, or a nodule. It may or may not contain an air/fluid level, and it is surrounded by a wall of varied thickness but usually greater than 3 mm in diameter (Fig. 1-54). Pathologically a cavity results from the expulsion of a necrotic part of the lesion into the bronchial tree. This may result in an air/fluid level that forms a straight line that is parallel to the bottom of the film (Fig. 1-55). An air/fluid level implies communication with the bronchial tree provided there has been no penetration of the chest wall. It usually also indicates liquifaction necrosis as would be seen in pyogenic infection due to a lung abscess. Fluid-filled cysts cannot be distinguished on plain radiographs from solid-mass lesions. However, on CT they may have low attenuation close to that of water (0 HU). However, cysts may contain fluid that is hemorrhagic or high in protein content, in which case they will appear as soft-tissue density on CT. On MR scans cysts containing hemorrhagic or proteinaceous fluid will usually appear bright on T1-weighted sequences and relatively heterogeneous on T2-weighted images, unlike "spring water" cysts that will have very low signal intensity on T1-weighted images and very bright signal intensity on T2-weighted images (Fig. 1-6).

The thickness and irregularity of the wall of a cavity or abnormal space as well as the location and the number of such spaces is important in differential diagnosis. For example, septic pulmonary infarcts associated with intravenous drug abuse are usually multiple, thick walled, and occur in the lower-lung zones peripherally (Fig. 1-56). CT may be particularly helpful in characterizing abnormal spaces in the lung, particularly in regard to their number and internal architecture.

Congenital cysts

Most congenital spaces in the lung are cysts. They are discussed in more detail in Chapter 2. Most arise from the primitive foregut. Examples include bronchogenic and esophageal duplication cysts (Fig. 1-53) in the mediastinum and intrapulmonary abnormalities such as cystic adenomatoid malformation and pulmonary sequestration as well as intrapulmonary bronchogenic cysts.

Acquired cysts and cavities

Infection   Cavities may develop in pyogenic and nonpyogenic infections, and thin-walled cysts called pneumatoceles are a complication of some infections. Pneumatoceles are particularly seen in children following staphylococcal pneumonia, but they can also be identified in adult AIDS patients with *Pneumocystis carinii* pneumonia (Fig. 1-57). They are usually thin walled and do not contain air/fluid levels. Pneumothorax is an asso-

ciated complication. Such cysts eventually resolve in the majority of patients.

Pyogenic abscesses develop as a result of liquifaction necrosis caused by bacteria. Lung abscesses are most frequently associated with aspiration and anaerobic pneumonia produced by mouth organisms. However, pyogenic abscesses can also be seen in staphylococcal, *Klebsiella*, and streptococcal pneumonia. If the abscess does not communicate with the bronchial tree it will appear as a water or soft-tissue density mass surrounded by pneumonia, but occasionally a solitary isolated mass is visualized. When bronchial communication occurs, an air/fluid level develops as the purulent material is drained through the bronchial tree (Fig. 1-55). Because lung abscesses are roughly spherical, the air/fluid level will be of equal dimensions or length on views obtained 90° to each other, that is, PA and lateral chest radiographs. This is in contradistinction to an empyema that may contain an air/fluid level if there is a bronchopleural fistula. Air/fluid levels in the pleural space typically have different lengths on views obtained at 90° to each other (i.e., PA and lateral).

The most classic example of nonpyogenic cavitary lesions are the cavities associated with tuberculosis. These usually have thick but rather smooth walls (Fig. 1-54). They are located in the apical and posterior segments of the upper lobes or the superior segments of the lower lobes. Similar cavities may occur in other granulomatous infections, particularly fungal infections. In immunocompromised patients invasive fungi, particularly aspergillus, may be associated with ischemic necrosis and the development of cavities with air crescents (Fig. 1-58). Echinococcal infection in the lung produces cystic lesions with thin walls. These cysts contain air, but there may be three individual layers of the wall present. As the inner cyst wall collapses the debris may float on the air/fluid level causing a "water-lily" sign. (See Chapter 3 on infections.)

Vasculitis and granulomatoses   Cavities may be identified in a group of diseases often referred to as vasculitis and granulomatosis. These include Wegener's granulomatosis, lymphomatoid granulomatosis, and other types of vasculitis. Necrobiotic nodules may be seen in rheumatoid lung disease. It is unusual for these cavities to contain air/fluid levels.

Neoplasms   A neoplasm in the lung may cavitate when it outgrows its blood supply. However, cavitation is most frequently identified with squamous-cell carcinoma either primary in the lung, or metastatic. Such cavities are usually thick walled (Fig. 1-59). Metastatic neoplasms usually arise from squamous-cell tumors of the head, neck, and cervix. It is not possible to distinguish cavitary neoplasms from other causes of cavitation.

Posttraumatic pneumatoceles   Posttraumatic pneumatoceles occur secondary to either penetrating or

Text continued on page 58.

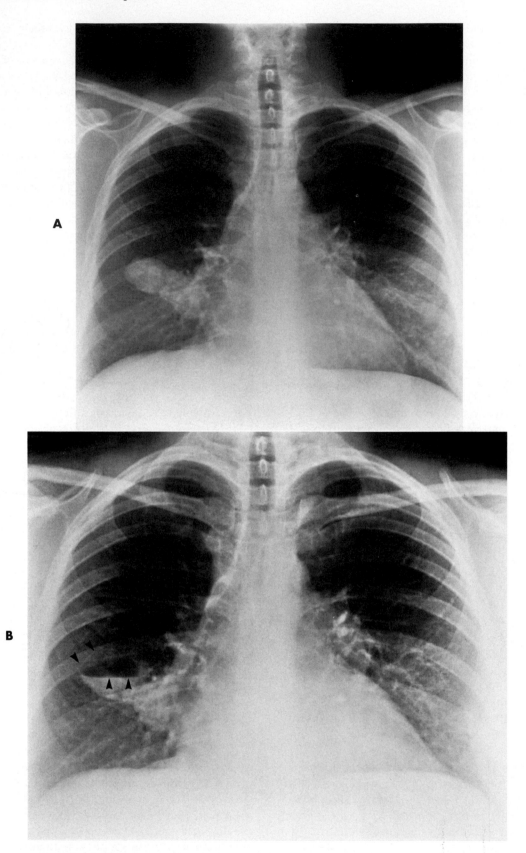

Fig. 1-53.   Bronchogenic cyst. **A,** PA view shows an ovoid opacity that represents the fluid-filled cyst in the right lung. **B,** After a needle biopsy an air/fluid level is seen and a small, thin wall superiorly (*arrowheads*).

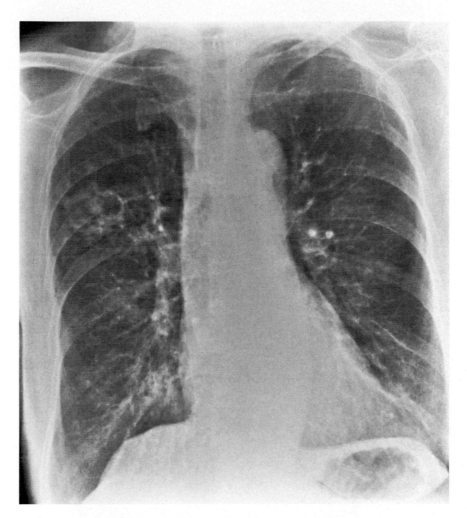

Fig. 1-54.   Cavity secondary to tuberculosis. There is a thick-walled multiloculated cavity in the right upper lobe.

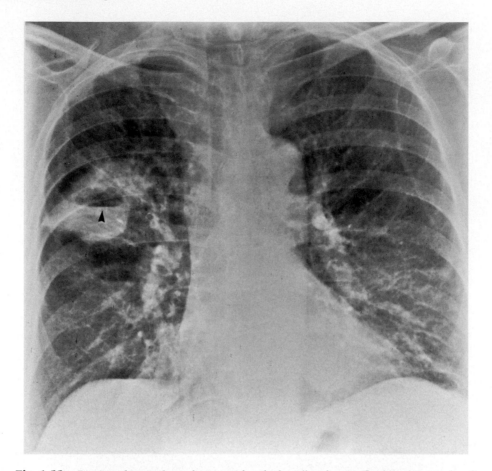

Fig. 1-55.   PA view shows a lung abscess with a thick wall and an air/fluid level (*arrowhead*).

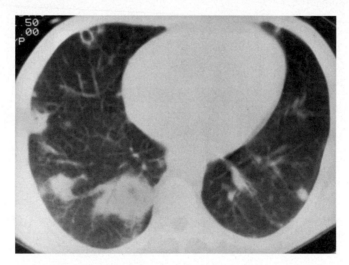

Fig. 1-56.   Septic infarcts. CT scan shows multiple nodules many of which are peripheral and some that are cavitary in the lower lung zones.

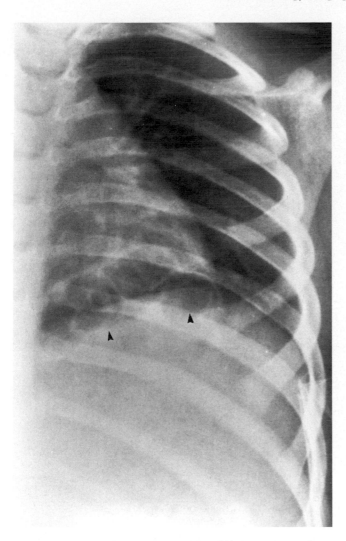

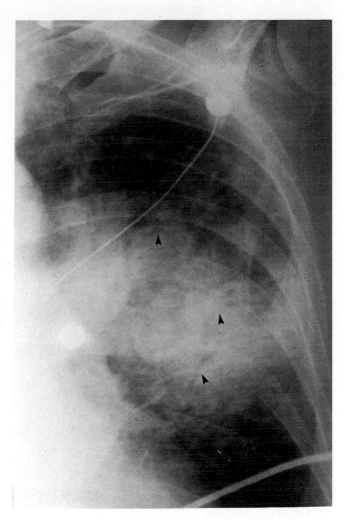

Fig. 1-57.   Pneumatoceles. Coned down PA view shows multiple thin-walled pneumatoceles above the left hemidiaphragm (*arrowheads*) in a child following staphylococcal pneumonia.

Fig. 1-58.   Invasive aspergillosis. In the left lung there are confluent large nodules that contain a rim of air ("air crescent" sign) (*arrowheads*).

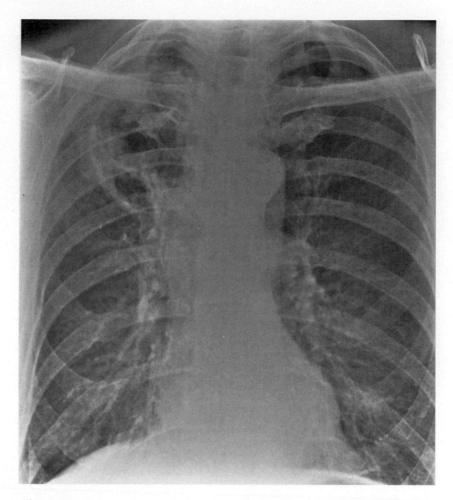

Fig. 1-59.   Lung carcinoma. Cavitary squamous carcinoma in the right upper lobe.

nonpenetrating trauma and result from laceration of the lung parenchyma (Fig. 1-60). They are usually unilateral and peripheral in location at the site of injury. Traumatic lung cysts may be filled with blood initially. However, communication with the bronchus may occur creating an air/fluid level. These pneumatoceles usually resolve in a few weeks, whereas hematomas may require months to resolve.

Pulmonary infarcts   Pulmonary infarcts rarely undergo cavitation. However, if there is associated infection, usually as a result of septic emboli, then cavitation may occur (Fig. 1-56). The classic features consist of ill-defined cavities at the bases of the lungs. Septic infarcts occur in intravenous drug abusers with tricuspid endocarditis or in patients with other causes of right-sided endocarditis, for example, congenital valve anomalies or indwelling catheters.

Blebs and bullae   Bullae are air-containing spaces within the lung parenchyma that measure more than a centimeter in diameter when distended and have a wall thickness of less than 1 mm (Fig. 1-61). They result from obstruction to air flow and are associated usually with emphysema. A bleb is a gas-containing space within the

visceral pleura of the lung. Radiologically it appears as a sharply demarcated thin-walled lucency contiguous with the pleura, usually at the lung apex. A bleb can be considered a bulla located in the visceral pleura outside the internal capsule of the lung.

Bronchiectasis   Cystic or saccular bronchiectasis may produce an appearance of multiple cystic spaces in the lung (Fig. 1-62). On standard films these cysts are usually associated with other signs of bronchiectasis such as bronchial-wall thickening seen en face or end on. If the bronchiectasis is diffuse, the lungs will be overinflated. In addition these cystic structures are usually more marked in the medial third of the lung along the bronchovascular bundles.

Diffuse infiltrative lung disease (honeycombing)   There are a number of interstitial lung diseases that may be associated with cyst formation in the lung. These may be thin-walled cysts that occur secondary to bronchiolar obstruction such as in lymphangioleiomyomatosis or histiocytosis X. Honeycombing refers to thick-walled cystic structures that are produced secondary to dissolution of alveolar walls and fibrosis with architectural distortion. This appearance occurs as part

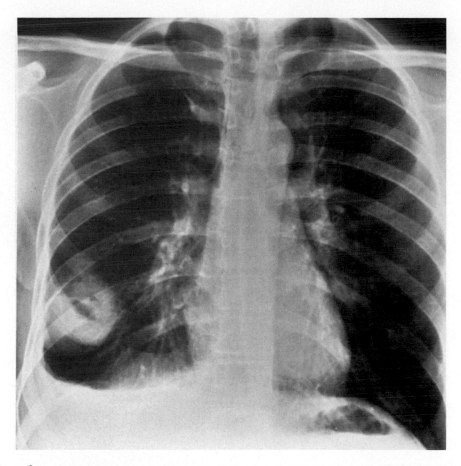

Fig. 1-60.   Lung laceration or posttraumatic pneumatocele. PA view shows a partially air-containing rounded opacity located peripherally with a small right effusion. Patient was involved in a motor vehicle accident.

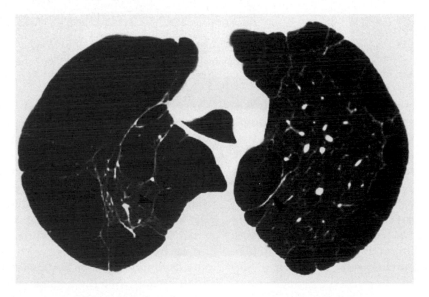

Fig. 1-61.   Bullae. There are multiple bullae with thin walls in both lungs (*arrowheads*).

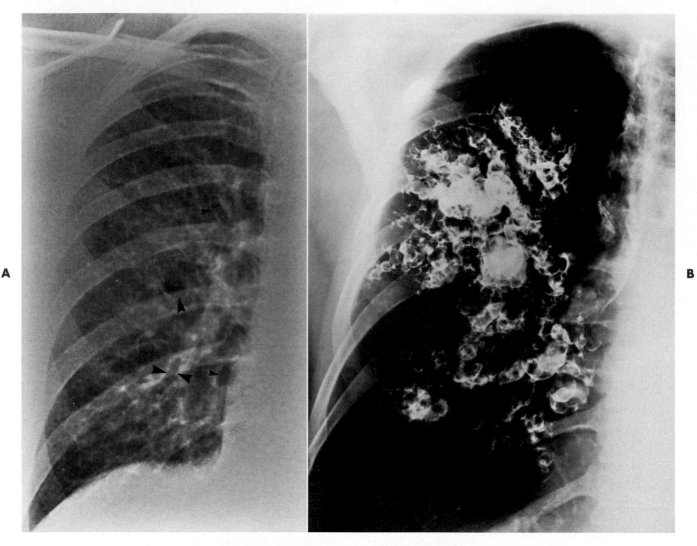

Fig. 1-62. Bronchiectasis. **A,** PA view shows multiple central cystic structures with bronchial wall thickening (*arrowheads*). **B,** A bronchogram in which contrast is introduced into the bronchial tree shows markedly dilated saccular bronchi (cystic bronchiectasis).

of the end-stage lung discussed previously, which represents the final common pathway of diffuse fibrotic diseases.

Radiographically honeycombing appears as closely approximated ring shadows usually less than 1 cm in diameter with walls that are 2 to 3 mm thick. It is usually associated with a coarse reticular pattern in the lung (Fig. 1-33). On high resolution CT these spaces typically line up one on top of the other in the subpleural or peripheral zones of the lung and are associated with traction bronchiectasis and architectural distortion of the lung.

Intrathoracic Air Trapping

Intrathoracic air trapping produces changes in radiographic density resulting in increased lucency in the lung. Air trapping is a relatively common condition. It may be localized or generalized as in chronic obstructive pulmonary disease. Air trapping may be difficult to detect on routine chest radiographs, which are conventionally obtained at full inspiration (Fig. 1-63). Air trapping only becomes apparent on expiratory chest radiographs. It results not only in increased luceny of the affected lung or portion of the lung but also in alteration in lung volume. The overall size of the lung that air traps may be equal to, smaller than, or larger than the contralateral normal lung on the inspiration radiograph, but on expiration the area containing trapped air will maintain its size while the normal lung will become smaller. This will result in signs of overexpansion of that portion of the lung that is trapping air. The signs include shift of the mediastinum away from the involved side and failure of elevation of the ipsilateral hemidiaphragm. The area of trapping may also appear relatively lucent when compared with the more normal lung. Air trapping may

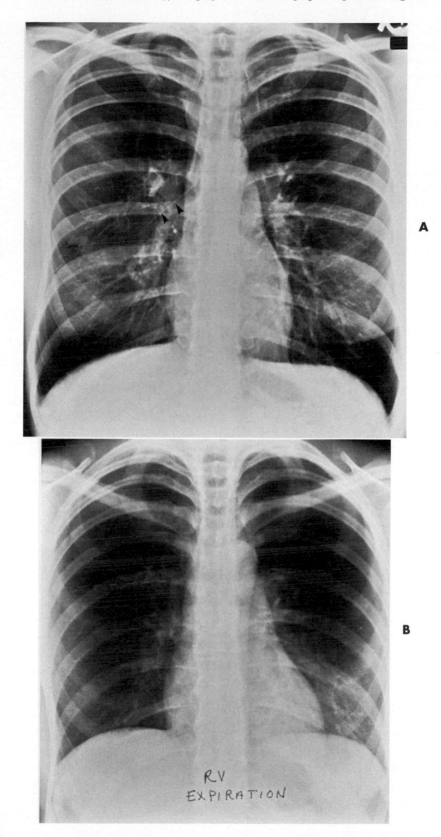

Fig. 1-63. Air trapping in the right lower lobe. **A,** PA view at inspiration shows a slightly small right lower lobe. The major fissure is depressed (*arrowheads*). **B,** On expiration the right lower lobe traps air. It is more lucent than the left base and the right hemidiaphragm is now lower than the left. Bronchiolitis obliterans.

involve an entire lung, lobe, or segment or it may be more patchy and occur at the lobular level.

Etiologies of air trapping include obstruction of a central bronchus by endobronchial or exobronchial lesions such as tumors or foreign bodies. The airway or bronchus is usually of sufficient diameter to allow air to enter during inspiration. However, during expiration when the bronchus decreases in caliber, air trapping occurs. Air trapping can also occur distal to complete airway obstruction because of collateral air drift through intraalveolar connections (pores of Kohn) and intraacinar connections (canals of Lambert), which permit air to pass from the normal portions of the lung to those distal to completely obstructed airways thus keeping these obstructed areas inflated. Collateral air drift occurs when fissures are incomplete.

Areas of air trapping may appear more lucent on standard chest radiographs obtained at inspiration (total lung capacity). This is because such areas are relatively oligemic with reduced pulmonary blood flow secondary to alveolar hypoxia. Blood flow is then diverted to the more normal areas of the lung. You must distinguish such areas due to air trapping from other causes of a radiolucent lung or lobe (Box 1-12). These other causes include: (1) technical factors; (2) chest-wall abnormalities; and (3) pulmonary vascular disease. Technical factors that may produce unilateral hyperlucency include grid cutoff, misalignment of the x-ray beam, and anode heel effect. A few degrees of rotation of the patient may also produce a difference in the relative density of the two hemithoraces. The most common chest-wall abnormality associated with unilateral hyperlucency is mastectomy. However, rare congenital anomalies such as absence of the pectoralis muscle or stroke, which produces unilateral atrophy of chest-wall muscles, may be responsible. There are a number of primary intravascular conditions that may cause hyperlucency of the lung or a portion of the lung, for example, pulmonary emboli. However, such disorders do not cause air trapping. Vascular causes of hyperlucency can be distinguished from air trapping by an expiration film.

As mentioned previously expiratory chest radiographs are the simplest and easiest method for demonstrating air trapping. Expiration films however are usually not sensitive in detecting generalized obstructive pulmonary disease such as emphysema. Limitation in the movement of the diaphragm can only be appreciated in the moderate to severe stages of the disease. In children or patients who are unable to cooperate, fluoroscopy of the chest may be helpful in demonstrating air trapping. Dynamic changes in volume with shift of mediastinal structures can be easily visualized.

There has been a great deal of recent interest in the use of CT for the identification of localized air trap-

---

Box 1-12 Unilateral Hyperlucency

TECHNICAL FACTORS

Grid cutoff
Anode heel effect
Rotation

CHEST WALL

Mastectomy
Absent pectoralis muscle

PLEURA

Pneumothorax

LUNG

Vascular conditions
  Congenital
    Absence of pulmonary artery
    Hypoplastic lung
      Congenital heart disease with abnormalities of
      pulmonary circulation
  Acquired
    Pulmonary embolus
    Tumor invading pulmonary artery
    Inflammatory stenosis (fibrosing mediastinitis)

AIRWAYS OR PARENCHYMAL ABNORMALITIES (AIR TRAPPING)

Large airway obstruction
  Foreign body
  Tumor
  Mucoid impaction
Small airways (bronchioles)
  Bronchiolitis obliterans (Swyer-James)
Peripheral lung
  Emphysema
  Bullae

---

ping. Such trapping occurs in diseases involving the small airways such as bronchiolitis obliterans (Fig. 1-64). HRCT findings include areas of decreased lung opacity that are usually patchy in distribution creating what has been called a pattern of "mosaic perfusion". The pulmonary vessels in the areas of decreased attenuation are decreased in caliber and there may be associated central bronchiectasis. Expiration HRCT scans can confirm focal areas of suspected air trapping. Marked lung inhomogeneity is usually seen on the expiration scans as the normal lung increases in attenuation, and the areas of air trapping remain relatively radiolucent or of low attenuation. A detailed discussion is provided in the chapter dealing with the airways (Chapter 13).

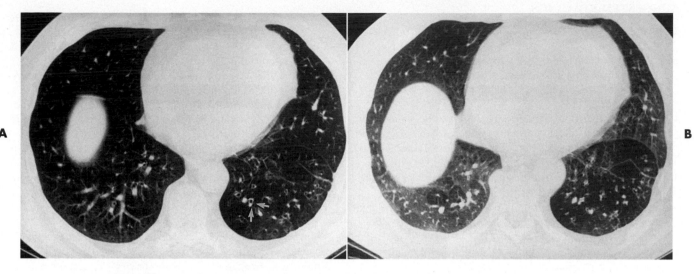

Fig. 1-64. CT of air trapping. **A,** Inspiration scan shows patchy variation in attenuation particularly in the left lower lobe where bronchiectasis is present (*arrowheads*). **B,** CT on expiration shows air trapping in the left lower lobe, which remains lucent, while most of the rest of the lungs increases in attenuation. A pattern of "mosaic perfusion" is seen in the right lower lobe.

Other Helpful Radiographic Signs of Disease

Localization of disease

The anatomic localization of disease is usually easily determined on standard PA and lateral chest radiographs. A classic radiographic sign that helps in the localization of disease processes that have caused an increase in opacification is the silhouette sign mentioned earlier (Figs. 1-38 and 1-39). Normally the mediastinal and diaphragmatic contours are visible because of their inherent contrast with the adjacent air-containing lung. When a lesion or opacity is situated in a portion of the lung adjacent to a mediastinal or diaphragmatic border, that border can no longer be seen. This sign is only apparent when structures have been adequately penetrated. An example of the use of the silhouette sign is in the differentiation of middle-lobe and lingular disease from lower-lobe disease. When disease processes involve the former lobes, the heart border will be obliterated. Obliteration of the posterior part of the aortic arch (the "aortic knob") on the left side is caused by disease in the apical posterior segment of the left upper lobe. It may be difficult on standard PA chest radiographs to identify minor degrees of consolidation or atelectasis in the basal segments of the lower lobes. Lack of visibility of the posterior portion of the hemidiaphragm in the lateral projection is often an important clue that you should look for to identify such disease (Fig. 1-39).

Distribution of disease within the lung

You should remember that the distribution of disease in the lungs may be a clue to diagnosis. Gravity is often an important factor. For example, aspiration pneumonia will typically occur in the posterior segments of the upper lobes and superior segments of the lower lobes when the patient is supine, and, similarly, when the patient is erect, the involvement will be in the basal segments of the lower lobes.

Because there is much more blood flow to the base of the lungs than the apices in the erect position, certain processes related to the pulmonary circulation occur at the bases, for example, pulmonary infarction is much more common in the lower lobes. Also metastatic lesions tend to occur at the bases.

Reactivation tuberculosis has an anatomic bias for the apices of the lung, particularly the apical and posterior segments of the upper lobes and superior segment of the lower lobes (Fig. 1-54). These are areas of the lung that are characterized by higher oxygenation with a high ventilation to perfusion ratio favoring the growth of mycobacteria.

A number of the diffuse lung diseases have an anatomic bias (Fig. 1-32). For example, idiopathic pulmonary fibrosis and fibrosis associated with collagen vascular disease as well as asbestosis tend to occur predominantly in the lower lung zones whereas upper-lobe predilection can be seen in diseases such as silicosis, sarcoidosis, and histiocytosis X.

SUGGESTED READINGS

Boyden EA: *Segmental anatomy of the lungs,* New York, 1955, McGraw-Hill.

Bragg DG, Freundlich IM: Cysts and cavities of the lung. In Freundlich IM, Bragg DG, editors: *Radiologic approach to diseases of the chest,* ed 2, Baltimore, 1977, Williams & Wilkins; pp. 119-130.

Crystal RG, Fulmer JD, Robers WC, et al: Idiopathic pulmonary fibrosis: clinical, histologic, radiographic, physiologic, scintigraphic, cytologic, and biochemical aspects, *Ann Intern Med* 85:769-788, 1976.

Doyle TC, Lawler GA: CT features of rounded atelectasis of the lung, *Am J Roentgenol* 143:225-228, 1984.

Felson B, Felson H: Localization of intrathoracic lesions by means of the postero-anterior roentgenogram: the silhouette sign, *Radiology* 55:363-368, 1950.

Felson B: The roentgen diagnosis of disseminated pulmonary alveolar diseases, *Semin Roentgenol* 2:3-21, 1967.

Flaherty RA, Keegan JM, Sturtevant HN: Post-pneumonic pulmonary pneumatoceles, *Radiology* 74:50-53, 1960.

Fleischner FG: Roentgenology of the pulmonary infarct, *Semin Roentgenol* 2:61-66, 1967.

Fleischner FG: The visible bronchial tree: a roentgen sign in pneumonic and other pulmonary consolidations, *Radiology* 50:184-190, 1948.

Fraser RG, Fraser RS, Renner JW, et al: The roentgenologic diagnosis of chronic bronchitis: a reassessment with emphasis on parahilar bronchi seen end-on, *Radiology* 120:1-8, 1976.

Fraser RG, Paré JAP, Paré PD, Fraser RS, Genereux GP: *Diagnosis of diseases of the chest,* ed 3, Philadelphia, 1989, WB Saunders, pp. 1-314 and 458-693.

Freundlich IM: Anatomy. In Freundlich IM, Bragg DG, editors: *Radiologic approach to diseases of the chest,* ed 2, Baltimore, 1997, Williams & Wilkins; pp. 31-48.

Freundlich IM: Pulmonary alveolar consolidation. In Freundlich IM, Bragg DG, editors: *Radiologic approach to diseases of the chest,* ed 2, Baltimore, 1977, Williams & Wilkins; pp. 89-100.

Freundlich IM: Pulmonary atelectasis. In Freundlich IM, Bragg DG, editors: *Radiologic approach to diseases of the chest,* ed 2, Baltimore, 1977, Williams & Wilkins; pp. 73-88.

Galvin JR, Gingrich RD, Hoffman E, et al: Ultrafast computed tomography of the chest, *Radiol Clin North Am* 32:775-793, 1994.

Gamsu G, Thurlbeck WM, Macklem PT, et al: Roentgenographic appearance of the human pulmonary acinus, *Invest Radiol* 6:171-176, 1971.

Genereux GP: CT of acute and chronic distal airspace (alveolar) disease, *Semin Roentgenol* 19:211-217, 1984.

Genereux GP: The end-stage lung: pathogenesis, pathology, and radiology, *Radiology* 116:279-284, 1975.

Glazer GM, Gross BH, Quint LE, et al: Normal mediastinal lymph nodes: number and size according to American Thoracic Society mapping, *Am J Roentgenol* 144:261-264, 1985.

Godwin JD, Vock P, Osborne DR: CT of the pulmonary ligament, *AJR* 141:231-236, 1983.

Godwin JD, Webb WR, Savoca CJ, et al: Review: multiple, thin-walled cystic lesions of the lung, *Am J Roentgenol* 135:593-604, 1980.

Greenspan RH, Curtis AM: Intrathoracic air trapping. In Freundlich IM, Bragg DG, editors: *Radiologic approach to diseases of the chest,* ed 2, Baltimore, 1977, Williams & Wilkins; pp. 195-210.

Groskin SA: *Heitzman's the lung: radiologic pathologic correlations,* ed 3, St. Louis, 1993, Mosby-Year Book; pp. 43-105.

Huang RM, Naidich DP, Lubat E, Schinella R, Garay SM, McCauley DI: Septic pulmonary emboli: CT-radiologic correlation, *AJR* 153:41-45, 1989.

Jardin M, Remy J: Segmental bronchovascular anatomy of the lower lobes: CT analysis, *AJR* 147:457-468, 1986.

Kalender WA: Technical foundations of spiral CT, *Semin Ultrasound CT MRI* 15(2):81-89, 1994.

Khoury MB, Godwin JD, Halvorsen RA Jr, et al: CT of obstructive lobar collapse, *Invest Radiol* 20:708-711, 1985.

Kuhlman JE, Fishman EK, Teigen C: Pulmonary septic emboli: diagnosis with CT, *Radiology* 174:211-213, 1990.

Kuhlman JE, Hruban RH, Fishman EK: Wegener granulomatosis: CT features of parenchymal lung disease, *J Comput Assist Tomogr* 15:948-952, 1991.

Kuhlman JE, Reyes BL, Hruban RH, Asken FB, Zerhouni EA, Fishman EK, Siegelman SS: Abnormal air filled spaces in the lung, *Radiographics* 13:47-75, 1993.

Libshitz HI: Intrathoracic lymph nodes. In Freundlich IM, Bragg DG, editors: *Radiologic approach to diseases of the chest,* ed 2, Baltimore, 1977, Williams & Wilkins; pp. 131-146.

Lien HH, Lund G: Computed tomography of mediastinal lymph nodes: anatomic review based on contrast enhanced nodes following foot lymphography, *Acta Radiol Diagn* 26:641-647, 1985.

Lubert M, Krause GR: Patterns of lobar collapse as observed radiographically, *Radiology* 56:165-168, 1951.

McLoud TC, Carrington CB, Gaensler EA: Diffuse infiltrative lung disease: a new scheme for description, *Radiology* 149:353-357, 1983.

McLoud TC, Meyer JE: Lymph node imaging of the thorax. In Clouse ME, Wallace S, editors: *Golden's diagnostic radiology: Lymphatic imaging: lymphography, computed tomography and scintigraphy,* ed 2, Baltimore 1985, Waverly Press; pp. 451-471.

McLoud TC: Diffuse infiltrative disease. In Putman CE, editor: *Pulmonary diagnosis, imaging, and other techniques,* New York, 1981, Appleton Communications; pp. 125-153.

Moore ADA, Godwin JD, Müller NL, et al: Pulmonary histiocytosis X: comparison of radiographic and CT findings, *Radiology* 172:249-254, 1989.

Muller NL: Computed tomography in chronic interstitial lung disease, *Radiol Clin North Am* 29:1085-1093, 1991.

Naidich DP, Khouri NF, Scott WW Jr, Wang KP, Siegelman SS: Computed tomography of the pulmonary hila: normal anatomy, *J Comput Assist Tomogr* 5:459-467, 1981.

Naidich DP, Khouri NF, Scott WW, et al: Computed tomography of the pulmonary hila: abnormal anatomy, *J Comput Assist Tomogr* 5:468-472, 1981.

Naidich DP, Khouri NF, Scott WW, et al: Computed tomography of the pulmonary hila: normal anatomy, *J Comput Assist Tomgr* 5:459-465, 1981.

Naidich DP, Zerhouni EA, Siegeleman SS: *Computed tomography and magnetic resonance of the thorax,* ed 2, New York, 1991, Raven Press: pp. 1-274.

Osborne D, Vock P, Godwin JD, Silverman PM: CT identification of bronchopulmonary segments: 50 normal subjects, *AJR* 142:47-52, 1984.

Proto AV, Ball JB Jr: Computed tomography of the major and minor fissures, *AJR* 140:439-448, 1983.

Proto AV, Speckman JM: The left lateral radiograph of the chest. I. *Med Radiogr Photogr* 55:30-42, 1979.

Proto AV, Speckman JM: The left lateral radiograph of the chest. II. *Med Radiogr Photogr* 56:38-50, 1980.

Reed JC, Madewell JE: The air bronchogram in interstitial disease of the lungs: a radiological-pathological correlation, *Radiology* 116:1-5, 1975.

Reich SB, Abouav J: Interalveolar air drift, *Radiology* 85:80-86, 1965.

Remy-Jardin M, Giraud F, Remy-Jardin J, Copin MC, Gosselin B, Duhamel A: Importance of ground-glass attenuation in chronic diffuse infiltrative lung disease, *Radiology* 189:693-698, 1993.

Robbins LL, Hale CH, Merrill OE: Roentgen appearance of lobar and segmental collapse of the lung: technique of examination, *Radiology* 44:474-471, 1945.

Robbins LL, Hale CH: The roentgen appearance of lobar and segmental collapse of the lung, II. The normal chest as it pertains to collapse, *Radiology* 44: 543-548, 1945.

Robbins LL, Hale CH: The roentgen appearance of lobar and segmental collapse of the lung, III. Collapse of an entire lung or the major part thereof, *Radiology* 45:23-26, 1945.

Robbins LL, Hale CH: The roentgen appearance of lobar and segmental collapse of the lung, IV. Collapse of the lower lobes, *Radiology* 45:120-127, 1945.

Robbins LL, Hale CH: The roentgen appearance of lobar and segmental collapse of the lung, V. Collapse of the right middle lobe, *Radiology* 45:260-266, 1945.

Robbins LL, Hale CH: The roentgen appearance of lobar and segmental collapse of the lung, VI. Collapse of the upper lobes, *Radiology* 45:347-355, 1945.

Rost RC, Proto AV: Inferior pulmonary ligament: computed tomographic appearance, *Radiology* 14:479-482, 1983.

Rouviere H: *Anatomy of the human lymphatic system.* Ann Arbor, 1938, Edwards Brothers.

Sandhu J, Goodman PC: Pulmonary cysts associated with PCP in patients with AIDS, *Radiology* 173:33-35, 1989.

Schneider HJ, Felson B, Gonzalez LL: Rounded atelectasis, *Am J Roentgenol* 134:225-229, 1980.

Sosman MC, Dodd GD, Jones WD, et al: The familial occurrence of pulmonary alveolar microlithiasis, *Am J Roentgenol* 77:947-952, 1957.

Swyer PR, James GCW: A case of unilateral pulmonary emphysema, *Thorax* 8:133-137, 1953.

Thurlbeck WM, Churg AM: *Pathology of the lung,* New York, 1995, Thieme Medical Publishers; pp. 589-737.

Thurlbeck WM, Muller NL: Emphysema: definition, imaging, and quantification, *AJR* 163:1017-1025, 1987.

Webb WR: High resolution computed tomography of obstructive lung disease, *Radiol Clin N Am* 32:745-757, 1994.

Webb WR, Glazer G, Gamsu G: Computed tomography of the normal pulmonary hilum, *J Comput Assist Tomogr* 5:476-484, 1981.

Webb WR, Jensen BG, Gamsu G, et al: Coronal magnetic resonance imaging of the chest: normal and abnormal, *Radiology* 153:729-735, 1984.

Webb WR: High resolution computed tomography of obstructive lung disease, *Radiol Clin N Am* 32:745-757, 1994.

Woodring JH, Fried M, Chuang VP: Solitary cavities of the lung: diagnostic implications of cavity wall thickness, *Am J Roentgenol* 135:1269-1274, 1980.

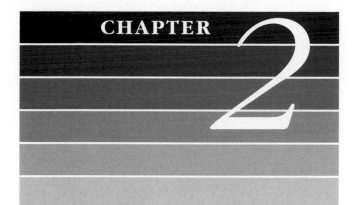

CHAPTER 2

Congenital Abnormalities of the Thorax

THERESA C. McLOUD

Several congenital abnormalities of the thorax have been described, but the majority are rare. Classification of these anomalies is difficult because the embryologic basis often is not clearly understood. A classification based on thoracic anatomic structures uses the following categories: (1) trachea, (2) bronchi, (3) lung, and (4) pulmonary vasculature. For congenital abnormalities involving the mediastinum, see Chapter 15. See Part III on Airways for a more comprehensive discussion of airways anomalies.

The diagnosis usually can be established noninvasively by means of standard radiographs, ultrasound (US), computed tomography (CT), and magnetic resonance imaging (MRI). A comprehensive listing of congenital abnormalities of the chest is provided in Box 2-1. In this chapter congenital abnormalities in adults are emphasized. (For those more commonly identified in infancy, please see Pediatric Radiology: THE REQUISITES.)

THE TRACHEA

The most common anomalies of the trachea include (1) congenital stenosis, (2) tracheomalacia, (3) congenital tracheobronchiomegaly, (4) aberrant tracheal bronchus, and (5) tracheoesophageal fistula.

Congenital Tracheal Stenosis

There are three patterns of congenital tracheal stenosis: (1) diffuse or generalized hypoplasia, (2) a funnel-like stenosis (the "carrot-shaped" trachea) often seen in association with an anomalous origin of the left pulmonary artery (Fig. 2-1), and (3) segmental stenosis. Either the diffuse or the funnel-like stenosis may be associated with absence of the posterior membranous wall due to complete ringlike tracheal cartilages.

Box 2-1 Congenital Abnormalities of the Thorax

TRACHEA

Tracheomalacia
Tracheal stenosis
Tracheal abnormalities in skeletal dysplasia syndromes
Tracheobronchomegaly
Tracheopathia osteoplastica
Intratracheal masses (hemangioma)
Tracheoesophageal fistula
Tracheal diverticulum

BRONCHI

Bronchial isomerism syndromes
Tracheal accessory bronchus
Bridging bronchus
Bronchomalacia
Bronchial atresia
Bronchiectasis
Congenital lobar emphysema

LUNGS

Horseshoe lung
Agenesis of the lung
Hypoplasia of lung
Congenital pulmonary lymphangiectasia
Pulmonary blastoma or hamartomas
Sequestration
Scimitar syndrome
Congenital cystic adenomatoid malformation
Bronchogenic cyst
Cystic fibrosis

VASCULAR ABNORMALITIES

Arteries

Absence of main pulmonary artery
Proximal interruption of the pulmonary artery
Anomalous origin of left pulmonary artery from right
Pulmonary artery stenosis or coarctation
Congenital aneurysm of pulmonary arteries
AV fistula

Veins

Hypogenetic lung—scimitar syndrome
Pulmonary varix
Anomalous pulmonary venous drainage

Lymphatics

Lymphangiectasis
Lymphangioma
   Localized
   Diffuse
Lymphangioleiomyomatosis

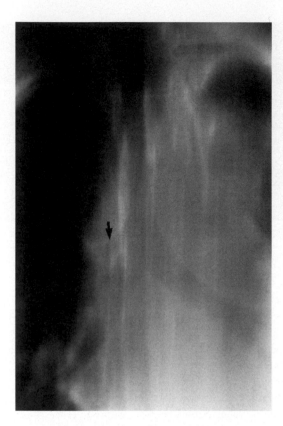

Figure 2-1. Congenital tracheal stenosis. AP tomogram shows a long funnel-shaped stenosis involving the intrathoracic trachea. The trachea has a more normal diameter above the carina. Note the tracheal bronchus to the right upper lobe *(arrow)*.

Tracheomalacia

Tracheomalacia is abnormal collapsibility of the trachea, which is due to softness or pliability of the tracheal cartilages. It may be either primary, associated with a localized absence of the tracheal cartilage, or secondary, as a result of external compression such as from an extrinsic mass. It is imperative to distinguish tracheomalacia from excessive collapse, which is secondary to abnormal expiratory pressures. For example, collapse of a long segment of the intrathoracic trachea may occur in late expiration in patients with asthma, chronic bronchitis, and bronchiolitis. Fluoroscopy and ultrafast computed tomography (CT) are excellent for evaluating tracheomalacia, both of which allow for real-time assessment of airway dynamics. A greater than 50% collapse of the tracheal diameter is considered abnormal (Fig. 2-2).

Congenital Tracheobronchomegaly (Mounier-Kuhn Syndrome)

Tracheobronchomegaly is characterized by loud, prolonged chronic cough with ineffective secretions, and recurrent bronchitis or pneumonia. The trachea demon-

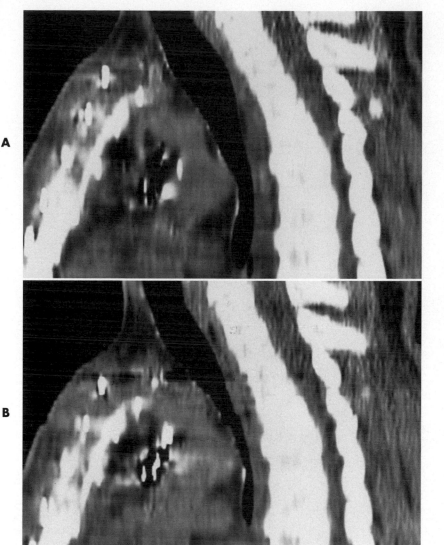

Figure 2-2 Tracheomalacia—shown by sagittal reformatted CT image. **A,** Inspiration. The trachea is of normal caliber. **B,** Expiration. There is excessive collapsibility of the trachea.

strates absence or atrophy of elastic fibers and thinning of muscle; airway dynamics are abnormal with dilation on inspiration and collapse on expiration. There are frequent saccular bulgings of the intercartilaginous membranes. You can establish the diagnosis on chest radiography when the transverse diameter of the trachea is greater than 25 mm and the diameters of the right and left main bronchi are greater than 23 and 20 mm, respectively (Fig. 2-3). CT will confirm the increased diameter of the trachea. Frequently there may be bronchiectasis in the lung parenchyma.

Aberrant Tracheal Bronchus

Rarely the right upper lobe bronchus or a segment of the right upper lobe bronchus may originate in the trachea (tracheal or preeparterial bronchus) (Fig. 2-4). This is usually of no clinical consequence, although following endotracheal intubation the balloon may inadvertently obstruct such a bronchus, causing right upper lobe atelectasis.

Tracheoesophageal Fistula

Congenital tracheoesophageal fistula is invariably a pediatric disease occurring in newborns and is most frequently associated with esophageal atresia. However, about 3% of all tracheoesophageal fistulas occur with an otherwise normal esophagus and patients may present in these instances in adult life. Roughly 75% will show communication with the trachea, and the remainder communicate with the major bronchi (Fig. 2-5). Patients usually have a history of recurrent pneumonias. The chest roentgenogram may show evidence of bronchiectasis. You can confirm the diagnosis by a contrast esophagram, which will often identify the fistula and show evidence of contrast material within the tracheobronchial tree and the lung.

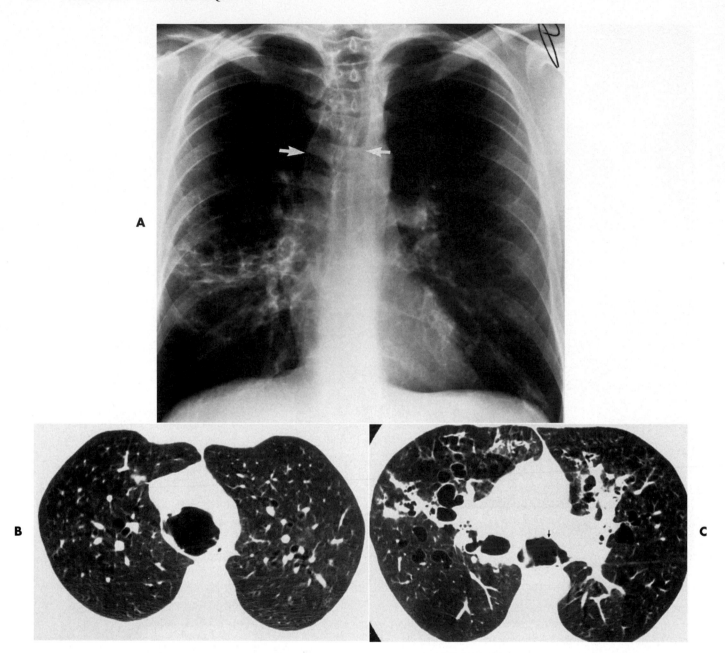

Figure 2-3 Congenital tracheobronchomegaly (Mounier-Kuhn syndrome). **A,** PA chest radiograph shows marked tracheal dilation (43 mm) *(arrows)*. There is also bronchiectasis in the right lung. **B,** CT scan confirms the large tracheal lumen. **C,** The dilation extends into the main bronchi, which exhibit saccular bulging of their walls *(arrow)*.

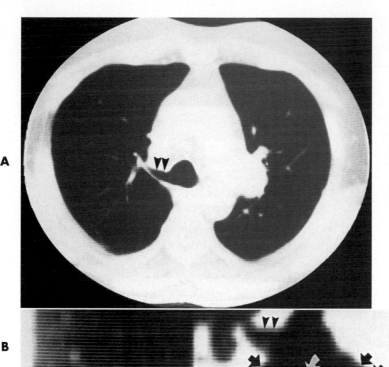

Figure 2-4 Tracheal bronchus. **A,** Axial CT showing the right upper lobe bronchus arising above the carina. **B,** Reformatted coronal CT image demonstrating the carinal spur *(curved white arrow)*, right and left main bronchi *(black arrows)*, and tracheal bronchus to the right upper lobe *(arrowheads)*.

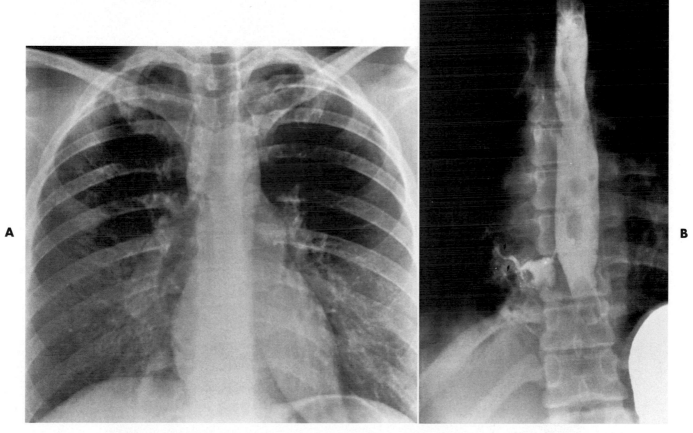

Figure 2-5 Congenital bronchoesophageal fistula in a 24-year-old woman with history of repeated pneumonias since childhood. **A,** PA chest radiograph shows patchy pneumonia in the right upper lobe and right base with right hilar and paratracheal adenopathy secondary to repeated infections. **B,** Barium esophagram demonstrates a fistula between the lower esophagus and a branch of the right lower-lobe bronchus *(arrows)*.

THE BRONCHI

Bronchial (Pulmonary) Isomerism Syndrome

Bronchopulmonary isomerism has an identical pattern of bronchial branching and an equal number of lobes in each lung. The anomaly may be isolated or associated with other anomalies. The bilateral right lung type may be associated with asplenia, and the bilateral left lung type may be associated with polysplenia.

Bronchial Atresia

This anomaly consists of atresia of a lobar or segmental bronchus with obliteration of the lumen and preservation of distal structures. The most common site is the left upper lobe, particularly the apical posterior segment. The right middle and upper lobes are less common. Mucus secreted within the airways distal to the atretic segment cannot pass the stenosis and accumulates as a mucous plug or mucocele. Collateral air drift keeps the lobe or segment inflated and it becomes hyperinflated as a result of expiratory air trapping. The chest radiograph shows an area of hyperlucency in the affected portion of the lung (Fig. 2-6). The mucocele will appear as an ovoid or branching structure at the hilar level. CT clearly demonstrates the mucoid impaction at the site of obstruction associated with lobar or segmental hyperinflation. There may be accompanying shift of the mediastinum and compression of the surrounding lung.

Congenital Bronchiectasis (Williams-Campbell Syndrome)

Congenital bronchiectasis is rare and its existence is controversial. It results from an intrinsic abnormality of cartilage. The cartilaginous deficiency occurs within the fourth- to sixth-order bronchi and is manifested by cystic bronchiectasis and pulmonary hyperinflation (Fig. 2-7). Bronchiectasis, which is acquired and secondary to chronic infection, may occur early in life as a result of other congenital, developmental, or genetic disorders. These conditions are listed in Box 2-2. (See Chapter 13 for further discussion.)

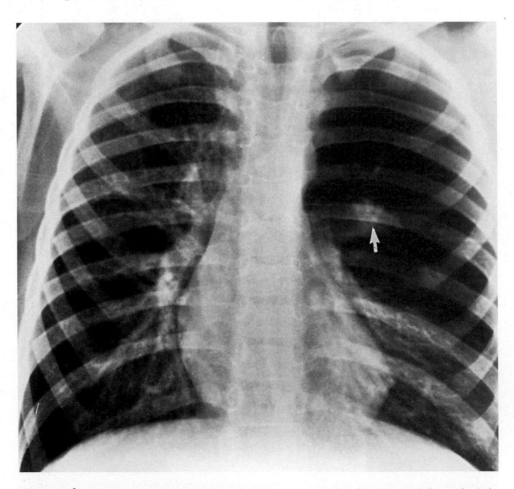

Figure 2-6 Bronchial atresia. AP radiograph shows an overinflated left upper lobe with slight mediastinal shift. The left perihilar opacity represents mucoid impaction distal to the atresia *(arrow)*.

LUNG

Pulmonary Agenesis and Hypoplasia

Pulmonary agenesis is a condition with total absence of the lung parenchyma and the vessels and bronchi distal to the carina. In pulmonary aplasia there is a rudimentary bronchus, which ends in a blind pouch without lung tissue or pulmonary vasculature. A decrease in the number or size of airways, vessels, and alveoli characterizes pulmonary hypoplasia. It may be primary or secondary to a number of pathogenetic mechanisms that may occur during gestation. These include decreased pulmonary vascular perfusion, oligohydramnios, or com-

---

Box 2-2   Bronchiectasis Associated with Developmental or Congenital Disorders

Congenital cystic bronchiectasis
Primary hypogammaglobulinemia
"Yellow nail" syndrome
Cystic fibrosis
Immotile-cilia syndrome (Kartagener's syndrome)

---

pression of the lung by a space-occupying mass within the pleural cavity (such as a congenital diaphragmatic hernia).

Agenesis, aplasia, and hypoplasia more frequently involve the right lung. In agenesis the radiograph shows complete absence of aerated lung in one hemithorax, with pronounced reduction in the volume of that hemithorax and associated shift of the mediastinum to the affected side (Fig. 2-8). There is usually pronounced compensatory overinflation of the contralateral normal lung. Pulmonary hypoplasia has similar findings because of volume reduction; however, there is a small lung on the affected side. In some cases it may be difficult on standard radiographs to distinguish severe pulmonary hypoplasia from aplasia or agenesis. In such instances, CT may be helpful in identifying either the absence or presence of the ipsilateral pulmonary artery and bronchus or the presence of a rudimentary bronchus in pulmonary aplasia. CT will also demonstrate rudimentary pulmonary tissue in the base of the hemithorax in severe pulmonary hypoplasia and a patent bronchus and accompanying pulmonary artery (Fig. 2-9).

Pulmonary hypoplasia must be differentiated from other conditions that may produce a small lung with markedly reduced volume of the hemithorax. These include total atelectasis of the lung, severe bronchiecta-

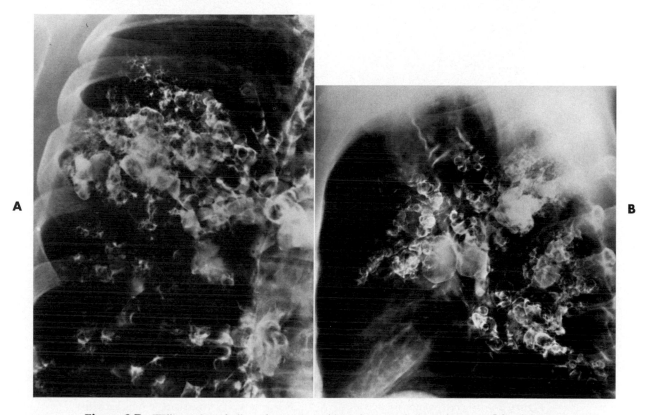

Figure 2-7   Williams-Campbell syndrome. PA and lateral views of a bronchogram of the right lung shows diffuse cystic bronchiectasis involving all lobes.

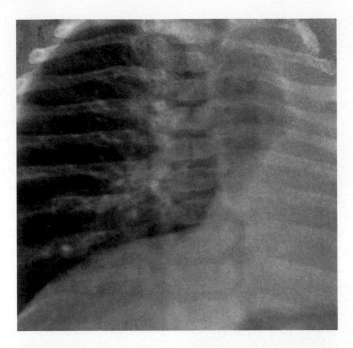

Figure 2-8 Pulmonary agenesis. AP radiograph of an infant shows complete absence of the left lung with pronounced mediastinal shift and overinflation of the right lung.

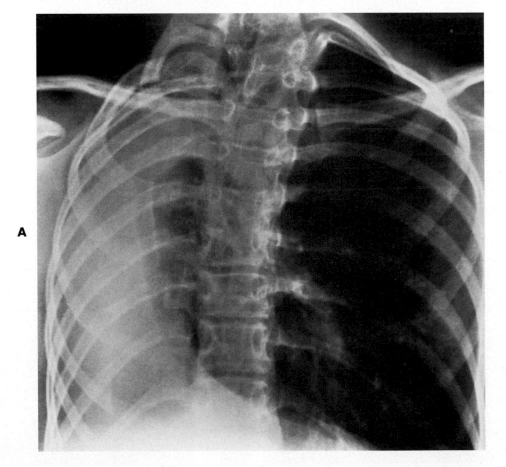

A

Figure 2-9 Severe pulmonary hypoplasia. **A,** PA chest radiograph suggests right lung agenesis.

Continued

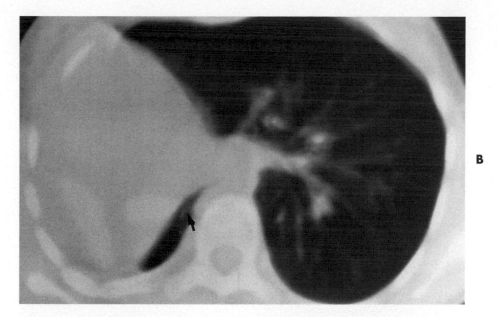

Figure 2-9, cont'd.   B, CT scan demonstrates rudimentary lung tissue at the right base, which contains pulmonary vessels *(arrow).*

sis with collapse, and advanced fibrothorax due to chronic pleural disease. CT is likely to be diagnostic in such cases.

Congenital Lobar Emphysema

The primary characteristic of congenital lobar emphysema is progressive overdistension of a lobe secondary to either an intrinsic bronchial obstruction due to a cartilage anomaly or deficiency or due to compression by an extrinsic vascular structure or mass (i.e., a bronchogenic cyst). In a minority of patients the hyperinflated lobe may be secondary to an abnormal increase in alveoli. The condition usually occurs in infants or young children. The left upper lobe is the most frequently affected, followed by the right middle lobe. The radiologic findings consist of overinflation of the affected lobe with varying degrees of mediastinal shift (Fig. 2-10). Occasionally the lobe may be opaque secondary to retained fetal lung fluid. The differential diagnosis includes (1) a foreign body in a older infant; (2) extraluminal compression of the bronchus by a bronchogenic cyst, teratoma, or other mass lesion; (3) bronchial atresia with overinflation; and (4) congenital lung cyst (Table 2-1). Acute cases of respiratory distress require surgical resection particularly in the neonatal period. However, the trend is toward supportive therapy because investigations show that these lesions may regress spontaneously without thoracotomy and lobar resection. A small percentage of cases are asymptomatic and may not be diagnosed until adult life.

Cystic Adenomatoid Malformation

Cystic adenomatoid malformation of the lung is a rare lesion that usually occurs in infancy with respiratory distress secondary to a space-occupying effect that compromises lung tissue. There are three types. Type I, the most common, is characterized by single or multiple large cysts of varying size measuring more than 2 cm in diameter. Type II consists of multiple small cysts of more uniform size not exceeding 2 cm in diameter, and type III consists of large, bulky, solid-appearing lesions that contain multiple microscopic-sized cysts.

The radiographic findings are variable and correlate with the type of lesion. Chest radiographs in the type I lesion typically show unilateral single or multiple air-filled cysts in the thorax of a neonate with respiratory distress (Fig. 2-11). The lesions may be very large and may occupy almost the entire lung, producing a mass effect with shift of the mediastinum and compression of the remaining lung. There may be a single dominant cyst surrounded by smaller cysts. If fluid is present, you can identify air-fluid levels on horizontal beam images. Type II lesions may show evidence of multiple small uniform cysts. A type III lesion usually appears as a solid intrathoracic mass or consolidation rather than as a cystic or air-filled structure.

The appearance on CT scanning is similar, and CT may document the number of cysts. Although cystic adenomatoid malformation has been considered a unilateral disease, CT has been reported to show evidence of bilateral involvement. CT imaging may be helpful in differentiating congenital cystic adenomatoid malformation from

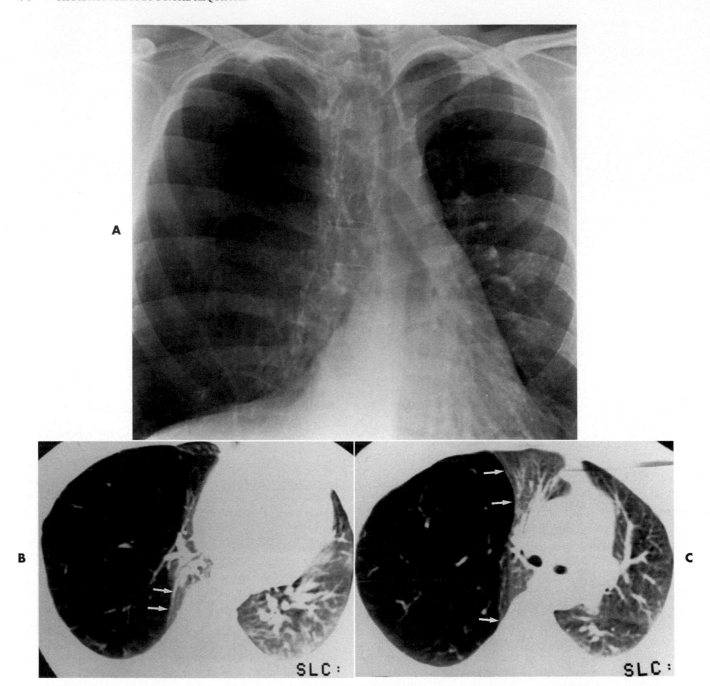

Figure 2-10   Congenital lobar emphysema (right middle lobe) in a 42-year-old man. **A,** PA chest radiograph shows pronounced overinflation of the right lung with mediastinal shift to the left. The vessels in the right lung are few in number and stretched, suggesting that the air-filled lung may represent only one lobe. **B & C,** CT scan demonstrates collapsed and compressed upper and lower lobes *(arrows)* and pronounced overinflation of the right middle lobe.

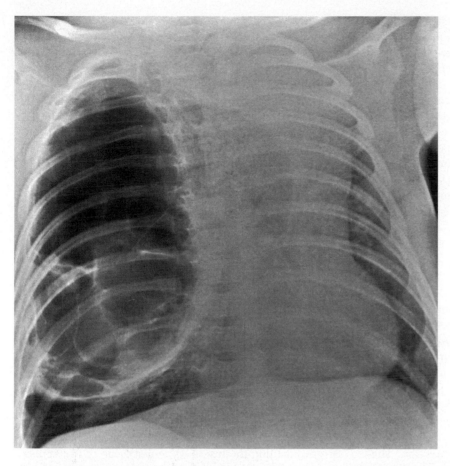

Figure 2-11 Cystic adenomatoid malformation Type 1. PA radiograph (magnification technique) shows multiple large air-filled cysts in the right lung with shift of the mediastinum to the left and compression to the remaining right lung above the diaphragm.

Table 2-1   Diagnosis of cystic or cystlike developmental lesions

Condition	Distinguishing Features
Congenital diaphragmatic hernia	Air-filled or contrasted-filled bowel loops above diaphragm.
Bronchogenic cyst	Usually mediastinal
	In lung—medial one third
	Usually opaque, occasionally air fluid level
	Marked displacement of lung and mediastinum not a feature
Congenital lobar emphysema	LUL, RML—no internal linear opacities
	Lucent usually
	Marked shift of mediastinum and compression of lung with mass effect
	If fluid-filled, may substitue CAM Type III
Cystic adenomatoid malformation	Lucent air-filled single or multiple cysts
	Mass effect
	Multiple internal linear opacities

other conditions. It can document the presence of air- or fluid-filled cysts, the extent of disease, and the amount of mass effect.

Roughly 80% of patients are under 6 months of age, although 17% of cases are reported in older children.

The definitive treatment is surgical excision. In neonates with severe respiratory distress, this lesion may constitute a surgical emergency.

Prognosis appears to be best in patients with type I lesions. If cysts are very large and interfere with normal pulmonary development, particularly if there is contralateral pulmonary hypoplasia, prognosis is poor.

Pulmonary Sequestration

Pulmonary sequestration consists of aberrant lung tissue that (1) has no normal connection with the bronchial tree or with the pulmonary arteries; or (2) is supplied by a systemic artery that usually arises from the aorta. It may be extralobar, contained within its own pleural envelope, or intralobar, contained within the substance of the lung (Table 2-2). Generally, sequestration is a congenital abnormality secondary to failure of obliteration of one of the systemic arterial connections to the base of the developing fetal lung. Controversy exists, however, particularly regarding intralobar sequestration, which may be acquired from chronic infection.

The arterial blood supply to the sequestered pulmonary tissue usually arises from the descending thoracic aorta, although the origin may be from the upper abdominal aorta or one of its major branches. The venous drainage of intralobar and extralobar sequestrations differ. Intralobar sequestration usually drains into a branch of the inferior pulmonary vein, creating a left-to-left shunt. Extralobar sequestration drains to the systemic veins, usually the azygos system.

Intralobar sequestration

Intralobar sequestrations are more common than the extralobar variety, and frequently these present in adult life either as an abnormality on a standard chest radiograph or as a cause of recurrent pneumonias. They almost invariably occur in the lower lobes in the area of the posterior basal segment. They affect the left side twice as frequently as the right. The radiographic appearance may vary, but there are two major patterns. These patterns depend on the degree of aeration and the presence or absence of associated infection. The lesion may appear as a solid-water density mass or area of consolidation, or alternatively it may appear as an air-containing single or multicystic lesion (Figs. 2-12 and 2-13). The air gains entry into the sequestered lung from the surrounding pulmonary tissue by means of collateral ventilation. If there is an infection, an air/fluid level may be seen. Both CT and MRI may be useful in evaluation. Contrast-enhanced CT (Fig. 2-13) and more frequently coronal MR show the abnormal systemic artery in the majority of cases. CT also demonstrates the internal architecture of the sequestration and its cystic components when present. Failure to identify a systemic artery on these examinations, however, does not exclude the diagnosis. Angiography will demonstrate the anomalous systemic vessel (Fig. 2-13).

Extralobar sequestration

Extralobar sequestration typically manifests in the newborn or early infancy. It is most often in the lower hemithorax between the lower lobe and the diaphragm, although it may occur within the substance of the diaphragm or in the mediastinum. Diagnosis can often be made without angiography by using CT and MRI, which may demonstrate the anomalous feeding and draining vessels.

On standard roentgenograms the extralobar sequestration usually appears as a single well-defined homogeneous area of increased opacity in the lower thorax close to the posterior medial hemidiaphragm. It occasionally appears as a small "bump" on the hemidiaphragm or inferior paravertebral region. There are no air bronchograms. The lesion is usually well defined and does not blend with the surrounding lung parenchyma. It may also occur in the mediastinum and in the pericardium or upper thorax, and rarely as a subdiaphragmatic mass. Occasionally there may be communication with the stomach or esophagus, and an esophagram is recommended to demonstrate the fistulous communication between the sequestration and the gastrointestinal tract. Aortography depicts the anomalous systemic artery or arteries feeding the lesion. Demonstration of the venous drainage may require selective angiography of the anomalous feeding vessels. Ultrasound may be useful in the diagnosis of pulmonary sequestration in neonates and infants with typical findings of a uniformly echogenic mass, occasionally with a hyperechoic rim. Duplex Doppler scanning and color Doppler flow imaging may be used to diagnose extralobar sequestration. Reports show aberrant arterial and venous structures supplying and draining these lesions. On CT images of the chest (Fig. 2-14) the lesions are usually homogenous well-defined masses of soft tissue attenuation, sometimes with areas of emphysema in the adjacent normal lung. CT may also demonstrate cystic areas within the sequestration.

Table 2-2 Pulmonary sequestration		
	Intralobar	**Extralobar**
Clinical Features	Adults	Infants
	Males and females equally	Males more than females
	Pneumonia or incidental finding	Asymptomatic or symptoms due to associated abnormalities
Location	60% left	90% left
	Posterior lower lobe	Above or below diaphragm
Arterial supply	Large vessel from aorta	Single or multiple systemic arteries
Venous drainage	Pulmonary vein	Systemic (azygos, hemiazygos, vena cava)
Connection with foregut	Rare	Occasionally
Pleura	No separate pleural covering	Separate pleural covering

Bronchogenic Cyst

Bronchogenic cysts are bronchopulmonary foregut malformations resulting from an abnormality of budding or branching of the tracheobronchial tree during embryologic development. Bronchogenic cysts are lined by pseudostratified ciliated columnar epithelium, and they usually contain smooth muscle, mucous glands, and cartilage. They may occur in either the mediastinum or, far less commonly, in the lung. They may be filled with either clear or mucoid material. (See Chapter 16, in which mediastinal bronchogenic cysts are discussed in more detail). The pulmonary variety typically occurs, in the lower lobes, usually in the medial third of the lung. They are sharply circumscribed, solitary, and typically round or oval; on standard chest roentgenograms (Fig. 2-15) they appear to be of soft tissue or unit density. The majority are asymptomatic but particularly the intrapulmonary cysts may become infected, resulting in communication with the tracheobronchial tree. This may lead to

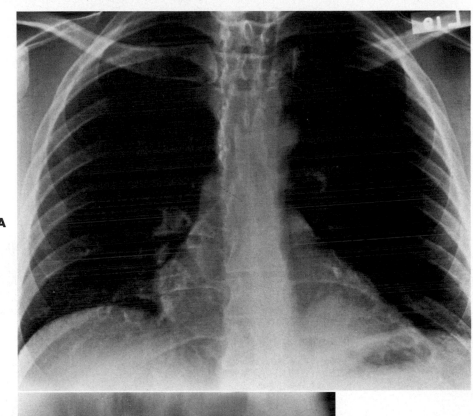

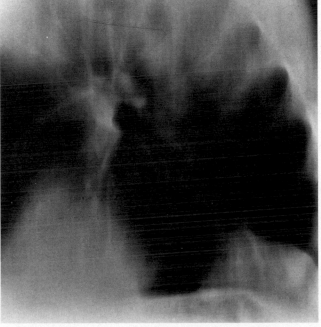

Figure 2-12 Intralobar sequestration. **A,** PA radiograph shows a solid masslike lesion in the left lower lobe abutting the diaphragm. **B,** Lateral tomogram confirms a well-defined mass posteriorly in the left lower lobe.

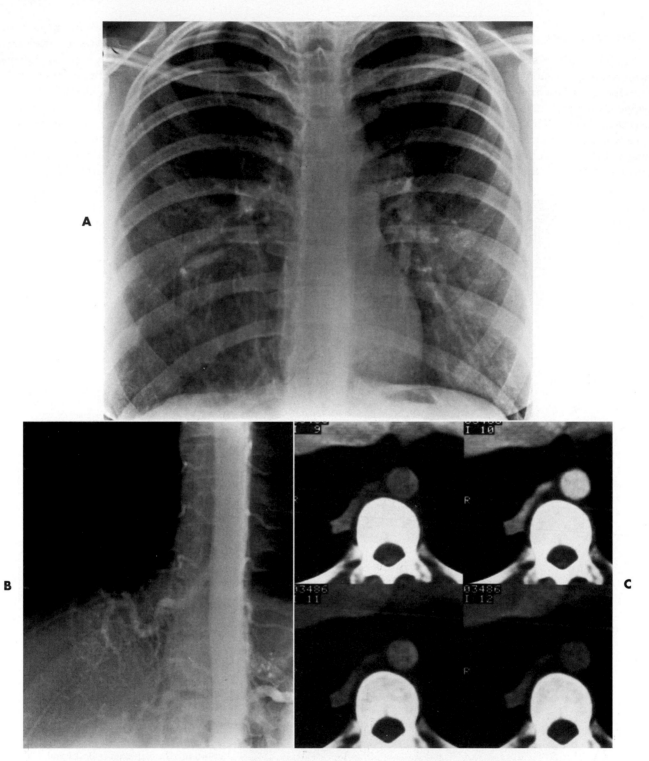

Figure 2-13   Intralobar sequestration (air-filled). **A,** PA radiograph. The pulmonary vessels at the right base display an abnormal course; this suggests they may be draped around a space-occupying but air-filled lesion. The right hemidiaphragm is slightly depressed, and the heart is shifted slightly to the left. **B,** Aortogram demonstrates a large single vessel arising from the distal aorta supplying a portion of the right lower lobe. **C,** Contrast-enhanced CT scan confirms the vascular supply.

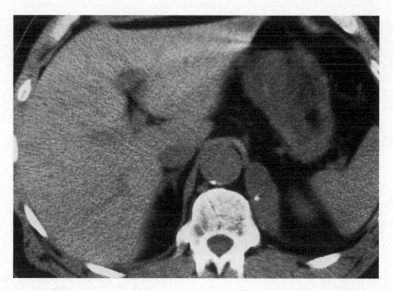

Figure 2-14 Extralobar sequestration. CT scan demonstrates a well-defined mass containing calcium abutting the left diaphragmatic crus.

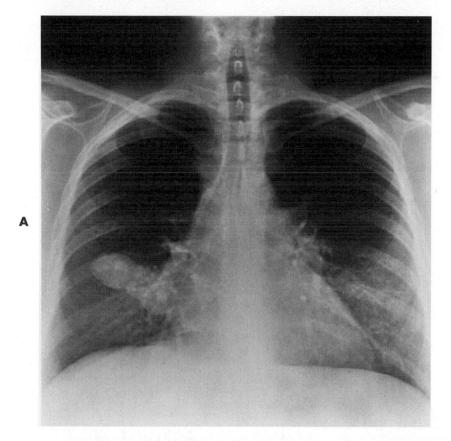

Figure 2-15 Bronchogenic cyst. **A,** PA chest radiograph shows a well-defined ovoid mass of soft tissue density in the medial third of the right lung.

Continued

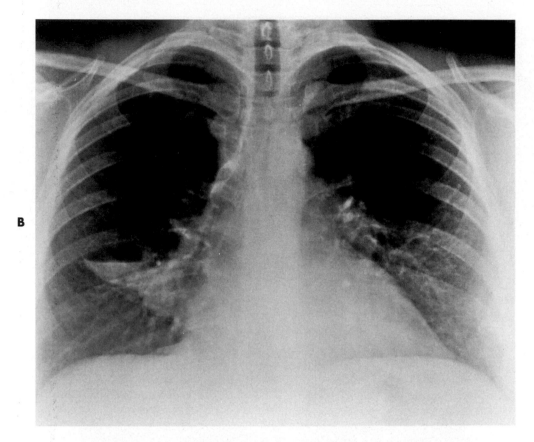

Figure 2-15, cont'd   **B,** Following needle aspiration biopsy, an air fluid is demonstrated and the wall appears very thin, consistent with a cyst.

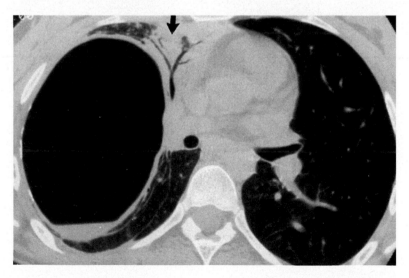

Figure 2-16   Infected bronchogenic cyst. CT scan demonstrates an air fluid in an infected bronchogenic cyst. There is evidence of pneumonia in the right middle lobe *(arrow).*

either the development of an air/fluid level or a surrounding consolidation in the lung parenchyma that will obscure the wall of the cyst (Fig. 2-16).

CT demonstrates a well-defined mass that may have variable CT densities depending on the nature of the fluid content. Roughly half the cysts have high attenuation greater than that of muscle because of mucoid content or hemorrhage (see Chapter 16, Mediastinum.) On MRI T1 images the lesions have the typical appearance of cysts with long T1 and T2 values. Cysts that contain mucus may have high signal intensity on T1-weighted images.

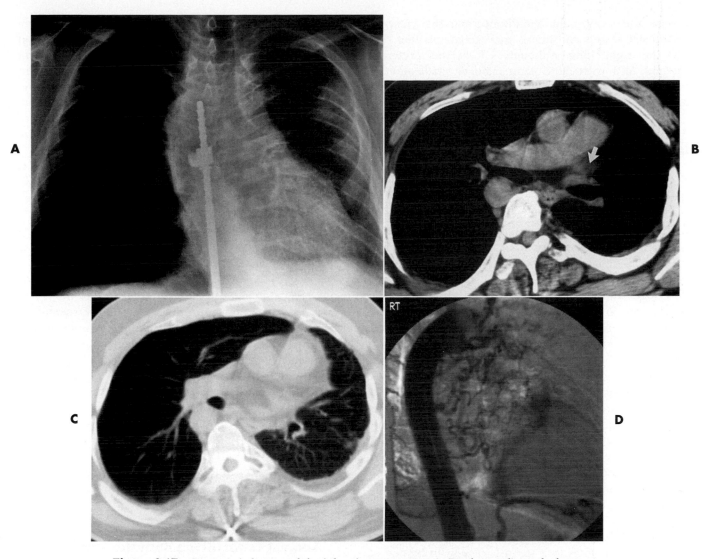

Figure 2-17 Congenital absence of the left pulmonary artery. **A,** PA chest radiograph shows a small left lung. There is scoliosis and a right aortic arch. **B,** CT scan demonstrates absence of the left pulmonary artery *(arrow)*. **C,** On the lung windows the pulmonary vessels appear small, and there is a fine reticular pattern suggesting collateral systemic vascular supply. **D,** Aortogram shows a right arch with enlarged bronchial and intercostal arteries supplying the left lung. Later films demonstrate retrograde flow from these vessels into more peripheral pulmonary arteries.

PULMONARY VESSELS

Anomalies of the Pulmonary Arteries

Absence of the main pulmonary artery and proximal interruption (absence of the right and left pulmonary arteries)

Absence of the main pulmonary artery frequently consists of atresia of the artery's proximal portion or of its entire length. The right and left main pulmonary arteries persist and connect to the aorta by a ductus.

Congenital unilateral absence of a pulmonary artery usually occurs with cardiac lesions, but it may be an isolated finding when it occurs on the right side.

Chest radiographic findings include evidence of a small lung as manifested by cardiac and mediastinal shift, absence of the pulmonary arterial shadow, elevation of the hemidiaphragm, and decrease in pulmonary vessels in the affected lung with oligemia (Fig. 2-17). There may be hyperinflation and herniation of the opposite lung across the midline. This entity must be distinguished from Swyer-James syndrome, which shares many of the radiographic features. This syndrome is due to bronchiolitis and is always associated with air trapping, which can be documented by either an expiration film or a ventilation perfusion scan. Absence of the right pulmonary artery can be confirmed with CT scanning (Fig. 2-17), which also reveals the small right hemithorax and the enlarged intercostal vessels and transpleural collaterals that supply the right lung. Although CT is the preferred method, MRI with either spin echo or gradient echo images also shows absence of the right pulmonary artery.

Anomalous origin of the left pulmonary artery from the right (pulmonary artery sling)

This is a relatively rare anomaly in which the left pulmonary artery arises from the right and courses to the left between the esophagus and trachea in its course to the left hilum. It may produce compression of both the right main bronchus and the trachea. It may occur as an isolated finding or be associated with congenital tracheal stenosis, particularly the type caused by complete or *O*-shaped cartilaginous rings, as described above. A barium swallow shows a focal impression on the anterior surface of the barium-filled esophagus in the region of the lower trachea. Diagnosis can be easily established with contrast-enhanced CT or MRI scans.

Pulmonary artery stenosis or coarctation

This is a rare anomaly characterized by single or multiple coarctations of the pulmonary arteries commonly with poststenotic dilation. The stenoses may occur anywhere in the pulmonary arterial tree. They may be short or long; unilateral or bilateral. This is usually associated with congenital cardiac or other anomalies.

The chest radiograph varies greatly in appearance depending on the stenoses' location and number. The pulmonary vasculature may appear normal, diminished, or increased. If there is a stenosis of a main branch of the pulmonary artery, the affected lung distal to the stenosis may show radiographic changes of diffuse oligemia and signs of pulmonary arterial hypertension and cor pulmonale.

Congenital Aneurysms of the Pulmonary Arteries

Congenital aneurysms of the pulmonary artery are rare and are usually associated with other pulmonary abnormalities such as arteriovenous fistulas or bronchopulmonary sequestration. When they occur in the central pulmonary arteries, they are usually associated with pulmonary valvular stenosis.

Anomalies of the Pulmonary Veins

Pulmonary Varix

A pulmonary varix is a rare localized enlargement of a segment of the pulmonary vein. It may be congenital or acquired. If acquired, it occurs secondary to prolonged pulmonary venous hypertension as seen in mitral stenosis. In the congenital variety the varix occurs in a pulmonary vein that drains normally into the left atrium. Pulmonary varices occur more frequently on the right side and are usually not associated with symptoms, although there are rare cases of hemoptysis or dysphagia due to pressure on the esophagus.

On standard radiographic films the varices appear as smooth rounded or lobulated masses of unit density frequently in the lower lung zones. On the right they may project behind the heart on the posteroanterior (PA) view, creating the impression of a solitary pulmonary nodule. On the lateral view they are localized posterior to the left atrium (Fig. 2-18).

Using dynamic enhanced CT or gradient echo MRI, one can easily identify the vascular nature of the lesion and its course draining into the left atrium. Dynamic CT demonstrates opacification during the venous phase. The most important differential diagnosis is an arteriovenous fistula. Dynamic CT scanning should allow differentiation by demonstrating the absence of an enlarged arterial feeding vessel, enhancement during the venous phase, and drainage of the varix into the left atrium. Pulmonary angiography is seldom necessary for diagnosis.

Anomalous Pulmonary Venous Drainage

This entity is discussed in detail in Chapter 9 of *Cardiac Radiology: The Requisites*.

Anomalies Involving Both the Arteries and Veins

Pulmonary Arteriovenous Fistulas

Pulmonary arteriovenous fistulas are abnormal communications between the pulmonary arteries and the pulmonary veins in which there is no capillary network that normally separates the arteries from the veins. There is a right to left shunt because blood passing through an arteriovenous fistula reaches the left atrium without being oxygenated. Pulmonary arteriovenous malformations may be single or multiple. They are "simple" if there is a single feeding artery and a single draining vein; they are complex if there are two or more feeding arteries and two or more draining veins. Between 40% and 60% of patients with arteriovenous fistulas in the lungs are patients with Osler-Weber-Rendu disease, characterized by both cutaneous and mucosal telangiectasias and occasionally AV fistulas in other organs.

Most patients are asymptomatic, but cyanosis, dyspnea, stroke, and brain abscess may occur as a result of the

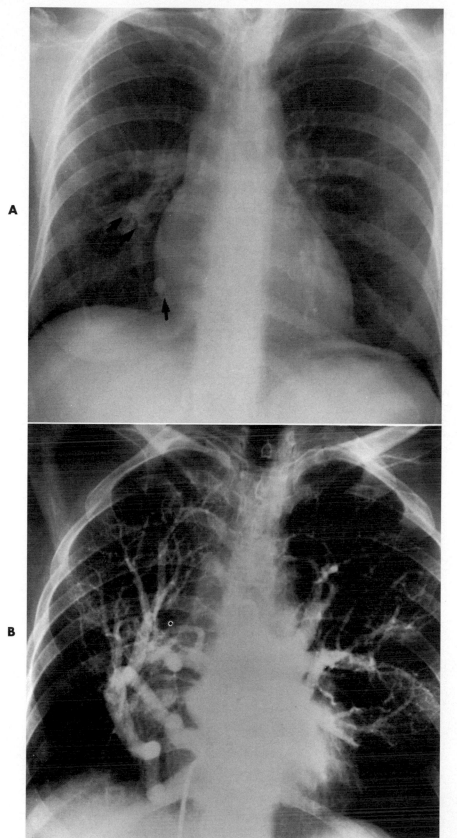

Figure 2-18   Pulmonary varix. **A,** PA chest radiograph shows a tubular and nodular opacity in the right lower lung zone *(arrows).* **B,** Venous phase of a pulmonary angiogram demonstrates a dilated tortuous pulmonary vein draining into the left atrium.

right to left shunt. Roughly 30% of the arteriovenous malformations in the lungs are multiple, and most occur in the lower lobes.

Standard chest radiographs show single or multiple well-defined nodules, which are often lobulated. These are typically in the medial third of the lung. Frequently the feeding artery and draining vein can be identified. The artery appears as a dilated vessel originating in the hilum, and the vein drains into the left atrium (Fig. 2-19, *A*).

Pulmonary angiography has been the method of choice for the identification of the size, number, and architecture of pulmonary venous malformations. The vast majority of patients receive pulmonary angiography because most of these lesions are now treated with therapeutic embolization; however, it is not essential for diagnosis. The typical morphology of these lesions allows identification with CT either with or without contrast injection (Figs. 2-19, *B* and 2-19, *C*). Dynamic contrast-enhanced CT is recommended. Rarely, thrombosis may lead to a lack of contrast enhancement. Spiral CT with 3-dimensional reconstruction is equivalent to angiography in both the detection of small arteriovenous malformations and in the delineation of the angioarchitecture, which is important prior to therapeutic embolization.

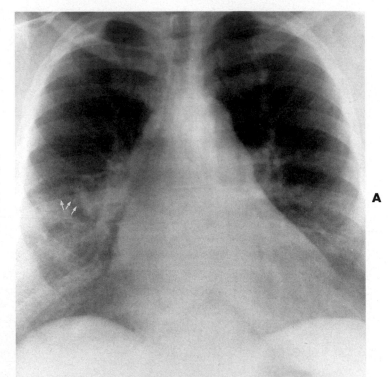

Figure 2-19 Pulmonary AV malformation. **A,** PA radiograph shows a tubular ringlike opacity lateral to the right hilum *(arrows)*. **B,** Contrast-enhanced CT scan demonstrates a tangle of vessels in the right lung. The feeding artery appears to arise from the interlobar branch of the right pulmonary artery *(arrows)*. **C,** The venous drainage is to the superior pulmonary vein *(arrows)*.

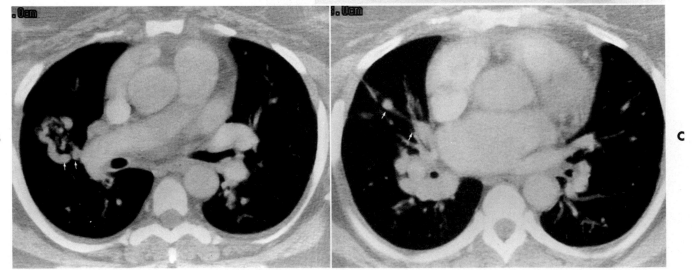

Congenital Hypogenetic Lung Syndrome (Scimitar or Congenital Pulmonary Venolobar Syndrome)

"Hypogenetic lung syndrome" or "congenital pulmonary venolobar syndrome" encompasses a constellation of congenital anomalies of the thorax that often occur together. The anomaly consists of hypoplasia of the right lung and of the right pulmonary artery. There is usually partial anomalous pulmonary venous return and partial or complete arterial supply to the affected lung from systemic vessels. There may also be absence of the inferior vena cava and duplication of the diaphragm (accessory diaphragm). Dextroposition of the heart occurs secondary to the hypoplasia of the right lung. The most constant feature is anomalous venous drainage with the entire right lung typically drained by a single vein that runs inferiorly parallel to the right border of the heart to join the inferior vena cava below the diaphragm. On the frontal radiograph this vein appears like a Turkish sword or scimitar (Fig. 2-20, A). Although the hypogenetic lung may occur occasionally on the left, the scimitar is almost exclusively right-sided. Other standard radiographic findings include a small ipsilateral thorax with decreased pulmonary vascularity on the involved side. The heart and mediastinum are shifted towards the involved side, and the heart border may be indistinct. On the lateral radiograph (Fig. 2-20, B) the cardiomediastinal shift produces a broad retrosternal band of opacity that may extend from the diaphragm to the apex of the involved hemithorax. This band is usually not an accessory diaphragm, which occurs in less than 10% of patients, and is a thin membrane fused anteriorly with the diaphragm that courses posterosuperiorly with the chest wall. It separates the right hemithorax into two parts, trapping part or all of the right middle or lower lobes below it. If the trapped lung is not aerated, it appears as a solid mass above the hemidiaphragm. If the lung is aerated, the accessory diaphragm appears as a fissurelike oblique line on the lateral radiograph. Aortography may be necessary to document the systemic arterial supply to the hypogenetic lung. CT may be useful in defining abnormalities of the central right pulmonary artery as well as the anatomy and course of the anomalous pulmonary "scimitar" vein. It may show enlarged inferior pulmonary veins coalescing within the right lower lobe.

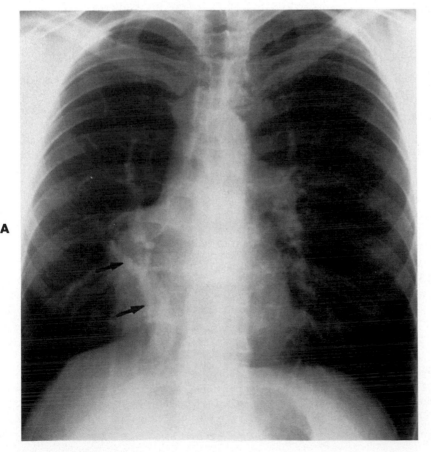

A

Figure 2-20 Venolobar or scimitar syndrome. **A,** PA chest radiograph shows a large vein *(arrows)* coursing toward the diaphragm. The heart border is indistinct.

Continued

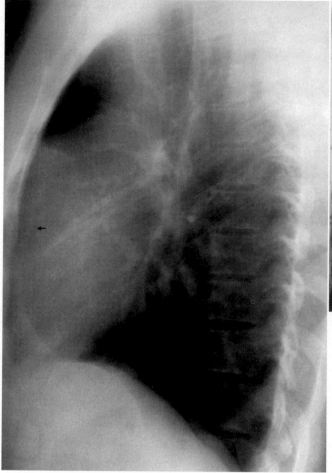

B

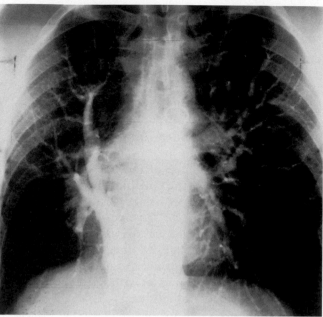

C

Figure 2-20, cont'd. B, Retrosternal opacity on lateral view *(arrow).* **C,** Venous phase of pulmonary angiogram confirms venous drainage of the right lung by means of a single large vein, which drains into the inferior vena cava.

Congenital Anomalies of the Lymphatics

There are four major types of developmental lymphatic disorders that involve the thorax: (1) pulmonary lymphangiectasis (see Pediatric Radiology:THE REQUISITES) characterized by a congenital anomalous dilation of the pulmonary lymph vessels; (2) localized lymphangioma, a cystic lesion occurring in the mediastinum;(3) diffuse lymphangioma, a proliferation of vascular spaces, mainly lymphatics, in which visceral and skeletal involvement are common; and (4) lymphangioleiomyomatosis, a diffuse infiltrative lung disease characterized by haphazard proliferation of smooth muscle in the lungs and dilation of lymphatic spaces. For lymphangioma see Chapter 13; for lymphangioleiomyomatosis—Chapter 7 on infiltrative lung disease.

SUGGESTED READINGS

Ben-Menachem Y, Kuroda K, Kyger ER et al:The various forms of pulmonary varices, *AJR* 125:881–889, 1975.

Carpenter BLM, Merten DF: Radiographic manifestations of congenital anomalies affecting the airway, *Radiol Clin North Am* 29:219–240, 1991.

Davis SD, Umlas SL: Radiology of congenital abnormalities of the chest, *Curr Opin Radiol* 4:25–435, 1992.

Fraser RG, Paré JAP, Paré PD et al: *Diagnosis of diseases of the chest,* Philadelphia, 1989, WB Saunders; pp 695–773.

Haddon MJ, Bowen A: Bronchopulmonary and neurenteric forms of foregut anomalies, *Radiol Clin North Am* 29:241–254, 1991.

Keslar P, Newman B, Oh KS: Radiographic manifestations of anomalies of the lung, *Radiol Clin North Am* 29:255–270, 1991.

Landing BH: Congenital malformations and genetic disorders of the respiratory tract, *Am Rev Respir Dis* 120:151–185, 1979.

Mata JM, Cáceres José, Lucaya J et al: CT of congenital malformations of the lung, *RadioGraphics* 10:651–674, 1990.

Morgan PW, Foley DW, Erickson SJ: Proximal interruption of a main pulmonary artery with transpleural collateral vessels: CT and MR appearance, *J Comput Assist Tomogr* 15:311–313, 1991.

Naidich DP, Zerhouni EA, Siegelman SS: *Computed tomography and magnetic resonance of the thorax,* New York, 1991, Raven Press; pp 503–556.

Panicek DM, Heitzman ER, Randall PA et al: The continuum of pulmonary developmental anomalies, *RadioGraphics* 7:474–772, 1987.

Remy J, Remy-Jardin M, Wattinine L et al: Pulmonary arteriovenous malformations: evaluation with CT of the chest before and after treatment, *Radiology* 82:809–816, 1992.

Rosado-de-Christenson ML, Frazier AA, Stocker JT et al: Extralobar sequestration: radiologic-pathologic correlation, *RadioGraphics* 13:425–441, 1993.

Scalzetti EM, Heitzman ER, Groskin SA et al: Developmental lymphatic disorders of the thorax, *RadioGraphics* 11:1069–1085, 1991.

White RI, Mitchell SE, Barth KH et al: Angioarchitecture of pulmonary arteriovenous malformations: an important consideration before embolotherapy, *Radiology* 140:681–686, 1983.

Woodring JH, Howard RS, Rehm SR: Congenital tracheobronchomegaly (Mounier-Kuhn syndrome): a report of 10 cases and review of the literature, *J Thorac Imaging* 6:1–10, 1991.

Woodring JH, Howard TA, Kanga JF: Congenital pulmonary venolobar syndrome revisited, *RadioGraphics* 14:349–369, 1994.

CHAPTER 3

Pulmonary Infections in the Normal Host

MEENAKSHI BHALLA
THERESA C. McLOUD

Pneumonia ranks fifth among the causes of death in the United States. A number of factors are responsible for this high mortality rate. These include 1) an increasing elderly population, (2) immunocompromised hosts in greater numbers, (3) new etiologic agents of pneumonia, (4) antibiotic-resistant organisms, and (5) unusual organisms acquired from international travel. The etiologic agent can reach the lungs by several routes. The most common is (1) inhalation of airborne droplets, followed by (2) aspiration of nasopharyngeal organisms, (3) hematogenous spread to the lungs from other extrathoracic sources of infection, (4) direct extension from a localized site of infection, and (5) infection from penetrating wounds.

Clinical features are important in the determination of the etiologic agent of pneumonia (Table 3-1). Community-acquired pneumonias occurring in previously healthy individuals are due to *Streptococcus pneumoniae* in the majority of cases (50% to 75%), *Mycoplasma pneumoniae,* viral organisms, or *Legionella pneumophila.* On the other hand, nosocomial pneumonias (pneumonias acquired in the hospital in patients who are already ill) are more likely to be due to gram-negative organisms or *Staphylococcus aureus.* Certain preexisting conditions are also associated with pneumonias due to specific organisms. For example, patients with altered states of consciousness or those in coma are more likely to develop aspiration and subsequently infections due to mouth organisms, that is, gram-negatives and anaerobes. *Staphylococcus aureus* infection can occur following influenza pneumonia; in patients with COPD, *Haemophilus influenzae* infection is common. Both *Staphylococcus aureus* and *Pseudomonas aeruginosa* organisms are common superinfectants in patients with cystic fibrosis.

CLASSIFICATION

The pathologic classification of pneumonias is based on the anatomic localization of the disease process. Categories include (1) lobar pneumonia, (2) bronchopneumonia or lobular pneumonia, (3) hematogenous bacterial infection, and (4) acute interstitial pneumonia.

Lobar Pneumonia

Pathologic features

This type of pneumonia results when inhaled organisms reach the subpleural zone of the lung and produce alveolar wall injury with severe hemorrhagic edema. This is followed by a rapid multiplication of organisms and invasion of the infected edema fluid by polymorphonuclear leukocytes. There is rapid spread through the terminal airways and pores of Kohn such that consolidation of an entire lobe or segment may occur. This process is now frequently aborted by administration of antibiotic therapy. The pattern is seen most frequently in pneumonias due to *Streptococcus pneumoniae,* the most common cause. *Klebsiella pneumoniae, Legionella pneumophila,* and *Mycoplasma pneumoniae* can also produce lobar consolidation.

Radiographic features

This type of pneumonia produces a pattern of confluent opacification frequently with air bronchograms (Fig. 3-1). The entire lobe may be involved, but more frequently because of early use of antibiotics the pneumonia will involve only one or more segments within a lobe (sublobar form). A lobar pneumonia may result in expansion of the lobe due to voluminous edema. This is usually caused by infection with *Klebsiella pneumoniae* (Fig. 3-2). The

---

Table 3-1 Summary of clinical clues to the etiology of pneumonia

Clinical Circumstance	Likely Causative Organisms
Previously well, community-acquired	50% to 75% due to *Streptococcus pneumoniae* (pneumococcus), *Mycoplasma pneumoniae,* virus, or *Legionella pneumophila*
Hospital-acquired, otherwise ill	Gram-negatives, including *Pseudomonas aeruginosa, Klebsiella pneumoniae, Escherichia coli,* and *Enterobacter* species; *Staphylococcus aureus;* less commonly pneumococcus and *Legionella*
Alcoholism	Pneumococcus most common; gram-negatives, anaerobes, and *S. aureus* frequent
Diabetes mellitus	Suspect gram-negatives and *S. aureus*
Altered consciousness, coma	Gram-negatives and anaerobes
Drug addiction	If not an AIDS patient, suspect staphylococcus and gram-negatives
Postinfluenza	*Staphylococcus aureus*
Chronic bronchitis with exacerbation	*Haemophilus influenzae* common
Cystic fibrosis	Mucoid *Pseudomonas aeruginosa*

From Woodring JH: Pulmonary bacterial and viral infections. In Freundlich IM, Bragg DG, editors: *A radiologic approach to diseases of the chest,* Baltimore, 1992, Williams & Wilkins.

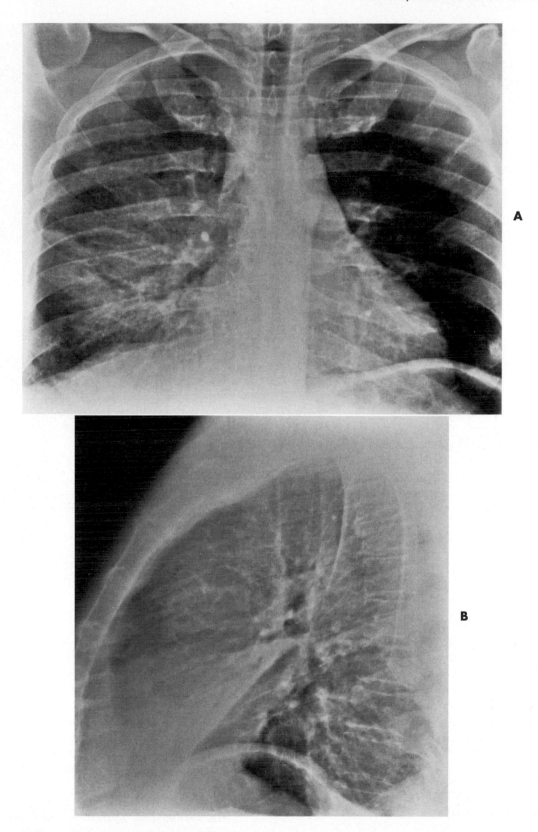

Figure 3-1. **A,** PA and, **B,** lateral views. Lobar consolidation involving the middle lobe. *Streptococcus pneumoniae* (pneumococcus).

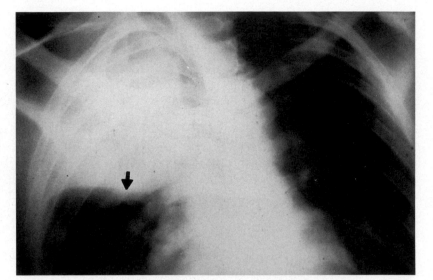

Figure 3-2. AP view of the patient with *Klebsiella* pneumonia shows homogeneous opacity of the right upper lobe with slight bulging of the minor fissure.

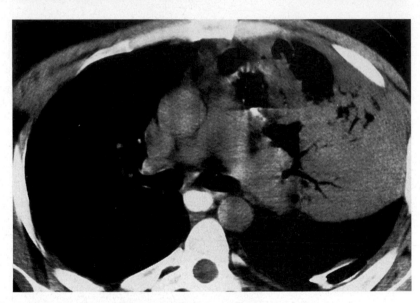

Figure 3-3. CT of pneumococcal left upper-lobar consolidation. There are clearly defined air bronchograms and evidence of cavitation.

enlargement of the lobe can be recognized radiographically by bulging of the interlobar fissures. Necrosis and cavitation with the development of a unique complication, pulmonary gangrene, may ensue. The CT features of lobar pneumonia are similar to those on standard radiography (Fig. 3-3). There is usually evidence of confluent opacification with air bronchograms. The air bronchograms are often more easily visualized with CT examination.

Table 3-2 summarizes these radiographic clues to the etiology of pneumonia.

Bronchopneumonia

Pathologic features

Bronchopneumonia (lobular pneumonia) results when organisms are deposited in the epithelium of peripheral airways, that is, either distal bronchi or bronchioles, resulting in epithelial ulcerations and formation of a peribronchiolar exudate. The inflammatory process spreads through the airway to involve the peribronchiolar alveoli, which become filled with edema and pus. Lobules may be affected in a patchy pattern initially, and further spread results in involvement of contiguous pulmonary lobules. Eventually a confluent bronchopneumonia may resemble lobar pneumonia. Offending organisms that produce this type of pathologic response include *Staphylococcus aureus,* gram-negative organisms, anaerobic bacteria, and *Legionella pneumophila.*

Radiographic features

The radiographic appearance of bronchopneumonia or lobular pneumonia is most frequently that of multiple ill-defined nodular opacities that are patchy but may eventually become confluent and produce consolidation with air-space opacification (Fig. 3-4). Such opacification may be multifocal and involve multiple

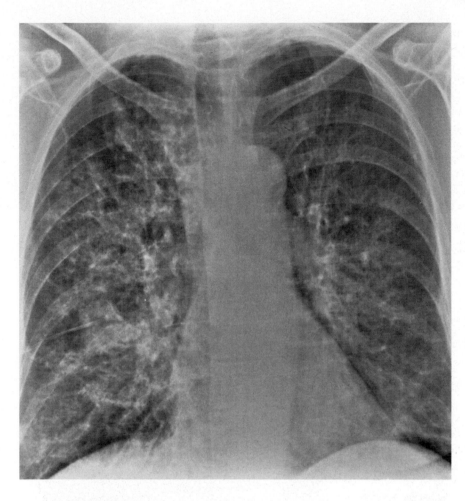

Figure 3-4. Bronchopneumonia. PA view demonstrates bilateral patchy and inhomogeneous opacities, which have become confluent in some areas. Viral influenza pneumonia.

Table 3-2   Summary of radiographic clues to the etiology of pneumonia

Radiographic finding	Likely causative organisms
"Round" pneumonia	Suspect *Streptococcus pneumoniae*
Complete lobar consolidation	*Streptococcus pneumoniae, Klebsiella pneumoniae,* and other gram-negative bacilli, *Legionella pneumophila,* and occasionally, *Mycoplasma pneumoniae*
Lobar enlargement	*Klebsiella pneumoniae,* pneumococcus, *Staphylococcus aureua, Haemophilus influenzae*
Bilateral pneumonia (bronchopneumonia)	Pneumococcus still common but suspect others including *S. aureus,* streptococci, gram-negative bacilli, anaerobes, *Legionella pneumophila,* virus, and aspiration syndromes
Interstitial pneumonia	Virus, *Mycoplasma pneumoniae,* and occasionally, *H. influenzae, S. pneumoniae,* and other bacteria
Septic emboli	Usually *S. aureus,* occasionally gram-negative bacilli, anaerobes, and streptococci
Empyema or bronchopleural fistula	*S. aureus,* gram-negative bacilli, anaerobes, and occasionally, pneumococcus; mixed bacterial infections common
Contiguous spread to chest wall	Actinomycosis; occasionally other bacteria or fungi
Cavitation	*S. aureus,* gram-negative bacilli, anaerobic bacteria, and streptococci; cavitation uncommon with *S. pneumoniae* or *L. pneumophila*
Pulmonary gangrene	*Klebsiella pneumoniae, Escherichia coli, H. influenzae, M. tuberculosis,* anaerobes, pneumococcus, or fungi
Pneumatoceles	*S. aureus,* gram-neagtive bacilli, *H. influenzae, M. tuberculosis,* and measles; pneumococcus rare.
Lymphadenopathy	*M. tuberculosis,* fungi, virus, *Mycloplasma pneumoniae,* common bacterial lung abscess, and rarely plague, tularemia, and anthrax
Fulminant course with ARDS	Virus, *S. aureus,* streptococci, *M. tuberculosis,* and *L. pneumophila*

From Woodring JH: Pulmonary bacterial and viral infections. In Freundlich IM, Bragg DG, editors: *A radiologic approach to diseases of the chest,* Baltimore, 1992, Williams & Wilkins.

lobes or may be diffuse. As the disease progresses, segmental and lobar opacification develops similar to a lobar pneumonia. Early necrosis and cavitation can occur. The nodular opacities of bronchopneumonia can be identified with facility on CT scans. The small nodules, usually less than 1 cm in diameter, represent peribronchiolar areas of consolidation or ground-glass opacity. They are called "acinar or air-space nodules," but these nodules histologically are peribronchiolar in location. They are ill-defined and may be of homogenous soft-tissue opacity and obscuring vessels, or they may be hazy and less dense so that adjacent vessels are clearly seen (ground-glass opacity). These nodules are usually centrilobular in location because of their proximity to small bronchioles.

Acute Interstitial Pneumonia

Pathologic features

This type of pneumonia is usually produced by viral organisms, which result in edema and mononuclear cell infiltration around the bronchi and bronchiolar walls and extend into the interstitium of the alveolar walls.

Radiographic features

Both a bronchopneumonia or an acute interstitial pneumonia may be seen with viral infections (Fig. 3-5). The radiographic appearance early on is that of thickening of end on bronchi and tram lines. However, this often evolves into a reticular pattern that may be seen extending outward from the hila.

Hematogenous Spread of Infection

Pathologic features

Hematogenous spread to the lungs from bacterial infection may occur, although this is unusual. One of the most frequent manifestations is septic infarcts. These usually originate from right-sided tricuspid endocarditis or infected thrombi within major systemic veins. This phenomenon is seen in intravenous drug abusers and patients with longstanding indwelling central catheters.

Radiographic features

Septic infarcts tend to be multiple and peripheral and to abut the pleural surface. They occur more frequently in the lower lobes. These nodules or wedge-shaped opacities may show evidence of cavitation (Fig. 3-6). CT may often demonstrate a vessel connected to the area of infarction. On CT images the septic infarcts appear as wedge-shaped peripheral opacities abutting the pleura. They may contain air bronchograms or rounded lucencies of air, sometimes referred to as pseudocavitation. True cavitation is also common.

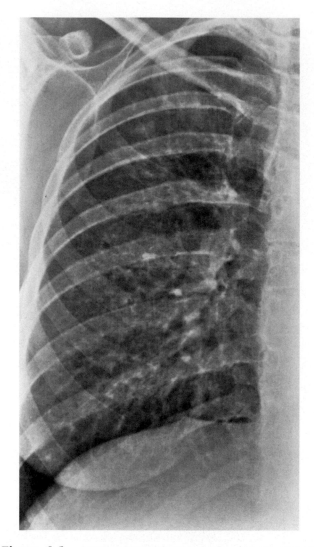

Figure 3-5. Acute interstitial pneumonia due to *varicella* (chickenpox). Coned-down view of the right lung demonstrates a fine reticulonodular pattern, which is more prominent centrally.

Occasionally septic bacterial infection may result in diffuse massive seeding of the lungs with a miliary, that is, a very small nodular pattern, although this is much more common with hematogenous dissemination of granulomatous infections.

COMPLICATIONS OF PNEUMONIA

See Box 3-1 for an outline of these complications.

Cavitation

Necrosis of lung parenchyma with cavitation (Fig. 3-7) may occur in pneumonia, particularly that produced by virulent bacteria, including *Staphylococcus aureus*, streptococci, gram-negative bacilli, and anaerobic bacteria. If the inflammatory process is localized, a lung

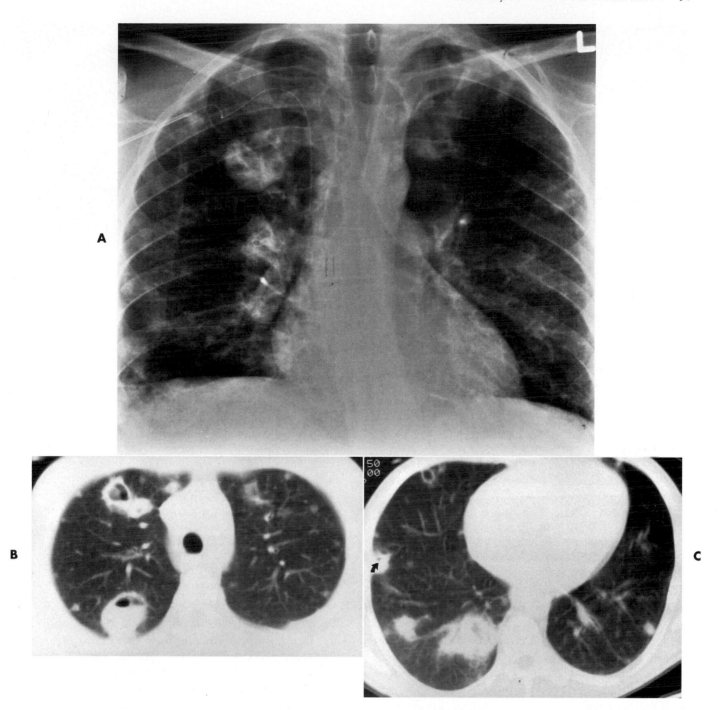

Figure 3-6.   Septic infarcts. Intravenous drug abuser. **A,** PA chest radiograph shows multiple bilateral cavitary nodules. **B,** and **C,** CT examination demonstrates that most of the infarcts are peripheral in location; some abut the pleura and occasionally are wedge-shaped. Both true and pseudocavities (*curved arrow*) are present.

Box 3-1 Complications of Pneumonia

CAVITATION

Organisms
  Staphylococcus aureus
  Streptococci
  Gram-negative bacilli
  Anaerobes
Types
  Lung abscess—single, well-defined mass often with
    air-fluid level
  Necrotizing pneumonia
    Small lucencies or cavities
  Pulmonary gangrene—sloughed lung

PNEUMATOCELES

Staphylococcus aureus
Children
Thin walls, multiple

ADENOPATHY

Common—granulomatous infections (TB, fungi)
Uncommon—most bacterial and viral infections

PLEURAL EFFUSIONS AND EMPYEMA

Common—40%
Parapneumonic
Empyema (BPF)

OTHER COMPLICATIONS

ARDS
Bronchiectasis
Slow resolution in elderly
Recurrent pneumonias

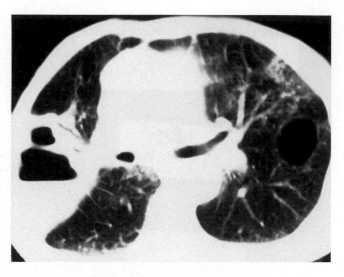

Figure 3-7. Cavitary pneumonia due to gram-negative organisms. CT shows two areas of cavitation with an air-fluid level in the more posterior, indicating bronchial communication.

Portions of dead lung may slough and form intracavitary masses.

Pneumatocele Formation

Pneumatoceles are usually associated with pneumonia caused by virulent organisms, the classical offender being *Staphylococcus aureus* (Fig. 3-10). These usually form subpleural collections of air, which result from alveolar rupture. Radiographically they appear as single or multiple cystic lesions with thin and smooth walls. They may show rapid change in size and location on serial radiographs.

Hilar and Mediastinal Adenopathy

Intrathoracic lymphadenopathy that can be recognized on standard films is uncommon in most bacterial and viral infections, some notable exceptions including *Mycobacterium tuberculosis, Pasteurella tularensis,* and *Yersinia pestis.* Adenopathy may also be associated with fungal infections or bacterial infections that are long standing or virulent, as in lung abscesses. CT may show slightly enlarged nodes (greater than 1 cm) in common bacterial infections that are not visible on standard radiography.

Pleural Effusions and Empyema

Pleural effusion is a common complication of pneumonia, occurring in about 40% of cases (Fig. 3-11). Most effusions are parapneumonic, but infection of the pleural space with empyema requiring drainage is an important but uncommon complication of some pneumonias. Empyemas can be recognized by the presence of gross

abscess will form. This is usually rounded and focal and appears as a mass (Fig. 3-8). With liquefaction of the central inflammatory process, a communication may develop with the bronchus; air will enter the abscess, forming a cavity. This often contains an air-fluid level. The walls of the cavity may be smooth, but more often they are thick and irregular.

Multiple small cavities or microabscesses may develop in a necrotizing pneumonia (Fig. 3-9). These are recognized as multiple areas of lucency within a consolidated lobe or segment. A similar appearance may be produced by consolidation superimposed on areas of preexisting emphysema. Finally, if the necrosis is extensive, arteritis and vascular thrombosis may occur in an area of intense inflammation, causing ischemic necrosis and death of a portion of lung. This is a particular complication of *Klebsiella* pneumonia and other pneumonias producing lobar enlargement. The radiographic features include multiple areas of cavitation often with air-fluid levels.

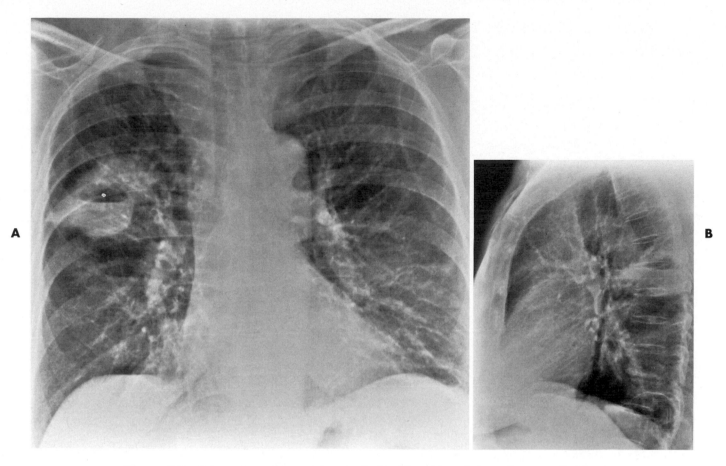

Figure 3-8. Primary lung abscess due to aspiration. PA and lateral views show a well-defined masslike opacity in the superior segment of the right lower lobe. There is cavitation with an air-fluid level and a thick wall.

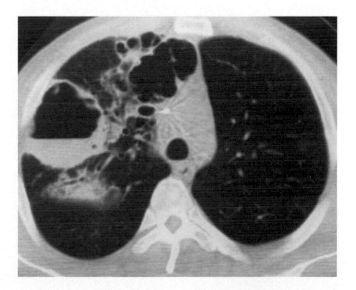

Figure 3-9. Microabscesses. *Pseudomonas* pneumonia, right upper lobe. There are multiple thin-walled multiloculated cavities with little surrounding parenchymal opacity.

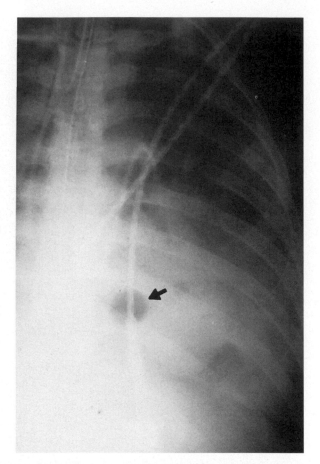

Figure 3-10.   Pneumatocele. Coned-down (AP) view of the chest in a patient with fulminant staphylococcal pneumonia shows rounded lucency in left lower lobe caused by a pneumatocele *(arrow)*.

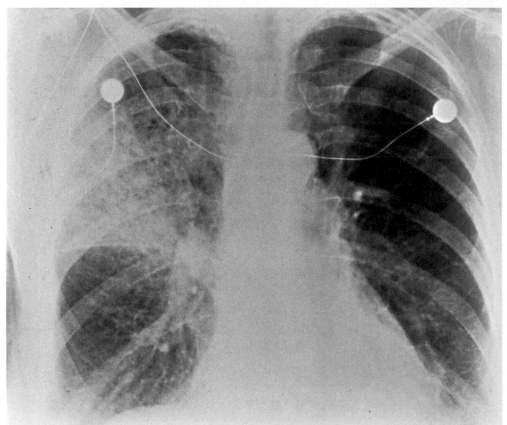

Figure 3-11.   Parapneumonic effusion (pneumococcal pneumonia). **A,** PA view shows right upper lobe consolidation.
Continued.

A

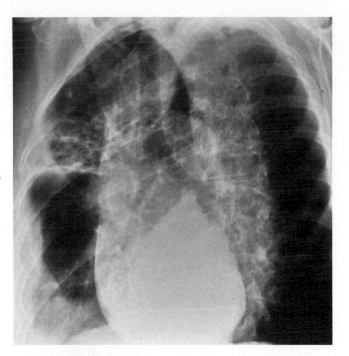

B

Figure 3-11, cont'd.   B, An oblique view two days later demonstrates a right effusion.

pus within the pleural space, by a white blood cell count in the pleural fluid of greater than 15,000/mm^3, by the presence of bacteria within the pleural fluid, or by a pH < 7.2. (See Chapter 18 for more detail on the pleural complications of pneumonia.)

Parenchymal necrosis in an underlying pneumonia may produce a fistula between the bronchus and the pleural space (bronchopleural fistula—BPF), and this will result in an empyema with an air-fluid level. Further discussion of these entities can be found in Chapter 18.

Other Complications

Rapidly progressive and fulminant bacterial or viral pneumonia may result in the adult respiratory distress syndrome. In the preantibiotic era, bronchiectasis was an extremely common complication of bacterial pneumonia, but the incidence of bronchiectasis has declined with the advent of antibiotics. Most pneumonias will clear rapidly within 2 or 3 weeks, but in elderly patients resolution may take 3 to 4 months. Necrotizing pneumonias also tend to resolve slowly. Recurrent pneumonias are frequently found in patients with predisposing factors such as chronic obstructive lung disease, bronchiectasis, alcoholism, and diabetes. Although recurrent or persistent pneumonia in the same location raises the possibility of an obstructing endobronchial lesion due to bronchogenic carcinoma, cancer accounts for less than 5% of such cases.

PNEUMONIAS CAUSED BY GRAM-POSITIVE BACTERIA

The most common gram-positive bacteria causing pneumonia include *Streptococcus pneumoniae* (pneumococcus), *Staphylococcus aureus,* and *Streptococcus pyogenes.*

Streptococcus Pneumoniae

Streptococcus pneumoniae or pneumococcus (Box 3-2) is responsible for a third to a half of community-acquired pneumonias in adults. These infections are more frequent in the winter and early spring. Pneumococcal pneumonia occurs in healthy people, but it is much more common in alcoholic, debilitated, and other immunocompromised individuals.

The radiographic features include consolidation that is usually unilateral although it may be bilateral and typically affects the lower lobes (Fig. 3-1). Although it is a lobar pneumonia, it is uncommon for the lobe to be completely consolidated. Cavitation is rare and large pleural effusions are infrequent. When present they suggest the development of empyema. Sometimes, especially in children, the pneumonia may have a rounded masslike appearance (Fig. 3-12). This is called a round pneumonia; it is due to centrifugal spread of the rapidly replicating bacteria by way of the pores of Kohn and canals of Lambert from a single primary focus in the lung.

Staphylococcus Aureus

Staphylococcus aureus (Box 3-3) is a gram-positive coccus in which the spherical organisms occur in pairs and clusters. This pneumonia rarely develops in healthy adults, but it is sometimes a complication of viral infections and is much more common in infants and children. In infants, unilateral or bilateral consolidation involving the lower lungs is the most frequent radiographic presen-

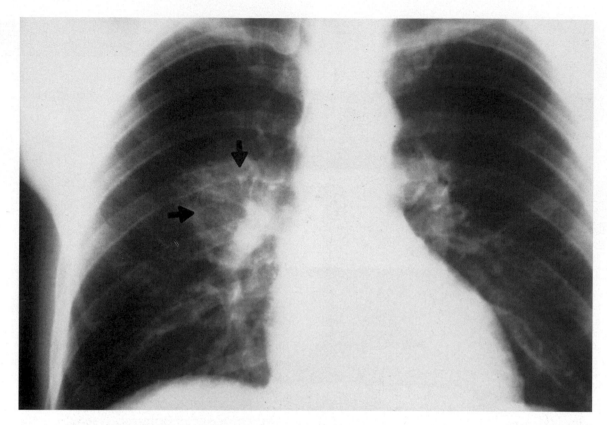

Figure 3-12.   Rounded pneumonia. PA chest radiograph of an adult patient shows an ill-defined rounded opacity in the superior segment of the right lower lobe (*arrows*) due to rounded pneumonia caused by pneumococcus.

Figure 3-13. *Staphylococcus aureus* abscess. Composite of four CT images of a patient with a left lower lobe staphylococcal abscess. Note the thick walls of the cavity (*closed arrows*) and the retained thick exudate in the center. Pockets of air in the peripheral regions of the cavity probably represent small pneumatoceles (*open arrows*). (Courtesy of Dorothy L. McCauley, M.D., New York University Medical Center, New York.)

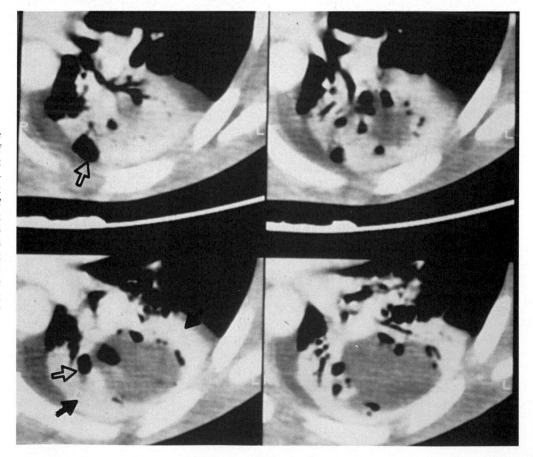

Box 3-3 *Staphylococcus aureus*

CHARACTERISTICS

Gram-positive coccus
Infants and children—more common
Postviral
Septic emboli
  Intravenous drug abusers
  Indwelling catheters

RADIOGRAPHIC FEATURES

Children
  Consolidation
  Lower lungs
  Pneumatoceles
Adults
  Bilateral
  Cavitation
  Empyema
Septic emboli
  Multiple
  Nodules or wedge-shaped opacities
  Peripheral, abut pleura
  Cavitation
  CT
  Pseudocavitation or true cavitation
  Feeding vessel

Box 3-4 *Streptococcus pyogenes*

CHARACTERISTICS

Gram-positive cocci
Uncommon, but occasionally epidemic

RADIOGRAPHIC FEATURES

Consolidation
Segmental
Lower lobes
Effusion

---

tation. Pneumatoceles, thin-walled cysts filled with air or partially filled with fluid, may develop and occasionally rupture into the pleural space, resulting in pneumothorax. In adults the disease is usually bilateral and preceded by an atypical pneumonia such as influenza. Cavitation is a frequent feature, and the cavities may be multiple, thick-walled, and irregular (Fig. 3-13). There is a high incidence of large pleural effusions, and empyema secondary to bronchopleural fistula is a common complication.

Staphylococcal infection in the lungs may occur by way of the hematogenous route. This is usually the result of septic emboli, which arise either in the central veins or as vegetations on cardiac valves, particularly in intravenous drug abusers and patients with indwelling intravenous catheters. The radiographic appearance is that of multiple nodular masses with or without cavitation as described above.

Streptococcus Pyogenes

Streptococci (Box 3-4) are gram-positive cocci that occur in pairs and chains. The pneumonia occasionally occurs in epidemic proportions. This form of pneumonia is much more rare than that caused by staphylococcus or pneumococcus.

The radiographic features include lower lobe consolidation often with a segmental distribution. Pleural effusions occur frequently, but localized empyema is unusual.

PNEUMONIAS CAUSED BY GRAM-NEGATIVE AEROBIC ORGANISMS

Pneumonias caused by gram-negative organisms usually are nosocomial pneumonias that affect hospitalized patients. These pneumonias tend to occur in patients maintained on artificial ventilators or in those who have intravenous catheters or a variety of other ancillary support systems. The incidence of gram-negative pneumonia acquired in the community is also increasing, and this may be related to the overgrowth of resistant organisms because of widespread use of broad-spectrum antibiotics.

Klebsiella Pneumoniae

Klebsiella pneumonia (Box 3-5) usually occurs in middle-aged or elderly patients, in those with underlying chronic lung disease, and in alcoholic individuals. Radiographic features consist of an upper lobar consolidation. Cavitation is frequent, and the lobar consolidation may lead to an expanded lobe with bulging interlobar fissures (Fig. 3-2). If necrosis is extensive, pulmonary gangrene as described above may develop.

Escherichia Coli

E. coli pneumonia (Box 3-6) may be caused by direct extension from the GI/GU tract across the diaphragm or secondary to a bacteremia. As is true of most of the gram-negative pneumonias, it is frequently characterized by the development of necrosis and multiple cavities. The lower lobes are more frequently involved.

Box 3-5 *Klebsiella pneumoniae*

CHARACTERISTICS

Middle-aged, elderly patients
Chronic lung disease and alcoholic patients

RADIOGRAPHIC FEATURES

Lobar consolidation
Bulging fissures
Cavitation
Pulmonary gangrene

Box 3-6 *Escherichia coli*

CHARACTERISTICS

Direct extension from GI/GU tract
Secondary to bacteremia

RADIOGRAPHIC FEATURES

Necrosis, multiple cavities
Lower lobes

Box 3-7 *Pseudomonas aeruginosa*

CHARACTERISTICS

Hospitalized, debilitated patients
Tracheostomy tubes and suction devices

RADIOGRAPHIC FEATURES

Lower lobes, consolidation
Rapid spread to both lungs
Multiple irregular nodules
Cavitation
Pleural effusions uncommon

Box 3-8 *Haemophilus influenzae*

CHARACTERISTICS

COPD
Bronchopneumonia

RADIOGRAPHIC FEATURES

Homogeneous, segmental
Lower lobes

Pseudomonas Aeruginosa

Pseudomonas aeruginosa pneumonia (Box 3-7) usually occurs in hospitalized patients, particularly those with debilitating disease (Fig. 3-9). Organisms often affect the lungs secondary to contamination of suction and tracheostomy devices. Radiographic features include a lower-lobe predilection. However, the consolidation may spread rapidly to affect both lungs. Pleural effusions are uncommon. Multiple irregular nodules may develop and are usually associated with bacteremia. These nodules may cavitate.

Haemophilus Influenzae

Haemophilus influenzae pneumonia (Box 3-8) usually develops in patients with chronic obstructive pulmonary disease. The appearance is typically that of a bronchopneumonia with homogeneous segmental opacities, usually in the lower lobes. Cavitation and pleural effusions are rare.

ASPIRATION PNEUMONITIS AND ANAEROBIC PNEUMONIA

Pulmonary aspiration (Box 3-9) is a very common clinical problem. Many conditions predispose to aspiration, including reduced levels of consciousness, alcoholism, drug addiction, esophageal disease, periodontal and gingival disease, seizure disorders, and nasogastric tubes.

Aspiration of particulate matter or foreign bodies may produce different clinical syndromes, depending on the size of the aspirated material and the level of airway obstruction. Large food particles or foreign bodies may be aspirated into the larynx and upper trachea resulting in the so-called "café coronary syndrome" due to acute upper airway obstruction. Such patients exhibit both respiratory distress and aphonia.

Chest radiographs are usually normal in patients who have aspirated foreign bodies. If the foreign body is opaque, it may be visible in the airways. Air trapping may occur if the foreign body causes airway obstruction of one of the major bronchi. This can be demonstrated by inspiratory and expiratory radiographs, decubitus views, or chest fluoroscopy. Occasionally complete obstruction of the bronchus results in atelectasis and, if the foreign body is unrecognized, the development of distal pneumonitis or bronchiectasis.

Ninety percent of aspiration pneumonias and lung abscesses are caused by anaerobic organisms. The pathogens include prevotella, bacteroides, fusobacterium, and peptostreptococcus. Because of the presence of oxygen in the lung, the progression of anaerobic infection is slow, beginning in the dependent lung zones. If the patient is in a supine position when the aspiration occurs, the superior segments of the lower lobes are

Box 3-9 Aspiration Pneumonitis and Anaerobic Pneumonia

CHARACTERISTICS
Common

Predisposing factors

Reduced consciousness
Alcoholism
Drug addiction
Seizures
Esophageal disease
Poor oral hygiene

CLINICAL SYNDROMES
"Café coronary" syndrome

Obstruction of larynx or upper trachea
Aphonia, respiratory distress, asphyxia

Bronchial obstruction

Aspiration pneumonitis or pneumonia

Mouth organisms
Slow progression

Aspiration gastric acid

Mendelson's syndrome

RADIOGRAPHIC FEATURES
Foreign body

Normal
Opaque foreign body in airway
Air trapping if bronchus obstructed
    Inspiratory-expiration radiographs
    Fluoroscopy
Atelectasis
Aspiration pneumonia
Location
    Superior segments lower lobes
    Posterior segments upper lobes
    Basilar segments lower lobes
Primary lung abscess
    Focal walled-off area of anaerobic pneumonia
    Superior segments lower lobes
    Thick-walled cavity
    Air-fluid level
    Rounded masslike lesion may precede cavitation
Aspiration pneumonitis
    No infection
    Patchy basilar opacities
Mendelson's syndrome
Aspiration of gastric acid
    Chemical pneumonitis and acute lung injury
    Diffuse consolidation resembling pulmonary edema

most commonly affected, the right side being more frequent than the left (Fig. 3-14). Aspiration can also occur into the posterior segments of both upper lobes. Chronic or recurrent aspiration, particularly in patients who are in the upright position, usually results in consolidation involving the basilar segments of the lower lobes. The middle lobe and lingula are very uncommon sites for aspiration pneumonia. Aspiration is the most common cause of a primary lung abscess (Fig. 3-8). A primary lung abscess refers to a focal walled-off area of anaerobic pneumonia with central liquefaction necrosis. It is most commonly identified in the superior segments of either lower lobe. Lung abscesses have a fairly thick wall and may or may not have an air-fluid level. A rounded masslike lesion may precede the development of cavitation.

Occasionally, aspiration of nontoxic material that contains insufficient bacteria to produce an infection or insufficient volume to produce atelectasis may occur. The radiographic appearance usually consists of basilar patchy opacities resembling atelectasis, and these clear within several days. Mendelson's syndrome is a specific form of aspiration that results from the aspiration of gastric acid. This event produces a chemical pneumonitis and acute lung injury. The radiographic manifestations of gastric aspiration are similar to those of noncardiogenic pulmonary edema. The distribution is usually diffuse.

ATYPICAL PNEUMONIA SYNDROMES (*LEGIONELLA, MYCOPLASMA,* AND *CHLAMYDIA*)

Atypical pneumonia syndrome (Box 3-10) describes pneumonias that either do not respond to antimicrobial therapy or do not have clinical features distinctive from the usual bacterial pathogens responsible for community-acquired pneumonias. Originally these atypical pneumonias were all thought to be due to viruses. However, other treatable organisms have emerged as important causes of atypical pneumonia. These include pneumonias caused by *Mycoplasma pneumoniae, Legionella pneumophila,* and *Chlamydia.* Such nonviral atypical pneumonias are for the most part readily treatable with antibiotics. Most patients with atypical pneumonia present with a nonspecific syndrome consisting of fever, usually without shaking chills; and nonproductive cough, headache, myalgias, and some degree of dyspnea. This is in contrast to the classic presentation of bacterial pneumonia, which is characterized by abrupt onset with fever, shaking chills, and purulent sputum, often with chest pain. As mentioned above, patients with the latter signs and symptoms usually have a bacterial pneumonia attributable to pneumococci, group A strepto-

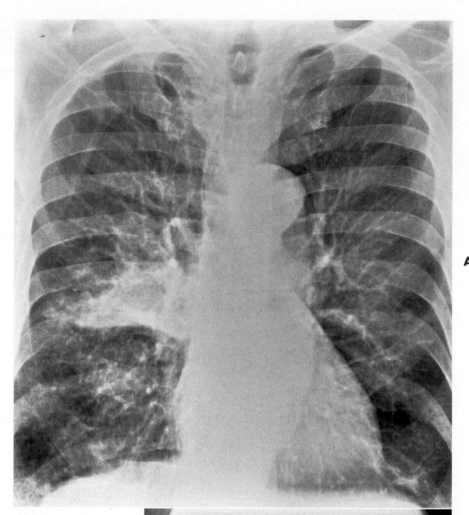

A

Figure 3-14.   Aspiration pneumonia in a patient with a history of seizures. PA and lateral chest radiographs demonstrate consolidation in the superior segment of the right lower lobe.

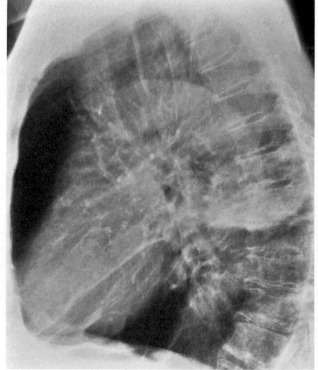

B

Box 3-10 Atypical Pneumonia Syndrome

ATYPICAL PNEUMONIA
Clinical features

Nonproductive cough
Fever
Dyspnea
Headache, myalgias
Extrapulmonary manifestations

Organisms

Legionella
Mycoplasma
Chlamydia
Viral

TYPICAL PNEUMONIA
Clinical features

Abrupt onset
Fever with chills
Productive cough
Purulent sputum
Chest pain

Organisms

Pneumococcus
Group A *Streptococcus*
Staphylococcus aureus
H. influenzae

Box 3-11 *Mycoplasma Pneumoniae*

CHARACTERISTICS

20% of pneumonias
Occurs most often in winter
Enclosed populations

RADIOGRAPHIC FEATURES

Diffuse
Reticulonodular pattern evolves to patchy
   consolidation
Hilar adenopathy (20%-40%)
Similar to viral infections

Box 3-12 Legionnaires' Disease

CHARACTERISTICS

Respiratory or systemic symptoms
Over age 60
Diarrhea common
Airborne spread through moist air exhaust or
   cooling towers
Diagnosis by serology with indirect fluorescent
   antibody

RADIOGRAPHIC FEATURES

Consolidation
Upper lobes
Rapid spread to other lobes

---

cocci, *Klebsiella, Staphylococcus aureus,* or *Haemophilus influenzae.* Many of the atypical pneumonias are associated with extrapulmonary manifestations. For example, diarrhea is a prominent part of both *Legionella* and *Mycoplasma* infection.

Mycoplasma Pneumoniae

Mycoplasma pneumoniae (Box 3-11) accounts for approximately 20% of all cases of pneumonia. It usually occurs during the winter months in enclosed populations; for example, college dormitories. The incubation period is 2 to 3 weeks and the onset is often insidious with low-grade fever and nonproductive cough. Extrapulmonary manifestations may include otitis and nonexudate pharyngitis as well as diarrhea.

The radiographic features are usually those of a fairly diffuse interstitial fine reticulonodular pattern. This may evolve to more patchy air space consolidation, particularly in the lower lobes (Fig. 3-15). Hilar adenopathy is seen in approximately 20% to 40% of patients. The radi-

ographic appearance is very similar to many viral infections. The diagnosis is made by serology.

Legionnaires' Disease

The first outbreak of Legionnaires' disease was recognized in Philadelphia at a Legionnaires' convention (Box 3-12).

Clinical features

Clinical features include (1) acute febrile illness without pneumonia, (2) systemic disease with primarily pulmonary manifestations, (3) a peak incidence in patients over the age of 60, (4) a predisposition in smokers and those with alcoholic liver disease, (5) high fever, shaking chills, and cough with small amounts of mucoid sputum, (6) pleuritic chest pain, (7) watery diarrhea in about a half of patients, and (8) headache. Transmission of the organism is airborne, usually through moist air exhaust or cooling towers.

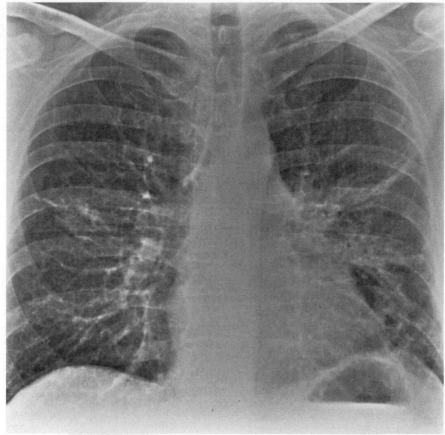

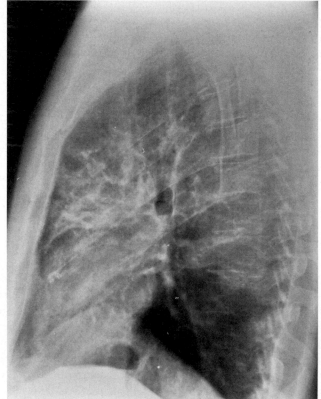

Figure 3-15. *Mycoplasma* pneumonia. There are patchy bilateral areas of inhomogeneous consolidation involving multiple lobes.

Radiographic features

The radiographic features often consist of segmental opacification and consolidation, particularly of an upper lobe. Rapid development of coalescence with complete consolidation of an involved lobe and rapid extension to adjacent lobes is common (Fig. 3-16). Parenchymal changes are extensive. Pleural effusions are uncommon. The diagnosis of Legionnaires' disease is usually made by serology using indirect fluorescent antibody. Direct identification of the organism may be confirmed by direct fluorescent antibody techniques (DFA) of properly collected specimens.

Chlamydia

Chlamydia, a long recognized cause of pneumonia in neonates, is an increasingly frequent cause of community-acquired atypical pneumonia in adult patients (Box 3-13). It is caused by the TWAR agent *(Chlamydia pneumoniae)*. *Chlamydia* pneumonia in the adult may occur in both compromised and noncompromised patients as an atypical pneumonia. The disease is characterized by fever and nonproductive cough. It is often preceded by a pharyngitis.

Radiographic features may be similar to *Mycoplasma* pneumonia. However, more commonly there is a localized area of consolidation in the middle or lower lobes, which may be patchy or homogeneous (Fig. 3-17).

Other Nonviral Atypical Pneumonias

There are a number of rather rare atypical nonviral pneumonias. These include psittacosis; Q fever, a rickettsial disease; and tularemia.

Chlamydia psittaci is the etiologic agent of psittacosis, which may be transmitted by any avian species and is also contracted by inhalation of infected aerosol material. The clue to the diagnosis is the history, which should include information about any contact with birds. Psittacosis usually mimics a standard bacterial pneumonia on chest radiography.

Coxiella burnetii is the etiologic agent of Q fever, which is a rickettsial disease. This is most common in the western and southwestern parts of the country and may be transmitted by infected dust from animals. The radiographic features are variable, but the most specific pattern simulates mycoplasma or viral pneumonia and usually consists of bilateral diffuse reticulonodular opacities.

Tularemia, another animal-associated, atypical pneumonia, is transmitted by tics in summer and rabbits in winter. There is an ulceroglandular form, which produces a skin papule that eventually ulcerates at the port of entry. Regional lymph nodes may become enlarged and eventually drain and ulcerate. In the typhoidal form, no portal of entry is apparent but patients are characteristically extremely ill with gastrointestinal syndromes. Pneumonia may occur with either of these presentations.

The most common radiographic feature is that of a localized and homogenous opacity, but lobar consolidation has also been reported. Occasionally, multiple lobes are involved. Bilateral hilar adenopathy is a characteristic but uncommon.

VIRAL PNEUMONIAS

Primary respiratory viruses (Box 3-14) include the parainfluenza and influenza group of viruses, respiratory syncytial virus (RSV), adenovirus, and picornavirus. The incidence of these infections varies with the age of the patient. For example, in children RSV is responsible for up to 85% of epidemic lower respiratory tract infections and up to 60% of all pneumonias; in adults the influenza and parainfluenza group are responsible for most of the epidemic viral pneumonias. These usually occur during late winter. Adenovirus and picornavirus cause nonepidemic respiratory infections. Other viruses such as cytomegalovirus produce pneumonia as part of a systemic infection.

In all cases, the infection usually begins in the larger central airways. At this stage the chest radiograph is frequently normal. The radiologic correlates of severe inflammation and edema of the bronchial walls include coarse reticular opacities in the form of rings and parallel lines (tram tracks) due to bronchial wall-thickening in the central perihilar lung zones. When the small airways are involved, a bronchiolitis develops. Involvement of terminal bronchioles may lead to airway obstruction. This is more likely to occur in infants and young children because the cross-sectional area of the airways is small. Diffuse overinflation and air trapping can be noted.

When the infection spreads to the alveoli, the disease is usually limited to the parenchyma around the terminal

---

Box 3-13 *Chlamydia* Pneumonia

CHARACTERISTICS

Chlamydia pneumoniae (TWAR agent)
Nonproductive cough
Preceding pharyngitis

RADIOGRAPHIC FEATURES

Localized consolidation lower lobes
Patchy or homogeneous

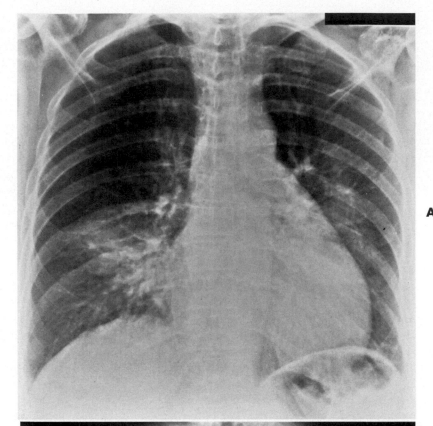

A

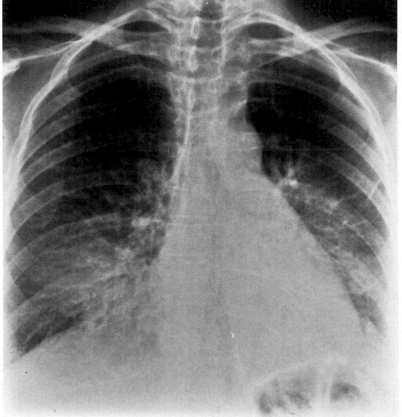

B

Figure 3-16. Legionnaires' disease. **A,** PA chest radiograph shows consolidation involving the right middle lobe and left mid lung zones. **B,** 24 hours later, the consolidation has become more extensive bilaterally.

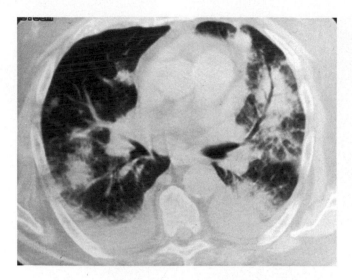

Figure 3-17. *Chlamydia* pneumonia. CT scan demonstrates bilateral patchy areas of consolidation.

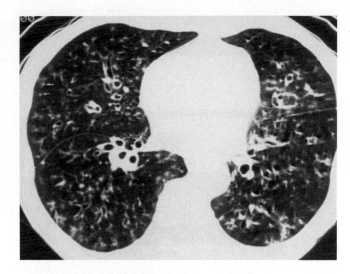

Figure 3-18. Tree-in-bud" appearance. Peripheral branching opacities (*large white arrow*) and centrilobular nodules 2 to 3 mm deep to the pleura can be identified (*small white arrows*). The appearance is due to small airways filled with secretions and inflammatory debris.

Box 3-14 Viral Pneumonias
CHARACTERISTICS **Viral organisms** Parainfluenza Respiratory syncytial virus (RSV) Adenovirus Picornavirus **RADIOGRAPHIC FEATURES** **Larger airways** Normal radiograph Tram tracks and ring shadows **Small airways (bronchiolitis)** Normal Overinflation and air trapping **Alveoli** Diffuse reticulonodular opacities Focal patchy consolidation

airways. In such instances the radiographic features in both children and adults usually consist of a diffuse reticulonodular pattern often with focal and patchy areas of consolidation (Fig. 3-4). Multiple lobes are usually involved. CT may reveal the anatomic localization of the disease. The bronchiolitis and surrounding inflammation produces nodular opacities, which are located in the center of the lobules. Branching centrilobular opacities

may simulate vessels and have often been referred to as the tree-in-bud appearance (Fig. 3-18).

Influenza

Influenza is one of the most frequently reported contagious diseases. Symptoms include fever, nonproductive cough, weakness, and myalgias. Most patients who develop severe pneumonia have underlying disease or superinfection with bacterial organisms.

Radiographic features are often due to complicating bacterial pneumonia. However, a diffuse reticulonodular pattern may be seen in infants and children with the disease.

Adenovirus

Adenovirus may occur in epidemic or pandemic proportions. When pneumonia develops there may be destructive changes involving the peripheral airways leading to chronic bronchitis, bronchiectasis, and bronchiolitis obliterans. Symptoms tend to persist after resolution of pneumonia. Radiographic features are very similar to pneumococcal pneumonia in pattern and distribution.

Respiratory Syncytial Virus

This virus, rarely reported in the adult, is the most prevalent respiratory viral pathogen in the first 6 months of life. It usually produces focal and diffuse bronchiolitis. If radiographs are abnormal they usually show increased

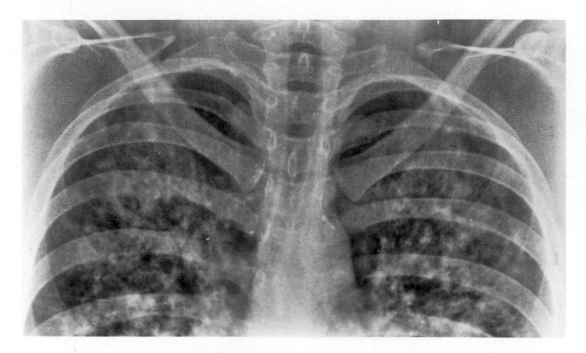

Figure 3-19.   Chickenpox—varicella pneumonia. Coned-down view of the upper lobes shows multiple ill-defined nodules in both upper lobes.

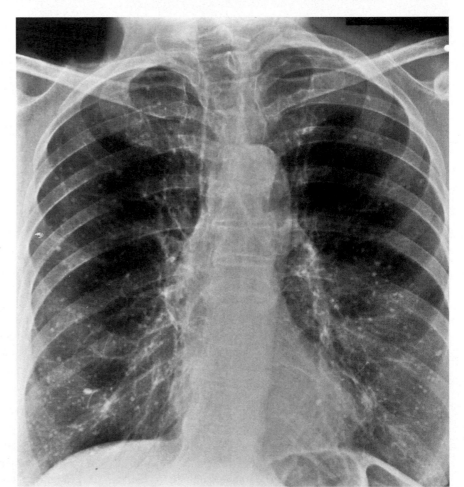

Figure 3-20.   Healed varicella pneumonia. There are multiple 1- to 3-mm calcified nodules in both lungs.

lung volumes and air trapping, and occasionally linear interstitial opacities may be identified.

Varicella-Herpes Zoster (Chickenpox)

Chickenpox infection may be responsible for severe pneumonia in the adult. The radiographic features are fairly characteristic. They consist of nodules ranging in size from 4 to 6 mm with ill-defined margins diffusely distributed throughout both lungs (Fig. 3-19). Radiographic resolution usually occurs over many weeks. One of the interesting sequelae of chickenpox pneumonia is the development of diffuse, discrete pulmonary calcifications that can be identified on routine radiographs obtained after the infection (Fig. 3-20). Histoplasmosis should be considered in the differential diagnosis of this appearance.

Cytomegalovirus

See Chapter 4 for a discussion of this topic.

Mononucleosis

The Epstein-Barr virus is the presumed etiologic agent for infectious mononucleosis. Although upper respiratory symptoms predominate, the patients may develop a nonproductive cough. The chest radiograph is usually normal, but occasionally pronounced hilar lymph node enlargement with an ill-defined diffuse reticular pattern in the lungs can occur.

GRANULOMATOUS INFECTIONS

Mycobacterial Disease

Mycobacteria are aerobic, nonmotile, nonspore-forming rods that have in common the characteristics of (1) staining bright red with carbol fuschin and (2) resistance to discoloration by strong acid solutions. The organisms are therefore referred to as "acid-fast" bacilli. There are a number of mycobacterial species, the most important include *M. leprae,* the cause of leprosy; *M. tuberculosis* and *M. bovis,* responsible for tuberculosis; and finally the nontuberculous mycobacteria that are important etiologic agents in the development of pulmonary disease.

Tuberculosis
Characteristics
In the latter part of the nineteenth century, tuberculosis (Box 3-15) was a leading cause of death in the United States. The advent of drug therapy and improved public health measures led to a steady decline in the incidence of tuberculosis following World War II until 1985. Since that year there has been a slow but steady increase in the incidence of tuberculosis. This is most likely related to the large number of cases associated with AIDS.

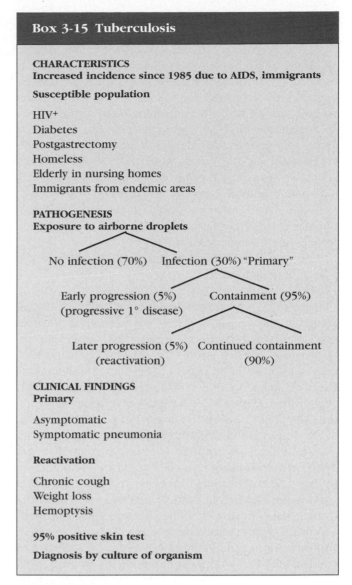

Box 3-15 Tuberculosis

CHARACTERISTICS
Increased incidence since 1985 due to AIDS, immigrants

Susceptible population

HIV+
Diabetes
Postgastrectomy
Homeless
Elderly in nursing homes
Immigrants from endemic areas

PATHOGENESIS
Exposure to airborne droplets

No infection (70%)   Infection (30%) "Primary"

Early progression (5%)   Containment (95%)
(progressive 1° disease)

Later progression (5%)   Continued containment
(reactivation)   (90%)

CLINICAL FINDINGS
Primary

Asymptomatic
Symptomatic pneumonia

Reactivation

Chronic cough
Weight loss
Hemoptysis

95% positive skin test

Diagnosis by culture of organism

Immigration into the United States of individuals from third world countries has also contributed to the increased prevalence of tuberculosis. In the United States tuberculosis is predominantly a disease of black and Hispanic men. The case rates for these men are twice as high as those for women, and similarly the case rate for white men is less than one fifth of that of nonwhite men. Other susceptible populations include the aged and the immunocompromised, particularly patients with AIDS.

Pathology and pathogenesis
Infection with tuberculosis occurs as the result of inhalation of airborne droplets containing the tubercle bacilli. The initial infection referred to as *primary* tuberculosis is most common in the lower lobes. The bacteria are ingested by macrophages and initially spread to local lymph nodes at this stage, and then they may disseminate throughout the body. The infection is usually contained if the host is immune competent. However, walled-off tubercle bacilli representing a

dormant focus of tuberculosis may activate under appropriate conditions. This may occur in the second type of tuberculosis referred to as *reactivation* or *post primary* tuberculosis. Such reactivation tuberculosis can occur any time after the primary infection, but the highest rate of reactivation occurs during the first and second years after initial infection. Reactivation tuberculosis usually involves the lung apex, but a dormant focus of tuberculosis may become active in other organs such as the bones, kidney, or brain. Clinically active disease may develop either at the time of primary TB infection (primary progressive tuberculosis) or when dissemination occurs (miliary tuberculosis). Clinical reactivation disease results when there is ineffective T-cell immune reaction.

The typical pathologic feature of tuberculosis is the caseating granuloma.

Clinical findings

In primary tuberculosis, patients are usually asymptomatic but may occasionally have a symptomatic pneumonia. Patients with acute or chronic reactivation tuberculosis usually present with a chronic cough, weight loss, and occasionally hemoptysis and dyspnea. The symptoms are often insidious. Ninety-five percent of patients with active tuberculosis will have a positive tuberculin skin test. The diagnosis must be made on the basis of culture of the organism, although the presence of acid-fast bacilli on smear from the sputum is strong presumptive evidence of tuberculosis. Classification of tuberculosis into primary or reactivation phases is based on the radiographic appearance. In third world countries and in the United States during the ninetieth and early twentieth centuries, primary tuberculosis was a disease of children, and reactivation tuberculosis was typically a disease of young adults. However, a significant change in the pattern of adult tuberculosis has occurred in the past several decades. There is now diminished exposure of children to TB, and when the disease occurs in adults it is often of the primary form. This has resulted in atypical radiographic manifestations of tuberculosis in adults, attributable to primary infection rather than reactivation of the disease.

Radiographic features

PRIMARY TUBERCULOSIS   There are several radiographic features of primary tuberculosis (Box 3-16). Primary tuberculous pneumonia can occur in any lobe of the lung but is more common at the lung bases (Fig. 3-21). In over a half of cases, the disease occurs in the lower lobes. One should consider any chronic consolidation, particularly in the bases of the lungs, as possibly suggestive of tuberculosis. Cavitation, though rare in primary tuberculosis, is more frequently reported in adults with the primary form of disease.

Mediastinal and *hilar adenopathy* is another feature of primary tuberculosis (Fig. 3-22). It may occur alone or in association with consolidation in the lung. It tends to

be particularly predominant in children. Computed tomography may be helpful in identifying and localizing adenopathy. On CT scans tuberculous adenopathy has a predilection for the right paratracheal, right tracheobronchial, and subcarinal regions. Occasionally atelectasis may occur secondary to extrinsic obstruction of a bronchus by enlarged lymph nodes. On CT scans obtained with intravenously administered contrast material, such nodes often demonstrate low-attenuation necrotic centers.

Pleural effusion due to tuberculous pleurisy, also a feature of primary infection, develops when subpleural foci of tuberculosis rupture into the pleural space. It presents 3 to 7 months after the initial exposure. Organisms are rarely found in the fluid, and the diagnosis must be confirmed with a pleural biopsy.

The *Ghon lesion* (Fig. 3-23) is a manifestation of primary tuberculosis, which usually occurs in childhood and is self-limited. The host defense mechanisms handle the initial infection and the area of consolidation in the lung slowly regresses to a well-circumscribed nodule. This nodule then shrinks and may disappear completely or remain as a solitary calcified granuloma. The adenopathy regresses as well and may also exhibit calcification (Rhanke complex).

REACTIVATION TUBERCULOSIS   *Reactivation tuberculosis* usually occurs in the apical and posterior segments of the upper lobes and in the superior segment of the lower lobes. It is characterized by chronic patchy areas of consolidation (Fig. 3-24). Cavitation is a hallmark of reactivation tuberculosis (Fig. 3-25). Cavities result when areas of caseation necrosis erode into the bronchial tree,

---

Box 3-16 Tuberculosis

RADIOGRAPHIC FEATURES

PRIMARY	REACTIVATION
Tuberculous pneumonia	**Apical and posterior segments, upper lobes, and superior segments, lower lobes**
Basilar consolidation	
Cavitation rare	
Mediastinal and hilar adenopathy	**Patchy areas of consolidation**
Children	**Cavitation**
Right side	
CT shows rim enhancement	**Bronchogenic spread**
	Chronic
Pleuritis	Fibronodular
	Fibrocalcific
Ghon lesion and Rhanke complex	Volume loss
	Bronchiectasis
Calcified	
Healed	

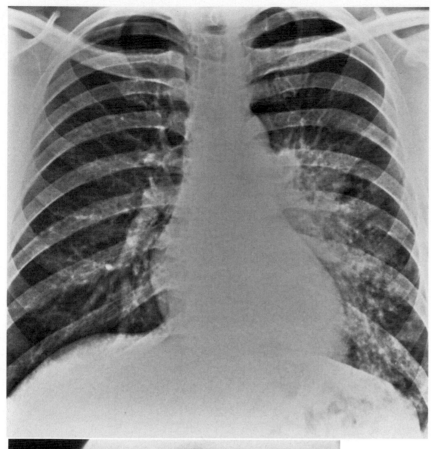

A

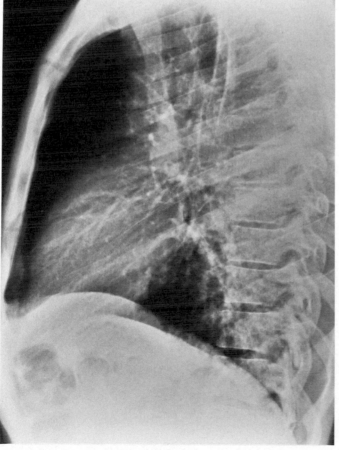

B

Figure 3-21. PA and lateral views. Primary tuberculous pneumonia. Patchy consolidation is present in the left lower lobe.

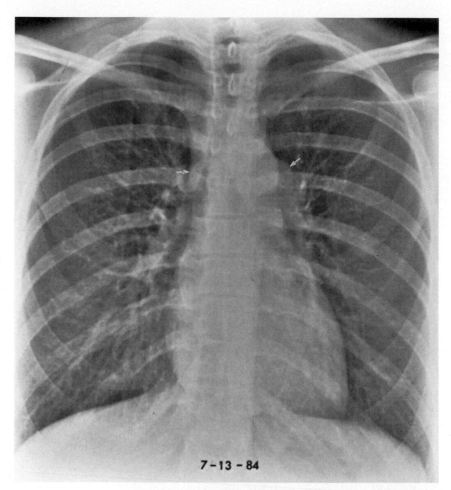

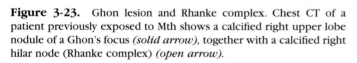

Figure 3-22. Mediastinal adenopathy in primary tuberculosis. Young black female presented with cervical adenopathy. PA chest radiograph shows enlargement of right paratracheal and left aorticopulmonary window nodes *(arrows).*

Figure 3-23. Ghon lesion and Rhanke complex. Chest CT of a patient previously exposed to Mth shows a calcified right upper lobe nodule of a Ghon's focus *(solid arrow),* together with a calcified right hilar node (Rhanke complex) *(open arrow).*

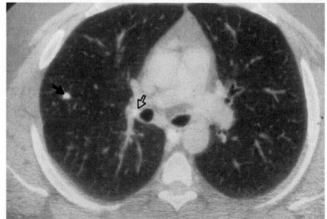

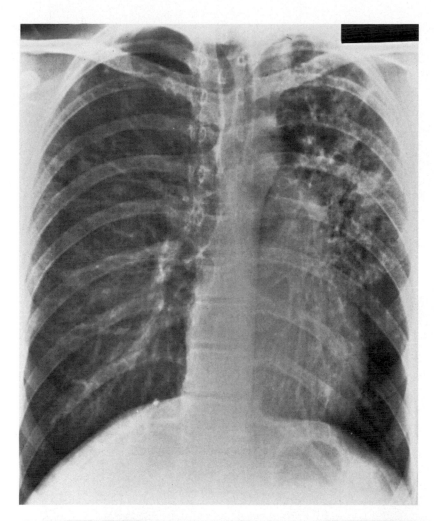

Figure 3-24. Reactivation tuberculosis. Patchy areas of consolidation involving the left upper lobe and superior segment of the left lower lobe. There is also evidence of some volume loss with shift of the trachea to the left, a common finding with Mtb infection even in the early stages of disease. Nodular lesions can be identified in the right upper lobe.

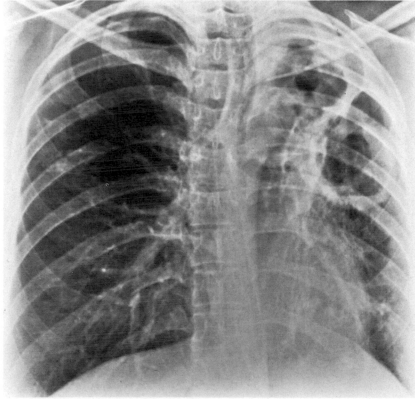

Figure 3-25. Cavitary tuberculosis. PA chest radiograph shows multiple cavities in the left upper lobe. A thick-walled cavity is present lateral to the left hilum. There is pronounced volume loss in the left upper lobe and apical pleural thickening.

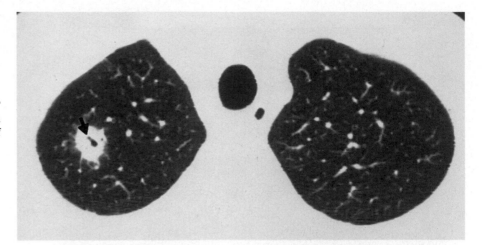

Figure 3-26. Cavitary tuberculosis. CT of a patient with reactivation TB showing a thick-walled cavity in the apical segment of the right upper lobe (*arrow*).

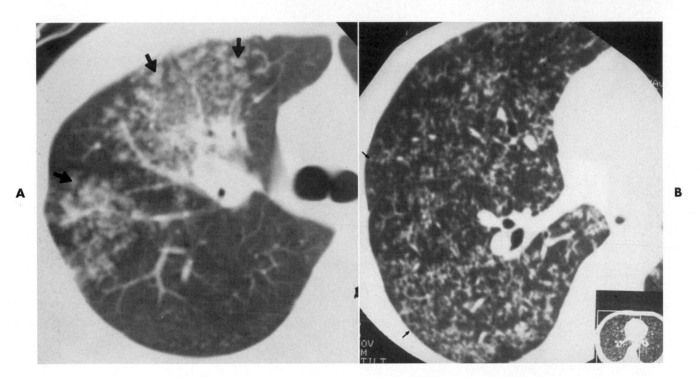

Figure 3-27. **A,** Bronchogenic spread of tuberculosis. CT shows a segmental distribution of confluent nodular opacities *(arrows)* in the right upper lobe. (Courtesy of Georgann McGuiness, M.D., New York University Medical Center, New York.) **B,** CT in another patient showing a typical "tree-in-bud" pattern. Centrilobular nodules and branching opacities can be identified close to the pleural surface (*arrows*).

expelling liquefied debris. CT is more sensitive than plain radiography in the detection of small cavities (Fig. 3-26). They may have either thick or thin walls, which can be either smooth or irregular. Bronchogenic spread of tuberculosis occurs when a cavity erodes into an adjacent airway and organisms spread endobronchially to other parts of the lung. The typical radiographic features (Fig. 3-27) consist of ill-defined nodules usually 5 to 6 mm in diameter. These are numerous and often bilateral. On CT the pattern of bronchogenic spread can easily be recognized by a tree-in-bud pattern. This consists of centrilobular branching linear opacities with or without the presence

of centrilobular nodules within 3 to 5 mm of the pleural surface or interlobular septa. This pattern is best appreciated on high-resolution CT. It is not specific for bronchogenic spread of tuberculosis and may occur in other inflammatory diseases involving the peripheral airways. The chronic lesion of reactivation tuberculosis usually consists of fibronodular opacities in the upper lobes, often with the presence of calcification (Fig. 3-28). This is usually associated with volume loss and retraction of the hila. Another feature of chronic reactivation tuberculosis is bronchiectasis. One should consider tuberculosis in the differential diagnosis of upper-lobe bronchiectasis. The

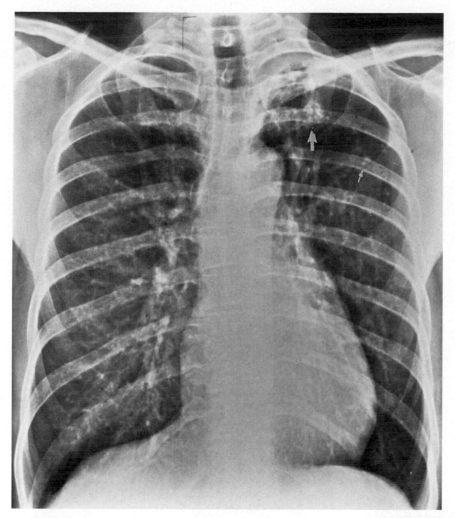

Figure 3-28. Fibrocalcific tuberculosis. PA chest radiograph demonstrates the features of chronic healed tuberculosis. There is apical pleural thickening and multiple calcified nodular and irregular opacities in the left upper lobe (*arrows*). Volume loss is not a prominent feature in this case. Although such an appearance suggests inactive disease, serial radiographs are necessary to determine stability. Viable organisms may be present, and the development of clinically active disease may rarely occur.

activity of tuberculous disease cannot be determined by radiographs; it is only confirmed by positive cultures. However, tuberculosis is considered radiographically stable if there has been no change over 6 months.

OTHER RADIOGRAPHIC FEATURES OF TUBERCULOSIS Unusual patterns of tuberculosis (Box 3-17) may occur in the patient who has altered host resistance to the primary infection. Miliary tuberculosis is a term used to define diffuse hematogenous dissemination of tuberculosis that has progressed when the host defense system is overwhelmed by massive hematogenous dissemination of organisms. It may occur anytime after the primary infection. The radiographic appearance (Fig. 3-29) is that of multiple tiny nodules in the interstitium of the lung measuring approximately 1 to 2 mm in diameter. CT may allow earlier detection than standard radiography (Fig. 3-30). Miliary disease takes up to 6 weeks to become apparent on plain radiographs.

Pneumothorax occasionally occurs secondary to tuberculosis. Tuberculosis may also cause ulceration of the bronchi, and advanced *endobronchial tuberculosis* may produce lobar atelectasis and strongly simulate a primary bronchogenic carcinoma of the lung. A local-

---

Box 3-17 Tuberculosis—Other Radiographic Features

MILIARY TUBERCULOSIS

Hematogenous dissemination
1-2 mm nodules, diffuse

PNEUMOTHORAX

ENDOBRONCHIAL TUBERCULOSIS

Lobar or segmental atelectasis

TUBERCULOMA

Single or multiple
>1 cm nodule

TUBERCULOUS EMPYEMA AND BRONCHOPLEURAL FISTULA

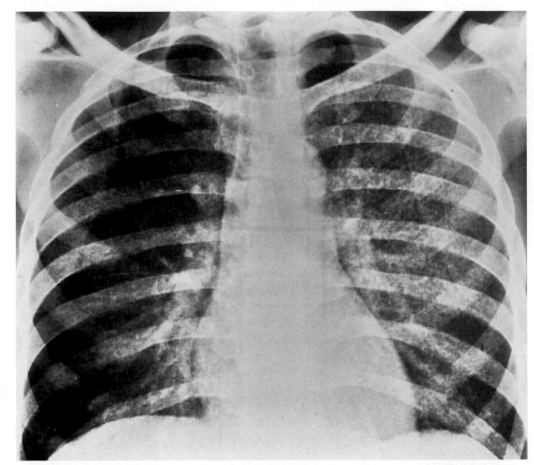

Figure 3-29. Miliary tuberculosis. PA chest radiograph demonstrates innumerable tiny 1- to 2-mm nodules in both lungs.

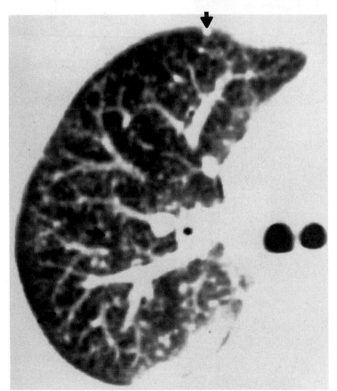

Figure 3-30. Miliary tuberculosis. CT findings. In contrast to bronchogenic spread, the nodules are diffuse and uniformly distributed (*arrows*).

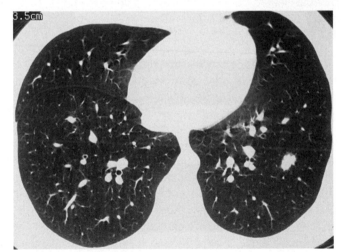

Figure 3-31. Tuberculoma. CT demonstrates a somewhat lobulated nodule in the left lower lobe. There was no evidence of calcification or other manifestations of tuberculosis in the lungs.

ized nodular focus of tuberculosis, referred to as a *tuberculoma* (Fig. 3-31), occurs in any portion of the lung and may be secondary to primary or reactivation tuberculosis. It is usually solitary, spherical, and smooth. It may contain a central calcification, but occasionally tuberculomas may be multiple and simulate metastatic disease.

Tuberculous empyema and *bronchopleural fistula* may develop secondary to a tuberculous pleural effusion. Such effusions can become loculated and remain quiescent for years.

Radiographic patterns of tuberculous disease in patients with the acquired immune deficiency syndrome may vary and are described in Chapter 4.

Nontuberculous mycobacterial infections

Characteristics   Some nontuberculous mycobacteria (Box 3-18) are pathogenic in humans. The most important of these organisms are *Mycobacterium avium intracellulare,* often commonly referred to as the MAC complex, and *Mycobacterium kanaseii.* These organisms often exhibit common features. They are usually found in the soil and water. Bronchopulmonary disease is caused by inhalation of the organisms, but no human-to-human transmission occurs. Unlike tuberculosis, nontuberculous mycobacterial infections present no evidence of a pattern of primary or reactivation disease. There are certain geographic areas of preponderance; for example, *M. kanaseii* is more prevalent in the western and southern United States, and *M. avium intracellulare* in the southeastern United States. There are three major clinical presentations that depend to some degree on the immune status of the host. [See Chapter 4 for description of MAC disease in AIDS patients.] In HIV-negative hosts, *M. avium intracellulare* typically affects male patients who are heavy smokers with underlying chronic obstructive pulmonary disease (COPD). Similar infections may occur in patients with silicosis or bronchiectasis. The radiographic features of both *M. kanaseii* and MAC in this group of patients are indistinguishable from tuberculosis. However, *Mycobacterium avium* complex lung disease may develop in older women who are considered immunologically competent and who do not have a background of COPD. This disease exists in a noncavitary form.

Because nontuberculous mycobacteria are common contaminants, the identification of invasive disease due to nontuberculous mycobacterial infection requires either (1) evidence of cavitation or progressive changes on chest radiographs, (2) at least two positive sputum cultures, or (3) evidence of mycobacteria on biopsy. It has long been believed that colonization by nontuberculous mycobacteria, particularly MAC, occurs in areas of preexisting lung disease such as bronchiectasis.

Radiographic features   The classic form of atypical mycobacterial infection produces features almost

COPD, chronic obstructive pulmonary disease.

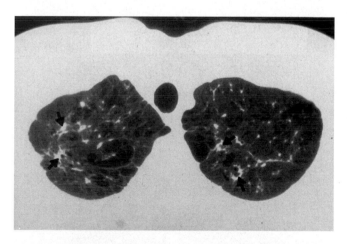

Figure 3-32.   Atypical mycobacterial infection. Chest CT in a patient with emphysema shows the appearance of "classic" atypical mycobacterial infection. There are biapical fibronodular opacities (*arrows*) accompanied by architectural distortion resembling the appearance of reactivation TB.

identical to reactivation tuberculosis (Fig. 3-32). Involvement occurs in the apical and posterior segments of the upper lobes and superior segment of the lower lobes. Cavitation is frequent and multiple cavities may be observed. The disease tends to be slowly progressive.

MAC lung disease occurring in older women who are usually nonsmokers without evidence of chronic obstructive pulmonary disease is noncavitary and is associated with bronchiectasis. The classic radiographic features are best appreciated on computed tomography (Fig. 3-33). The findings are those of cylindrical bronchiectasis associated with multiple small but focal lung nodules usually measuring approximately 5 mm in diameter. Any lobe may be involved, but the lingula and middle lobe have the highest prevalence. Occasionally air space disease may also be delineated. Evidence seems to indicate that patients with these findings are truly infected and not colonized with MAC and that the MAC infection causes the bronchiectasis rather than colonizing preexisting disease.

Fungal Diseases of the Lung

A wide variety of fungi may produce lung disease. These can be divided into two groups. Those that are truly pathogenic can produce pulmonary infection in normal hosts. These include *Histoplasma, Coccidioides, Blastomyces,* and *Cryptococcus.* A second group of fungi are secondary invaders or opportunistic organisms, which produce disease in immunosuppressed patients. The latter group include *Aspergillus, Candida, Cryptococcus,* and *Mucor.* This latter group is discussed in the chapter dealing with opportunistic pulmonary infections (Chapter 4).

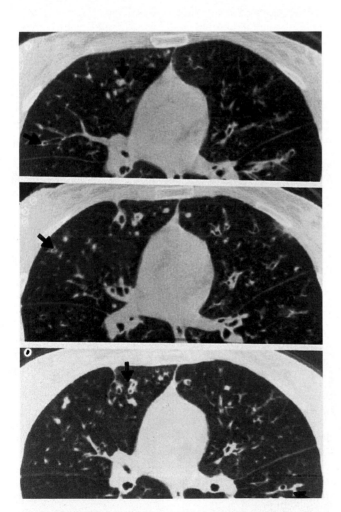

Figure 3-33. Mycobacterial avium complex infection. Three selected images from a chest CT of an elderly woman. Note scattered nodules and peripheral areas of bronchiectasis with mucous plugging (*arrows*).

Box 3-19 Histoplasmosis

CHARACTERISTICS
Dimorphic fungus

River valleys in United States

Soil excrement of birds or bats

ENDEMIC AREAS
80% infected

Most asymptomatic

PATHOGENESIS AND PATHOLOGY
Inhalation of spores
↓
Localized lung infection
↓
Hilar and mediastinal nodes
↓
Dissemination to liver and spleen
↙   ↘
Containment   Chronic cavitary lung infection

RADIOGRAPHIC FEATURES
Acute phase

Consolidation—segmental or sublobar
Ipsilateral mediastinal or hilar adenopathy

Epidemic form

Multiple nodules
± Adenopathy
Healed phase—calcification

Solitary histoplasmoma

Up to 4 cm
Central nidus of Ca^{++}

Chronic cavitary form—simulates TB

Additional features

Splenic calcification
Adenopathy—eventually calcifies
Broncholith
Fibrosing mediastinitis
Disseminated—miliary pattern

Histoplasmosis

Characteristics *Histoplasma capsulatum* (Box 3-19) is a dimorphous fungus that gains entry to the lung by inhalation. It is worldwide in distribution, and in the United States it occurs along river valleys, particularly the Ohio, Mississippi, and St. Lawrence. The organism exists in the soil, particularly when it is contaminated by the excrement of birds, such as pigeons, or bats. Many epidemics may occur when there is heavy exposure due to demolition or construction in areas containing such droppings, such as bat caves, chicken houses, or attics of old buildings. In edemic areas, up to 80% of the population may be infected, but most individuals are asymptomatic. Inhalation of spores results in a localized infection of the lung, which will then migrate to mediastinal and hilar lymph nodes and eventually to the spleen and liver. Usually the organisms are destroyed, and there is no residual of the initial infection, although a scar or calcification may occur. If individual foci of infection and necrosis persist, they may enlarge resulting in a chronic cavitary lesion indistinguishable from tuberculosis. Pathologically, well-defined granulomas may be found during the acute phase of disease in the lung, in the mediastinum, and in the various organs to which the organism disseminates. When healed these granulomas are small and densely calcified.

Outbreaks of histoplasmosis are usually associated with constitutional symptoms and nonproductive cough. Many such cases never come to medical attention.

Radiographic features There are a wide variety of radiographic manifestations of histoplasmosis. The acute phase of the disease is characterized by single or multiple areas of consolidation, which are usually segmental or sublobar in distribution. These may be accompanied by ipsilateral hilar or mediastinal adenopathy, and occasionally adenopathy alone may be the only finding. In the epidemic form of the disease, multiple discrete nodules may be seen throughout both lungs either alone or associated with hilar adenopathy (Fig. 3-34). They are usually 1 to 5 mm in diameter, discrete, and poorly marginated. With healing, these nodules may remain visible as multiple discrete calcified lesions less than a centimeter in diameter with or without calcified hilar lymph nodes (Fig. 3-35). A third radiographic pattern consists of a solitary granuloma or histoplasmoma, which is usually well defined and can range in size from several millimeters to 4 cm. It typically contains a central or target type of calcification. These usually occur in the lower lobes, and there may be associated smaller satellite calcified nodules.

There are a number of additional radiographic features that may be identified with *Histoplasma* infection. These include calcifications in the spleen, often best detected on computed tomography. As mentioned above, mediastinal lymphadenopathy is common either as a sole manifestation of histoplasmosis or accompanying pulmonary consolidation or nodules. Nodes frequently calcify as healing occurs. Such calcified lymph nodes may lead to two complications, broncholiths and fibrosing mediastinitis. Calcified lymph nodes may over time erode into a bronchus, producing broncholithiasis and its resulting symptom complex. Patients may have unexplained chronic cough and hemoptysis. CT can best identify the intrabronchial calcification that may be associated with distal atelectasis of a segment or lobe (Fig. 3-36). The other complication, fibrosing mediastinitis, is discussed in Chapter 17. This condition is caused by the effect of large calcified lymph nodes constricting and

A
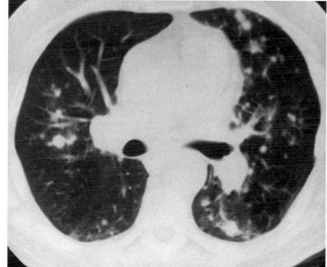

B
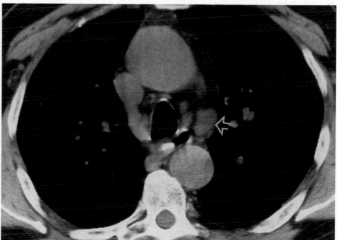

Figure 3-34.   Histoplasmosis (acute) seen on CT image. **A,** The lung windows demonstrate multiple bilateral pulmonary nodules. **B,** On the mediastinal windows there is adenopathy in the aorticopulmonary window (*arrow*).

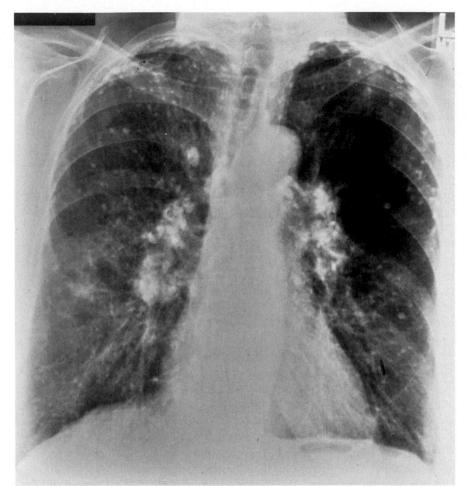

Figure 3-35. Healed histoplasmosis. There are multiple small calcified nodules in both lungs as well as densely calcified hilar and mediastinal nodes.

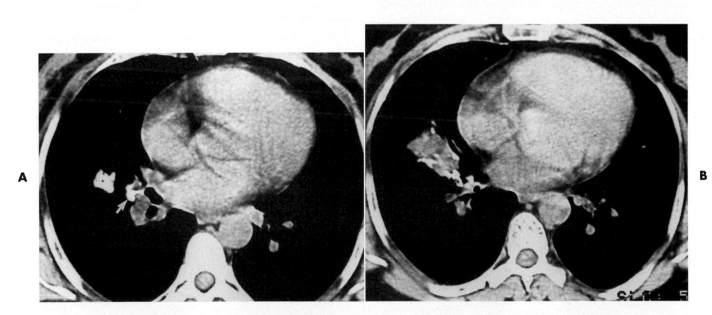

Figure 3-36. Broncholith with associated middle lobe collapse. CT demonstrates; **A,** a calcified broncholith obstructing the lateral segmental bronchus of the right middle lobe (*arrow*); **B,** areas of calcification in the partially collapsed lobe.

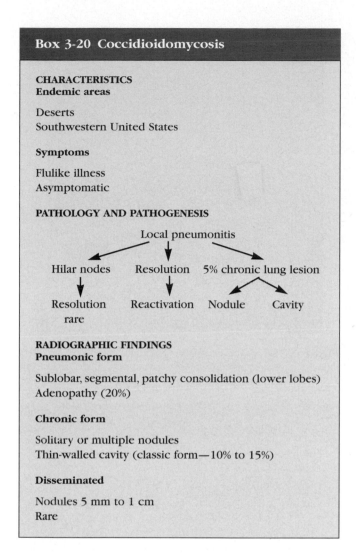

Box 3-20 Coccidioidomycosis

CHARACTERISTICS
Endemic areas

Deserts
Southwestern United States

Symptoms

Flulike illness
Asymptomatic

PATHOLOGY AND PATHOGENESIS

Local pneumonitis

→ Hilar nodes   → Resolution   → 5% chronic lung lesion

→ Resolution   Reactivation   Nodule   Cavity
rare

RADIOGRAPHIC FINDINGS
Pneumonic form

Sublobar, segmental, patchy consolidation (lower lobes)
Adenopathy (20%)

Chronic form

Solitary or multiple nodules
Thin-walled cavity (classic form—10% to 15%)

Disseminated

Nodules 5 mm to 1 cm
Rare

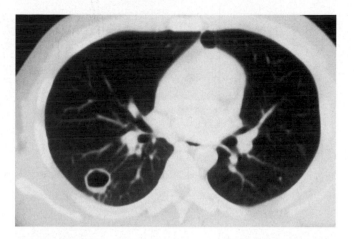

Figure 3-37. Coccidioidomycosis. CT demonstrates a relatively thin-walled cavity in the right lower lobe. The classic lesion of coccidioidomycosis has a paper-thin wall.

flulike illness. Acute severe disease may be associated with fever, cough, and pleuritic chest pain.

Pathology and pathogenesis With initial inhalation of the spores, a local response or pneumonitis occurs. The immune system eventually destroys the organism with resolution of the pneumonia. In about 5% of individuals there may be a chronic, often asymptomatic pulmonary lesion such as a pulmonary nodule or cavity. Similarly to tuberculosis, reactivation of the initial focus can occur. Dissemination of the organism to hilar and mediastinal nodes is common, and diffuse dissemination is rare but almost universally fatal.

Radiographic features The initial pneumonic form of the disease is characterized by an area of consolidation anywhere in the lung but most commonly in the lower lobes. It is usually either sublobar, segmental, or patchy. It may be bilateral. Hilar and mediastinal lymph node involvement occurs in about 20% of cases, and rarely it can be seen in the absence of the parenchymal consolidation. Most of these lesions resolve spontaneously without therapy.

The radiographic features of chronic coccidioidomycosis include either solitary or multiple nodules. These tend to cavitate rapidly, and typically the cavities have very thin walls (Fig. 3-37). The thin-walled cavity is the classic lesion of coccidioidomycosis, but it occurs in only 10% to 15% of cases. Disseminated coccidioidomycosis is extremely rare and is characterized radiographically by nodules ranging from 5 mm to 1 cm in diameter. A more classic miliary pattern can also be observed.

North American blastomycosis

Characteristics Blastomyces dermatitidis (Box 3-21) is a dimorphic fungus that grows in a mycelial form in the soil. Infection can occur either by inoculation of the skin or by inhalation of organisms into the lungs. The organism is endemic in North America, mostly in the

encasing important mediastinal structures, particularly the superior vena cava with resultant superior vena caval syndrome; the trachea; right main bronchus; and central pulmonary arteries. Compression of pulmonary veins may lead to venous infarcts in the lungs.

There is a rare chronic form of histoplasmosis that simulates tuberculosis. It usually consists of thin- or thick-walled cavities with patchy areas of consolidation, particularly involving the upper lobes with fibrosis and retraction. Disseminated histoplasmosis, which may occur in normal individuals, is much more common in immunosuppressed patients. Radiographically, the appearance is identical to miliary tuberculosis.

Coccidioidomycosis

Characteristics Coccidiodes immitis infection (Box 3-20) follows inhalation of infected spores in endemic areas, that is, the southwestern United States and Central and South America in desert areas. The clinical presentation is quite variable. Most individuals are asymptomatic or there may be a mild lower respiratory

Box 3-21 North American Blastomycosis

CHARACTERISTICS

Dimorphic—fungus
Wooded areas—hunters

RADIOGRAPHIC FEATURES

Patchy segmental or nonsegmented consolidation
Solitary or multiple nodules
Disseminated—miliary pattern

Box 3-22 Cryptococcus

CHARACTERISTICS

Spores in soil contaminated with pigeon and chicken
excreta
70% patients with clinical disease are immunocompromised hosts
CNS involvement

RADIOGRAPHIC FINDINGS

Single or multiple nodules >1 cm
Lower lobes

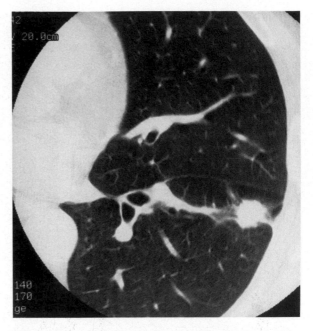

Figure 3-38. Cryptococcus in a patient with lymphoma. CT demonstrates an irregular nodule with a tag extending to the pleura.

Box 3-23 Candidiasis

CHARACTERISTICS
Candida albicans most common

Immunocompromised hosts

Exists in oropharynx

PATHOLOGY AND PATHOGENESIS
Mucous membranes and skin

Pulmonary

Aspirated organisms from oral cavity
Secondary to fungemia

RADIOGRAPHIC FINDINGS
Multiple, patchy, bilateral areas of consolidation

Multiple nodules ± cavitation

same areas where histoplasmosis occurs, but also in the in the southeastern United States. Blastomycosis is an infection associated with hunters because the organisms are prevalent in wooded areas.

Pathology and pathogenesis The organism is usually inhaled from the soil, and if the initial port of entry is the lung, a focal pneumonic process will occur. The disease can be self-limited or a disseminated form can occur.

Radiographic features The radiographic findings are nonspecific but consist of areas of inhomogeneous consolidation in a segmental or nonsegmental distribution in any area of the lung. The next most common manifestation is that of solitary and multiple pulmonary nodules. The solitary nodules may simulate bronchogenic carcinoma. These nodules can range from 3 to 6 mm in diameter. A third pattern results from disseminated disease and consists of a diffuse nodular or micronodular pattern.

Cryptococcus
Characteristics Cryptococcus neoformans (Box 3-22) is an encapsulated yeastlike fungus that exists in the soil and in the yeast form in humans. Often the soil may be contaminated by pigeon or chicken excreta. Seventy percent of individuals who have clinical disease are immunocompromised. (See Chapter 4 for more discussion.) The central nervous system is the most frequently affected site.

Radiographic features In the normal host the most common finding is that of single or multiple pulmonary nodules approximately 1 to 5 cm in diameter usually in the lower lobes (Fig. 3-38). Cavitation, lymph-node enlargement, and pleural effusion are all uncommon. Adenopathy is rarely identified. Characteristically the single or multiple nodules tend to abut the pleura.

Candidiasis
Characteristics Candidiasis (Box 3-23) may be caused by a group of various organisms in the *Candida* group of which *Candida albicans* is the most important species. *Candida albicans* lives in human and animal sources and

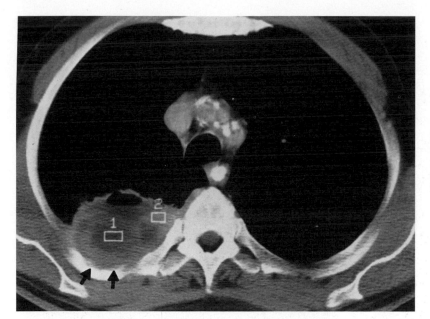

Figure 3-39. Actinomycosis. CT in a patient who developed an actinomycotic right upper lobe posterior segment necrotic consolidation after dental extraction. Note the erosion of the cortex of the overlying rib (*arrows*).

Box 3-24 Actinomycosis

CHARACTERISTICS
Rod-shaped bacterium, anaerobe

Mouth organisms

Poor oral hygiene

Forms

Cervicofacial
Gastrointestinal
Thoracic
    Focal abscess
    Invasion of chest wall

RADIOGRAPHIC FEATURES
Consolidation

Rounded abscess

Chest wall invasion (best seen on CT)

Bone destruction
Osteomyelitis and periostitis
Pleural effusion

Radiographic features The radiographic findings are usually nonspecific. Although most fungal diseases, particularly in immunocompromised hosts, are characterized by multiple nodules with cavitation, *Candida* pneumonia is more likely to produce areas of consolidation that are multiple and patchy and involve both lungs. Cavitation and hilar adenopathy are very rare, and pleural effusion occurs in approximately 25% of cases.

Actinomycosis
Characteristics *Actinomyces* (Box 3-24) is actually a rod-shaped bacterium rather than a fungus, but it is often considered a fungus, both because of its clinical presentation and radiographic findings. The organism is found in the mouth, and pulmonary infection usually occurs in people with extensive dental caries and poor oral hygiene. Involvement is secondary to aspiration of these organisms. There are three forms of actinomycosis: the cervicofacial, gastrointestinal, and thoracic. The hallmark of the pulmonary disease is a focal abscess with extension to the chest wall, with secondary complications such as osteomyelitis, bronchopleural fistula, and even pericarditis. The organism is an anaerobe, and anaerobic cultures must be obtained to confirm the diagnosis. Typical sulfur granules may be identified on pathologic specimens.

Radiographic features The radiographic features initially consist of an area of consolidation in the lung. This may become rounded and suggestive of an abscess. Classic signs include extension of the disease process into the chest wall with bone destruction and osteomyelitis (Fig. 3-39). Chest wall invasion is best appreciated on CT scanning. Pleural effusions are also moderately common. Invasion of the ribs or vertebral bodies characteristically causes bone destruction and fairly extensive reactive periostitis.

may be a normal inhabitant of the oral pharynx. As a result, short of an open-lung biopsy, the true invasiveness or pathogenicity of this organism when recovered from the sputum is difficult to determine. It is an unusual infection found in immunocompromised individuals.

Pathology and pathogenesis The most common sites of infection are the mucous membranes and skin. Pulmonary candidiasis is unusual but may occur as a primary infection of the lungs, presumably secondary to aspiration of the organisms from the oral cavity. In most immunocompromised patients, pulmonary infection accompanies a diffuse widespread fungemia.

Nocardiosis

Characteristics *Nocardia* (Box 3-25) is a gram-positive organism, and although it is classified as a bacterium, it shares many features with fungal disease. It is weakly acid-fast and can be confused with mycobacteria or *Legionella.* It is similar to *Actinomyces,* but the disease usually occurs in immunocompromised patients rather than in normal hosts. (See Chapter 4.)

Radiographic features Focal consolidation is said to be the most common finding, although often the disease appears as single or multiple nodules with cavitation. Unlike aspergillosis, progression of disease usually is rather slow. Chest wall involvement may occur but is rare.

Aspergillosis

Aspergillus (Table 3-3) is also a dimorphic fungus of which there are many species, the most common being *Aspergillus fumigatus. Aspergillus* grows widely in soil and water and decaying vegetation as well as animal material. Aspergillosis occurs in several different forms in the lung. These include (1) noninvasive (mycetoma) and semiinvasive aspergillosis, (2) invasive aspergillosis, and (3) allergic bronchopulmonary aspergillosis. The type of involvement depends on the immune status of the host. Infection is initiated by the inhalation route, and *Aspergillus* spores may exist in the mouth and airways of normal hosts. Immunocompetent or mildly immunosuppressed patients may acquire mycetomas or semiinvasive aspergillosis, whereas those who are severely immunosuppressed develop invasive aspergillosis. Allergic bronchopulmonary aspergillosis usually occurs in asthmatic patients.

Aspergilloma or Mycetoma (Noninvasive Aspergillosis)

CHARACTERISTICS The most common radiographic form of aspergillosis is the mycetoma or fungus ball. The fungus ball consists of aspergillus hyphae, mucus, and cellular debris developing within a preexisting cyst, cavity, bulla, or in an area of bronchiectasis. It grows as a saprophytic organism and as a rule is noninvasive. A high incidence of mycetoma has been noted in patients with sarcoidosis and cystic fibrosis. Symptoms usually include hemoptysis, which may be life-threatening.

RADIOGRAPHIC FEATURES The radiographic appearance of a fungus ball or mycetoma can be quite characteristic (Fig. 3-40). Typically there is a solid round opacity within a cavity or thin-walled cyst. Air may dissect into the solid mass creating an "air crescent." In the majority

---

Box 3-25 Nocardiosis

CHARACTERISTICS

Gram-positive, acid-fast bacterium
Immunocompromised hosts

RADIOGRAPHIC FINDINGS

Single or multiple nodules ± cavitation
Slow progression
Focal consolidation

Table 3-3 Aspergillosis

Aspergilloma or Mycetoma	Semiinvasive Aspergillosis	Invasive Aspergillosis	Allergic Bronchopulmonary Aspergillosis
CHARACTERISTICS	**CHARACTERISTICS**	**CHARACTERISTICS**	**CHARACTERISTICS**
Fungus ball	Mildly immuno-suppressed hosts	Immunocompromised hosts	Hypersensitivity reaction to aspergillus in mucous plugs

Preexisting
  Cavity
  Bulla
  Bronchiectasis
Saprophytic
Sarcoidoisis, cystic fibrosis
Hemoptysis
	Focal consolidation → cavity → air crescent → thick-walled cavity → fungus ball	Granulocytopenia	Mucoid impaction
			Asthmatic patients

RADIOGRAPHIC FEATURES	**RADIOLOGY**	**RADIOLOGY**	**RADIOGRAPHIC FEATURES**

Round opacity within cyst or cavity
Air crescent
Mobile
Pleural thickening
	Cavity ± fungus ball
	Air crescent
	Pleural thickening
		Single or multiple nodules
		Cavitation
		Air crescent
		"Halo" sign on CT
			Mucoid impaction
			  Central branching opacities
			  Central bronchiectasis
			Lobar consolidation
			Chronic
			  Upper lobe scarring and bronchiectasis

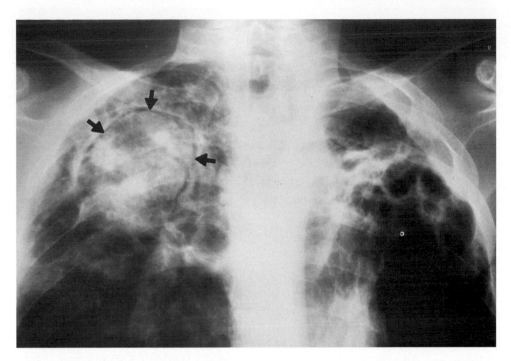

Figure 3-40.   Fungus ball or mycetoma due to aspergillus. Coned-down PA view of the chest of a patient with biapical fibrocavitary tuberculosis accompanied by volume loss. There is a mass in a large right upper-lobe cavity with air dissecting into the cavity producing "air crescents" (*arrows*).

of cases the fungus ball is mobile, and changes in position occur with changes in body posture. Extensive pleural thickening at the apex of the thorax frequently accompanies the development of a mycetoma. In making the differential diagnosis one should consider both necrotizing squamous-cell carcinoma or an intrapulmonary abscess.

No treatment is necessary in asymptomatic individuals, but in those who develop severe hemoptysis there are several therapeutic options. One is an interventional radiologic technique that consists of embolization of bronchial arteries that supply the cavity. Direct installation of amphotericin B in the form of a paste inserted through a percutaneous catheter into the cavity has been successful in some cases.

Semiinvasive aspergillosis

CHARACTERISTICS   Semiinvasive aspergillosis occurs in mildly immunosuppressed patients such as those with alcoholism, chronic debilitating illness, or advanced malignancy. The lesion usually begins as a focal consolidation in the apex of one or both lungs that progresses over a period of months to become cavitary. It may form a "crescent" of air (air crescent) similar to that seen in a mycetoma. A thick-walled cavity, which later becomes thin-walled and contains a fungus ball, is then formed.

RADIOGRAPHIC FEATURES   The appearance may be identical to a mycetoma. It consists of a cavity with or without a fungus ball and air crescent, or it may be a localized area of consolidation. Extensive pleural thickening can also be identified.

Invasive aspergillosis   The features of invasive aspergillosis are described in chapter 4 dealing with pulmonary infections in the immunocompromised patient.

Allergic bronchopulmonary aspergillosis (see Chapter 13 on Airways)   This disease occurs almost exclusively in asthmatic individuals. *Aspergillus* spores contained within mucous plugs in the tracheobronchial tree incite an allergic reaction. The syndrome consists of blood eosinophilia with positive precipitins and marked elevation of IgE antibodies. Large masses of mucus and aspergillus hyphae can become trapped in the airways, producing mucoid impaction of the bronchi.

RADIOGRAPHIC FEATURES   The most characteristic pattern is that of mucoid impaction of the bronchus. Central branching opacities sometimes termed finger-in-glove or V pattern, are identified. A more extensive description is provided in Chapter 13. Usually atelectasis distal to the areas of mucoid impaction does not occur because of collateral air drift. Air trapping may be identified. Lobar consolidation may occasionally be present. As the mucous plugs are expectorated, areas of central bronchiectasis can be identified, particularly on CT scans. Patients usually respond to steroids, but in the chronic form of the disease, scarring and upper-lobe bronchiectasis are prominent features.

Mucormycosis

Characteristics   Mucormycosis, almost exclusively a disease in immunocompromised patients, is discussed in Chapter 4.

PROTOZOAN AND OTHER PARASITIC INFECTIONS

In the United States, parasitic infection of the lung is rare. Pneumonia is due to a hypersensitivity reaction to the organisms, or it is secondary to systemic invasion of the lungs and pleura.

Pneumocystis Carinii

This pneumonia is discussed in Chapter 4 dealing with pneumonias in the immunocompromised patient.

Toxoplasmosis

Toxoplasma gondii pulmonary involvement usually develops as part of a more generalized disease. The congenital variety is the most common and results from transmission of the organism from mother to fetus. It is associated with a consolidative and hemorrhagic pneumonia in neonates. In adults, toxoplasmosis, like pneumocystosis, occurs in patients who are immunocompromised. The radiographic appearance is that of fairly diffuse reticulonodular opacities.

Echinococcus

Characteristics

Echinococcus granulosus (Box 3-26), the cause of most cases of human hydatid disease, occurs in two forms: pastoral and sylvatic, which differ in both definitive and intermediate hosts and in geographic distribution. The pastoral variety is more common and occurs in sheep, cows, or pigs as the intermediate hosts, and in dogs as the definitive host. It is particularly common in sheep-raising areas. The sylvatic variety has as the definitive host the dog, wolf, or arctic fox. Approximately 65% to 70% of *Echinococcus* cysts occur in the liver and 15% to 30% in the lungs. The hydatid cyst itself is composed of two layers, an exocyst and an endocyst. Daughter cysts may be formed within the endocyst. Cysts may rupture in the lung parenchyma with resulting intense inflammation. Rupture into the bronchus may result in severe hypotensive shock.

Radiographic features

Echinococcus cysts are usually well-circumscribed spherical or oval masses that may be single or multiple (Fig. 3-41). They are usually located in the lower lobes. If communication develops between the cysts and the bronchial tree, air may enter between the pericyst and exocyst, producing the appearance of a thin crescent of air around the periphery of the cyst sometimes called the meniscus or crescent sign. Bronchial com-

---

Box 3-26 *Echinococcus*

CHARACTERISTICS
Forms

Pastoral
  Sheep-raising areas
  Sylvatic
  Dog, wolf, arctic fox—definitive hosts

Sites of involvement

1. Liver—65%-70%
2. Lung—15%-30%

Cysts

Structure
  Endocyst
  Exocyst
  Daughter cysts
Complications
  Rupture—local inflammation
  Anaphylaxis

RADIOGRAPHIC FEATURES

Single or multiple
Spherical
Lower lobes
"Meniscus" or "crescent" sign
Air-fluid level—"water lily" sign
No Ca^{++}

---

munication occurs directly into the endocyst. Occasionally both an air-crescent sign and air-fluid level can be identified. The membrane of the cyst, which has ruptured into the bronchial tree, may float on the fluid within the cyst, giving rise to the classic "water lily" sign. CT can distinguish cystic from solid lesions and may identify the pathognomonic features in ruptured or complicated hydatid cysts, such as the presence of daughter cysts and endocyst membranes. Calcification of a pulmonary hydatid cyst is very rare.

Amebiasis

Characteristics

Pulmonary amebiasis is rare and is usually a sequela of hepatic or gastrointestinal involvement. Amebiasis is caused by the protozoan *Entamoeba histolytica*. This organism causes dysentery and is worldwide in distribution. Pleuropulmonary complications usually occur when the liver is involved. Patients present with right upper quadrant and right-sided pleuritic chest pain.

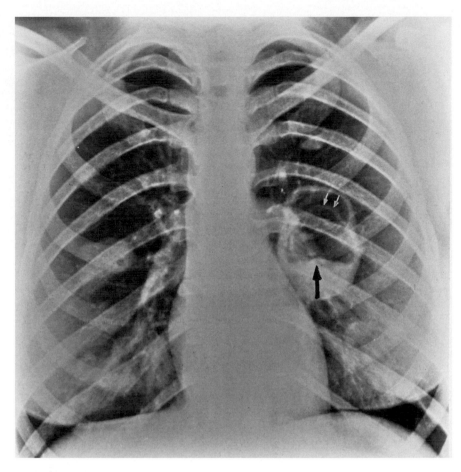

Figure 3-41. Echinococcus cysts. There are multiple nodules in both lungs, some of which are cavitated. A meniscus or crescent can be identified (*small arrows*) in the large cyst in the left lung, which also displays an air-fluid level and "water lily" sign (*black arrow*).

Radiographic features

The common radiographic features are right-sided pleural effusion with basal consolidation. Involvement of the lung may occur secondary to rupture of an amebic abscess in the liver. Occasionally areas of consolidation in the right lower lobe may progress to abscess formation with cavitation.

Schistosomiasis

Schistosomiasis is a common disease in many areas of the world including Central and South America, the Middle East, and Far East. The intermediate host of this parasite is the snail. Humans contact the parasites in water where the parasites penetrate the skin, reach the circulation, and eventually grow in the mesenteric or pelvic venous plexes where they mature into adult worms and lay eggs. Pulmonary symptoms may occur during the larval migration phase in the lungs due to a hypersensitivity reaction. A progressive diffuse endarteritis and thrombosis may result from impaction of ova in the pul-

monary circulation, with the eventual development of pulmonary arterial hypertension.

Pathology and pathogenesis

Pathologic changes in the lungs occur as the result of deposition of eggs or ova, which are released directly into the systemic venous blood or occasionally into the portal system where eggs can reach the lungs through anastomotic channels as the liver becomes cirrhotic. The embolized ova become impacted in pulmonary arterioles and then extruded into the surrounding tissue. This causes an obliterative arteriolitis, which can result in increased pulmonary artery pressure. The ova may mature into adult worms in the lungs and can cause lung damage.

Radiographic features

Pulmonary arterial hypertension is the most frequent finding in pulmonary schistosomiasis (Fig. 3-42). The appearance consists of dilation of the central pulmonary arteries with rapid tapering. The passage of larva through the pulmonary capillaries can cause a transitory

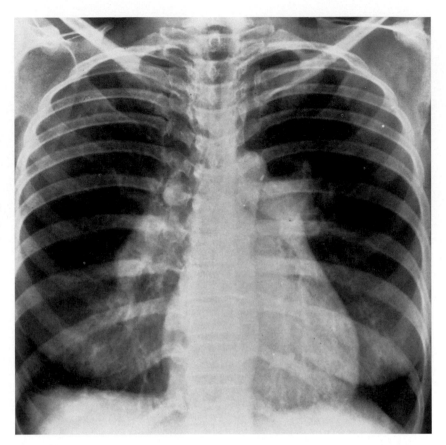

Figure 3-42. Pulmonary arterial hypertension in pulmonary schistosomiasis. There is dilation of central pulmonary arteries. The patient was a 48-year-old Puerto Rican woman with proven schistosomiasis, cirrhosis, and portal hypertension.

eosinophilic pneumonia simulating Löeffler's syndrome. This is characterized by the presence of peripheral areas of consolidation.

Other Metazoan Infections

Infection of the lungs may occur with a number of worms including ascariasis, strongyloidiasis, trichinosis, ancylostomiasis (hookworm disease), and filaria (tropical eosinophilia). Most of these organisms produce hypersensitivity reactions in the lungs similar to Löeffler's syndrome. (See Chapter 9 for further discussion.)

SUGGESTED READINGS

Aquino S, Gamsu G, Webb WR et al: Tree-in-bud pattern: frequency and significance on thin section CT, *J Comput Assist Tomogr* 20:594-599, 1996.

Berkmen YM: Aspiration and inhalation pneumonias, *Semin Roentgenol* 15:73-84, 1980.

Cantanzaro A: Pulmonary coccidioidomycosis, *Med Clin North Am* 64:461-465, 1980.

Christensen EE, Dietz GW, Ahn CH et al: Pulmonary manifestations of *Mycobacterium intracellulare*, *Am J Roentgenol* 133:59:1979.

Comstock GW: Epidemiology of tuberculosis, *Am Rev Respir Dis* 125(3):8-16, 1982.

Dalhoff K, Maass M: *Chlamydia pneumoniae* pneumonia in hospitalized patients, *Chest* 110:351-356, 1996.

Davies SF: An overview of pulmonary fungal infections, *Clin Chest Med* 8(3):495-512, 1987.

Des Prez RM, Goodwin RA Jr: *Mycobacterium tuberculosis*. In Mandell GL, Douglas RG Jr, Bennet J, editors: *Principles and practice of infectious diseases*, ed 2, New York, 1985, Churchill Livingstone; pp 1383-1412.

Drutz DJ: *Coccidioidal pneumonia*. In Pennington JE, editor: *Respiratory infections—diagnosis and management*, ed 3, New York, 1994, Raven Press; pp 569-597.

Edelstein PH, Meyer RD: *Legionella pneumonias*. In Pennington JE, editor: *Respiratory infections—diagnosis and management*, ed 3, New York, 1994, Raven Press; pp 455-484.

Eisenstadt J, Crane LR: *Gram-negative bacillary pneumonias*. In Pennington JE, editor: *Respiratory infections—diagnosis and management*, ed 3, New York, 1994, Raven Press; pp 369-406.

Epstein DM, Kline LR, Albelda SM et al: Tuberculous pleural effusions, *Chest* 91:106-110, 1987.

Fairbank JT, Mamourian AC, Dietrich PA et al: The chest radiograph in Legionnaires' disease: further observations, *Radiology* 147:33-34, 1983.

Finegold SM: *Aspiration pneumonia, lung abscess, and empyema*. In Pennington JE, editor: *Respiratory infections—diagnosis and management*, ed 3, New York, 1994 Raven Press; pp 311-322.

Flynn MW, Felson B: The roentgen manifestations of thoracic actinomycosis, *Am J Roentgenol Radium Ther Nucl Med* 110:707-716, 1970.

Fraser RG, Paré JAP, Paré PD, Fraser RS et al: *Diagnosis of diseases of the chest,* ed 3, Philadelphia, 1989, WB Saunders; pp 774-1115.

Gefter WB, Weingard TR, Epstein DM et al: Semi-invasive pulmonary aspergillosis: a new look at the spectrum of aspergillus infections of the lung, *Radiology* 140:313-321, 1981.

Gefter WB: The spectrum of pulmonary aspergillosis, *J Thorac Imaging* 7(4):56-74, 1992.

Genereux GP, Stilwell GA: The acute bacterial pneumonias, *Semin Roentgenol* 15:9-16, 1980.

Goodwin RA Jr, DesPrez RM: *Histoplasma capsulatum.* In Mandell GL, Douglas RG Jr, Bennett J, editors: *Principles and practice of infectious diseases,* ed 2, New York, 1985, Churchill Livingstone; pp 1468-1479.

Greendyke WH, Resnick DL, Harvey WC: The varied roentgen manifestations of primary coccidioidomycosis, *Am J Roentgenol* 109:491-499, 1970.

Halvorsen RA, Duncan JD, Merten DF et al: Pulmonary blastomycosis: radiologic manifestations, *Radiology* 150:1-5, 1984.

Hartman TE, Swensen SJ, Williams DE: *Mycobacterium avium-intracellulare* complex: evaluation with CT, *Radiology* 187:1-4, 1992.

Janower ML, Weiss EB: Mycoplasmal, viral, and rickettsial pneumonias, *Semin Roentgenol* 15:25-34, 1980.

Kauffman RS: Viral pneumonia. In Pennington JE, editor: *Respiratory infections—diagnosis and management,* ed 3, New York, 1994, Raven Press; pp 515-532.

Khoury MB, Goodwin JD, Ravin CE et al: Thoracic cryptococcosis: immunologic competence and radiologic appearance, *Am J Roentgenol* 142:893-896, 1984.

Kroboth FJ, Yu VL, Reddy SC et al: Clinicoradiographic correlation with the extent of Legionnaire disease, *AJR* 141:263-268, 1983.

Kuhlman JE, Deutsch JH, Fishman EK et al: CT features of thoracic mycobacterial disease, *Radiographics* 10:413-431, 1990.

Kuhlman JE, Fishman EK, Teigin C: Pulmonary septic emboli: changes with CT, *Radiology* 174:211-213, 1990.

Landay MJ, Christensen EE, Bynum LJ et al: Anaerobic pleural and pulmonary infections, *AJR* 134:233-240, 1980.

Luby JP: Pneumonia caused by *Mycoplasma pneumoniae* infection, *Clin Chest Med* 12(2):237-244, 1991.

Lynch DA, Simone PM, Fox MA et al: CT features of pulmonary *Mycobacterium avium* complex infection, *J Comput Assist Tomogr* 19:353-360, 1995.

Malo JL, Hawkins R, Pepys J: Studies in chronic allergic bronchopulmonary aspergillosis. I. Clinical and physiological findings, *Thorax* 32:254-257, 1977.

McGarry T, Giosa R, Rohman M et al: Pneumatocele formation in adult pneumonia, *Chest* 92:717-720, 1987.

Miller WT, MacGregor RR: Tuberculosis: frequency of unusual radiographic findings, *Am J Roentgenol* 130:867-875, 1978.

Miller WT, Miller WT Jr: Tuberculosis in the normal host: radiological findings, *Semin Roentgenol* 23:109-118, 1993.

Miller WT: Granulomatous infections of the lung. In Freundlich IM, Bragg DG, editors: *A radiologic approach to diseases of the chest,* Baltimore, 1992, Williams & Wilkins.

Miller WT: Pulmonary infections. In Taveras JM, Ferrucci JT, editors: *Radiology: diagnosis-imaging-intervention,* vol 1, Philadelphia, 1988, JB Lippincott.

Miller WT: Spectrum of pulmonary non-tuberculous mycobacterial infection, *Radiology* 191:343-350, 1994.

Moore EH: Atypical mycobacterial infection in the lung: CT appearance, *Radiology* 187:777-782, 1993.

Newman GE, Effman EL, Putman CE: Pulmonary aspiration complexes in adults, *Curr Probl Diagn Radiol* 11(4):1-47, 1982.

Ort S, Ryan JL, Barden G et al: Pneumococcal pneumonia in hospitalized patients' clinical and radiological presentations, *JAMA* 249:214-218, 1983.

Patz EF, Goodman PC: Pulmonary cryptococcosis, *J Thorac Imaging* 7(4):51-55, 1992.

Petty TL: Adult respiratory distress syndrome, *Semin Respir Med* 3:219-224, 1982.

Putman CE: Infectious pneumonias—including aspiration states. In Putman CE, Ravin CE, editors: *Textbook of diagnostic imaging,* ed 2, Philadelphia, 1994, WB Saunders; pp 495-525.

Rohlfing BM, White EA, Webb WR et al: Hilar and mediastinal adenopathy caused by bacterial abscess of the lung, *Radiology,* 1978.

Ruben FL, Nguyen MLT: Viral pneumonitis, *Clin Chest Med* 12(2):223-235, 1991.

Rubin SA, Winer-Muram HT: Thoracic histoplasmosis, *J Thorac Imaging* 7(4):39-50, 1992.

Sanders WE Jr: *Other mycobacterium species.* In Mandell GL, Douglas RG Jr, Bennett JE, editors: *Principles and practice of infectious diseases,* ed 2, New York, 1985, Churchill Livingstone; pp 1413-1430.

Stead WW: Tuberculosis among elderly persons: an outbreak in a nursing home, *Ann Intern Med* 94:606, 1981.

Woodring JH, Rehm SR, Broderson H et al: Pulmonary aspiration of gastric contents, *J KY Med Assoc* 83:299-306, 1985.

Woodring JH, Vandiviere HM, Fried AM et al: Update: the radiographic features of pulmonary tuberculosis, *AJR* 146:497-506, 1986.

Woodring JH: Pulmonary bacterial and viral infections. In Freundlich IM, Bragg DG, editors: *A radiologic approach to diseases of the chest,* Baltimore, 1992, Williams & Wilkins.

CHAPTER 4

Pulmonary Infection in the Immunocompromised Host (Non-AIDS) and Pulmonary Disease in AIDS

MEENAKSHI BHALLA
THERESA C. McLOUD

PULMONARY INFECTIONS IN THE IMMUNOCOMPROMISED PATIENT (NON-AIDS)

The compromised host may be defined as an individual with altered defense mechanisms or immunity. Non-HIV positive immunocompromised hosts include patients with hematologic malignancies such as lymphoma and leukemia; recipients of organ transplants; patients treated aggressively with cytotoxic drugs for solid tumors; and those receiving high-dose corticosteroid therapy for collagen vascular and other disorders.

The lung is a frequent target of infection in the immunocompromised host, and mortality associated with pulmonary disease is often as high as 40% to 50%. Infection is the most frequent cause of the radiographic abnormality; however, other conditions such as extension of malignancy (for example, lymphoma or metastases), drug reactions, or other noninfectious processes may be diagnostic possibilities (Table 4-1). Unfortunately, noninvasive diagnostic methods such as sputum smears and cultures that are used for evaluation of pneumonia are less useful in the immunocompromised host. The clinician must therefore choose between using invasive techniques to determine the exact cause of the pneumonia or employing empirically chosen therapy. The former choice is not without hazard in debilitated patients; the latter is complicated by the broad range of possible causes and appropriate therapies. The radiologist plays an important role. It involves (1) detection of an abnormality on the chest roentgenogram; (2) analysis of the radiographic features with regard to diagnosis and choice of an appropriate interventional technique; (3) performance of percutaneous needle biopsy of focal lesions when appropriate; and (4) monitoring response to therapy and the development of complications. Although the radiographic features in most opportunistic infections are relatively nonspecific, there is a general correlation between the type of radiographic pattern and the microorganism producing the pneumonia. There are three major patterns used for classification: (1) lobar or segmental consolidation, (2) nodules with rapid growth and/or cavitation, and (3) diffuse lung disease.

Table 4-1   Radiographic patterns in HIV-negative immunocompromised patients with pulmonary disease

Lobar or Segmental Consolidation	Nodules with Rapid Growth ± Cavitation	Diffuse Lung Disease

• Organisms—bacteria
   • Gram-negative organisms
   • Gram-positive organisms
   • *Legionella pneumophila*
 • Radiographic features
   • Lobar or segmental
   • Frequent caviation
 • Diagnosis
   • Sputum smear and culture
   • Serology—*Legionella*
 • Differential diagnosis
   • Neoplasm
     • Lymphoma
	• Organism
	   • Fungi
	   • Nocardia
	   • *Legionella* (Pittsburgh agent)
	   • *Staphylococcus aureus* (septic infarcts)
	 • *Aspergillus*
	   • Characteristics
	     • Invasive—blood vessels— infarction
	     • Neutropenia
	   • Radiographic features
	     • Nodules
	     • Cavitation
	     • "Air crescent" sign
	     • "Halo sign" on CT
	 • Mucormycosis
	   • Diabetes, leukopenia
	   • Blood vessel invasion
	   • Radiographic appearance identical to *Aspergillus*
	 • Diagnosis
	   • Invasive procedure—TBB, TNB
	 • Differential diagnosis
	   • Metastases
	   • Lymphoma
	   • Lymphoproliferative disease
		• Causes
		   • Infection
		     • *Pneumocystis carinii*
		     • Virues (CMV)
		   • Cytotoxic drug reactions
		   • Lymphangitic spread of tumor
		   • Radiation pneumonitis
		   • Nonspecific interstitial pneumonitis
		 • *Pneumocystis carinii* pneumonia
		   • Characteristics
		     • 40% diffuse pneumonias in immunocompromised hosts
		     • Acute and fulminating
		   • Radiographic findings
		     • Central perihilar linear opacities → diffuse consolidation
		     • CT—ground-glass opacification
		   • Diagnosis
		     • BAL
		 • Cytomegalovirus
		   • Organ transplants
		   • Diffuse nodular or linear pattern on radiograph

BAL, bronchoalveolar lavage; *CMV,* cytomegalovirus; *TBB,* transbronchial biopsy; *TNB,* transthoracic needle biopsy.

Radiologic Patterns

See Table 4-1 for a summary of radiographic patterns in HIV-negative immunocompromised patients with pulmonary disease.

Lobar or segmental consolidation (bacterial pneumonia)

Causes Bacteria are the most common infectious agents invading the lungs of immunocompromised hosts. Colonization of the oral pharynx by altered flora in the presence of reduced lung defense mechanisms leads to a preponderance of gram-negative bacillary pneumonias. They include *Klebsiella, Enterobacter, Pseudomonas, Escherichia coli, Proteus,* and *Serratia.* Among gram-positive organisms, staphylococci are the most common.

The radiographic features include localized dense consolidation, which may be lobar or segmental. Cavitation is a frequent feature. Cavities may be solitary, but frequently you can identify many small microabscesses. Patchy multilobar pneumonia may also occur. Effusions if present are typically small, and empyemas are unusual. Occasionally, the chest roentgenogram may be normal, especially in the setting of neutropenia. You can

diagnosis bacterial pneumonia by isolation and culture of these organisms from sputum samples or by observing a clinical response to empirically chosen antibiotics.

Legionnaires' disease bacterium *(Legionella pneumophila)* and Pittsburgh pneumonia agent are causes of acute bronchopneumonia in the immunocompromised host, particularly in renal transplant patients. The clinical and radiographic appearance of *Legionnella pneumophila* in these patients is usually identical to that seen in the normal host. Multilobar consolidation is frequent. However, the Pittsburgh agent *(Legionnella micdadei)* typically produces circumscribed areas of pneumonia creating a nodular appearance on the chest radiograph (Fig. 4-1).

Tuberculosis occurs with increased frequency in certain subgroups of immunosuppressed patients. However, in most reported series of pneumonias the presence of mycobacterial disease in immunocompromised hosts is low. Tuberculosis, when it occurs in this setting, does carry a high fatality rate. The radiologic features of pulmonary tuberculosis are usual and consist of apical and posterior segmental disease in the upper lobes with or without the development of cavitation. In the differential diagnosis you should consider infection with atypical mycobacteria.

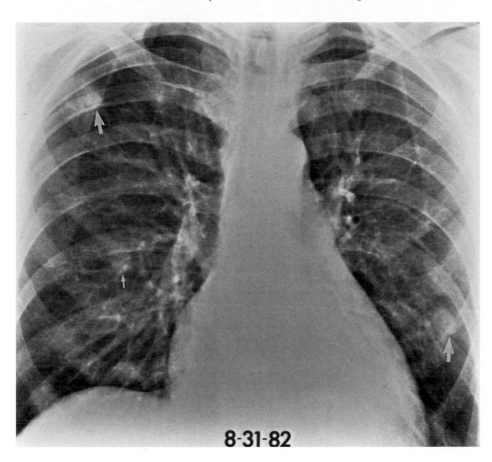

8-31-82

Fig. 4-1. *Legionella micdadei* pneumonia. A PA chest radiograph shows multiple nodules in both lungs *(arrows)*.

Differential Diagnosis There is a limited differential diagnosis of lobar or segmental consolidation in the immunosuppressed patient. Lymphoma involving the lung parenchyma may appear as a localized air space or alveolar consolidation with prominent air bronchograms. This appearance may signal relapse after treatment, and hilar and mediastinal adenopathy may not be present.

Nodules with rapid growth and/or cavitation (fungal pneumonias)

Causes Multiple nodules with rapid growth and/or cavitation is a frequent feature of fungal infection in the compromised host. This group includes pneumonias produced by *Nocardia*, although *Nocardia asteroides* is a higher transitional form of bacterium. The fungi most frequently isolated include the commensals such as *Aspergillus, Candida, Mucor,* and true pathogenetic fungi such as *Cryptococcus*. Fungal pneumonia characteristically develops in patients with hematologic malignancies who are neutropenic from cytotoxic drugs or who are receiving or have just completed a course of broad-spectrum antibiotics for fever of unknown cause.

Aspergillus pneumonia is the most common fungal pulmonary infection in immunosuppressed patients. *Aspergillus* causes an invasive necrotizing pneumonia secondary to invasion of blood vessels with accompanying pulmonary infarction. The roentgenographic features consist of multiple nodular areas of consolidation often abutting the pleural surfaces (Fig. 4-2). These frequently cavitate and may show crescentic radiolucencies around the parenchymal opacities (the "air crescent" sign) that may mimic mycetoma. This sign can also be identified on CT studies (Fig. 4-3). Another characteristic finding is a pulmonary mass surrounded by a zone of lower attenuation with ground-glass opacification (the "halo" sign), probably produced by adjacent hemorrhage. The diagnosis of *Aspergillus* pneumonia usually requires invasive procedures such a needle aspiration or open-lung biopsy.

Pulmonary disease caused by *Mucor* is clinically and radiographically indistinguishable from that caused by *Aspergillus*. It is frequently seen in patients with lymphoproliferative disease, leukopenia, and diabetes, and detected in patients after antibiotic usage. The organism likewise has a predilection for blood-vessel invasion and pulmonary infarction (Fig. 4-4).

Primary candidal pneumonias are rare in immunosuppressed patients; the lung is more likely to be involved during a disseminated fungemia. Invasive biopsy is usually required for diagnosis. The radiologic appearance is nonspecific, and there may be areas of airspace consolidation or nodular opacities.

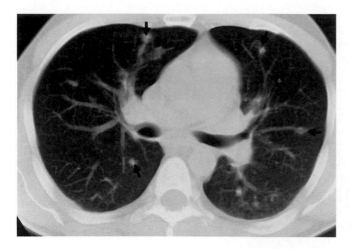

Fig. 4-2. Invasive aspergillosis. There are multiple bilateral nodules *(arrows)*. Blood vessels can be identified leading to the nodules in some instances.

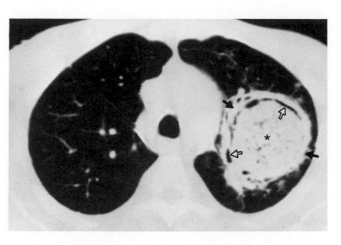

Fig. 4-3. Invasive aspergillosis. CT in an immunocompromised patient. A rim of air in the periphery, that is, an air crescent *(open arrows)* separates the central amorphous infarcted lung *(asterisk)* from the rim of inflamed viable lung *(black arrows)*. This appearance is often seen as the patient's white cell count is recovering.

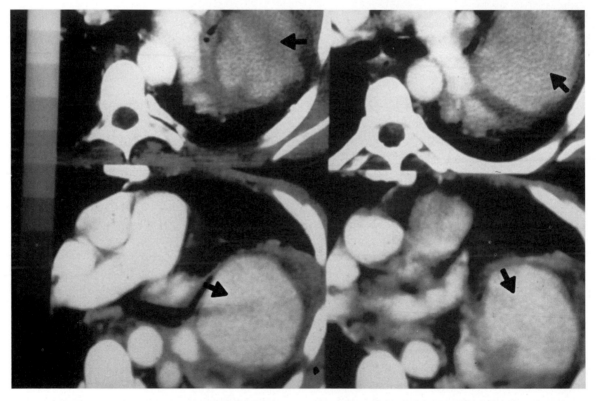

Fig. 4-4. Mucormycosis. Composite of four CT images of an immunocompromised patient who developed mucormycosis and mycotic aneurysm *(arrows)* of the pulmonary artery in the left lung. (From Bhalla M: Cross-sectional imaging of pulmonary vascular and perfusion abnormalities. In Taveras JM, Ferrucci JT, editors: *Radiology: diagnosis-imaging-intervention,* Philadelphia, 1987, JB Lippincott. Courtesy of E.A. Kazerooni.)

Cryptococcal pneumonia, much less common than *Aspergillus* pneumonia, generally occurs in patients with defective cellular immunity rather than in neutropenic hosts. Disseminated disease with central nervous system involvement is the rule, and neurologic symptoms may first call attention to the presence of cryptococcal disease. The radiographic manifestations consist of single or multiple nodules with or without cavitation. Well-defined lobar or segmental consolidation is infrequent. *Cryptococcus* may be isolated from the sputum or more fre-

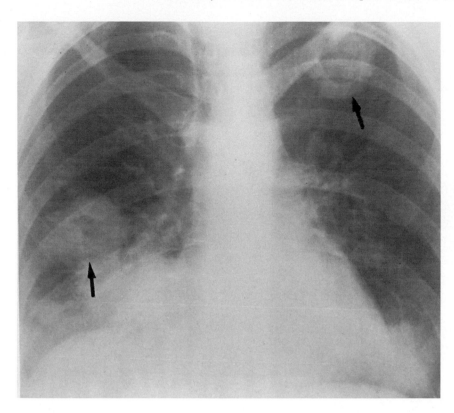

Fig. 4-5. Nocardiosis. Patient on high-dose steroids. There are multiple nodules. Some are cavitated *(arrows)*.

quently from the cerebrospinal fluid on lumbar puncture. In some cases a lung biopsy is required.

Nocardia asteroides is an opportunistic bacterium that causes pneumonia in the compromised host in diseases and conditions in which cellular immunity is depressed. Antecedent corticosteroid therapy is a common history, but white blood cell counts are often normal. *Nocardia* generally does not cause a fulminant, rapidly progressive pulmonary infection. The usual radiologic appearance is that of single or multiple nodules with or without cavitation (Fig. 4-5). They may extend to the pleural surface with associated pleural effusion or chest-wall invasion. The diagnosis can occasionally be made on sputum smears or cultures, but invasive procedures are usually required.

Differential Diagnosis The differential diagnosis of the radiographic appearance of multiple nodules in the immunocompromised host is rather limited. Such an appearance may be produced by metastatic disease or occasionally by lymphoma involving the lung parenchyma. In both instances, rapid growth is usually not a feature. Transplant recipients who receive cyclosporin as a principal immunosuppressive agent may develop an unusual lymphoproliferative disorder in the lung. This usually presents 4 to 6 months after transplantation, although its appearance may be delayed as long as 2 years. The pulmonary manifestations include either a solitary mass or multiple pulmonary nodules often associated with hilar adenopathy. Involvement of multiple organs frequently occurs. The radiographic abnor-

malities often regress after the reduction of immunosuppression.

Diffuse lung disease

Causes A radiologic pattern of diffuse infiltration of the lungs in the immunocompromised host can be produced by a number of microorganisms, the most common of which are the protozoan (now considered a fungus) *Pneumocystis carinii* and a variety of viral agents including *Herpes zoster,* as well as cytomegalovirus. A diffuse interstitial pattern can also be seen as a result of nonspecific interstitial pneumonitis, cytotoxic drug reactions, radiation pneumonitis, or lymphangitic spread of tumor.

Pneumonia caused by *Pneumocystis carinii* currently is the most common cause of diffuse pneumonia among immunocompromised patients. It accounts for approximately 40% of diffuse pneumonias in compromised hosts. Once classified as a protozoan, the organism is now considered to be a fungus. The pneumonia it produces is acute and fulminating. The classic radiographic manifestation is initially a central, bilateral, perihilar, and linear process that progresses over 3 to 5 days to a homogeneous diffuse alveolar consolidation (Fig. 4-6). Hilar adenopathy and pleural effusion are distinctly unusual. Computed tomography (CT), particularly high-resolution CT, may show areas of disease due to *Pneumocystis carinii* pneumonia when the standard chest radiograph is normal. Involved areas of the lung show "ground-glass" opacification without obliteration of normal pulmonary vessels. Because it is not possible

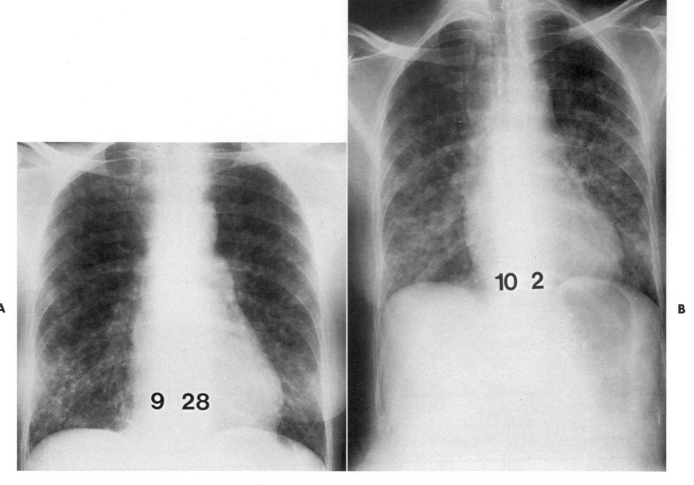

Fig. 4-6. *Pneumocystis carinii* pneumonia in a renal transplant patient. **A,** The original radiograph shows a diffuse reticulonodular pattern more pronounced at the bases. **B,** In 4 days progression has occurred with a more confluent, consolidative pattern.

to culture these organisms, the diagnosis depends on morphologic identification of *Pneumocystis* in respiratory secretions obtained by bronchoalveolar lavage or from lung tissue.

Viral pneumonias generally have not been common in immunocompromised patients. Usually these viral infections are caused by members of the *Herpes* group, either *Herpes zoster* or *Herpes simplex*. However, organ transplant recipients are at high risk for viral pneumonia. By far, the most common agent of viral pneumonia in these patients is cytomegalovirus (CMV). Radiographically, CMV pneumonia is characterized by a symmetric diffuse bilateral linear or nodular pattern (Fig. 4-7). It may begin in the lower lobes peripherally and extend superiorly and centrally. Occasionally, unilateral consolidation or a solitary nodule may be identified. Confirmation of the diagnosis usually requires lung biopsy with identification of characteristic intranuclear inclusion bodies or isolation of virus directly from lung tissue.

Differential Diagnosis The noninfectious etiologies that produce fever and interstitial disease in immunocompromised hosts include lymphangitic spread of tumor, radiation pneumonitis, drug-induced lung toxicity, and the rather ill-defined entity, "nonspecific interstitial pneumonitis."

Diagnostic and therapeutic approach

Two major factors help to narrow the differential diagnosis of fever and new lung disease in the compromised host: (1) the underlying disease process and the risk factors attendant on it and its therapy, and (2) radiographic patterns of the new lung disease. When these considerations are taken into account and a noninvasive workup is carried out, many patients may be successfully managed without an invasive procedure.

Standard chest radiography is the basic imaging technique used to detect and evaluate respiratory disease in the immunocompromised patient. In many instances,

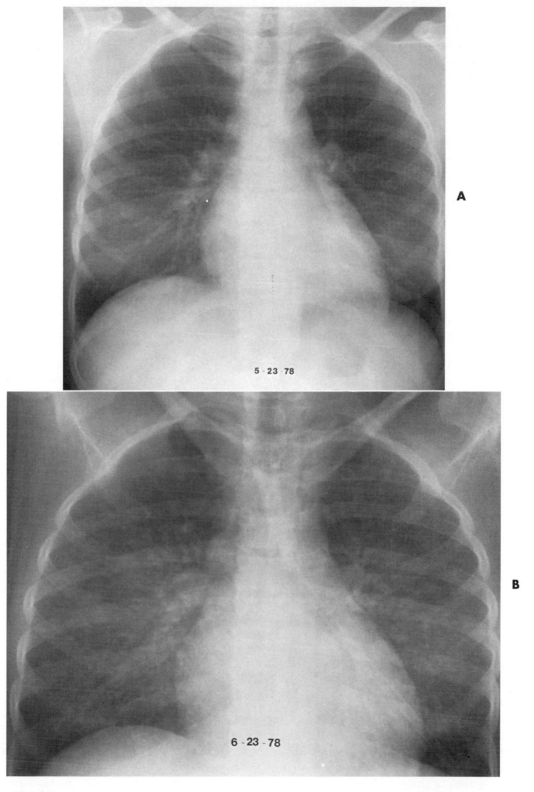

Fig. 4-7. Cytomegalovirus pneumonia. Renal transplant patient. **A,** Baseline radiograph is normal. **B,** PA radiograph one month later demonstrates bilateral reticulonodular opacities in both lungs.

however, CT may provide additional useful information. CT is more sensitive than standard radiography in identifying the number of lesions in the lungs. In the immunocompromised host, focal abscesses may be identified on CT in areas that are difficult to evaluate with plain radiographs; these areas include the apical, retrocardiac, and subdiaphragmatic lung. CT also provides a cross-sectional mapping of the extent of the disease; in the immunocompromised patient with diffuse lung disease, this may be useful, particularly as a guide to transbronchial or open-lung biopsy.

When bacterial infection is clinically suspected, especially if there is a focal area of lobar or segmental consolidation noted on the radiograph, empiric broad-spectrum antibiotic coverage is recommended for the first 48 hours. If after that time there is no response and if the patient's clinical status will permit an invasive procedure, a lung biopsy or lavage is frequently performed. Such a procedure should be carried out even sooner if there are nodules or cavitary lesions likely to be the result of fungal infection. Fungal and peripheral lesions are best approached by percutaneous needle biopsy; larger areas of consolidation by either needle biopsy or transbronchial biopsy with the use of a fiberoptic bronchoscope. You, therefore, perform an important function in the diagnostic approach to focal lesions in the lung either solid or cavitary. For percutaneous biopsy, thin-walled 18–22 gauge needles are preferred. You can perform needle aspiration biopsies either under fluoroscopic or CT guidance. Such procedures, however, are contraindicated in immunocompromised patients with low platelet counts.

Pneumocystis carinii pneumonia is one of the leading diagnostic possibilities when bilateral diffuse disease is present on the chest roentgenogram. An empiric course of trimethoprim sulfamethoxazole can be employed, but often a specific diagnosis is required. Bronchial lavage or, less frequently, transbronchial and video-assisted lung biopsy are the preferred approaches.

PULMONARY DISEASE IN AIDS (TABLE 4-2)

Epidemiology

There are currently over 500,000 cases of AIDS in the United States. Worldwide, by the year 2000 another 30 to 40 million cases are anticipated to develop, and 90% of these will be in developing countries. The Center for Disease Control defines active cases of AIDS by HIV seropositivity plus a number of accompanying conditions including opportunistic infections, HIV encephalopathy, and the "wasting" syndrome. The definition also includes HIV seropositivity plus pulmonary tuberculosis, recurrent bacterial pneumonias, invasive cervical carcinoma, and a CD4 cell count less than 200 mm².

See Table 4-2 for a summary of radiographic patterns in AIDS pulmonary disease.

Pulmonary Diseases

Major categories of disease involving the lungs include infections; neoplastic entities, such as Kaposi's sarcoma and lymphoma; and lymphoproliferative disorders.

Infections

Infections in AIDS are outlined in Box 4-1.

Fungal The most common infection is *Pneumocystis carinii* pneumonia (PCP). This organism is now recognized as a fungus rather than a protozoan. Sixty percent to 85% of HIV-positive patients will develop PCP, and most will have a CD4 count less than 200 mm². The diagnosis can often be made on induced sputum samples or bronchoalveolar lavage. Extrapulmonary dissemination can occur especially in patients maintained on PCP prophylaxis. Radiographic features include most commonly a diffuse reticular or consolidative process, which may be perihilar (Fig. 4-8). The CT appearance as mentioned above usually consists of diffuse ground-glass opacities, which may be identified even when the radiograph is normal (Fig. 4-9). Atypical manifestations include nodules, focal lesions, adenopathy, and miliary disease. Cystic lung disease occurs in at least 10%, and pneumothorax may be a complicating factor (Figs. 4-10 and 4-11).

Other fungal infections are rare and account for less than 5% of pneumonias in HIV-positive patients. They include infections with *Cryptococcus, Candida, Histoplasma, Aspergillus,* and *Coccidioides,* and they often reflect disseminated disease. Radiologic findings are nonspecific, and pleural effusions are common as is adenopathy, which is rare with PCP and bacterial pneumonias. Cryptococcal infection is the fourth most common opportunistic infection and the most common fungal infection, involving 6% to 13% of AIDS patients. Meningoencephalitis is the most common form, and the lungs are the most common site of extra central nervous system (CNS) involvement. Radiologic features include discrete nodules with or without cavitation. Pleural effusions are common, and adenopathy may occur. Histoplasmosis is important in the HIV-positive patient in endemic areas. *Histoplasma* lung disease usually represents a disseminated infection, and the typical radiographic findings are those of a miliary pattern.

Bacterial Bacterial pneumonias occur in 5% to 30% of AIDS patients. Pathogens are of the common types seen in the general population. Community-acquired organisms such as pneumococcus and *H. influenzae,* as well as *Staphylococcus* and gram-negative bacteria, are identified. Two episodes of bacterial pneumonia within a 12-month period in an HIV-positive patient defines the

Box 4-1 Infections in AIDS

PNEUMOCYSTIS CARINII Pneumonia
Characteristics

Fungus
60% to 85% of HIV+
CD4 <200
Incidence decreasing because of prophylaxis

Radiologic Features

Diffuse reticular or consolidative process
"Ground-glass" early on CT
Atypical features
  Nodules
  Adenopathy
  Miliary disease
Cysts

FUNGAL INFECTIONS
Characteristics

Less than 5% of pneumonias
Cryptococcus most common
  Central nervous system involvement

Radiographic Features

Nodules with or without cavitation
Pleural effusions
Adenopathy
Disseminated disease
  "Miliary" pattern, histoplasmosis

BACTERIAL PNEUMONIAS
Characteristics

5% to 30% of AIDS patients
Pneumococcus, *H. influenzae, Staphylococcus,* gram-
  negatives

Radiographic Features

Focal consolidation

MYCOBACTERIAL INFECTIONS
Tuberculosis
Characteristics

10% have CD4 <200 m³
  Occasionally multidrug resistant
  Dissemination common

Radiographic features

CD4 <200 m³
  Adenopathy (CT-enhancing rim)
  Basilar consolidation
CD4 >200 m³
  Pattern of reactivation
  Disseminated—miliary pattern

Mycobacterium avium Complex (MAC)
Characteristics

  Disseminated disease
  Severe immunodeficiency
  5% pulmonary involvement

Radiographic features

  Adenopathy
  Nodules
  Focal consolidation—cavitation

VIRAL PNEUMONIAS
CMV
Characteristics

  Usually not sole pulmonary pathogen

Radiographic findings

  Diffuse reticulonodular opacities
  CT
    "Ground-glass"
    Linear opacities
    Consolidation

Table 4-2 Radiographic Patterns in AIDS Pulmonary Disease

Diffuse Infiltrative Disease		Nodules		Effusion			Adenopathy			Focal or Lobar Consolidation	
Common	Less Common	Common	Less Common	Common	Less Common	Uncommon	Common	Less Common	Uncommon	Common	Uncommon
PCP	Disseminated	KS	KS	Bacterial	PCP		MTb	Fungal	PCP	Bacterial	PCP
LIP	MTb, MAC	Septic	MTb	pneumonia	Viral		KS	MAC	Viral	pneumonia	MAC
KS	Viral	emboli	Lymphoma	MAC	Fungal			Lymphoma	LIP	MTb	
	Disseminated	MTb							(± cavitation)		
	fungal	Fungal							Fungal		
	Strongyloides	Lymphoma							(± cavitation)		

KS, Kaposi's syndrome; *LIP,* lymphocytic interstitial pneumonitis; *MAC, Mycobacterium avium* complex; *MTb, Mycobacterium* tuberculosis; *PCP, Pneumocystis carinii* pneumonia.

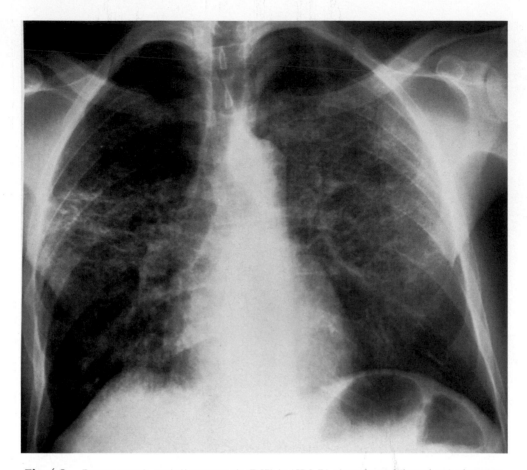

Fig. 4-8. *Pneumocystis carinii* pneumonia (PCP) in AIDS. PA view shows bilateral reticular opacities fanning out from the hila to the periphery.

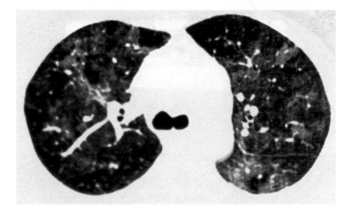

Fig. 4-9. PCP pneumonia in an AIDS patient. There are diffuse patchy ground-glass opacities. Note that the pulmonary vessels can still be identified in the areas of opacification.

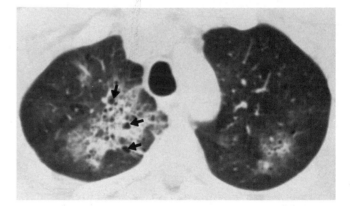

Fig. 4-10. PCP pneumonia. CT of a patient with *Pneumocystis* pneumonia. There are small cysts in the more severely affected right upper lobe *(arrows)*. (Courtesy of Georgann McGuiness, M.D., New York University Medical Center, New York.)

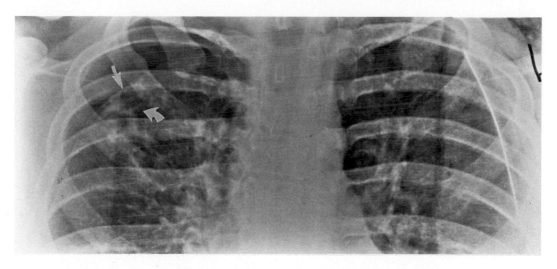

Fig. 4-11. Pneumothorax complicating PCP pneumonia. There is a right apical pneumothorax *(arrow)*. Multiple cysts can be identified in the underlying lung *(curved arrow)*.

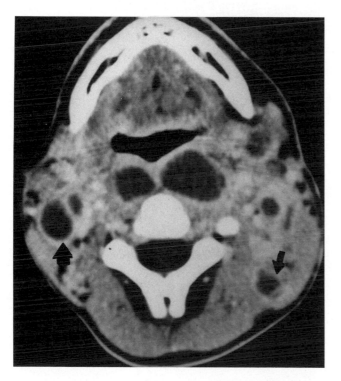

Fig. 4-12. Tuberculous adenopathy in AIDS. Severely immuno-compromised patient (CD4 count = 100). Contrast-enhanced CT of the neck shows multiple enlarged nodes with enhancing rims and necrotic centers *(arrows)*.

presence of AIDS. CD4 counts <200 m³ are associated with a 20% incidence of recurrent pneumonia.

Mycobacterial infections can be seen with either tuberculosis or *Mycobacterium avium-intracellulare* (MAC) organisms. Seventy percent of HIV⁺ patients with tuberculosis (TB) have CD4 counts <200 m³. Drug prophylaxis (INH) is effective in preventing TB in the HIV-positive patient. The radiologic pattern depends on early versus late onset relative to waning immunity. In the late stages of full-blown AIDS, features are similar to primary TB with adenopathy and lower-lobe disease. Miliary dissemination is common. On CT the adenopathy often is characterized by an enhancing rim with a necrotic center (Fig. 4-12). In patients with CD4 counts higher than 200, an upper-lobe distribution similar to classic reactivation TB is frequently identified (Fig. 4-13). MAC is a disseminated disease in AIDS. Only 5% have pulmonary involvement. Radiologic manifestations include adenopathy, nodules, and focal consolidation with cavitation.

Viral Viral infections are a rare cause of significant clinical disease in HIV⁺ patients. Most are due to cytomegalovirus (CMV) and are usually a reactivation of latent infection. CT findings include ground-glass attenuation, dense consolidation, bronchial wall thickening or bronchiectasis, and diffuse linear opacities.

Neoplasm

Neoplasms in AIDS are outlined in Box 4-2.

Kaposi's sarcoma Kaposi's sarcoma is the most common malignancy in AIDS patients. It is much more common in the homosexual population. A third of AIDS patients with Kaposi's sarcoma will have pulmonary involvement, and in 10% to 15% of cases it is clinically apparent. It is almost always associated with mucocutaneous involvement. Radiographic features include two major patterns: (1) perihilar interstitial disease, and (2) multiple nodules (Fig. 4-14). Pleural effusions are common, and adenopathy is a frequent feature. On high-resolution CT (HRCT) the pattern consists of an axial distribution of nodular or more confluent opacities, with thickening of the bronchovascular bundles.

Lymphoma Lymphoma seen in AIDS patients is usually disseminated at the time of diagnosis involving the CNS, liver, or gastrointestinal tract. It is usually extranodal

Text continued on p. 149

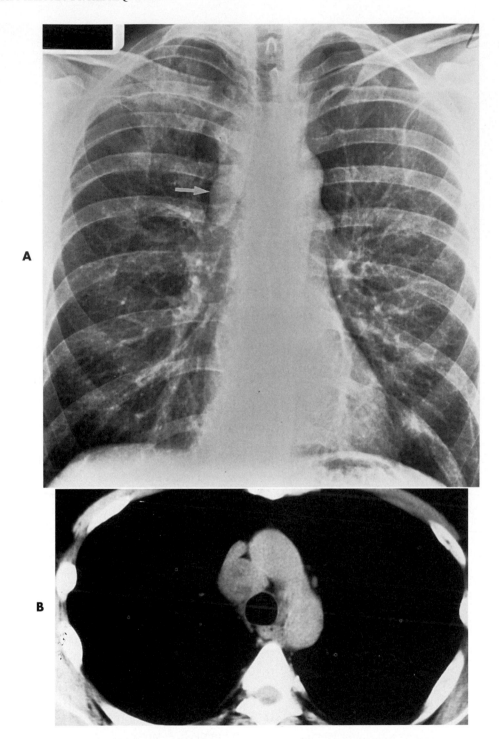

Fig. 4-13.   Tuberculosis in an AIDS patient. **A,** The standard radiograph demonstrates right apical opacity. There is also right paratracheal adenopathy *(arrow)*. **B,** The adenopathy is confirmed on a CT scan. CD4 count was 350.

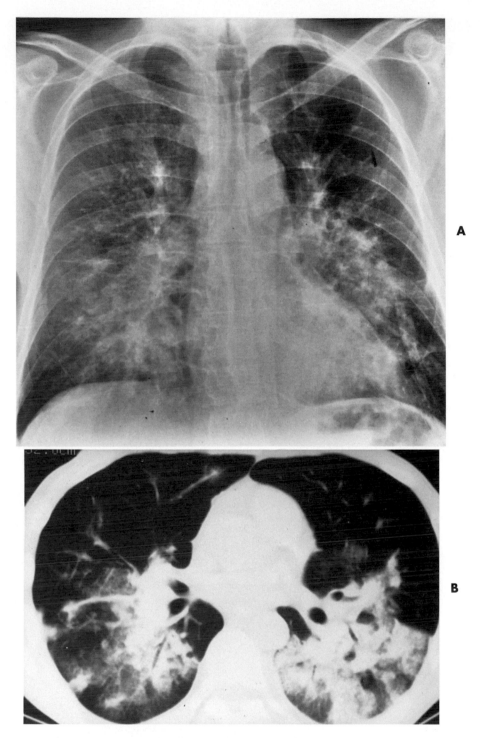

Fig. 4-14.   Kaposi's sarcoma. **A,** Standard PA radiograph demonstrates a diffuse abnormality characterized by central confluent opacities and ill-defined nodules. **B,** CT shows the central distribution of tumor, which is spreading from the hila along the bronchovascular bundles.

Box 4-2 Neoplasms in AIDS

KAPOSI'S SARCOMA
Characteristics

Most common malignancy
Homosexual population
Mucocutaneous involvement

Radiographic Features

Perihilar interstitial disease (CT—axial nodular
    thickening)
Multiple nodules
Pleural effusion

LYMPHOMA
Characteristics

Disseminated disease
Extranodal
B-cell

Radiographic Features

Bilateral diffuse opacities
Discrete nodules
Pleural effusion
Adenopathy less common

Box 4-3 Lymphoproliferative Disorders in AIDS

LYMPHOCYTIC INTERSTITIAL PNEUMONITIS
Characteristics

Diffuse lymphoid hyperplasia in lungs
Children

Radiographic Features

Diffuse small nodules

NONSPECIFIC INTERSTITIAL PNEUMONITIS

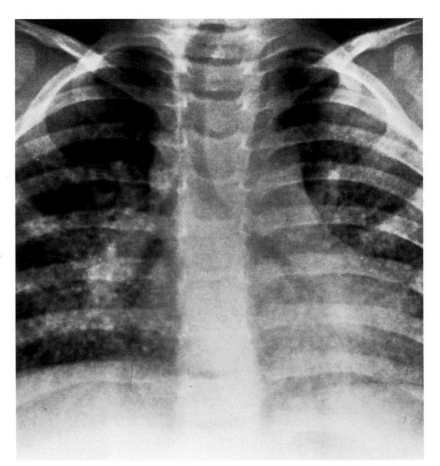

Fig. 4-15. Lymphocytic interstitial pneumonitis in a child with AIDS. There are diffuse small nodules present bilaterally.

in distribution, and 25% of patients have thoracic involvement. The prognosis is extremely poor. It is typically a B-cell lymphoma, associated with Epstein-Barr virus. Radiologically it may present as nonspecific bilateral diffuse opacities, discrete nodules, or pleural effusions. Mediastinal adenopathy may occur, but it is less common than in non-AIDS patients.

Lymphoproliferative disorders

These include lymphocytic interstitial pneumonitis (LIP) or nonspecific interstitial pneumonitis, outlined in Box 4-3.

LIP is a diffuse pulmonary disorder characterized by infiltration of the interstitium by lymphocytes, plasma cells, and histiocytes. It is thought to represent a lymphoid hyperplasia in response to chronic antigenic stimulus by the HIV virus. It is much more common in children. Radiologic findings include a diffuse pattern with nodules of less than 3-mm or a reticulonodular pattern (Fig. 4-15). Less common is patchy airspace disease. LIP is steroid-responsive and not premalignant.

Nonspecific interstitial pneumonitis is a benign, mononuclear-cell, interstitial process with no identifiable pathogens. The diagnosis is made by lung biopsy, and the course is usually benign.

SUGGESTED READINGS

Albelda SM, Talbot GH, Gerson SL et al: Pulmonary cavitation and massive hemoptysis in invasive pulmonary aspergillosis. Influence of bone marrow recovery in patients with acute leukemia, *Am Rev Respir Dis* 131:115-118, 1985.

Bergin CJ, Wirth RL, Berry GJ et al: *Pneumocystis carinii* pneumonia: CT and HRCT observations, *J Comput Assist Tomogr* 14:756-759, 1990.

Castellino RA, Blank RN: Etiologic diagnosis of focal pulmonary infection in immunocompromised patients by fluoroscopically guided percutaneous needle aspiration, *Radiology* 132:563-567, 1979.

Curtis AM, Smith GJW, Ravin CE: Air crescent sign of invasive aspergillosis, *Radiology* 133:17-21, 1979.

Fanta CH, Pennington JE: Fever and new lung infiltrates in the immunocompromised host, *Clin Chest Med* 2:19-25, 1981.

Goodman PC, Broaduss VC, Hopewell PC: Chest radiographic patterns in the acquired immunodeficiency syndrome, *Am Rev Respir Dis* 129:365, 1984.

Kuhlman JE, Kavuru M, Fishman EK et al: *Pneumocystis carinii* pneumonia: spectrum of parenchymal CT findings, *Radiology* 175:711-714, 1990.

Lerner PI: Pneumonia due to *Actinomyces, Propionibacterium* and *Nocardia.* In Pennington JE, ed: *Respiratory infections—diagnosis and management,* ed 3, New York, 1994, Raven Press; pp 615-631.

McGuinness G, Scholes JV, Garay SM et al: Cytomegalovirus pneumonitis: spectrum of parenchymal CT findings with pathologic correlation in 21 AIDS patients, *Radiology* 192:451-459, 1994.

McLoud TC, Naidich DP: Thoracic disease in the immunocompromised patient, *Radiol Clin North Am* 30(3):525-554, 1992.

McLoud TC: Pulmonary infections in the immunocompromised host, *Radiol Clin North Am* 27:1059-1066, 1989.

Ognibene FP, Pass HI, Roth JA et al: Role of imaging and interventional techniques in the diagnosis of respiratory disease in the immunocompromised host, *J Thorac Imaging* 3(2):1 20, 1988.

Patz EF, Goodman PC: Pulmonary cryptococcosis, *J Thorac Imaging* 7(4):51-55, 1992.

Sider L, Gabriel H, Curry DR et al: Pattern recognition of the pulmonary manifestations of AIDS on CT scans, *Radiographics* 13:771-784, 1993.

Singer C, Armstrong D, Rosen RP et al: Diffuse pulmonary infiltrates in immunosuppressed patients: prospective study of 80 cases, *Am J Med* 66:110-114, 1979.

CHAPTER 5

Radiography in the Critical Care Patient

BEATRICE TROTMAN-DICKENSON

The interpretation of the chest radiograph in the intensive care patient is a challenging exercise. A wide-spectrum of pulmonary and pleural abnormalities may occur, and their radiographic appearance is complicated by several coexisting pathologies. Unravelling the various components is hindered by the supine projection of the majority of the radiographs, the variability of serial radiographs due to technique, and the multitude of tubes, lines, and other devices partially obscuring the underlying lungs.

For a safe and logical approach you should first determine the nature and location of all the support devices such as tubes and lines (Table 5-1). Incorrect position-ing is an important cause of morbidity. Then a systematic review of the lungs, pleura, and mediastinum ensures that you make all the important observations. Interpretation may be difficult, because the radiographic features are often nonspecific. It is therefore very important that you have as much clinical information as possible and the aid of prior radiographs. Additional radiographic studies such as decubitus views, ultrasound, or computed tomography will often help you clarify a difficult interpretation or a suspected clinical problem.

SUPPORT DEVICES

Endotracheal Tube

Malposition occurs in about 15% of placements, with emergency intubation having the highest complication rates. Physical examination is an unreliable guide to correct tube location and a chest radiograph is required for confirmation. You can determine correct placement of the endotracheal tube by the location of the tube tip relative to the carina. Ideally the tip should be between 5 to 7 cm of the carina, with the head in the neutral position, that is, inferior border of the mandible projected over the C5 and C6 vertebra. During flexion and extension of the cervical spine the tip of the endotracheal tube may vary by a distance of 2 cm. The endotracheal tube should be at least 3 cm distal to the cords. Too high a location may result in inadvertent extubation or may damage to the vocal cords. Too low a position results in endo-bronchial intubation, right more frequent than left (Fig. 5-1). This may result in overinflation and possibly pneu-mothorax on the intubated side and atelectasis of the opposite lung.

Esophageal intubation may be recognized by the margins of the endotracheal tube lying lateral to the tracheal air column and gaseous gastric distention. A right posterior oblique chest radiograph will displace

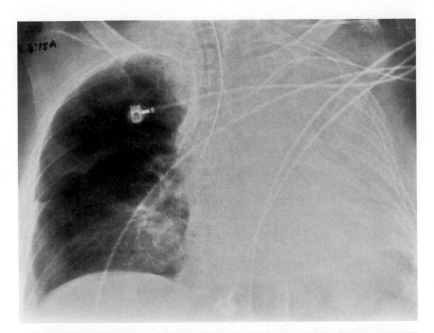

Fig. 5-1. Right main-bronchus intubation. The endotracheal tube lies within the right main bronchus, resulting in complete collapse of the left lung. There is right lower-lobe pneumonia.

Tube/Line	Location
Table 5-1 Correct Positioning for Tubes and Lines	
Endotracheal tube	5–7 cm above carina
Nasogastric tube	Sideholes/tip below left hemidiaphragm in stomach
Central venous pressure catheter	Superior vena cava
Pulmonary artery line	Pulmonary artery within 2 cm of hilum
Intraaortic counterpulsation balloon catheter	Just below superior aortic knob countour
Cardiac pacemaker (right ventricular lead)	PA view—projected over cardiac apex; lateral—lies anterior and inferior (behind sternum)
Automatic implantable cardioverter defibrillation device	Proximal lead—superior vena cava; distal lead—right ventricle; patch—left chest wall or on pericardial surface
Pleural drainage tubes	Midaxillary, 6th-8th interspace directed anterior-superiorly (pnx) directed posterior-inferiorly (effusion)

the trachea to the right of the esophagus and will allow you to recognize the esophageal intubation (Fig. 5-2). The optimal width of the tube should be one half to two thirds the width of the tracheal lumen, and the inflated cuff should not distend the tracheal wall. Following a tracheostomy, the tube tip is ideally situated between one half to two thirds of the distance from the stoma to the carina. The width of the tube should be approximately two thirds the width of the trachea and the tip should not be wedged against the tracheal wall.

Tracheal laceration due to the endotracheal tube may result in pneumomediastinum, pneumothorax, and/or subcutaneous emphysema. The tip of the endotracheal tube may be seen to be deviated to the right of the tracheal lumen. Inflation of the cuff by more than 2.8 cm (normal diameter 2 to 2.5 cm) is suspicious for tracheal laceration as is identification of the lower margin of the cuff at less than 1.3 cm from the tube tip (normal dis-

tance 2.5 cm). Tracheal stenosis may occur at the tracheostomy stoma or at the endotracheal tube tip (Fig. 5-3). At the stoma, stenosis is due to granulation tissue formation or fibrosis with destruction of the tracheal cartilage. At the cuff site, stenosis is secondary to a circumferential scar varying between 1 and 4 cm in length, typically 1.5 cm below the stoma.

Nasogastric Tube and Feeding Tube (Box 5-1)

Incorrect positioning of a nasogastric tube is the most common tube complication (Fig. 5-4). Radiographic confirmation of correct positioning is mandatory before suction or feedings begin. The tube may be seen lodged within the tracheobronchial tree or coiled with the larynx or pharynx. More commonly the tube lies too high in the esophagus above the gastroesophageal junction (Fig. 5-5). On many tubes the side holes extend for a distance of 10 cm from the tip, and therefore at least 10 cm

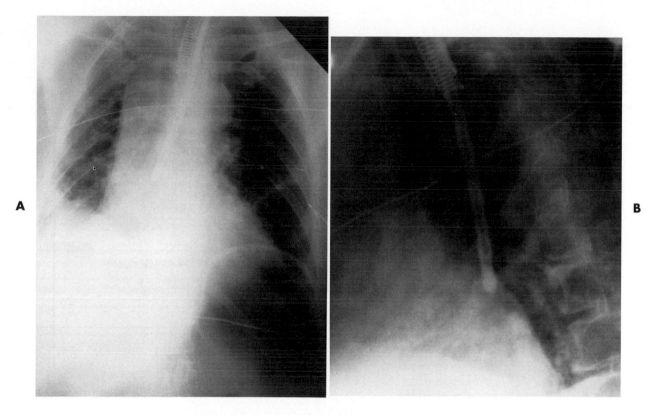

Fig. 5-2.   Endotracheal tube intubation of the esophagus. **A,** AP radiograph reveals an endotracheal tube lying adjacent and parallel with an esophageal stethoscope. There is gross gastric gaseous distension. **B,** An oblique lateral radiograph confirms the esophageal intubation with the endotracheal tube.

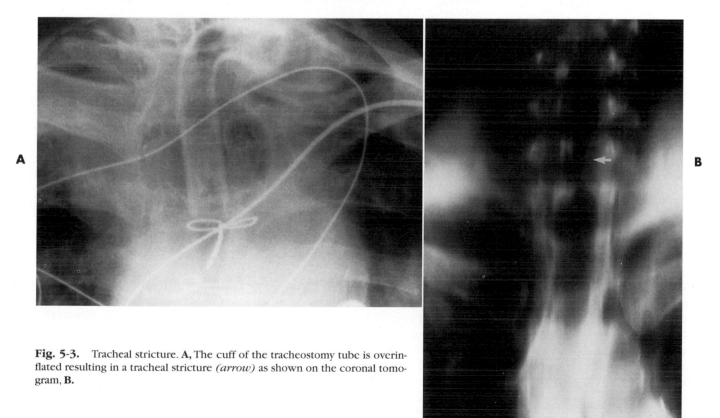

Fig. 5-3.   Tracheal stricture. **A,** The cuff of the tracheostomy tube is overinflated resulting in a tracheal stricture *(arrow)* as shown on the coronal tomogram, **B.**

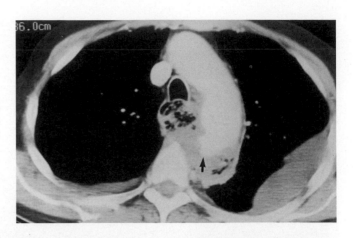

Fig. 5-4. Esophageal perforation due to a nasogastic tube. **A,** Contrast-enhanced CT demonstrates a complex paraesophageal mass containing air and representing a mediastinal abscess. The abscess invades the posterior wall of the aortic arch, resulting in a mycotic aneurysm *(arrow)*. There are bilateral pleural effusions.

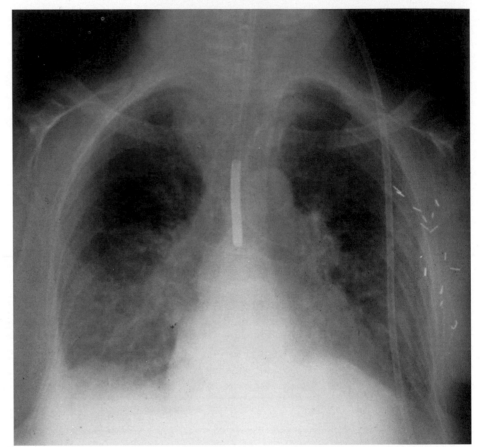

Fig. 5-5. Intrathoracic nasogastric tube. The nasogastric tube lies too proximal, with the tip lying within the midesophagus. There is bilateral lower-lobe consolidation due to an aspiration pneumonia. Left axillary surgery has been performed.

of tubing should be seen within the stomach. Side holes above the gastroesophageal junction predisposes to the risk of aspiration of gastric contents. Feeding tubes should be positioned in the duodenum to reduce the risk of gastroesophageal reflux of feedings and aspiration. The entroflex tube is inserted over a wire; perforation of the esophagus or stomach is a potential hazard. Also the stiff stylet may inadvertently enter the lung and cause a pneumothorax (Fig. 5-6).

Such complications associated with the nasogastric and feeding tube are listed in Box 5-1.

Central Venous Catheter

Central venous catheters are used routinely in the management of critically ill patients for venous access and measurement of intravascular blood volume (central venous pressure). As many as 40% of catheters are malpositioned. The catheters are usually placed either by way of the subclavian or internal jugular vein. The optimal site for the catheter tip is within the superior vena cava, identified on the frontal view as at the level of the first anterior intercostal space. A catheter within the brachiocephalic veins will produce inaccurate CVP mea-

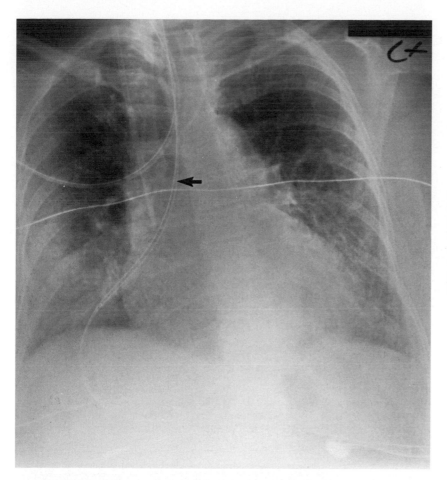

Fig. 5-6. Endobronchial enterflex feeding tube. The guide wire and feeding tube have passed through the right main bronchus *(arrow)* into the lower-lobe bronchus and out through the diaphragmatic pleura. A follow-up radiograph showed a right pneumothorax. A right internal jugular catheter sheath lies with the tip within the SVC.

Box 5-1 Nasogastric and Feeding Tube

COMPLICATIONS

Aspiration pneumonia
Pulmonary abscess
Pneumothorax
Esophageal or gastric perforation

---

surements due to interference by the proximal venous valves, while positioning within the right atrium is associated with an increased risk of cardiac perforation and arrhythmias. A catheter that follows a left anterior paramediastinal course is most likely in a left-sided superior vena cava (Fig. 5-7). This venous anomaly occurs in 0.3% of the population and is usually associated with a right-sided superior vena cava. The left superior vena cava drains into the right atrium by way of the coronary sinus (Fig. 5-8). Catheter placement in an arterial vessel is usually clinically suspected because of the pulsatile flow through the catheter. This may be confirmed on the chest radiograph by the course of the catheter following the major arterial vessels.

Pneumothorax is a common complication of line insertion, occuring in up to 5% of patients, particularly following a subclavian approach. The pneumothorax is often difficult to detect clinically, and a chest radiograph with the patient preferably erect should be obtained after every line insertion. The pneumothorax may be evident immediately, hours or, rarely, days after insertion. Examination of the lung and pleura opposite to the line insertion is important because bilateral punctures may have been attempted.

Inadvertent puncture of the subclavian or carotid artery may result in an extrapleural hematoma, recognized as a small apical opacity or as mediastinal widening due to more extensive bleeding. Rarely, a pseudoaneurysm of these vessels may form (Fig. 5-9).

Ectopic infusion of fluid into the mediastinal or pleural space through inadvertent placement of a line outside of a vein produces a radiograph suggestive of significant intrathoracic bleeding. The diagnosis is suggested by the temporal relationship to the catheter insertion and is confirmed by thoracocentesis.

Catheter fragmentation with subsequent central venous embolization is estimated to occur in 1% of catheter placements (Fig. 5-10). Many cases are unrecognized clinically and may be detected by the astute radiologist. The fragments typically migrate through the central veins and right heart chambers and into the pulmonary artery and its branches. Death, arrythmias, cardiac or ves-

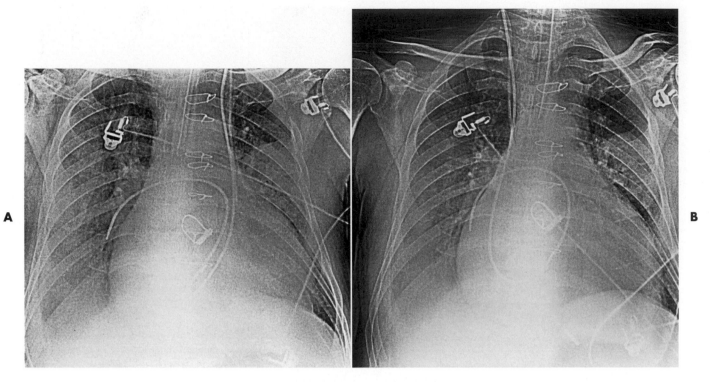

Fig. 5-7. Left-sided superior vena cava with right superior vena cava. **A,** The pulmonary artery catheter has entered a left SVC and passed through the coronary sinus into the right atrium and out into the right pulmonary artery. **B,** In the same patient a right internal jugular approach demonstrated a right SVC. (Digital radiographs.)

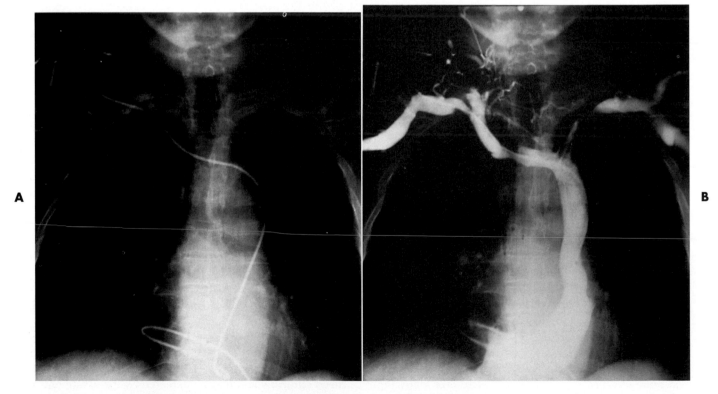

Fig. 5-8. Left-sided superior vena cava with absent right superior vena cava. **A,** PA radiograph reveals a right pacing lead introduced with a right subclavian approach crossing the midline and descending along the left mediastinal border before crossing over to the right at the base of the heart. **B,** Venogram confirms an absent right superior vena cava, with the subclavian veins draining into a left SVC and then into the coronary sinus.

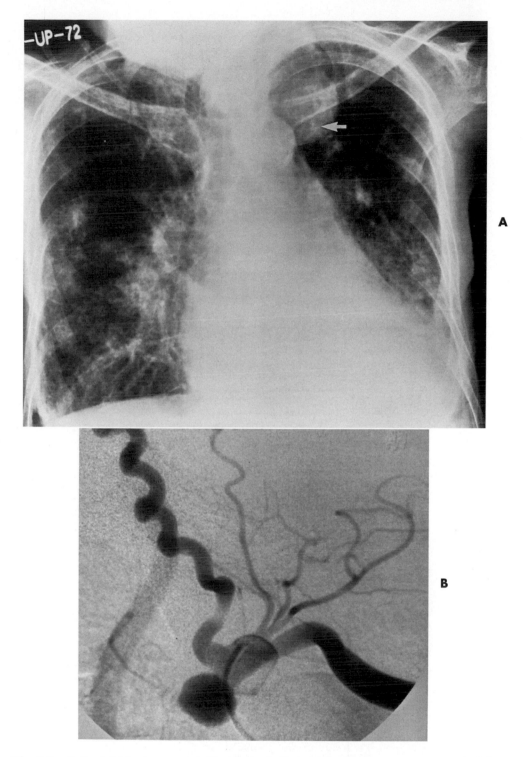

Fig. 5-9.   Left subclavian aneurysm. **A,** PA radiograph shows a large homogenous opacity in the left upper thorax *(arrow)* following attempted central-line placement. The patient has a staphylococcal pneumonia and cardiomegaly. **B,** An angiogram with a selective injection into the origin of the left subclavian artery demonstrates an aneurysm, which was subsequently embolized.

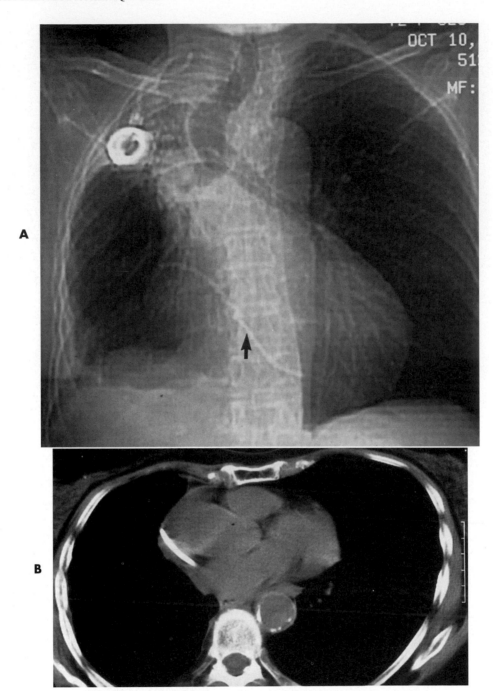

Fig. 5-10.   Intracardiac catheter fragment. **A,** An intravenous port catheter is positioned through the right subclavian vein. The catheter has fractured, and the distal fragment has migrated into the right atrium *(arrow).* **B,** Confirmed on the CT scan. The fragment was removed percutaneously through the right femoral vein with an angiographic snare.

sel perforation, sepsis, mycotic aneurysm, and pulmonary emboli may result. In many cases, percutaneous retrieval devices will successfully remove the fragment.

Complications of line insertion in part reflect the expertise of the operator. For this reason, the femoral vein approach has gained popularity. There is obviously no risk of a pneumothorax, access is direct and therefore technically easier, and the puncture site is readily com-pressible. Bleeding from an inadvertent puncture of the femoral artery is easily controlled. Concern over the potentially increased risk of infection and thrombosis using this approach has proved unwarranted.

Percutaneous intravascular central catheters (PICC) are particularly useful for long-term access. They are of small size (2 to 5F in diameter) and are routinely placed by way of the antecubital veins. Because of their fine cal-

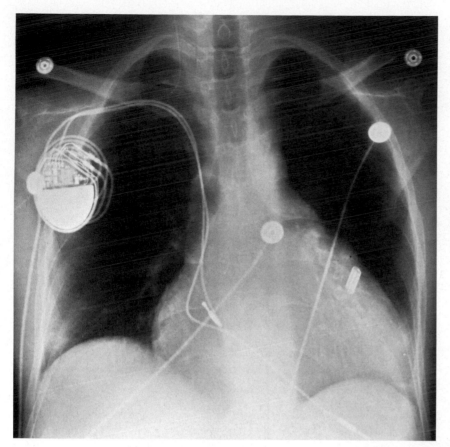

Fig. 5-11. Incorrect position of PICC catheter. The catheter tip lies within the right internal jugular vein. There is a right-sided permanent pacemaker with atrial and ventricular leads.

iber, they may be difficult to visualize radiographically, particularly in the mediastinum. There is obviously no risk of a pneumothorax, and the risk of infection and thrombosis is low. These lines are very flexible and may become displaced; you should therefore regularly review routine radiographs (Fig. 5-11).

Hickman lines are increasingly used in patients following organ transplantation or for prolonged chemotherapy, because of the low incidence of line infections. These catheters are inserted surgically by way of the subclavian vein and are positioned in the distal superior vena cava or proximal right atrium. The catheter may become pinched at the junction of the clavicle and the first rib, resulting in difficult infusions (when the arms are down), thrombosis, or catheter fragmentation.

Complications associated with the central venous catheter are reviewed in Box 5-2.

Pulmonary Artery Catheter

Pulmonary artery catheters are frequently used to monitor the hemodynamic status of critically ill patients to aid in the differentiation of cardiogenic and noncardiogenic pulmonary edema. The complication rate of these catheters is low, but the complications may be fatal. The catheter is typically inserted through the subclavian or internal jugular vein and "floated" distal to the

---

Box 5-2   Central Venous Catheter Complications

TECHNIQUE

Inaccurate readings
Catheter fragmentation

CARDIAC

Arrythmias
Peripheral venous thrombosis
Vascular or cardiac perforation

PLEURAL

Extrapleural hematoma
Pneumothorax
Hemothorax

SEPSIS

Septic emboli
Mycotic aneurysm

---

pulmonic valve to lie within the right or left main pulmonary artery. An inflatable balloon at the catheter tip is used to obtain a pulmonary capillary wedge pressure that reflects left atrial pressure and left-end diastolic volume. Balloon inflation is required only at the time of

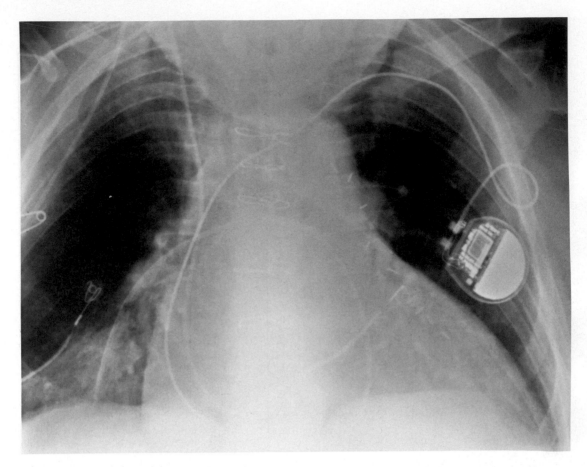

Fig. 5-12. Pulmonary artery catheter-induced hemorrhage. The catheter tip, lying in a segmental basal branch of the pulmonary artery, is too distal. The surrounding air-space opacification represents hemorrhage. There is a permanent left single pacemaker in situ with a single right-ventricular pacing lead.

obtaining measurements and may be radiographically visible as a 1-cm round lucency at the catheter tip. On inflation, the catheter floats distally into a smaller arterial vessel; when the balloon is deflated the tip should lie in the right or left pulmonary artery within 2 cm of the hilum. Coiling or looping of the catheter within the atrium or ventricle may cause arrhythmias, for example, right bundle branch block, complete heart block, and tricuspid valve rupture.

Pulmonary infarction is the most common serious complication; it results from either the too-peripheral location of the catheter or the too-prolonged inflation of the balloon in a major peripheral pulmonary artery. The resultant obstruction to distal flow is due either to the catheter itself or to clot formation on or around the catheter tip. The extent of the infarct is determined by the size and distribution of the occluded vessel. Typically, infarction is recognized as patchy consolidation involving the region of the lung peripheral to the catheter. Management requires removal of the catheter, a frequently sufficient treatment.

Pulmonary hemorrhage, another complication, has a similar radiographic appearance and is more common in patients with pulmonary arterial hypertension and in those receiving anticoagulation (Fig. 5-12). It may be due to pseudoaneurysm formation, a rare but potentially fatal complication resulting from rupture of the pulmonary artery (Fig. 5-13). You should suspect a pseudoaneurysm of the pulmonary artery in any patient with a Swan-Ganz catheter who develops hemoptysis or unexplained cardiorespiratory distress. A contrast-enhanced CT scan will demonstrate the aneurysm often surrounded by air-space opacification due to alveolar hemorrhage. Selected patients may then require angiography and embolization, or a thoracotomy. Other complications include bronchial-arterial fistula and uncontained pulmonary artery rupture.

Intraaortic Counterpulsation Balloon Catheter

The intraaortic counterpulsation balloon catheter (IACB) device is used to improve cardiac function following cardiac surgery or in the treatment of cardiogenic shock. The catheter has a 26- or 28-mm inflatable balloon at its tip. The balloon is inflated during diastole and

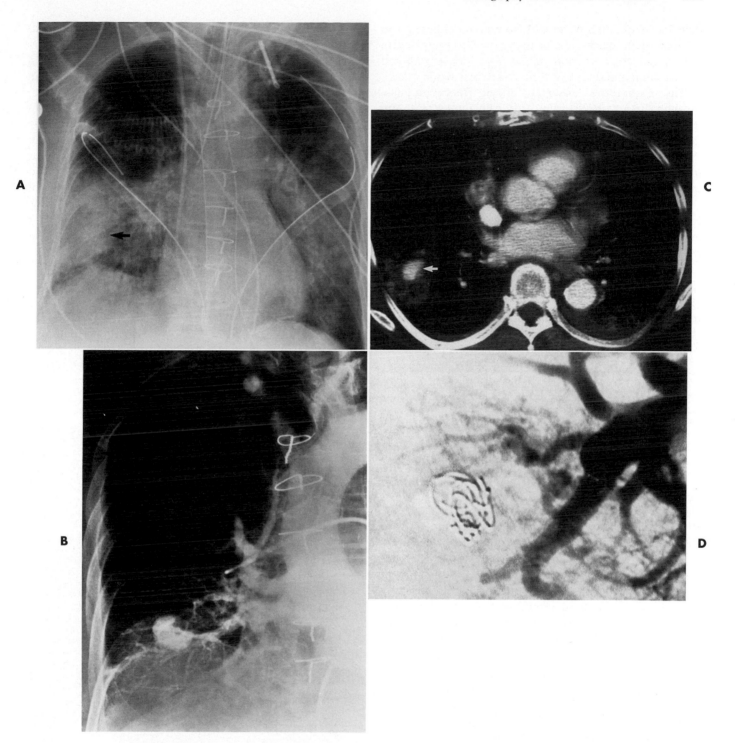

Fig. 5-13. Pulmonary artery aneurysm. **A,** The supine AP radiograph reveals a densely opacified area in the periphery of the right lower lobe *(arrow)* with an absence of air bronchograms. A Swan-Ganz catheter lies in the proximal right pulmonary artery. **B,** Contrast-enhanced CT image at the level of the left atrium demonstrates an aneurysm of a basal segmental branch of the right pulmonary artery *(arrow)* with surrounding hemorrhage. **C,** An angiogram confirmed this finding, and the aneurysm was successfully occluded by embolization with coils. **D,** The aneurysm was attributed to pulmonary artery catheter-induced rupture from too distal intraoperative placement.

deflated in systole in time with an electrocardiogram to coincide with every cycle or every third to fourth cycle the overall effect is increased oxygen delivery to the myocardium and decreased left-ventricular work.

The catheter is inserted either percutaneously through the femoral artery or surgically directly into the thoracic aorta. The tip is usually identified by a small radioopaque rectangular marker and should lie distal to the left subclavian artery just below the superior contour of the aortic knuckle. Even with a correctly positioned catheter the ostia of the mesenteric and renal arteries may be crossed. If the catheter is advanced too far it may obstruct the left subclavian or carotid artery, increasing the risk of cerebral embolism (Fig. 5-14). If the balloon lies too low, counterpulsation is less effective. Aortic dissection is a complication of insertion (Fig. 5-15). Patients with a tortuous aorta or extensive atherosclerotic disease are most at risk. You can suspect the diagnosis by the loss of contour of the descending thoracic aorta on the plain radiograph, and confirm it by aortography or contrast-enhanced CT.

Cardiac Pacemaker and Automatic Implantable Cardioverter Defibrillation Device

Pacemakers are used for a variety of conduction abnormalities. The most commonly used pacemaker has a right ventricular lead. Insertion is by a transvenous approach with the electrode lying along the base of the right ventricle with the tip directed toward the apex. On the frontal radiograph the pacemaker lead is projected to the left of the midline at the ventricular apex. On the lateral view the lead lies anteriorly and inferiorly. A lead directed upward and laterally on the frontal radiograph and posteriorly on the lateral view lies within the coronary sinus. Ideally there should be a slight bend in the lead just proximal to the tip as a result of entrapment within the right ventricular trabeculae.

Fractures of the lead commonly occur at three locations: near the tip, near the pacemaker box, and at the venous access site. Sharp angulation, fixation, or flexion of the lead increases the risk of fracture. Myocardial perforation is uncommon and is recognized by the projection of the electrode tip beyond the cardiac border. The majority of perforations are clinically insignificant, but a pericardial effusion or a tamponade may result.

The automatic implantable cardioverter defibrillator (AICD) is used to prevent sudden death caused by ventricular fibrillation. The system is comprised of a pulse generator and electrodes for both arrhythmia sensing and the delivery of pacing and defibrillator pulses to the myocardium. The AICD may be inserted either through a thoracotomy or with transvenous electrodes inserted through the subclavian or cephalic vein. Two electrodes are required: (1) the proximal lead, positioned in either the brachiocephalic vein or the superior vena cava, and (2) the distal lead, positioned within the right ventricle. The electrodes may be on a single lead or on two separate leads (Fig. 5-16). If transvenous leads alone are insufficient to generate defibrillation, a subcutaneous patch can be inserted surgically along the left lateral chest wall or on the pericardium. Malfunction of the system is tested by routine device interrogation and chest radiography with frontal and lateral views. Fractures or retraction of the leads are uncommon, but the consequences may be fatal. Early detection of dislodgement allows repositioning before the electrode becomes adherent to the venous endothelium or endocardium.

Complications associated with the cardiac pacemaker and the AICD are listed in Box 5-3.

Pleural Drainage Tubes

Pleural drainage tubes are used to evacuate air and or fluid. To relieve a simple pneumothorax, the tube should be positioned near the lung apex and directed anterosuperiorly. To drain pleural fluid, the tube should be posi-

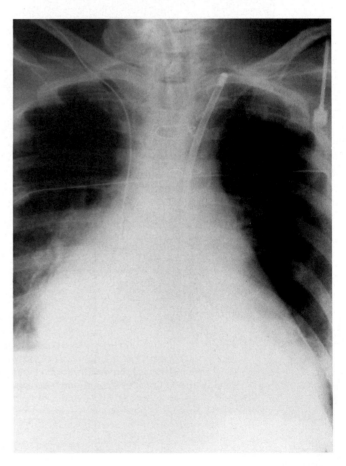

Fig. 5-14. IAB—too high. Catheter tip lies in origin of left carotid artery.

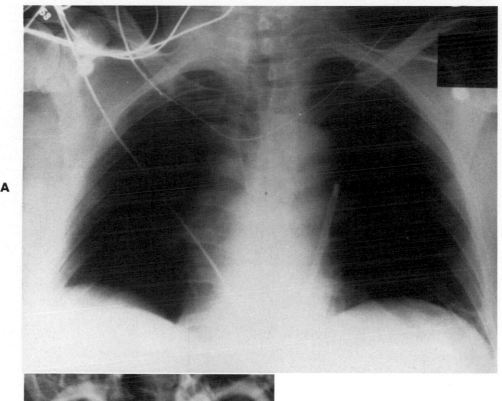

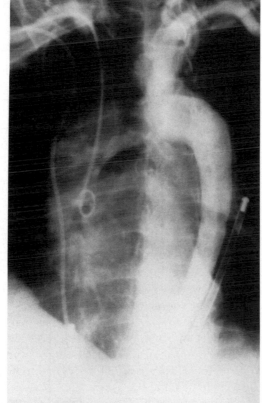

Fig. 5-15. Aortic dissection by an IAB. **A,** The intraaortic ballon catheter has an oblique course with the tip overlying the region of the left pulmonary artery lateral to the aortic contour. **B,** An arch angiogram reveals aortic dissection, with the catheter lying outside the opacified true lumen lying within the nonopacified false lumen of the dissection.

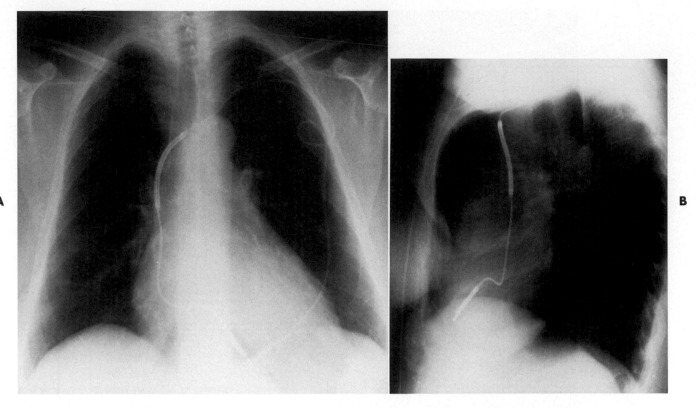

Fig. 5-16.   AICD electrode. PA and lateral radiograph show a single transvenous lead with an electrode at the level of the superior vena cava and another in the right ventricle. In this patient a patch over the left ventricle was not clinically necessary.

Box 5-3   Cardiac Pacemaker and AICD

CARDIAC PACEMAKER
Complications

Fracture of pacing lead
Pneumothorax
Pericardial effusion
Cardiac rupture

AICD
Complications

Fracture of lead
Retraction of lead

AICD, automatic implantable cardioverter defibrillator.

---

tioned posteroinferiorly through the 6th to 8th intercostal spaces in the midaxillary line. Loculated pleural air and fluid collections may require multiple drains positioned under radiologic guidance. Complications of tube drainage include bleeding due to the laceration of an intercostal artery and laceration of the liver, spleen, or stomach due to perforation through the diaphragm. Intraparenchymal placement may lead to hematoma, parenchymal laceration, and bronchopleural fistula.

Malfunction of the tube may occur from incorrect positioning within the extrapleural soft tissues or within the fissures. Failure to drain may be due to blockage of the tube from blood or debris or to adhesions and multiloculation of the collection. Too-rapid reexpansion of the underlying lung may result in unilateral pulmonary edema.

PULMONARY DISEASE

Atelectasis

Atelectasis, a common finding in the critically ill patient, represents areas of nonaerated lung usually due to retained secretions. The extent may vary from linear bands of subsegmental atelectasis to more extensive patchy opacification representing segmental atelectasis to lobar collapse (Table 5-2). You may see air bronchograms, and the appearance is often indistinguishable from pneumonia. The presence of fever is not helpful, because it may be present in both conditions. However, atelectasis is usually basal with a predominance in the left lower lobe particularly following cardiac surgery (Fig. 5-17). Typically, atelectasis appears and resolves more rapidly than pneumonia and is associated with volume loss.

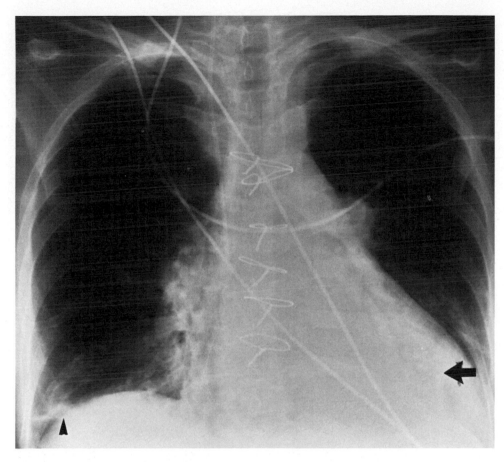

Fig. 5-17.   Atelectasis. PA radiograph in a patient with postoperative coronary artery bypass grafts shows left lower-lobe partial atelectasis *(arrow)* and right basal subsegmental atelectasis *(arrowhead)*. Mild cardiomegaly is noted.

Table 5-2	Atelectasis: distribution versus radiographic appearance
Distribution	**Radiographic appearance**
Subsegmental	Linear, bandlike
Segmental	Focal segmental opacification
Partial	Patchy opacification resembling pneumonia
Lobar	Dense homogenous opacity conforming to lobe with signs of volume loss (see Chapter 1)

Table 5-3	Aspiration versus radiologic outcome
Type	**Radiologic outcome**
Acidic gastric contents	Pulmonary edema
Bland fluids, small volume	Usually normal
Food, oral pathogens	Pneumonia

Aspiration

Aspiration is also a common complication and is often unrecognized clinically. The radiographic appearance is determined by the volume and nature of the aspirate as well as by the position of the patient. Aspiration occurs into the dependent regions of the lung, and with the patient in the supine position this will involve the posterior segments of the upper lobes and the superior and occasionally basal segments of the lower lobes (Fig. 5-18). Three types of aspirate have been described with differing radiologic outcomes (Table 5-3). The aspiration of acidic gastric contents produces a chemical pneumonitis resembling pulmonary edema. The onset of symptoms is rapid within minutes; these are associated with severe bronchospasm and hypotension. Fever and a leucocytosis are common. The chest radiograph shows bilateral perihilar opacification. Clinical and radiographic resolution usually occurs within a couple of days. The aspiration of innocuous fluids such as blood or water is rarely clinically significant unless the fluid volume is large. The radiograph is typically normal, while the aspiration of

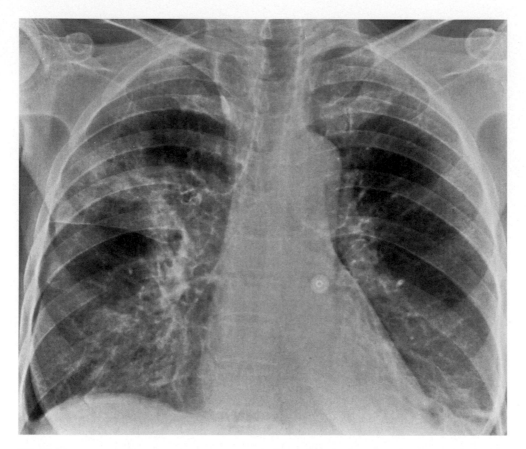

Fig. 5-18. Aspiration pneumonia. PA radiograph shows right upper-lobe and bilateral lower-lobe consolidation representing aspiration into the dependent regions of the lungs.

food or oral pathogens results in an aspiration pneumonia with the typical appearance of persistent air-space opacification in the dependent regions of the lung.

Pneumonia

Pneumonia is an important complication, but it can be difficult to diagnose clinically (Table 5-4). Fever and a leucocytosis may be absent, or the white count may be elevated from a number of other causes. The radiographic appearance may be similar to that of atelectasis, or pulmonary edema. Atypical pulmonary edema due to underlying emphysema or asymmetric clearing is particularily confusing. In the presence of adult respiratory distress syndrome (ARDS), the diffuse air-space opacification of the noncardiogenic edema may mask the appearance of a pneumonia. In addition, the presence of positive sputum cultures may be misleading, merely representing colonization rather than infection.

Nosocomial bacterial pneumonia complicates the clinical course of up to 40% of ventilated patients with a mortality rate as high as 80%. Nosocomial pneumonia is more likely to be complicated by either empyema or a pulmonary abscess than is a community-acquired infection. Colonization of the oropharyngeal and endotra-

Table 5-4   Air-space opacification: radiographic distribution versus etiology

Radiographic distribution	Etiology
Diffuse, symmetrical, perihilar May be dependent	Cardiogenic pulmonary edema
Patchy, asymmetric, peripheral Dependent, air bronchograms	Noncardiogenic pulmonary edema (ARDS)
Patchy, asymmetric, peripheral Nondependent	Bronchopneumonia
Patchy, asymmetric Dependent	Aspiration pneumonia
Peripheral, wedge-shaped, cavitation	Septic infarcts

cheal tube by pathogenic bacteria occurs early, usually within 24 hours of intubation. The reliability of cultures from aspirated or expectorated tracheal secretions is low, and protected brush catheter specimens obtained through a bronchoscope are essential for an accurate diagnosis of a lower respiratory-tract infection.

Septic pulmonary emboli may arise from an infected catheter, an abscess, endocarditis, or pulmonary or urinary tract infection. The classic appearance of septic

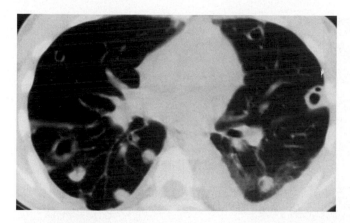

Fig. 5-19. Septic emboli. CT scan through the mid chest shows multiple peripheral rounded pulmonary opacities, some of which are cavitating. This represents pulmonary infarcts in differing stages of evolution.

Table 5-5   Radiographic Features of Cardiac versus Noncardiac Edema

Signs	Cardiac	Renal	ARDS*
Cardiomegaly	Present	Present	Absent
Vascular redistribution	Present	Absent	Absent
Widened vascular pedicle	Present	Present	Absent
Pleural effusions	Present	Present	Absent
Kerley lines	Present	Present	Absent
Peribronchial cuffing	Present	Present	Absent
Air-space opacification	Diffuse perihilar	Central perihilar	Patchy peripheral

infarcts is of peripheral wedge-shaped opacities and nodules with or without cavitation. These may be seen on the plain radiograph but are best demonstrated on computed tomography (Fig. 5-19). Other radiographic features include the presence of bilateral patchy parenchymal opacification, which progresses slowly or more rarely occurs rapidly, mimicking pulmonary edema.

Pulmonary Thromboembolism

The incidence of pulmonary thromboembolism as a complication of hospitalization is reported as occurring in only 0.2% of patients. The true incidence is probably much higher. Many thromboembolic episodes are unrecognized as supported by autopsy studies that report the incidence as ranging from 5% to over 50% of postmortem studies. The plain radiographic features, ventilation perfusion scans, and pulmonary angiography are discussed elsewhere.

Pulmonary Edema

The chest radiograph provides an assessment of the systemic blood volume, pulmonary blood volume, pulmonary vascular flow patterns, and extravascular water. The aim is to differentiate cardiogenic from noncardiogenic pulmonary edema due to fluid overload (renal) or increased permeability edema (ARDS) (Table 5-5). In the critical-care setting this is often difficult.

Serial change in the width of the vascular pedicle (width of the superior mediastinum extending from the right lateral border of the superior vena cava at the point at which it crosses the right main bronchus to the left lateral margin demarcated by the outer border of the left subclavian artery as it arises from the aortic arch) reflects circulating blood volume and provides a useful assessment of the patient's fluid status. In 95% of normal individuals, the vascular pedicle measures between 38 and 58 mm.

Because of the wide normal range, comparison of serial radiographs in an individual patient is more useful than an absolute measurement. However similar radiographic positioning is required, and portable supine radiographs are rarely directly comparable. In fluid overload, the vascular pedicle typically increases in size, while in cardiogenic edema only half the patients will have an abnormally wide vascular pedicle. Patients with permeability pulmonary edema (ARDS) will have a normal or small pedicle.

You can assess central venous pressure by observing the relative width of the azygous vein seen end-on at the right tracheobronchial angle. The azygous vein responds directly to right atrial pressure rather than to changes in circulating blood volume. This vein normally measures less than 1 cm on radiograph taken with the patient erect. Enlargement may be physiological, as with the patient in the supine position and in pregnancy because of increased venous return or pathology such as in congestive cardiac failure.

You can estimate pulmonary blood flow by assessing the caliber of the pulmonary vessels. In congestive cardiac failure the arteries and veins dilate and the nondependent vessels enlarge disproportionally. On the erect radiograph, this is seen as an increased diameter of the upper-zone vessels relative to that of the lower-lobe vessels (cephalization). In the radiograph with the patient supine this gradient will be anteroposterior and cannot be appreciated unless a CT is performed. Arterial enlargement alone can be assessed on the supine radiograph. Normally the size ratio between a pulmonary artery and its accompanying bronchus is 1:1, and an increase in this ratio indicates increased pulmonary flow. This is seen in fluid overload and left-ventricular failure.

The Swan-Ganz catheter provides a reliable physiologic measurement of cardiac function. As the pulmonary capillary wedge pressure increases, transudation of fluid into the interstitium occurs with accumulation of fluid around

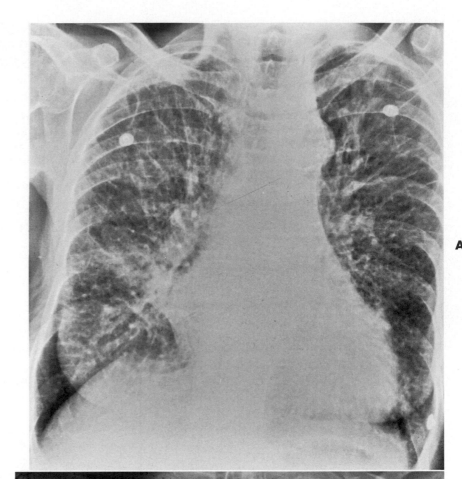

A

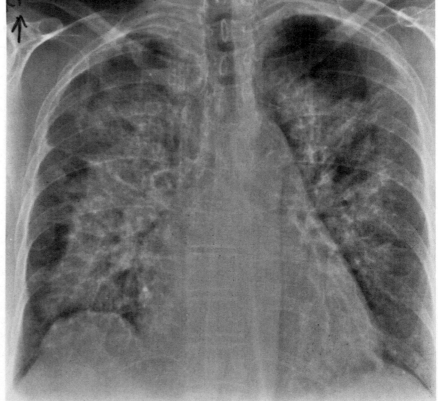

B

Fig. 5-20. Cardiogenic pulmonary edema. **A,** Interstitial pulmonary edema. PA radiograph reveals multiple linear opacities throughout both lungs. These lines are comprised of long septal perihilar opacities (Kerley A) and short peripheral lines (Kerley B). **B,** Alveolar pulmonary edema. PA radiograph demonstrates a "bat's wing" pattern of perihilar consolidation surrounded by a radiolucent peripheral zone of normal lung. Cardiomegaly is noted in both cases.

the pulmonary vessels and bronchi. Radiographically, the vessels appear indistinct as a result of the perivascular cuffing, and the bronchial walls are thickened from peribronchial cuffing. Fluid accumulates within the interlobular septa and is seen as fine linear horizontal opacities extending to the pleural surface (Kerley B lines) or as perihilar linear opacities that are longer and central (Kerley A lines). Further increases in wedge pressure result in alveolar pulmonary edema with a perihilar "bat's wing" distribution to the air-space opacification (Fig. 5-20).

The distribution of the air-space opacification of pulmonary edema is usually symmetrical. Atypical patterns are seen in chronic underlying lung disease, for example, chronic obstructive pulmonary disease where the edema may be patchy or linear and asymmetric. Asymmetric pulmonary edema is usually due to gravity and therefore patient position, but it may occur following aspiration or thoracocentesis. The latter is due to the too-rapid reinflation of a collapsed lung. Pulmonary edema of the remaining lung is a well-recognized complication following pneumonectomy.

The posttherapeutic "lag phase" phenomenon describes the discrepancy between the improving pulmonary capillary wedge pressure and the lack of radiographic resolution. This occurs because although the wedge measurements may have returned to normal, it may still take hours or days for the reabsorption of large amounts of extracellular fluid and therefore clearing of the radiographic abnormality. This phenomenon is frequently seen in patients with left-sided heart failure.

Permeability edema (e.g., ARDS) results from the accumulation of a proteinaceous fluid in the extravascular space due to increased microvascular permeability. The major radiologic feature is patchy peripheral alveolar opacification. Interstitial pulmonary edema does form but is masked by the air-space opacification. The heart size is normal and pleural effusions are usually absent.

Adult Respiratory Distress Syndrome

Adult respiratory distress syndrome (ARDS) is a clinical diagnosis of acute respiratory failure characterized by profound hypoxia associated with a chest radiograph demonstrating widespread pulmonary opacification with air bronchograms. The risk factors for developing ARDS include multiple trauma, fat emboli, sepsis, severe pneumonia, aspiration of gastric contents, and multiple transfusions. Often more than one risk factor is present. The ini-

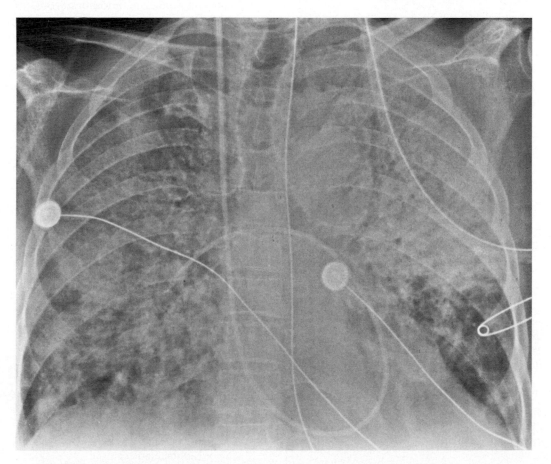

Fig. 5-21.   ARDS. AP radiograph in an elderly woman reveals widespread consolidation with air bronchograms. The heart size is normal. There are no pleural effusions.

tiating event may have occurred hours or days before as with sepsis or fat emboli, or the ARDS may have developed acutely, as following gastric aspiration. The resultant diffuse alveolar damage produces a generalized permeability defect producing noncardiogenic pulmonary edema.

The radiographic appearance is frequently distinguishable from other causes of pulmonary edema. The distribution of the consolidation is more peripheral, and air bronchograms are a prominent feature (Fig. 5-21A). In contrast to cardiogenic, uremic, and hypervolemic edema, the vascular pedicle is not widened and cardiomegaly and upper-lobe vessel diversion is absent. When visualized, the upper-lobe vessels are constricted rather than dilated. Septal lines are usually absent as are pleural effusions. The lung volumes are reduced, although because of mechanical ventilation this may not be apparent. Barotrauma with pneumothorax and pneumatocele formation is a frequent complication due to the reduced lung compliance and the prolonged assisted mechanical ventilation requiring high peak end-expiratory pressure (PEEP). Recovery may be complicated by the development of fibrosis and cystic lung destruction (Fig. 5-21B).

ABNORMAL AIR COLLECTIONS

Subcutaneous Emphysema

Barotrauma from prolonged or high-pressure ventilation may result in subcutaneous emphysema, pulmonary interstitial emphysema (PIE), pneumomediastinum, and recurrent pneuomothoraces (Fig. 5-22). Subcutaneous emphysema confined to the cervical region suggests possible injury to the upper airway or esophagus during intubation. Subcutaneous emphysema along the chest wall should alert the observer to the presence of a pneumothorax, with the lateralization indicated by the distribution of the emphysema. A continuous increase in the volume of subcutaneous air adjacent to a chest tube indicates a malfunctioning tube or improper wound dressing.

Pneumothorax

On a radiograph with the patient erect, the pneumothorax edge is readily identified as an well-defined white line (pleural edge) with an absence of vessels superiorly and laterally. On the radiograph with the patient supine, pleural air preferentially collects anteriorly and surrounds the anterior mediastinal structures (Box 5-4). A suprahilar pneumothorax outlines the superior vena cava and azygos veins on the right and subclavian artery and superior pulmonary veins on the left. An infrahilar pneumothorax produces the deep sulcus sign with sharp delineation of the costophrenic sulcus and adjacent diaphragmatic and cardiac contours (Fig. 5-23). A large supine pneumothorax may result in hyperlucency of the affected hemithorax compared with the opposite lung. Decubitus views with the side of interest uppermost will confirm the diagnosis.

A subpulmonic pneumothorax (Box 5-5) appears as a hyperlucent upper quadrant of the abdomen and visualization of the superior contour of the diaphragm. A deep costophrenic sulcus is also seen. Visualization of both the anterior and posterior diaphragmatic surfaces may be seen and is known as the double diaphragm sign. The central infracardiac aspect of the diaphragm is normally not visible, but it can be seen in pneumomediastinum or pneumoperitoneum. Loculated pneumothoraces can be difficult to identify in the supine patient, and in selected patients a CT scan is indicated for diagnosis and drainage.

Pulmonary Interstitial Emphysema

Pulmonary interstitial emphysema (PIE) represents air dissecting around the pulmonary veins and lymphatics. Air may dissect along the axial interstitium medially, resulting in pneumomediastinum, which is rarely clinically significant, and pneumothorax. Radiographically, PIE (Box 5-6) is recognized as lucent streaks radiating from the hilum in a nonbranching disorganized pattern,

---

Box 5-4 Radiographic Signs of Supine Pneumothorax (Anteromedial)

SUPRAHILAR

Right pneumothorax outlines
    Superior vena cava
    Azygous vein
Left pneumothorax outlines
    Left subclavian artery
    Superior pulmonary veins

INFRAHILAR

Sharp delineation
    Costophrenic "deep sulcus sign"
    Diaphragmatic contour
    Cardiac contour
    Pericardial fat pad

Box 5-5 Radiographic Signs of Subpulmonic Pneumothorax

Hyperlucent upper-abdominal quadrant
Deep costophrenic sulcus (deep sulcus sign)
Sharp diaphragmatic contour
Double diaphragm sign

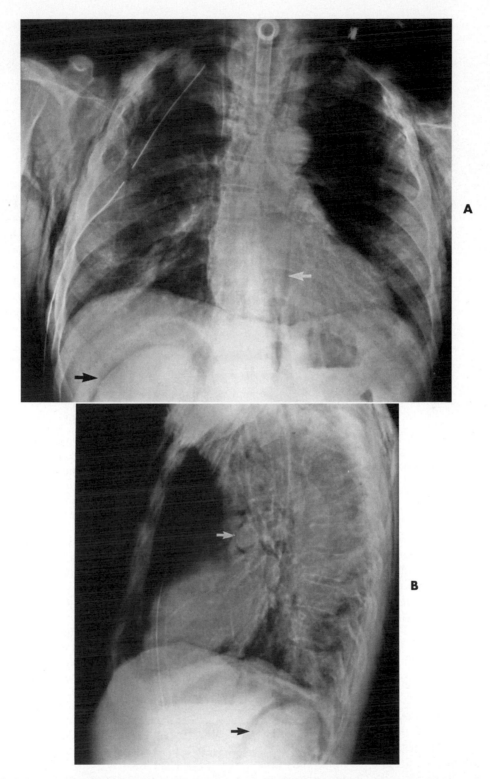

Fig. 5-22. Abnormal air collections. Subcutaneous emphysema with pneumomediastinum and pneumoperitoneum. **A,** AP radiograph in a trauma patient reveals extensive subcutaneous emphysema. Pneumomediastinum outlines the contours of the aorta and pulmonary arteries *(white arrows).* There is pneumoperitoneum with retroperitoneal air outlining the renal contours *(black arrows),* **B.**

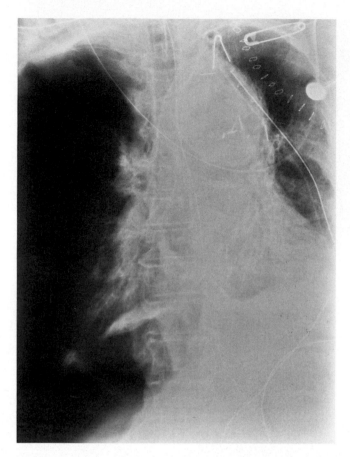

Fig. 5-23. Tension pneumothorax with subpulmonic component. A supine AP radiograph in a ventilated patient following aortic-dissection repair reveals a large right pneumothorax with contralateral mediastinal displacement. There is a subpulmonic distribution to the pneumothorax as shown by a deep sulcus sign.

most readily seen against a background of consolidation, for example, ARDS. Larger radiolucencies seen in a perihilar or subpleural distribution represent air cysts (less than 5 mm) or pneumatoceles. Subpleural cysts predispose to an increased risk of pneumothorax.

Pneumomediastinum

Pneumomediastinum is usually a benign condition but may be the consequence of airway or esophageal rupture. Radiographically pneumomediastinum is seen as air outlining the contours of the mediastinal structures, specifically the medial border of the superior vena cava, the great vessels of the arch, around the pulmonary arteries, and along the thoracic aorta. Pneumothorax and pneumopericardium may be indistinguishable from pneumomediastinum. Decubitus views will differentiate between these air collections, as air in the pleural space will rise to the highest point and air within the pericardium will also change to a nondependent location around the heart while pneumomediastinum remains unaltered in configuration.

Box 5-6 Pulmonary Interstitial Emphysema

Linear and mottled radiolucencies
Air cysts (<5 mm)
Pneumatoceles

PLEURAL FLUID COLLECTIONS

Plain radiographs sometimes supplemented by decubitus views are usually sufficient to document a pleural effusion. Ultrasound is reserved for patients in whom diagnostic uncertainty persists and for guidance of drainage procedures, while CT is particularly valuable in the presence of complex pleural-pulmonary disease. With CT you will frequently be able to distinguish between a pulmonary abscess and an empyema and to delineate the contours of a multiloculated collection (see Chapter 18 on Pleura).

SUGGESTED READINGS

Cascade PN, Kazerooni EA: Aspects of chest imaging in the intensive care unit, *Crit Care Clin* 10:2, 247-263, 1994.

Drucker EA, Brooks R, Sweeney MO et al: Malfunction of implantable cardioverter defibrillators placed by a nonthoracotomy approach: frequency of malfunction and value of chest radiography in determining the cause, *AJR* 165:275-279, 1995.

Fraser RG, Pare JAP, Pare PD: *Pulmonary hypertension and edema. Diagnosis of diseases of the chest,* ed 3, vol 3, Philadelphia, 1991, WB Saunders.

Goodman RG, Kuzo RS (eds): Intensive care radiology (review), *Radiol Clin North Am,* 34(1):1-190, 1996.

Goodman RG, Putman CE (eds): *Critical care imaging,* ed 3, Philadelphia, 1992, WB Saunders.

Lefcoe MS, Fox GA, Leasa DJ et al: Accuracy of portable chest radiography in the critical care setting: diagnosis of pneumonia based on quantitative cultures obtained from protected brush catheter, *Chest* 105:885-887, 1994.

McCarroll KA (ed): Imaging in the intensive care unit, *Crit Care Clin* 10:2, 1994.

Milne ENC, Pistolesi M, Miniati M et al: The radiologic distinction of cardiogenic and noncardiogenic edema, *AJR* 144:879, 1985.

Talgiabue M, Casella TC, Zincone GE et al: CT and chest radiography in the evaluation of adult respiratory distress syndrome, *Acta Radiol* 35:230-234, 1994.

Zarshenas Z, Sparschu RA: Catheter placement and misplacement, *Crit Care Clin* 10(2):416-435, 1994.

Ziter FMH Jr, Westcott JL: Supine subpulmonary pneumothorax, *AJR* 137:699-701, 1981.

CHAPTER 6

Thoracic Trauma

BEATRICE TROTMAN-DICKENSON

Chest injuries are responsible for 25% of all trauma-related deaths. Traditionally these injuries are classified as "blunt trauma" if the chest wall remains intact and "penetrating" if the chest wall is breached. Blunt trauma is more common and is frequently due to motor vehicle accidents. These injuries are related to the deceleration force at impact. In penetrating injury the major risk is to mediastinal vascular structures.

The plain chest radiograph is the initial investigation for all cases of trauma. The aim is to identify life-threatening complications from trauma or from injudicial placement of tubes and lines during resuscitation (Box 6-1). Computed tomography (CT) has an important secondary role. Its primarily use is to clarify an abnormality suspected on the plain radiograph.

INJURIES TO THE CHEST WALL

Rib Fractures

Injuries to the chest wall, rib fractures in particular, are common. The complications of rib fractures (e.g., pneumothorax, splenic rupture) are considered important rather than the injury itself. You will not always detect rib fractures on the initial radiograph because an undisplaced fracture or costovertebral separation is difficult to identify. Multiple rib views are unnecessary because the treatment for clinically suspected rib fractures is the same, whether they are demonstrated radiographically or not. In children, rib fractures are uncommon because of the elasticity of the cartilage. The presence of multiple fractures of varying age with prominent callus suggests the possibility of child abuse. In adults, multiple bilateral healed or healing fractures are often associated with alcoholism.

The site of the rib fractures is an important guide to the direction and severity of the trauma and the nature of possible complications (Table 6-1).

Fractures of the first three ribs indicate relatively severe trauma and may be associated with airway, spinal, or vascular injury (Fig. 6-1). Ninety percent of patients with tracheobronchial injury will have rib fractures at this site. Only 3% to 15% of patients with upper rib fractures will have brachial plexus or vascu-

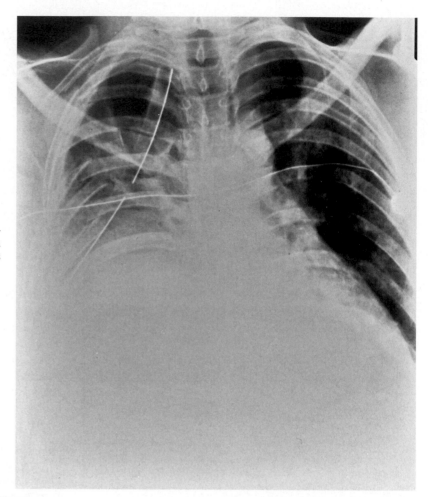

Fig. 6-1 Upper rib fractures. A PA erect chest radiograph reveals multiple right upper rib fractures and a right basal pleural effusion. A right pneumothorax has resolved following tube placement.

Box 6-1 Life-Threatening Injuries

Tracheal rupture
Tension pneumothorax
Hemothorax
Cardiac tamponade
Aortic transection

Table 6-1 Rib Fractures

Location	Associations or Complications
First three pairs	Spinal or vascular injury, tracheobronchial rupture
Last three pairs	Hepatic, splenic, renal injury
Multiple sites	Flail chest
Multiple healed, adult	Alcoholism
Multiple healed, child	Child abuse

lar injury; therefore, you should not perform angiography routinely, but reserve it for selected patients. Fractures of the lower three ribs should raise the suspicion of splenic, hepatic, or renal trauma (Fig. 6-2). These should be further evaluated with abdominal CT (Fig. 6-3).

Several plain chest radiographic findings may indicate splenic trauma. Displacement of the gas-filled fundus of the stomach medially and anteriorly by hematoma and the loss of definition of the left hemidiaphragm indicating diaphragmatic rupture are signs suggesting a probable splenic injury.

Multiple rib fractures involving more than two contiguous ribs at more than one site on each rib constitutes a flail chest (Fig. 6-4). Severe respiratory compromise may develop as a result of the paradoxic movement of the flail segment during respiration.

Extrapleural hematomas frequently accompany rib fractures. On the chest radiograph, the hematoma may appear as a focal lobulated opacity that has a convex margin with the lung. It fails to alter configuration with changes in patient position. Extrapleural hematoma at the apices may be due to hemorrhage from subclavian vessels and on the left side aortic tear from the initial

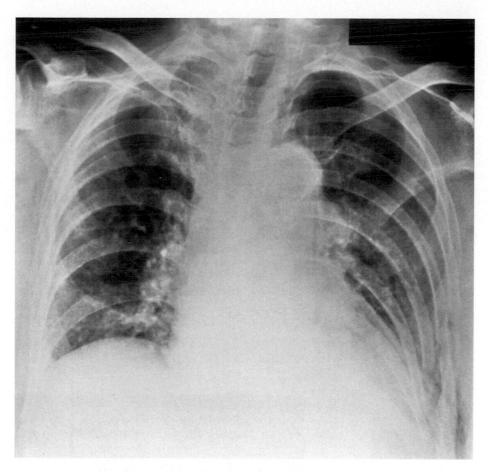

Fig. 6-2   Lower rib fractures. A supine AP radiograph reveals multiple lower-left rib fractures and subcutaneous emphysema along the lower lateral left chest wall. The left hemidiaphragm is not seen because of a pleural effusion and left lower-lobe atelectasis. Evaluation for splenic trauma is mandatory.

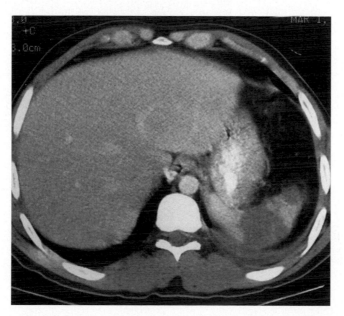

Fig. 6-3   Splenic laceration. Contrast-enhanced CT scan through the upper abdomen shows multiple low-density lesions within the spleen due to the lacerations. There is a small left pleural effusion posteriorly.

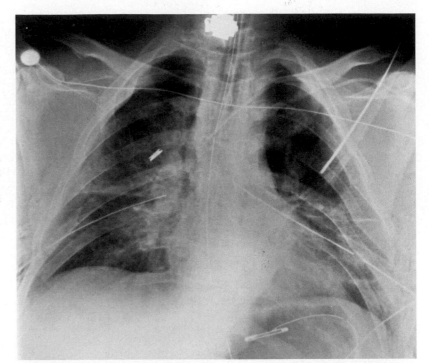

Fig. 6-4   Flail chest. Supine AP radiograph reveals multiple left-rib fractures with fractures occurring at more than one point on several contiguous ribs. There is a small right pneumothorax and widespread pulmonary contusion.

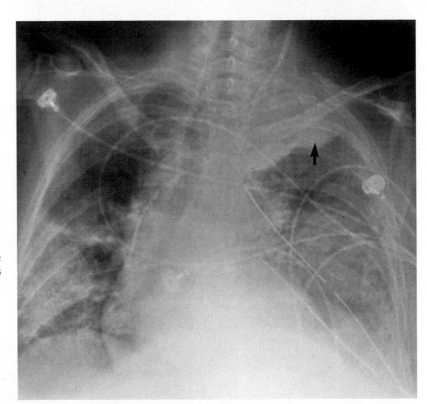

Fig. 6-5   Left extrapleural hematoma (*arrow*). Due to an internal jugular central-line placement. There is extensive pulmonary opacification due to contusion.

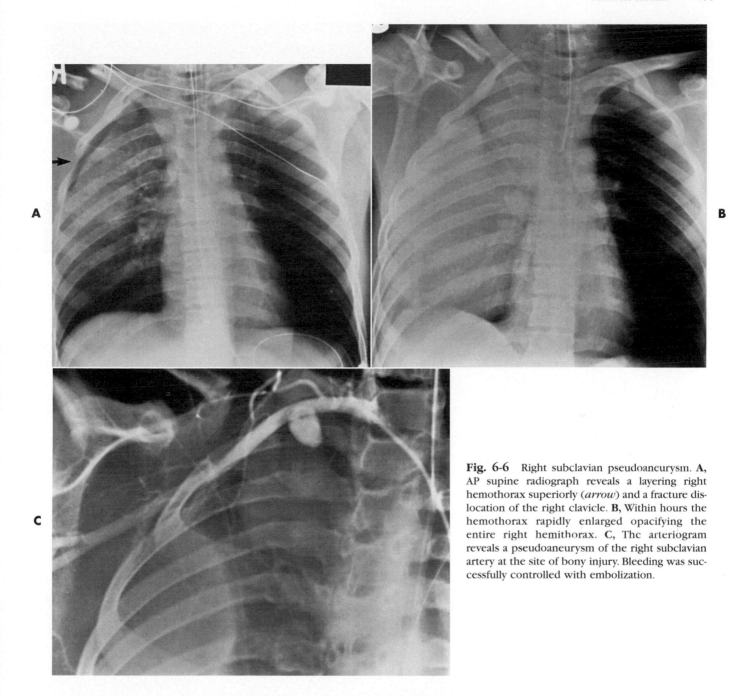

Fig. 6-6   Right subclavian pseudoaneurysm. **A,** AP supine radiograph reveals a layering right hemothorax superiorly (*arrow*) and a fracture dislocation of the right clavicle. **B,** Within hours the hemothorax rapidly enlarged opacifying the entire right hemithorax. **C,** The arteriogram reveals a pseudoaneurysm of the right subclavian artery at the site of bony injury. Bleeding was successfully controlled with embolization.

trauma or bleeding secondary to central line placement (Fig. 6-5). Hemorrhage from intercostal vessels may result in a rapidly developing hemothorax and exsanguination. Angiography and treatment with embolization is life saving (Fig. 6-6).

Sternal Fractures

Sternal fractures occur in less than 10% of major thoracic trauma patients. Sternal injury may be associated with trauma to the mediastinal vascular structures or myocardial contusion. The diagnosis is most easily identified on the lateral radiograph (Fig. 6-7). Sternoclavicular

dislocations are difficult to identify on the plain radiograph, but CT more readily demonstrates them. The majority are due to an anterior dislocation and are of little clinical significance. Posterior dislocation is more serious because of injury to the adjacent mediastinal vessels, trachea, and esophagus.

Spinal Injury

Spinal injury is frequent in high-velocity trauma. Up to 30% of patients with significant thoracic injuries will have spinal trauma. Over 60% of fracture dislocations in the thoracic spine are associated with complete neuro-

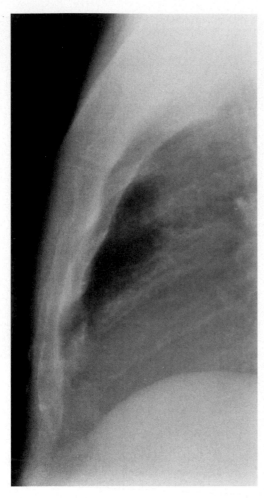

Fig. 6-7 Sternal fracture. A lateral chest radiograph reveals a fracture with deformity of the sternum distal to the manubrial-sternal junction.

Fig. 6-8 Spinal fracture. CT scan (bone windows) reveals an unsuspected oblique fracture through the transverse process of the thoracic vertebra and a fracture through the adjacent left posterior rib. A small right pleural effusion is seen.

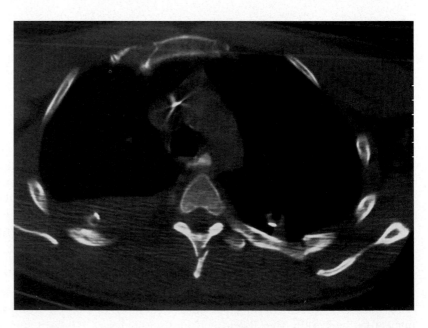

logic defects, compared with 32% in the cervical spine and 2% in the lumbar spine (Box 6-2). Early identification of the bony abnormality may prevent irreversible and potentially devastating cord injury. You should obtain penetrated views on the frontal radiograph and cross-table lateral radiographs in all patients with severe trauma. Selected patients may require a CT or MRI (Fig. 6-8). The majority of fracture dislocations will be at the thoracolumbar junction. Multiple fractures are found in 10% of patients. Eighty percent of these injuries will be non-contiguous. The radiologic features include abnormal vertebral shape, location, size, and density. The "rule of two's" applies (Box 6-3).

INJURY TO THE TRACHEA AND MAJOR AIRWAYS

Tracheobronchial Rupture

Tracheobronchial rupture (TBR) is associated with a high incidence of injury to the upper bony thorax. The tear may be partial or complete. The diagnosis is frequently delayed, resulting in tracheal or bronchial stenosis from partial healing. The early diagnostic features include persistent severe pneumomediastinum, subcutaneous emphysema, and pneumothorax (Box 6-4). Unusual signs of rupture include the "fallen lung" sign, "bayonet deformity" of the trachea, and ectopic endotracheal-tube or balloon-cuff position.

Bronchial Rupture

Bronchial rupture occurs within 2.5 cm of the carina in 80% of patients. Right-sided rupture is more common than left sided, and the majority of patients will develop a pneumothorax. Pneumomediastinum, however, may be the only finding, particularly with injury to the left main bronchus, which has a longer mediastinal (extrapleural) course. Following partial bronchial rupture, a pneumothorax develops that is usually large and fails to resolve, despite tube drainage, implying a persistent air leak. The fallen lung sign occurs with complete disruption of the main stem bronchus (Fig. 6-9). The lung falls inferiorly and laterally to the base of the hemithorax in contrast to a pneumothorax from a partial bronchial tear, where the lung collapses medially and centrally. As with partial rupture the lung fails to reexpand on tube drainage.

Box 6-4 Rupture of Trachea/Major Bronchus
Pneumomediastinum Persistent pneumothorax despite drainage Fallen lung

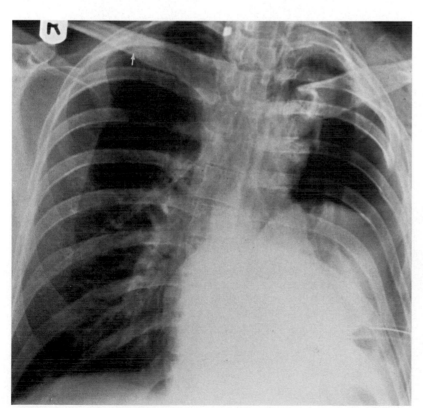

Fig. 6-9 Fallen lung—rupture of the left main bronchus. Erect AP radiograph reveals a large left pneumothorax persisting despite tube drainage. There is a small right apical pneumothorax (*arrow*) and subcutaneous emphysema in the left chest wall. There are multiple left rib fractures and left sternoclavicular dislocation.

ESOPHAGEAL RUPTURE

Esophageal disruption is uncommon following blunt trauma; iatrogenic causes such as endoscopic dilation of a stricture are more likely. Severe pneumomediastinum is a manifestation of rupture. Other findings include pneumothorax, left pleural effusion, and mediastinal widening due to hemorrhage or mediastinitis. Leakage of oral contrast detected by a contrast swallow or by thoracic CT confirms the diagnosis.

PLEURAL ABNORMALITY

Pneumothorax

A pneumothorax occurs twice as often in patients with blunt trauma than in those with a penetrating injury. The identification of even a small pneumothorax is important because a rapid increase in size of the pneumothorax may occur in mechanically ventilated patients with disastrous results. Because most chest radiographs are performed with the patient in the supine position, it may be difficult to recognize even a large pneumothorax. Air collects in the most nondependent regions; therefore, in the supine position air collects in an anterior and often inferior location (Box 6-5; Fig. 6-10). Recognition of a pneumothorax on an erect radiograph is much easier (Fig. 6-11). The identification of a pleural edge with absence of lung vessels laterally is diagnostic. A tension pneumothorax is a medical emergency (Box 6-6; Fig. 6-12). Pneumothoraces are frequently associated with severe extrathoracic trauma. A

Box 6-5   Identifying Pneumothorax: Helpful Radiographic Features (Supine)

Deep sulcus sign
Hyperlucency of hemithorax
Double diaphragmatic contour
Sharp mediastinal and cardiac contours (e.g., right cardiophrenic region and cardiac apex)

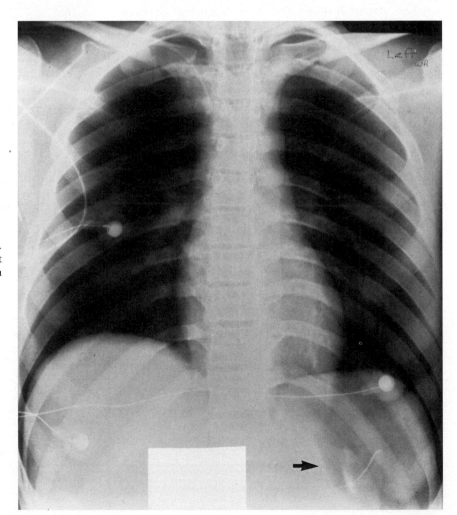

Fig. 6-10   Pneumothorax—supine radiograph. AP radiograph in a ventilated patient with right central line illustrates the deep sulcus sign (*arrow*) of a supine left pneumothorax.

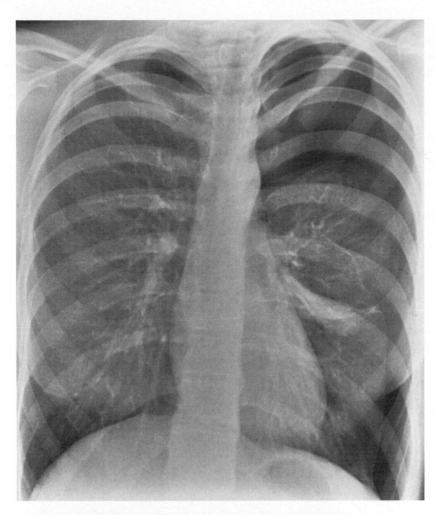

Fig. 6-11 Pneumothorax—erect radiograph. PA radiograph demonstrates a large left pneumothorax.

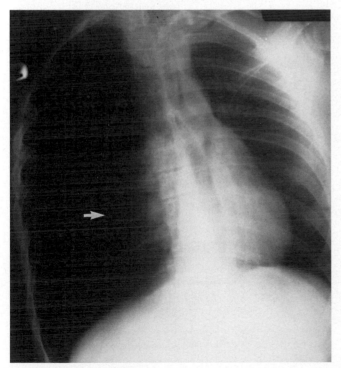

Fig. 6-12 Tension pneumothorax. PA radiograph reveals a large right pneumothorax (*arrow* marks pleural edge) with flattening of the right hemidiaphragm and contralateral mediastinal displacement.

recent study demonstrated a pneumothorax in 52% of patients with closed head injury. You should always review the lung bases on abdominal CT scans because you will often identify an unsuspected pneumothorax.

Pneumomediastinum

Pneumomediastinum is a frequent finding following blunt trauma. The most common cause is disruption of the lung parenchyma and interstitial dissection of air due to sudden chest compression followed by reexpansion. It is often associated with a pneumothorax. It may be seen in association with TBR, although TBR accounts for less than 1.5% of cases. Radiographically, you see a thin radioopaque line parallel with the mediastinal contour and extending to the midhemidiaphragm (Fig. 6-13). The line represents visualization of the parietal pleura as a

result of the adjacent air lucency. Pneumomediastinum is most clearly seen on the left, creating a sharply defined aortic contour that can often be followed into the abdomen, along with a continuous diaphragm sign seen underlying the cardiac contour. The air may dissect superiorly into the neck through the fascial planes, inferiorly into the retroperitoneum, and around the intraperitoneal structures or subcutaneously (Fig. 6-14). Pneumomediastinum alone is rarely clinically significant, although it may be exacerbated by positive pressure ventilation.

Pleural Effusions

Following trauma the majority of pleural collections are due to hemorrhage. Surgery is required in less than 10% of cases of hemothorax. The principle indication is bleeding at a rate of greater than 200 ml/hour or an effusion of greater than 1 liter at presentation. A rapidly expanding pleural effusion is most likely arterial in origin and may be life-threatening. The cause is usually due to laceration of intercostal arteries or to internal mammary or large mediastinal vessels. Bleeding from a systemic vessel results in a continually expanding hemothorax despite the quantity of blood already present. The admission radiograph may show complete opacification of the hemithorax with contralateral mediastinal displacement

---

Box 6-6 Signs of Tension Pneumothorax
Flattening of ipsilateral hemidiaphragm
Spreading of the ipsilateral ribs
Contralateral mediastinal displacement

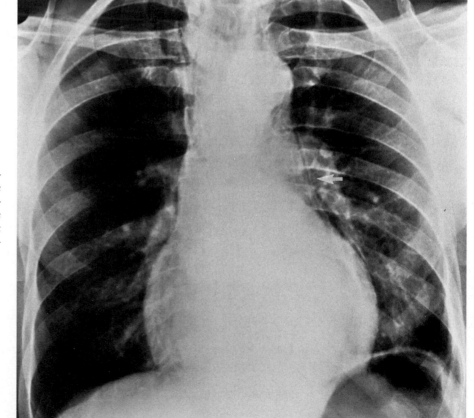

Fig. 6-13 Pneumomediastinum. PA radiograph reveals a thin radioopaque line (*arrow*), which parallels the left mediastinal border extending from the level of the aortic knob around the superior cardiac border. There is a small right apical pneumothorax.

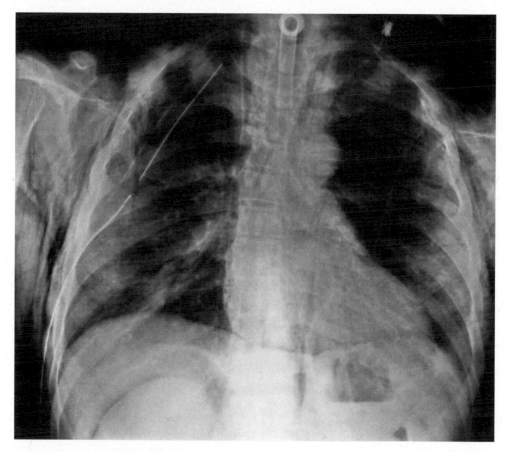

Fig. 6-14 Pneumomediastinum and pneumoperitoneum. AP radiograph in a ventilated patient demonstrates extensive subcutaneous emphysema. The pneumomediastinum outlines the descending thoracic aorta and extends through the aortic hiatus into the abdomen. Retroperitoneal air outlines the kidneys. The right pneumothorax has resolved on drainage.

due to the large volume of hemorrhage (Fig. 6-6). Venous hemorrhage is usually self-limiting as the expanding hemothorax compresses the underlying lung causing pulmonary tamponade and therefore hemostasis. The hemothorax is visualized as opacification of the pleural space to varying degrees with a well-defined meniscus (Box 6-7). A hemothorax may result from laceration of the pleura by fractured ribs (occurring with or without a pneumothorax) or from closed-chest trauma without evidence of rib fractures. Hemothorax from aortic rupture is common and invariably left-sided; it should not be erroneously attributed to left-sided rib fractures. A left-sided pleural effusion or hydropneumothorax frequently develops following rupture of the esophagus. Identification of ingested material within the pleural fluid is diagnostic.

On the erect radiograph, an uncomplicated pleural effusion demonstrates a well-defined superior border, convex downward with widening of the lateral pleural stripe and blunting of the costophrenic sulcus. On the supine radiograph, the pleural effusion layers in the dependent part of the pleural space, resulting in uniform opacification of the hemithorax. This is most easily recognized with unilateral collections.

Subpulmonic effusions may collect in the erect patient with elevation and flattening of the hemidiaphragm. The diaphragmatic contour loses the usual midpoint peak, which is displaced laterally. Fluid may collect in the mediastinal pleura, causing a paraspinal opacity or may track into the fissure.

The presence of air within the effusion may result from a traumatic pneumothorax or a bronchopleural fistula.

Loculated Pleural Collections

Loculated pleural collections may be subtle and, when bilateral, difficult to identify in the supine patient. CT or ultrasound, which can be performed at the bedside, will confirm the clinical suspicion and permit accurate tube placement.

Rupture of the Thoracic Duct

Rupture of the thoracic duct is rare and is usually the result of a penetrating injury. Treatment is surgical liga-

Box 6-7   Differentiation of Pleural Effusions
Rapid onset, minutes, life-threatening—Arterial injury Slowly progressive, hours, self-limiting—Venous injury Chylous, several days, chronic—Thoracic duct injury

tion of the duct. The chylous effusion typically develops over several days and may become very large. The chylous nature of the fluid may not be readily appreciated in the fasting patient or when the fluid is blood-stained; in these instances, a high degree of suspicion is required to make the diagnosis.

PULMONARY PARENCHYMAL INJURY

Pulmonary parenchymal injury may be widespread and bilateral. It is usually most severe at the sites of skeletal injury. In most patients the pulmonary injury resolves without complication. Its presence alone is not an indication for thoracic CT.

Contusion

Contusion (hemorrhage) is the most frequent complication and is usually radiographically evident within 6 hours of trauma. Initial clearing is rapid and may be complete within 24 to 48 hours, but more typically it resolves over 72 hours. Radiographically, contusions appear as nonsegmental homogenous opacities, which are frequently peripheral in location (Fig. 6-15). They may or may not be associated with fractures. The contusions may be multifocal, solitary, unilateral, or bilateral. Air bronchograms are an atypical finding because the bronchi are filled with blood. Air-space opacification that is slow to resolve or increases in extent suggests an additional complication such as infection, pulmonary edema, or adult respiratory distress syndrome (ARDS).

Laceration

More severe trauma causes disruption of the parenchyma, which results in laceration. Pulmonary lacerations are a frequent accompaniment to contusion and may initially be masked by the surrounding hemorrhage. Radiographically an ovoid radiolucency with a surrounding pseudomembrane is seen forming a pneumatocele (Fig. 6-16A). This appearance is most easily recognized on CT. Hemorrhage into the cavity produces a hematoma, which may be associated with an air-crescent sign around the blood clot (Fig. 6-16B) or an air/fluid level (Fig. 6-17). Pneumatoceles are usually small, less than 5 mm, but lesions greater than 10 mm may occur. Typically, lacerations resolve slowly over weeks but the hematoma may produce a solitary nodule or mass that persists for months. In the absence of the salient history, the latter may be mistaken for a carcinoma (Fig. 6-18). Other complications of laceration include bronchopleural fistula and infection, which may require surgical intervention.

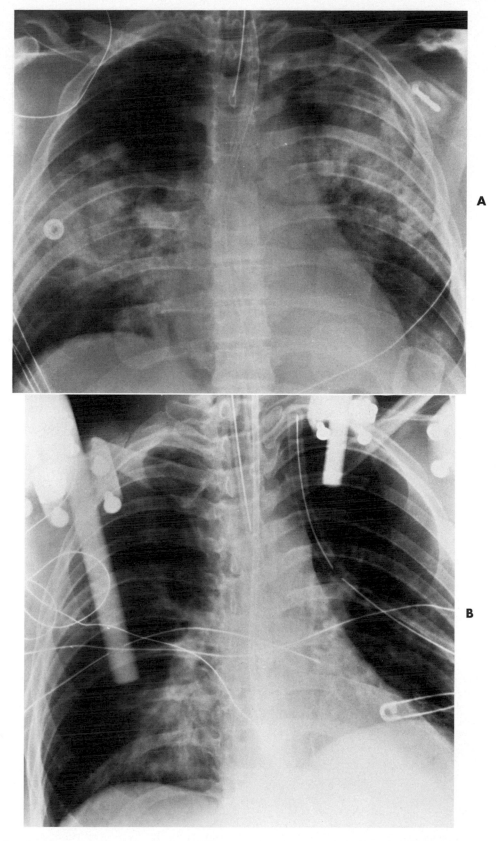

Fig. 6-15 Pulmonary contusion. **A,** Admission radiograph reveals extensive bilateral air-space opacification and a fracture dislocation of the right clavicle. **B,** Six days later there has been significant clearing of the pulmonary contusion with persistent right lower-lobe opacification due to atelectasis. There has been interval placement of a left-chest tube.

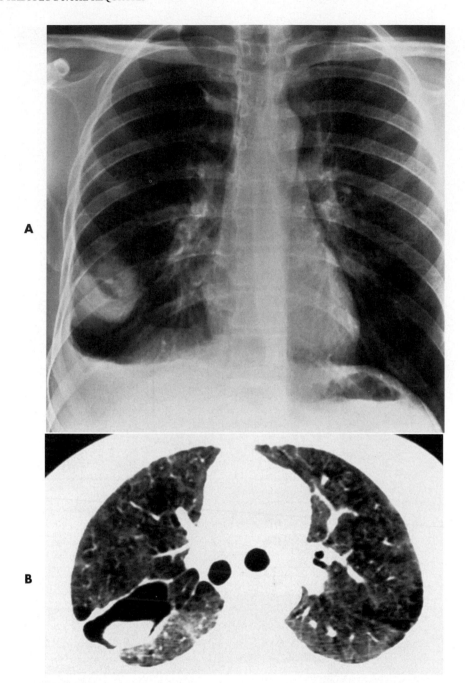

Fig. 6-16 Pulmonary laceration containing hematoma. **A,** PA chest radiograph reveals a right lower-lobe rounded opacity with a central lucency and a small right pleural effusion. The appearance mimics a pulmonary abscess or tumor. The history of recent right-sided trauma provides the diagnosis. **B,** CT scan at the level of the carina (lung windows) showing a large pneumatocele in the right upper lobe abutting the fissure. The cavity contains a hematoma, which may persist for months and resemble a pulmonary tumor.

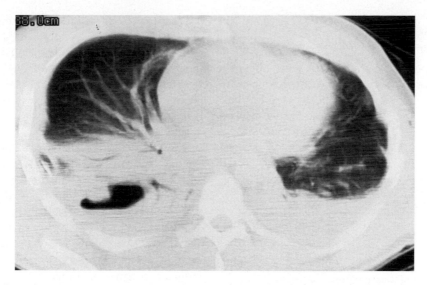

Fig. 6-17   Pulmonary laceration containing an air-fluid level. The CT scan reveals a large ovoid pneumatocele within the right lower lobe. The cavity contains an air-fluid level and is surrounded by densely consolidated lung representing extensive hemorrhage. There are bilateral pleural effusions.

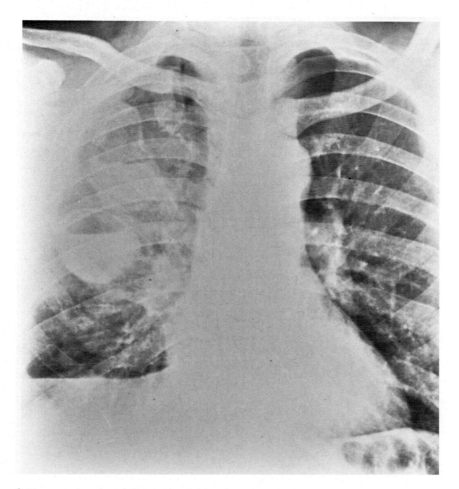

Fig. 6-18   Cavitating pulmonary lesions. PA radiograph demonstrates multiple cavities with air fluid levels within the right lung. The patient had been involved in an MVA months earlier.

DIAPHRAGMATIC RUPTURE

Diaphragmatic rupture is associated with severe injury and a high mortality secondary to the associated injuries (Box 6-8). The diaphragm is typically torn in the area of the central tendon or musculotendinous insertion and is usually left-sided. Rupture into the pericardium is rare.

Box 6-8 Diaphragmatic Rupture

70% involve the left hemidiaphragm
50% are missed clinical diagnosis
50% have no initial radiologic findings
50% are identified at exploratory surgery

Diaphragmatic rupture is often a missed diagnosis but is more readily recognized if the injury is recent and the tear is large and left-sided (Fig. 6-19). A delayed diagnosis is associated with morbidity and mortality from bowel strangulation and obstruction. The radiographic features are typically subtle. However, the demonstration of a gas-containing abdominal viscus within the thorax by a contrast swallow provides the definitive diagnosis (Fig. 6-20). Other signs include a nasogastric tube coiled in the hemithorax, an apparent elevation of the hemidiaphragm with loss of contour, contralateral mediastinal displacement, and a left pleural effusion. Herniation of abdominal viscera such as the liver or spleen may be more difficult to recognize (Fig. 6-21). Many of these features may be mimicked or masked by traumatic lung cysts, pulmonary contusion, atelectasis, pleural effusions, or a chronic hiatal hernia.

Text continues on p. 193

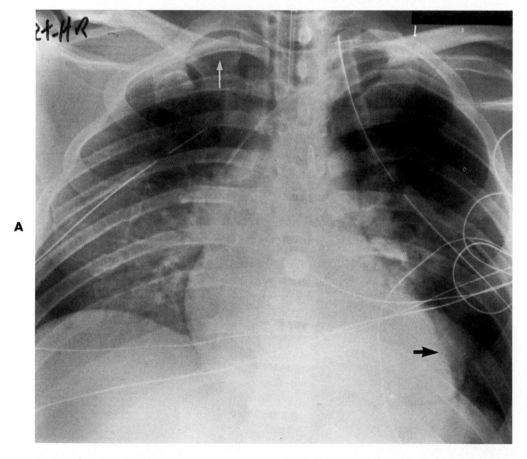

Fig. 6-19 Left diaphragmatic rupture—admission radiograph. **A,** Supine radiograph reveals a dense left retrocardiac opacity (*black arrow*) with an oblique contour. The left diaphragmatic contour is absent medially. In addition there are multiple bilateral rib fractures and a small right apical pneumothorax (*white arrow*). There is right lower-lobe and left perihilar opacification representing contusion.

Continued

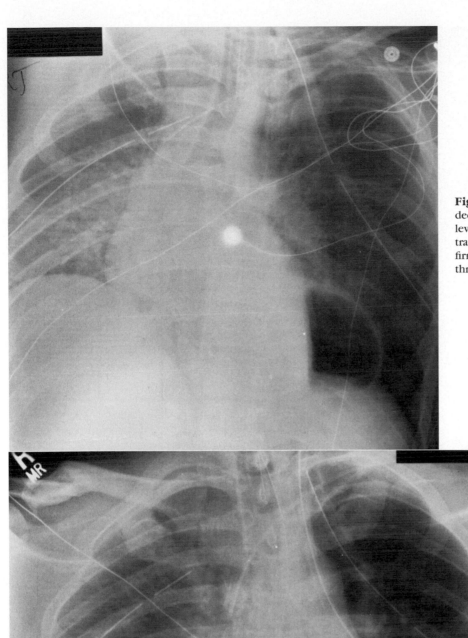

Fig. 6-19, cont'd. B, A right-side-down decubitus radiograph demonstrates an air-fluid level in the left retrocardiac region. **C,** A contrast study through the nasogastric tube confirms intrathoracic herniation of the stomach through a partial left-diaphragmatic tear.

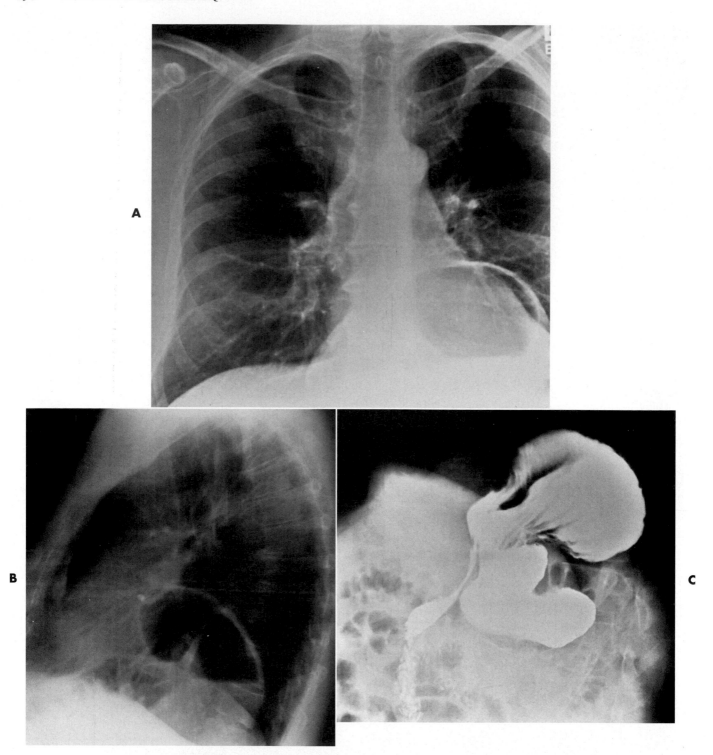

Fig. 6-20   Left diaphragmatic rupture—delayed diagnosis. **A,** An erect PA radiograph reveals a large air/fluid behind the heart. The left hemidiaphragm is obscured. **B,** The lateral radiograph demonstrates the presence of folds and an air/fluid level within the retrocardiac lucency. **C,** A barium study confirms intrathoracic herniation of the fundus of the stomach due to a ruptured left diaphragm.

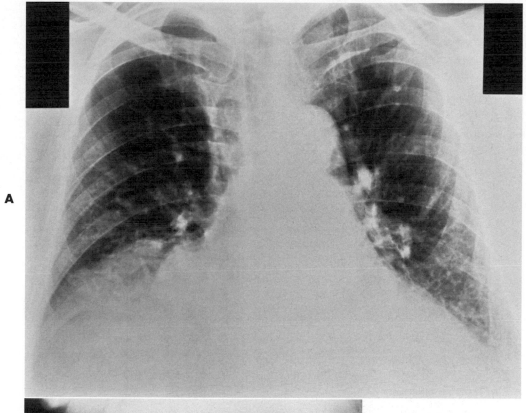

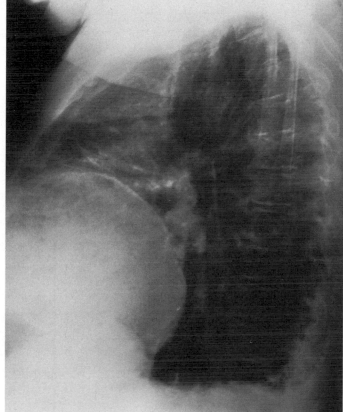

Fig. 6-21 Right diaphragmatic rupture—delayed diagnosis. **A,** PA radiograph demonstrates opacification of the right inferior hemithorax with loss of the cardiac and diaphragmatic contours. The cardiac silhouette is enlarged. **B,** Lateral radiographs show the opacity to lie anteriorly overlying the cardiac contour. The opacity is well defined and of mixed density with areas of lucency.   *Continued*

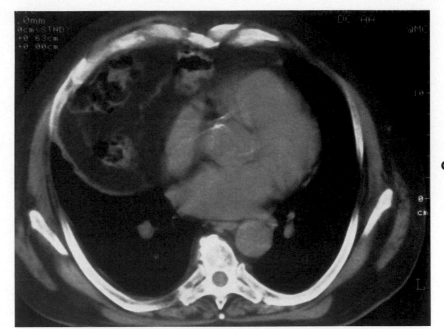

Fig. 6-21, cont'd   C, The CT scan through the lung bases shows the opacity to be due to herniation of mesenteric fat and large bowel through a right diaphragmatic tear. The mesentery surrounds the right cardiac contour.

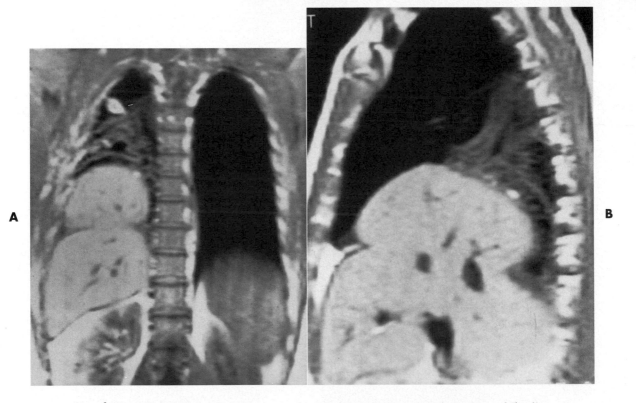

Fig. 6-22   MRI diaphragmatic rupture. **A,** Coronal image demonstrates herniation of the liver through a tear in the right hemidiaphragm. **B,** Lateral image reveals the size and location of the tear. There is also consolidation of the right lower lobe and fluid within the horizontal fissure.

Ultrasonography, CT, and MRI have all been used to document diaphragmatic rupture. Ultrasound is often limited by the presence of bowel gas. CT is useful in confirming the herniation of abdominal viscera, but it cannot identify the actual site of the tear. MRI with its ability to image in multiple planes allows recognition of the site of rupture (Fig. 6-22). Intrathoracic splenosis is a curious complication of diaphragmatic rupture. Fragments of the ruptured spleen may implant within the pleural cavity, enlarge, and produce an intrathoracic mass. A radionucleotide splenic scan will confirm the etiology of the mass.

LUNG HERNIATION/TORSION

Herniation of lung through the chest wall due to separation of the ribs and injury to the intercostal muscles is an infrequent complication and is of little clinical significance. Lung torsion, however, is a surgical emergency. Torsion of either a lobe or the complete lung may occur and result in pulmonary infarction. Fortunately, this injury is extremely rare; it is, however, more likely to occur in children. Recognition of torsion may be very difficult. It is suspected when a collapsed or consolidated lung lies in an unusual position and there is malposition of the hilar structures, fissures, or the pulmonary vessels. Serial radiographs may be diagnostic because they demonstrate the changing position of a readily identifiable opacity (Fig. 6-23).

TRAUMA TO THE AORTA

Causes and Survival

Motor vehicle accidents (MVA) are a common cause of deceleration injury to the thoracic aorta. Following complete transection, the majority of victims will die at the site of the accident. The survivors have incomplete tears with the surrounding adventitia maintaining the integrity of the aorta (Box 6-9). The typical site of injury is at the aortic isthmus, the transition zone between the relatively mobile aortic arch and the tethered aortic root and descending thoracic aorta. Without surgical repair, over half these patients will succumb within the first 24 hours. Untreated, the majority of the survivors will die in the following weeks. Only 2% survive long-term with a pseudoaneurysm (Fig. 6-24).

Box 6-9 Aortic Rupture Survival

80% succumb immediately (complete transection)
50% of those surviving (incomplete tears), if untreated, will rupture within 24 hours
2% of survivors succumb every hour
2% survive long-term with a pseudoaneurysm

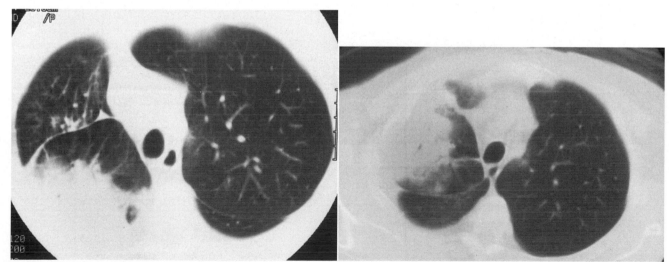

Fig. 6-23   Pneumonia in the right upper lobe, which is posterior on the supine CT scan, **A,** and moves anteriorly on the prone scan, **B.** The rapid change in location is due to lung torsion.

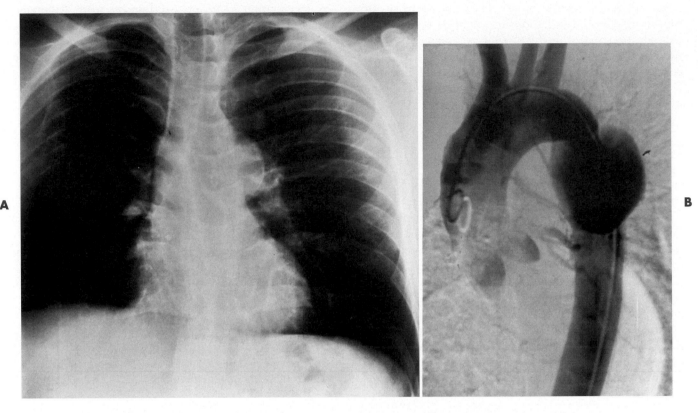

Fig. 6-24 Pseudoaneurysm of the aortic arch. **A,** PA radiograph demonstrates an enlarged contour to the aortic knob with curvilinear calcification. **B,** An arch angiogram demonstrates a pseudoaneurysm of the arch at the level of the ligamentum arteriosum. The patient had been in an MVA many years ago.

Box 6-10   Plain Radiographic Findings of Aortic Rupture

Mediastinal width increased
>8 cm
>25% thoracic diameter at arch
Effacement of aortic arch contour
Left apical cap or pleural effusion
Deviation of trachea and nasogastric tube to the
right
Depressed left main bronchus

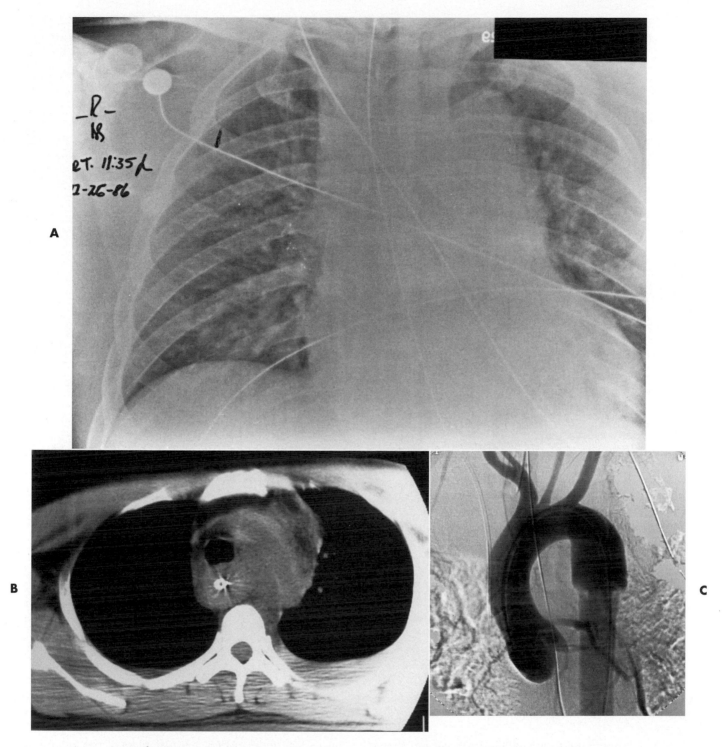

Fig. 6-25   Aortic transection. **A,** AP reveals a widened mediastinium, a left apical extrapleural cap, and displacement of the csophagus to the right. **B,** CT demonstrates mediastinal hematoma. **C,** Arch angiogram demonstrates the typical appearance of a tear at the ligamentum arteriosum.

Radiographic Findings

Plain film findings (Box 6-10), although highly sensitive, are not very specific (Fig. 6-25A) and may be difficult to interpret. If possible, obtain an erect radiograph. The AP supine projection magnifies the medi-

astinum and may cause apparent rather than real mediastinal widening. Layering pleural effusions are more difficult to recognize and may obscure mediastinal contours.

Aortography is mandatory in any patient with plain radiographic features suggestive of transection or in

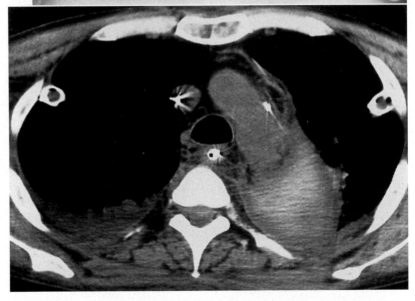

Fig. 6-26 Aortic tear—contained rupture. **A,** AP supine radiograph reveals a widened left superior mediastinum. The aortic knob is obscured. There is widespread patchy air space opacification representing extensive contusion. **B,** Contrast-enhanced CT scan demonstrates a large periaortic hematoma of high attenuation representing active bleeding. The posterior arch of the aorta has an irregular ill-defined contour. The appearance represents a contained aortic rupture. There are bilateral pleural effusions. Angiography confirmed the aortic tear.

patients with a normal chest radiograph who were involved in high-speed deceleration accidents (Fig. 6-25B).

Many of these angiograms will be normal, and therefore some physicians advocate the use of contrast-enhanced CT to select patients for aortography. It has been suggested that patients without CT-documented hematoma do not need angiography because an aortic tear is then very unlikely. However, aortic tears have been demonstrated in patients with a normal CT. Also of note, the mediastinal hematoma may prove to be due to bleeding from mediastinal veins or sternal or spinal injury rather than to aortic injury (Fig. 6-26).

More recently, aortic tears have been directly identified with helical contrast-enhanced CT of the thorax (Fig. 6-27). This diagnostic technique, although promising, is still under review because tears of the ascending aorta are not always identified.

CARDIAC INJURY

Pneumopericardium

This complication is usually the result of penetrating trauma. Pneumomediastinum may lead to pneumopericardium from air tracking along the adventitia of the

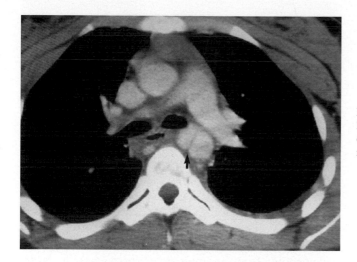

Fig. 6-27 CT diagnosis of aortic tear. Contrast-enhanced study at the level of the main pulmonary artery demonstrates an anterior and subcarinal mediastinal hematoma and a tear through the descending thoracic aorta (*arrow*).

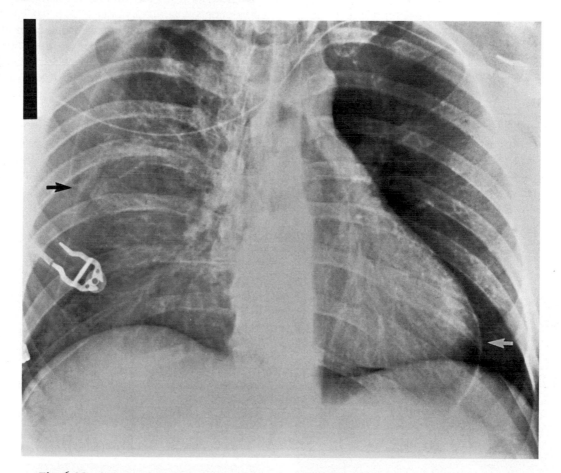

Fig. 6-28 Pneumopericardium. AP supine radiograph demonstrates air around the apex of the left ventricle (*white arrow*). There is a moderate right pneumothorax (*black arrow*).

pulmonary veins and into the pericardial space. Radiographically, air is seen outlining the cardiac contour extending to the pericardial reflection at the level of the origin of the aortic great vessels (Fig. 6-28). Unlike in pneumomediastinum, air in the pericardium will alter with the position of the patient. Pneumopericardium is rarely clinically significant, although there are reports of tamponade following tension pneumopericardium.

Hemopericardium

Hemopericardium may occur as a result of blunt trauma, but it more typically follows a penetrating injury

(Fig. 6-29). Cardiac tamponade may develop and rapidly become life-threatening. The chest radiograph may demonstrate a normal cardiac contour, and therefore a high index of clinical suspicion is required to make the diagnosis. The diagnosis is more readily made if the cardiac size is large or increasing on serial radiographs. Echocardiography will rapidly confirm the presence of pericardial fluid. CT will not only demonstrate the high density of the fluid but will also confirm the clinical findings of tamponade by showing periportal edema and distention of the inferior vena cava and the hepatic and renal veins.

Pericardial rupture is rare and usually fatal. The diaphragmatic or mediastinal pleurae may also be involved. Left-sided pericardial-pleural rupture can result in herniation of an abdominal viscus into the pericardial cavity. Pneumothorax and pneumopericardium are associated findings.

Myocardial Contusion

Cardiac contusion is common and is frequently asymptomatic. Most cases go unrecognized. Cardiac monitoring will identify contusion-related arrhythmias. Radionuclide ventriculography will detect wall-motion abnormality. Right ventricular dysfunction is most common and is explicable by its immediate retrosternal location. The ventricular dysfunction is usually reversible unless myocardial infarction has occurred.

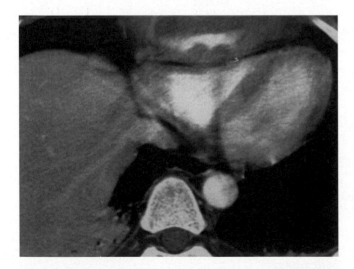

Fig. 6-29 Intrathoracic hematoma following a stabbing. Contrast-enhanced CT scan through the base of the heart demonstrates a large anterior intrathoracic hematoma compressing the right ventricle. The high density within this hematoma represents active bleeding. A hemopericardium is excluded. A chest-wall hematoma at the stab wound site is seen.

INDIRECT PULMONARY COMPLICATIONS OF TRAUMA

Adult Respiratory Distress Syndrome

ARDS, characterized by widespread pulmonary opacification, is associated with hypoxia and decreased lung compliance requiring mechanical ventilation. The syndrome is due to noncardiogenic pulmonary edema, which may progress to pulmonary fibrosis in severe cases. The initial chest radiograph is frequently normal. A characteristic delay of up to 12 hours from the clinical onset of respiratory failure to the appearance of radiographic abnormalities is well recognized. Progressive opacification from an interstitial appearance to widespread consolidation develops (Fig. 6-30). The consolidation involves all lung zones extending from the apex to the lung bases and to the extreme periphery of each lung. Fluctuation in the parenchymal opacification is not as rapid as in cardiogenic pulmonary edema. The heart size is usually normal, and pleural effusions are not a major feature.

Interstitial emphysema leading to tiny cysts and larger pneumatoceles and pneumothorax are frequent complications. The severity of ARDS varies from complete recovery within days, to prolonged assisted ventilation over months with residual permanent lung damage, to death from respiratory failure. Pulmonary edema from fluid overload, pneumonia, and atelectasis may complicate the syndrome.

Fat Embolism Syndrome

Fat embolism is common, but fortunately, fat embolism syndrome is rare (Box 6-11). It is most likely to occur after severe bony injury. The syndrome encompasses pulmonary and systemic manifestations involving the brain, kidneys, and skin. Fat emboli are thought to originate at the site of fractures and to enter the intramedullary veins. The circulating fat globules are

---

Box 6-11   Diagnosis—Fat Embolism Syndrome

Severe bony injury
Hypoxia, tachypnea
Widespread pulmonary opacification
Fat globules in sputum, urine
Petechia in skin and optic fundi
Delirium, convulsions, coma

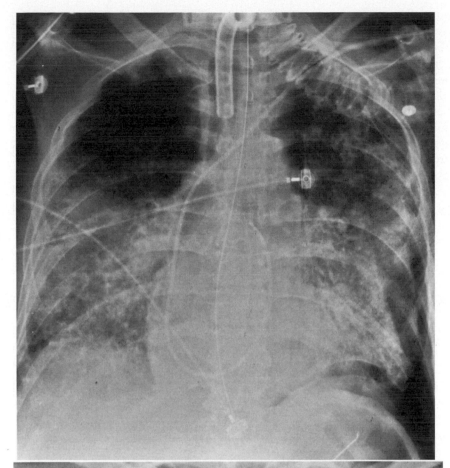

Fig. 6-30 ARDS—barotrauma. **A,** Supine AP radiograph in a ventilated patient reveals widespread pulmonary opacification with air bronchograms and a left pneumothorax with a subpulmonic component. In addition, there is left subcutaneous emphysema. **B,** One month later the airspace process has almost cleared, revealing fibrosis particularly within the left upper lobe. A right pneumothorax has resolved on tube drainage.

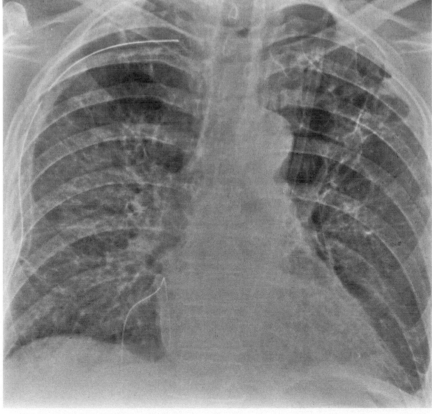

then trapped within the pulmonary vasculature. This causes obstruction and chemical injury from the released fatty acids. The resultant endothelial damage leads to leakage of fluid, hemorrhage, and inflammation. There is a typical lag time of 12 to 72 hours before the syndrome develops. This allows you to differentiate it from the other complications of trauma that usually present immediately. Fat embolism syndrome is a cause of ARDS. Therefore, the identification of fat globules allows the differentiation of this cause of ARDS from the many others. Prevention of fat embolism syndrome includes early immobilization of fractures and the recognition that patients with closed fractures are most at risk.

SUGGESTED READINGS

Daffner R: *Imaging of vertebral trauma,* Rockville, Ill, 1988, Aspen.

Dee PM: The radiology of chest trauma (review), *Radiol Clin North Am* 30:291-306, 1992.

Fraser RG, Pare JAP, Pare PD: *Diagnosis of diseases of the chest,* vol IV, ed 3, Philadelphia, 1991, WB Saunders; 2481-2518.

Gavant ML, Menke PG, Fabian T: Blunt traumatic aortic rupture detection with helical CT of the chest, *Radiology* 197:125-133, 1995.

Groskin SA: Selected topics in chest trauma (review), *Radiology* 183:605-617, 1992.

Kerns SR, Gay SB: Computed tomography of blunt trauma, *AJR* 156:273-279, 1990.

Mirvis SE, Templeton P: Imaging in acute thoracic trauma (review), *Semin Roentgenol* 27:184-210, 1992.

Murphey M, Batmitzky S, Bramble J: Diagnostic imaging of spinal trauma, *Radiol Clin North Am* 27:855-872, 1989.

Richardson P, Mirvis SE, Scorpio R: Value of CT in determining the need for angiography when the findings of mediastinal hematoma on chest radiographs are equivocal, *AJR* 156:273-279, 1991.

Stark P, Jacobson F: Radiology of thoracic trauma (review), *Curr Opin Radiol* 4(5):87-93, 1992.

Trerotola SC: Can helical CT replace aortography in thoracic trauma? (editorial), *Radiology* 197:13-15, 1995.

CHAPTER 7

Chronic Diffuse Infiltrative Lung Disease

THERESA C. McLOUD

A large number of chronic diseases may produce diffuse infiltration of the lung. Some are primarily lung disorders, and some others are manifestations of diseases arising elsewhere. Although these disorders have frequently been referred to as interstitial lung diseases, many also involve the alveolar spaces, and the designation "chronic diffuse infiltrative" is now widely accepted. Over 150 such disorders have been described, and a comprehensive list is provided in Box 7-1. Despite the large number, approximately 15 to 20 constitute 90% of such disease states, and these are the entities that will be discussed in this chapter. For pneumoconioses and vascular disorders, please see Chapters 8 and 9.

CLINICAL PRESENTATION

Patients usually present (Box 7-2) with dyspnea as the predominant symptom. Frequently on physical examination the only finding is dry rales or crackles. Physiologically, the abnormalities primarily affect gas exchange and result in hypoxemia. There may be reduced lung volumes that result in a restrictive pattern on pulmonary function tests.

The standard chest radiograph still remains the basic, and in some cases the only, imaging technique that is useful. The chest radiograph, however, is often nonspecific. In recent years the development of high-

Box 7-1 Diffuse Infiltrative Lung Diseases

INFECTIONS

Viral and mycoplasma pneumonia
Miliary tuberculosis
Fungal
Parasitic

IMMUNOLOGIC AND CONNECTIVE TISSUE DISORDERS

Progressive systemic sclerosis
Lupus erythematosis
Rheumatoid lung
Dermatomyositis
Ankylosing spondylitis
Drug reactions
Chronic eosinophilic pneumonia
Wegener's granulomatosis
Idiopathic pulmonary hemorrhage
Goodpasture's syndrome

ENVIRONMENTAL

Allergic alveolitis—hypersensitivity pneumonitis
Silicosis
Coal worker's pneumoconiosis
Asbestosis
Berylliosis
Other pneumoconioses

CHRONIC INTERSTITIAL PNEUMONIAS AND PULMONARY FIBROSIS

Usual (idiopathic pulmonary fibrosis)
Desquamative interstitial pneumonitis
Lymphocytic interstitial pneumonitis
Secondary to radiation
Secondary to neurofibromatosis

SARCOIDOSIS

OTHER SPECIFIC DISORDERS

Histiocytosis X (Langerhans histiocytosis)
Lymphangioleiomyomatosis
Gaucher's disease
Pulmonary alveolar microlithiasis
Pulmonary alveolar proteinosis
Amyloidosis

NEOPLASTIC

Metastatic carcinoma, lymphangitic carcinomatosis
Bronchioloalveolar carcinoma
Leukemia
Lymphoma

CARDIOVASCULAR

Pulmonary edema
Hemosiderosis, chronic passive congestion

PULMONARY VASCULAR DISEASE

Venoocclusive
Arteriolitis
Fat embolism
Embolism from oily contrast media
Multiple emboli and idiopathic pulmonary hypertension

Box 7-2 Clinical Presentation

Dyspnea
Dry rales or crackles
Reduced lung volumes
Evaluations
    Chest radiograph
    CT
    Gallium scan

resolution computed tomography (HRCT) has resulted in markedly improved diagnostic accuracy in chronic diffuse infiltrative lung disease. The following are the main technical components: (1) 1.5- to 2-mm-thick sections, (2) use of high-resolution algorithm, (3) targeted reconstruction to a single lung (optional), (4) prone scans to evaluate early or minimal basal disease. Prone scans are necessary to distinguish dependent atelectasis, a physiologic phenomenon, which usually occurs posteriorly in the basal areas of the lungs from true early infiltrative lung disease. Gallium scanning has also been used in the evaluation of infiltrative lung disease and is discussed in more detail in Nuclear Medicine: The Requisites.

PATTERN RECOGNITION

Classification

Pattern recognition in diffuse infiltrative lung disease has been the subject of controversy for many years. Traditional interpretation of chest radiographs separates these processes into two groups, (1) those diseases that radiographically appear to involve the terminal air spaces or alveoli, and (2) those that appear to involve the interstitium. However, there are number of problems that limit this approach to differential diagnosis. First, many pulmonary diseases produce pathologic changes in both compartments and second, disease processes that are pathologically classified as interstitial may produce an alveolar pattern on the radiograph. A graphic or morphometric classification is a better approach and is enumerated in Box 7-3. The patterns are described as nodular, irregular or linear, cystic, ground-glass, and parenchymal consolidation. Most of these patterns can be readily identified on standard radiographs, but ground-glass and cystic disease are much more readily appreciated on HRCT. Many diseases demonstrate more than one pattern (Box 7-3).

Pattern Characteristics

The nodular pattern (Fig. 7-1) is composed of multiple small nodules that may range from 1 mm to 1 cm in size. Irregular linear opacities (Fig. 7-2) frequently form a reticular pattern that may be fine or coarse. There are generally two types of cystic patterns: thin-walled cysts (Fig. 7-3) and honeycombing. Honeycomb spaces are generally 1 cm or less in diameter with relatively thick walls (>2 mm) and are a pathologic correlate of end-stage lung with fibrosis (Fig. 7-2). Ground-glass attenuation is a term used almost exclusively with CT. It consists of an amorphous opacification or increase in attenuation, which is of mild severity and is not sufficient to obliterate the pulmonary vessels. On the other hand, parenchymal consolidation, which has been previously referred to as alveolar or air-space disease, is characterized by dense opacification often with air bronchograms (Fig. 7-4). This opacification obliterates the pulmonary vasculature. Septal lines are a common feature of many infiltrative lung disorders but are particularly predominant in lymphangitic spread of carcinoma and in congestive heart failure.

You should also consider a number of other features in the differential diagnosis. These include distribution of disease, pleural abnormalities, the size of the lungs, the presence of pulmonary arterial hypertension, and mediastinal and hilar adenopathy.

Zonal Distribution

There are zonal preferences in the lungs (Box 7-4), although when many diseases become severe they are often diffuse. For example, histiocytosis, sarcoidosis, silicosis, and coal worker's pneumoconiosis typically favor the upper lobes, whereas idiopathic pulmonary fibrosis and fibrosis associated with collagen vascular disease tend to be a lower-zone phenomenon. Pleural disease may take one of several forms (Box 7-5). Pneumothorax may be seen as a complication of any cause of end-stage lung, but it may be identified early in the course of such

---

Box 7-3 Patterns of Opacities in Infiltrative Lung Disease

NODULAR OR RETICULAR NODULAR PATTERN (SMALL ROUNDED OPACITIES)

Silicosis
Coal worker's pneumoconiosis
Hypersensitivity pneumonitis
Histiocystosis X
Lymphangitic carcinomatosis
Sarcoidosis*
Pulmonary alveolar microlithiasis

LINEAR PATTERN (SMALL IRREGULAR, RETICULAR OPACITIES)

Idiopathic pulmonary fibrosis (UIP) (IPF)*
Chronic interstitial pneumonias (DIP, LIP, BIP)
Sarcoidosis
Radiation fibrosis
Fibrosis associated with collagen vascular disease
Asbestosis
Drug reactions
Lymphangitic carcinomatosis

CYSTIC PATTERN

IPF (honeycombing)
Lymphangioleiomyomatosis
Histiocytosis X

GROUND-GLASS ATTENUATION

Hypersensitivity pneumonitis
DIP
Alveolar proteinosis*
IPF

PARENCHYMAL CONSOLIDATION (AIR-SPACE OR ALVEOLAR DISEASE)

Bronchiolitis obliterans organizing pneumonia
Chronic eosinophilic pneumonia
Bronchioloalveolar carcinoma
Lymphoma
Alveolar proteinosis
Vasculitis
Pulmonary hemorrhage

SEPTAL LINES

Lymphangitic carcinomatosis
CHF—interstitial edema

---

* Pattern that is predominant or usually associated with specific disorder *BIP,* bronchiolitis with interstitial pneumonia; *CHF,* congestive heart failure; *DIP,* desquamative interstitial pneumonitis; *IPF,* idiopathic pulmonary fibrosis; *LIP,* lymphocytic interstitial pneumonitis; *UIP,* usual interstitial pneumonitis.

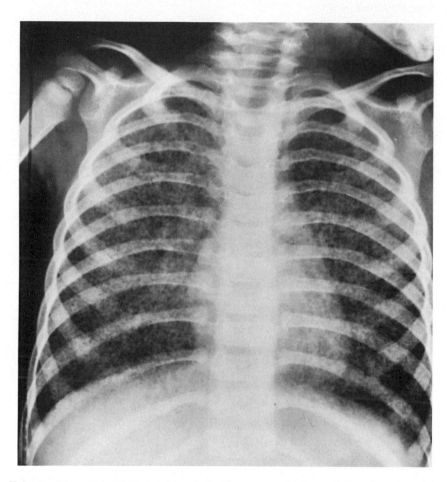

Fig. 7-1   Nodular pattern. Miliary tuberculosis. There are multiple small (1 to 3 mm) nodules distributed diffusely throughout the lungs.

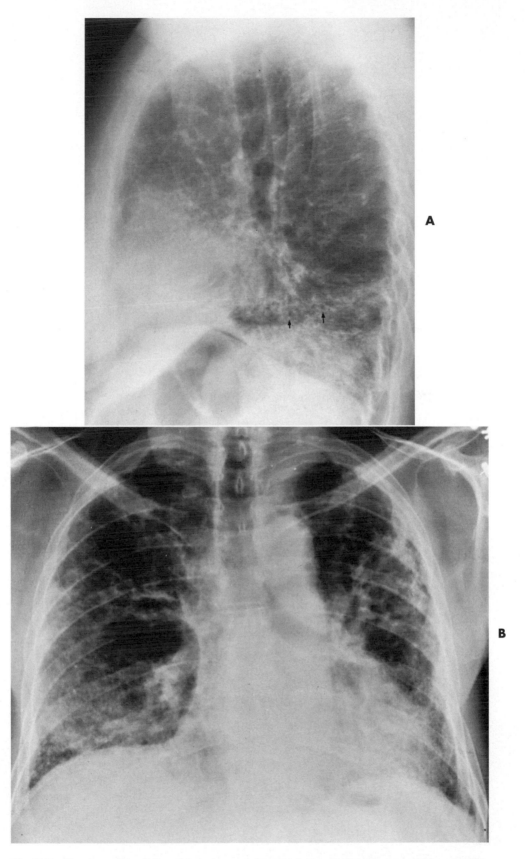

Fig. 7-2   Linear opacities. Idiopathic pulmonary fibrosis. **A,** Lateral film. There are linear opacities at the bases posteriorly of medium coarseness. There is also a suggestion of honeycombing (*arrows*). **B,** PA view in another patient shows coarse linear opacities distributed more diffusely.

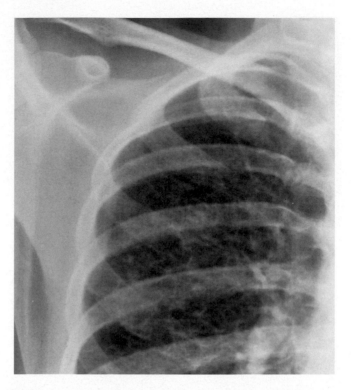

Fig. 7-3 Thin-walled cysts. Histiocytosis X. Thin-walled cysts can be identified in the upper lobes.

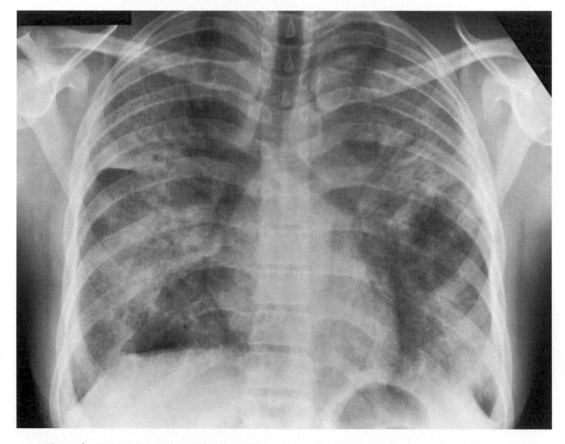

Fig. 7-4 Parenchymal consolidation (air-space or alveolar disease). There is confluent diffuse consolidation. Air bronchograms can be identified in the right upper lobe. This is a nice example of an alveolar pattern in a patient with interstitial lung disease (sarcoidosis).

Box 7-4   Zonal Preference

UPPER ZONES

Silicosis
Coal worker's pneumoconiosis
Sarcoidosis
Ankylosing spondylitis
Histiocytosis X

LOWER ZONES

Chronic interstitial pneumonias
IPF
Asbestosis
Fibrosis due to collagen vascular disease

CENTRAL

Pulmonary edema
Pulmonary alveolar proteinosis
Some lymphangitic tumors (Kaposi's)
Lymphoma

PERIPHERAL

Chronic interstitial pneumonias, IPF
Bronchiolitis obliterans-organizing pneumonia
Chronic eosinophilic pneumonia

IPF, idiopathic pulmonary fibrosis.

Box 7-6   Adenopathy

STANDARD RADIOGRAPHS

Silicosis
Sarcoidosis
Lymphoma
Lymphangitic carcinomatosis

CT (MORE SENSITIVE IN DETECTION OF ADENOPATHY)

Idiopathic pulmonary fibrosis
Hypersensitivity pneumonitis
Fibrosis associated with collagen vascular disease
Lymphangioleiomyomatosis

Box 7-5   Pleural Disease

PNEUMOTHORAX

Lymphangioleiomyomatosis
Histiocytosis X
End-stage honeycombing

PLEURAL EFFUSION

Lymphangioleiomyomatosis
Collagen vascular disease
Lymphangitic carcinomatosis
Pulmonary edema

PLEURAL THICKENING

Asbestosis (plaques or diffuse)
Collagen vascular disease

Box 7-7   Lung Volumes

REDUCED

Idiopathic pulmonary fibrosis
Chronic interstitial pneumonias
Asbestosis
Collagen vascular disease

NORMAL

Sarcoidosis
Histiocytosis

INCREASED

Lymphangioleiomyomatosis

mildly enlarged lymph nodes in idiopathic pulmonary fibrosis; hypersensitivity pneumonitis; fibrosis associated with the collagen vascular diseases; and lymphangioleiomyomatosis.

The size of the lung, that is, the lung volumes, may also be a clue to differential diagnosis (Box 7-7). The fibrotic disorders are characterized by marked restriction and small lungs will invariably be seen in idiopathic pulmonary fibrosis and related disorders. On the other hand, histiocytosis X and sarcoidosis in the early stages are usually associated with normal lung volumes, but lymphangioleiomyomatosis produces air trapping with large lung volumes. Finally, pulmonary arterial hypertension usually indicates end-stage disease with pronounced obliteration of the pulmonary vasculature. Except for pulmonary vascular diseases, signs of pulmonary arterial hypertension are rarely identified.

diseases as histiocytosis X and lymphangioleiomyomatosis, in which there is a high prevalence. Similarly, pleural effusions and diffuse thickening are often associated with collagen vascular disease and asbestos exposure. Pleural plaques, a fairly unique feature, are produced almost exclusively by asbestos exposure. Adenopathy (Box 7-6), which is recognized on standard radiographs, is associated with silicosis and sarcoidosis, lymphangitic carcinomatosis, and lymphoma. CT is more sensitive in the identification of adenopathy and may demonstrate

HIGH-RESOLUTION CT FEATURES OF CHRONIC INFILTRATIVE LUNG DISEASE

The five classifications of patterns of diffuse infiltrative lung disease on HRCT are: (1) linear or reticular opacities, (2) nodular opacities, (3) cystic lesions, (4) ground-glass opacification, and (5) parenchymal consolidation (alveolar or air-space disease). Webb and colleagues describe such HRCT findings in diffuse lung disease further in their work (see Suggested Readings).

Reticular or Linear Opacities

Reticular opacities are generally due to interstitial thickening by cells, fluid, or fibrous tissue (Box 7-8).

Axial interstitial thickening

Thickening of the axial interstitium (the interstitium that is peribronchovascular in location) (Fig. 7-5) occurs in many chronic infiltrative lung diseases such as lymphangitic spread of carcinoma, pulmonary fibrosis, and sarcoidosis. It is manifested by both bronchial-wall thickening and apparent enlargement of central pulmonary vessels. The thickening may be smooth or nodular. You must distinguish this appearance from a primary airway problem, bronchiectasis. In bronchiectasis, the bronchi will show evidence of bronchial-wall thickening, but the bronchi in addition will be dilated and larger than adjacent pulmonary artery branches. This will result in the appearance of large ring shadows. In patients with isolated bronchiectasis, there will be no other signs of infiltrative lung disease.

Septal thickening (interlobular septal thickening)

Thickening of the interlobular septa (Fig. 7-6) is common in many infiltrative lung diseases. In the peripheral lung it appears as 1- to 2-cm lines that extend perpendicularly from the pleural surface into the substance of the lung. In the more central portion of the lung the thickened septa can outline the secondary pulmonary lobules, producing polygonal structures that are 1 to 2.5 cm in diameter. These structures typically have a central dot that represents the pulmonary artery. Occasionally you can identify lines 2.5 cm in length that outline more than one lobule, particularly in the periphery of the lung. These have been called "parenchymal bands" and "long lines."

Centrilobular abnormalities

Prominence of the central dot (Fig. 7-6) within the secondary pulmonary lobule (the centrilobular vessel) may occur in a number of infiltrative lung diseases. The

---

Box 7-8 High-resolution CT—Linear Opacities

Thickening of bronchovascular bundles (axial)
Interlobular septal thickening (septal lines)
Intralobular interstitial thickening
Honeycombing
Subpleural lines
Centrilobular abnormalities

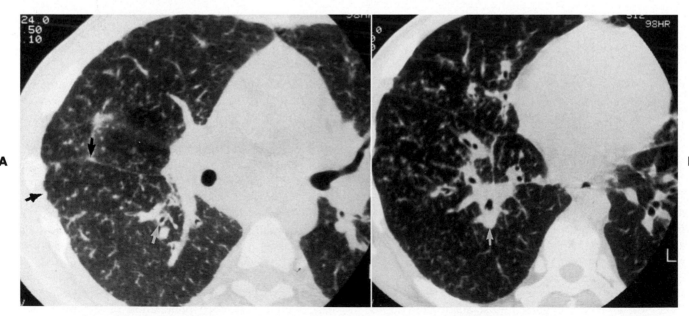

A   B

Fig. 7-5 Axial interstitial thickening. Sarcoid. **A,** There is bronchial wall-thickening (*white arrow*). Small nodules are seen subpleurally along the fissures and lateral chest wall (*black arrows*). **B,** The central pulmonary vessels appear enlarged (*arrows*).

intralobular bronchiole often becomes visible when there is centrilobular thickening. Centrilobular abnormalities can also be seen in patients with diseases of the peripheral airways, that is, the bronchioles.

Intralobular interstitial thickening

Involvement of the interstitium within the lobule either around the central artery and bronchiole or related to the interlobular septum may produce a fine reticular pattern within the lobule itself (Fig. 7-7). This usually extends from the centrilobular vessel peripherally to join a thickened septum.

Subpleural lines

A subpleural line may be defined as a curvilinear opacity less than 1 cm from the pleural surface. It parallels the pleura and is a few millimeters thick. First described in

asbestosis, this finding can occasionally be seen in normal lungs and is due to dependent atelectasis.

Nodules and Nodular Opacities

Some authors have attempted to differentiate interstitial from airspace or acinar nodules on HRCT. Because the anatomy of the secondary pulmonary lobule can be readily observed on HRCT, this distinction may often be possible even though overlap in the appearance of interstitial and alveolar nodules occurs and many disease processes involve both compartments.

Interstitial nodules

Interstitial nodules (Fig. 7-8) tend to be well defined and can be seen in numerous infiltrative lung diseases. They may be located in the axial interstitium along the

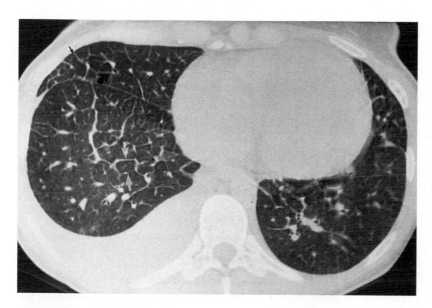

Fig. 7-6 Septal thickening. Pulmonary venoocclusive disease. Central septal lines outline the secondary pulmonary lobule, which appears as a polyhedral structure (*white arrows*). Peripheral septal lines lie perpendicular to the pleural surface (*black arrow*). Central dot in the lobule is prominent, and the intralobular bronchiole is visible (*curved black arrow*).

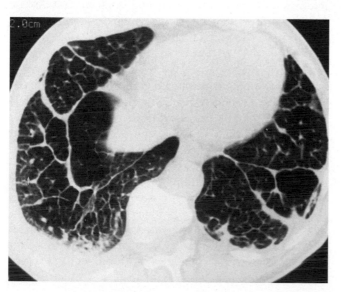

Fig. 7-7 Intralobular interstitial thickening. Idiopathic pulmonary fibrosis. A fine reticular pattern is seen within a secondary pulmonary lobule on the right (*small white arrow*).

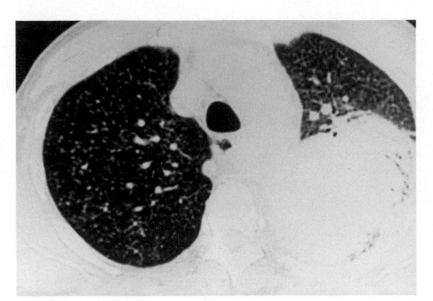

Fig. 7-8 Interstitial nodules. Miliary tuberculosis. In the right upper lobe there are multiple small well-defined nodules.

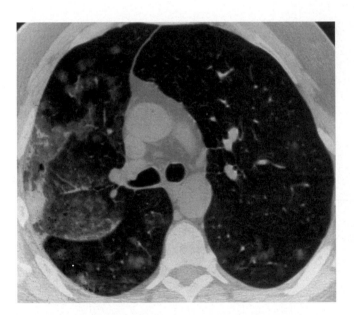

Fig. 7-9 Air-space nodules. Bronchioloalveolar carcinoma. Ill-defined nodules up to one centimeter are identified in both lungs. There is also ground-glass opacification and more confluent consolidation in the right lung.

peribronchovascular bundles, in the interlobular septa in a subpleural location adjacent to fissures, and in the central portion of the secondary pulmonary lobule.

Air-space nodules

You frequently find ill-defined nodules ranging from 6 mm to 1 cm in diameter in association with air-space consolidation around the peripheral bronchioles, particularly around the terminal bronchiole in the center of the secondary pulmonary lobule. These are not truly acinar but may be considered "air-space" nodules (Fig. 7-9). They may be associated with more confluent areas of air-space consolidation with air bronchograms. Such nod-

ules may be seen in patients with lobular pneumonia, endobronchial spread of tuberculosis, and bronchioloalveolar carcinoma.

Masses of fibrosis or conglomerate masses

Large masses of fibrous tissue may occur, usually in the central or axial interstitium (Fig. 7-10). They are usually associated with architectural distortion and volume loss. They typically produce traction bronchiectasis centrally in the bronchi that they encompass. This appearance is typical for silicosis and for coal worker's pneumoconiosis, but it may also occur in endstage sarcoidosis.

The Cystic Pattern

The cystic abnormalities include honeycombing, traction bronchiectasis, lung cysts, and cavitary nodules. For findings related to emphysema and small airways disease (such as bronchiolitis, which may cause decreased lung opacity), see Chapters 10 and 13.

Honeycombing

Honeycombing is produced pathologically by the dissolution of alveolar walls with the formation of randomly distributed air spaces that are lined by fibrous tissue. Honeycombing represents an end-stage lung that is destroyed by fibrosis. The typical appearance of honeycombing is that of thick-walled cystic spaces that are usually less than a centimeter in diameter (Fig. 7-11). Honeycombing typically is in the peripheral portions of the lungs subpleurally, particularly in idiopathic pulmonary fibrosis. It is often accompanied by other signs of infiltrative lung disease, particularly the patterns associated with reticular opacities and architectural distortion.

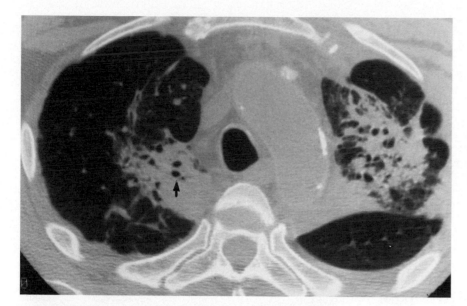

Fig. 7-10   Masses of fibrosis. End-stage sarcoid. There are large masses of fibrous tissue centrally in the upper lobes associated with traction bronchiectasis (*arrow*).

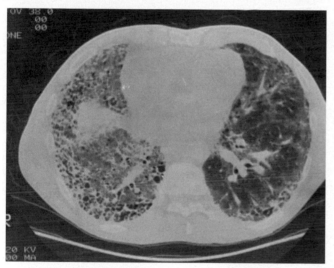

Fig. 7-11   Honeycombing. Idiopathic pulmonary fibrosis. Thick-walled cystic spaces can be seen subpleurally in the bases.

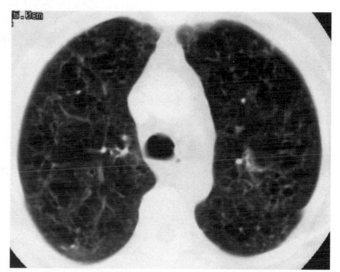

Fig. 7-12   Lung cysts. Histiocytosis X. Thin-walled, air-containing cysts in the upper lobes. There is no evidence of architectural distortion or fibrosis.

Traction bronchiectasis

Traction bronchiectasis (Fig. 7-10) is a phenomenon that occurs in the presence of severe lung fibrosis and distortion of lung architecture, in which the fibrous tissue produces traction on the bronchial walls, resulting in irregular bronchial dilation. It usually involves the more central bronchi.

Lung cysts

On HRCT, the term "lung cyst" refers to a thin-walled (usually <2 mm), well-defined and circumscribed air-containing lesion that is 1 cm or more in diameter (Fig. 7-12). You can readily differentiate such cysts from honeycombing because of their thinner walls and also from lack of other signs of fibrosis. Emphysematous bullae are focal areas of emphysema measuring a centimeter or more in diameter and having a wall less than a millimeter in thickness. Although they may be difficult to distinguish from true lung cysts, they are most frequently associated with other signs of extensive emphysema.

Cavitary nodules

Cavitary nodules have much thicker and more irregular walls than lung cysts. Among the infiltrative lung diseases they are typically seen in histiocytosis X.

Ground-Glass Opacity

Ground-glass opacity is defined as an ill-defined area of increased attenuation in the lung that does not

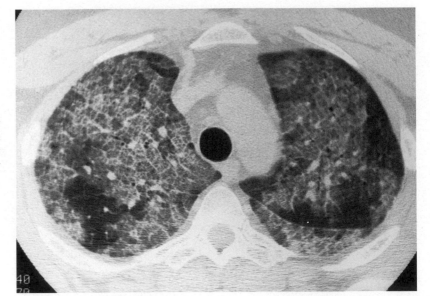

Fig. 7-13 Ground-glass opacification. Pulmonary alveolar proteinosis. There is increased attenuation in the lungs bilaterally, but the pulmonary vessels are not obscured. There is also prominent septal thickening.

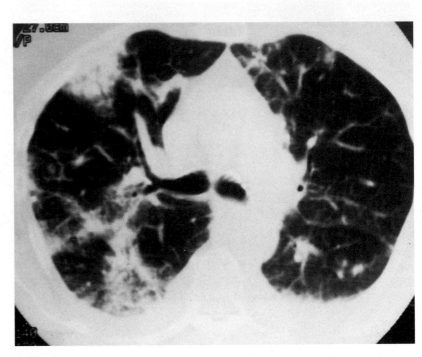

Fig. 7-14 Air-space consolidation. Bronchiolitis obliterans-organizing pneumonia. Patchy areas of consolidation containing air bronchograms are seen in the lungs peripherally.

obscure the underlying vessels (see discussion of air-space consolidation) (Fig. 7-13). Ground-glass opacity may occur as a predominant finding, or it may be associated with other patterns. Physiologically it may be due either to disease in the interstitium with alveolar wall thickening or disease in the alveoli of minimal severity, or to a combination of both.

Ground-glass opacity usually reflects an ongoing and potentially treatable process such as active alveolitis in desquamative interstitial pneumonitis or an active infection such as *Pneumocystis carinii* pneumonia. Pulmonary edema and hemorrhage may produce similar ap-

pearances. Areas showing ground-glass opacification are good sites for lung biopsy because they are more likely to yield active diagnostic material.

Air-Space Consolidation

Air-space consolidation is increased opacification that results in the obscuration of vessels and is frequently characterized by the presence of air bronchograms (Fig. 7-14). Disease processes producing such an appearance usually are characterized by a replacement of alveolar air by fluid, cells, or other material.

Box 7-9 Sarcoidosis

CHARACTERISTICS

Etiology—unknown
Pathology—noncaseating granulomas
Clinical
    20 to 40 years of age
    50% asymptomatic
    Elevated angiotensin-converting enzyme levels

RADIOGRAPHIC FEATURES

Symmetrical adenopathy
Nodular or reticular nodular opacities
Upper lung zones
Fibrosis
    Upper lobes, hilar retraction
    Bullae

HIGH-RESOLUTION CT

Nodular thickening along lymphatics
    Axial
    Interlobular septa, fissures, subpleural zones
Fibrosis
    Reticular—axial
    Upper lobes—architectural distortion
    Fibrotic masses
    Traction bronchiectasis
Differential diagnosis
    Granulomatous infections
    Silicosis—progressive massive fibrosis

DISEASES CHARACTERIZED BY A NODULAR OR RETICULONODULAR PATTERN

Sarcoidosis

Sarcoidosis (Box 7-9) is difficult to define, but it is a systemic disorder of unknown cause characterized pathologically by widespread noncaseating granulomas. Such granulomata are not unique to sarcoidosis and may appear in many other conditions. The diagnosis therefore must be based on consistent clinical and laboratory findings, tissue biopsy, and exclusion of other diseases, particularly granulomatous infections. The noncaseating granulomas may resolve spontaneously or may progress to fibrosis.

Most patients are young (20 to 40 years of age), and at least one half are asymptomatic. The disease is more frequent in blacks. When symptoms occur they are usually systemic rather than respiratory.

Radiographic findings

The chest radiograph is abnormal in more than 90% of patients. Lymph node enlargement, parenchymal abnormalities, or a combination of the two constitute the major radiographic changes. Intrathoracic lymphadenopathy appears in 75% to 85% of patients with sarcoidosis at some time during the course of their disease. On the initial chest radiograph, approximately one half of the patients will have this finding exclusively; the other half will have lymphadenopathy plus parenchymal disease. Bilateral hilar adenopathy is the most frequent finding and occurs in up to 98% of cases with nodal enlargement (Fig. 7-15). Bilateral symmetrical mediastinal adenopathy is also frequent. The parenchymal lung disease in sarcoidosis typically consists of a nodular or a reticulonodular pattern, which is more predominant in the upper lung zones (Fig. 7-16). It is common for the adenopathy to decrease as the parenchymal disease becomes worse. In about 25% of patients the radiographic findings may be atypical and can include diffuse air-space disease or large parenchymal nodules simulating cannonball metastases.

Sarcoid granulomas are distributed primarily along the lymphatics (1) in the peribronchovascular bundles emanating from the hila in an axial distribution, and (2) to a lesser extent in the interlobular septa and subpleural lymphatics both peripherally and along the fissures. This distribution is much more easily recognized on HRCT than on plain radiographs. On HRCT (Fig. 7-5) the classic pattern consists of small nodules identified along the axial interstitium, that is, emanating out from the hila along the bronchovascular bundles, within the interlobular septa, adjacent to the major fissures, and in the subpleural regions. The nodules may vary from 2 mm to 1 cm in diameter. Confluence of granulomas may result in large opacities with ill-defined contours, some of which may appear nodular and others of which may contain air bronchograms.

Approximately 20% of patients with radiographic evidence of interstitial lung disease will develop fibrosis. The fibrosis in sarcoidosis is quite characteristic (Fig. 7-17). It is typically identified in the upper lobes, which show evidence of hilar retraction and bullae. The fibrosis is more pronounced in the apical and posterior portions of the upper lobes and the superior segments of the lower lobes. On HRCT (Figs. 7-10 and 7-18) you can recognize the fibrosis as irregular reticular opacities, which are usually more predominant along the bronchovascular bundles. Loss of volume in the upper lobes with distortion of lung architecture occurs. Large masses of fibrous tissue may develop centrally along the perihilar bronchi and vessels, particularly in the upper lobes; this is often associated with traction bronchiectasis. Given this appearance you must also consider silicosis and tuberculosis in the differential diagnosis.

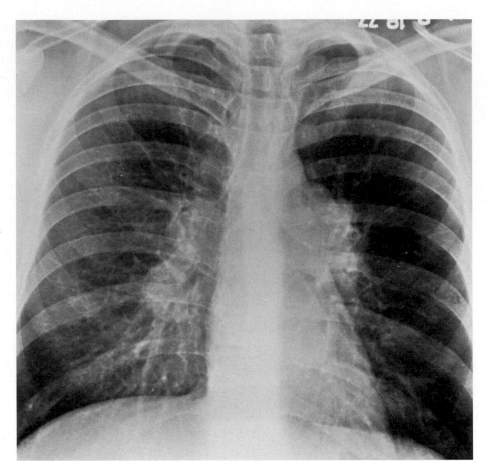

Fig. 7-15 Sarcoidosis. Bilateral symmetric hilar adenopathy.

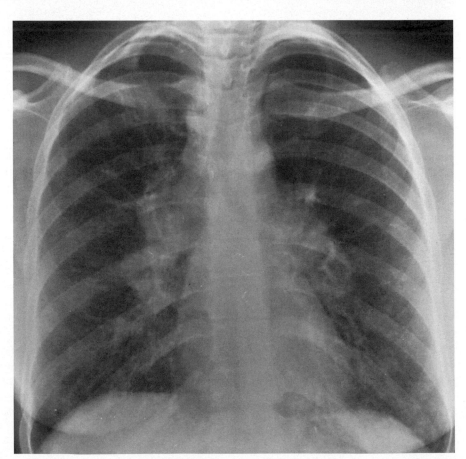

Fig. 7-16 Sarcoidosis. Adenopathy and parenchymal disease. There is evidence of a typical distribution of adenopathy, right paratracheal and bilateral hilar ("1, 2, 3" sign). There are linear and nodular opacities, particularly at the bases.

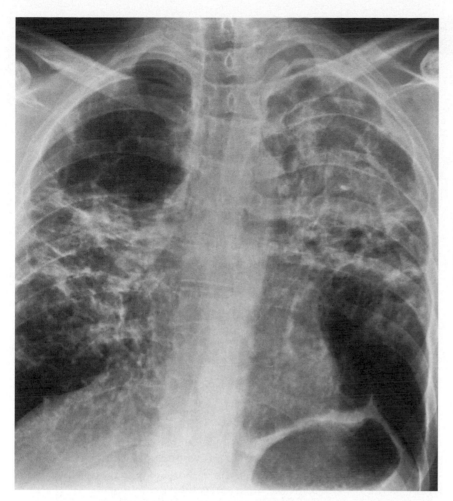

Fig. 7-17 End-stage sarcoidosis. PA chest radiograph shows right perihilar and left upper lobe fibrosis with straightening of the left main bronchus due to hilar retraction. There are bullae in the right upper lobe.

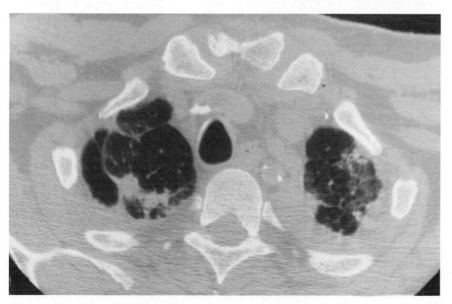

Fig. 7-18 End-stage sarcoidosis. High-resolution CT shows coarse linear opacities in both upper lobes with multiple bullae.

Box 7-10   Lymphangitic Carcinomatosis

CHARACTERISTICS

Sites: colon, lung, breast, stomach

RADIOGRAPHIC FEATURES

Reticular-nodular
Adenopathy
Effusions

HIGH-RESOLUTION CT

Nodular axial thickening
Septal thickening
Nodular thickening of fissures
Polygonal structures
Normal lung architecture

DIFFERENTIAL DIAGNOSIS

Lymphoma
Sarcoidosis
Kaposi's sarcoma

Other imaging modalities

Gallium citrate (Ga-67) has been used to assess activity in sarcoidosis. There is observable uptake both in the lymph nodes and the lung parenchyma. (See Nuclear Medicine: The Requisites.) There are no specific laboratory tests for the diagnosis of sarcoidosis, although elevation of angiotensin-converting enzyme (ACE) in the serum of patients with active sarcoidosis is common, but there may also be elevation of ACE levels in other diseases. Diagnosis is usually made by bronchoscopy with transbronchial biopsy, which has an extremely high yield because of the close relationship of the noncaseating granulomas to the peripheral bronchi. The prognosis of sarcoidosis is related to the findings on chest radiograph at the time of the initial presentation. The majority of patients with adenopathy alone will clear completely, but approximately 15% to 25% of patients with parenchymal abnormalities on the initial chest radiograph will develop progressive pulmonary fibrosis.

Lymphangitic Carcinomatosis

Pulmonary lymphangitic carcinomatosis (Box 7-10) is characterized by metastatic tumor involving the lymphatic system of the lungs. It occurs most commonly in patients with carcinomas of the lung, breast, stomach, and colon, and in those with metastatic adenocarcinoma from unknown primary sites. Patients usually have dyspnea and dry cough.

Standard radiographic findings

On standard chest radiographs you may observe a constellation of findings (Fig. 7-19). These include diffuse reticular nodular or linear opacities, septal lines, hilar and mediastinal adenopathy, and pleural effusions. Frequently there are only one or two of these features, and the signs are often nonspecific. HRCT provides more specific findings (Fig. 7-20). The pattern is related to the distribution of lymphatics in the lung. Features include the following: (1) smooth or nodular axial interstitial thickening along the bronchovascular bundles, (2) septal thickening, (3) smooth or nodular thickening of the fissures, (4) normal lung architecture, (5) identification of polygonal structures (secondary pulmonary lobules). Given the correct clinical history in a symptomatic patient, these findings are virtually pathognomonic. One of the most characteristic findings is the observance of polygonal arcades or polygons, seen in about 50% of patients with lymphangitic spread of carcinoma (Fig. 7-20B). These structures usually contain a central dot that is visible on HRCT. The appearance is caused by the presence of thickened interlobular septa surrounding secondary lobules, seen in cross section. The central dot represents the intralobular central artery branch surrounded by axial interstitium that is thickened by tumor.

Differential diagnosis

In the differential diagnosis, you will have to consider other diseases that may be characterized by nodules, septal thickening, and an axial distribution, that is, those diseases that have a perilymphatic distribution of abnormalities. These include sarcoidosis, lymphoma when it involves the lung, and Kaposi's sarcoma.

The most effective means of making the diagnosis is transbronchial biopsy with use of the fiberoptic bronchoscope. As in sarcoidosis, the proximity of the lesions to the bronchi results in high diagnostic accuracy rates.

DISEASES CHARACTERIZED BY AN IRREGULAR LINEAR PATTERN

There is a linear or a reticular pattern of opacities in a large number of diffuse infiltrative lung diseases. The most important of these are the chronic interstitial pneumonias and idiopathic pulmonary fibrosis (Boxes 7-11 and 7-12).

Chronic Interstitial Pneumonias and Idiopathic Pulmonary Fibrosis

Terminology

The terminology used to describe these diseases is somewhat confusing. In the 1950s this disorder or group of disorders was referred to as the Hamman-Rich syndrome, which was characterized by rapidly progressive interstitial fibrosis. In the 1960s Liebow described several chronic interstitial pneumonias as a group of disorders of known or unknown etiology characterized by an inflammatory process in the alveolar walls with a strong

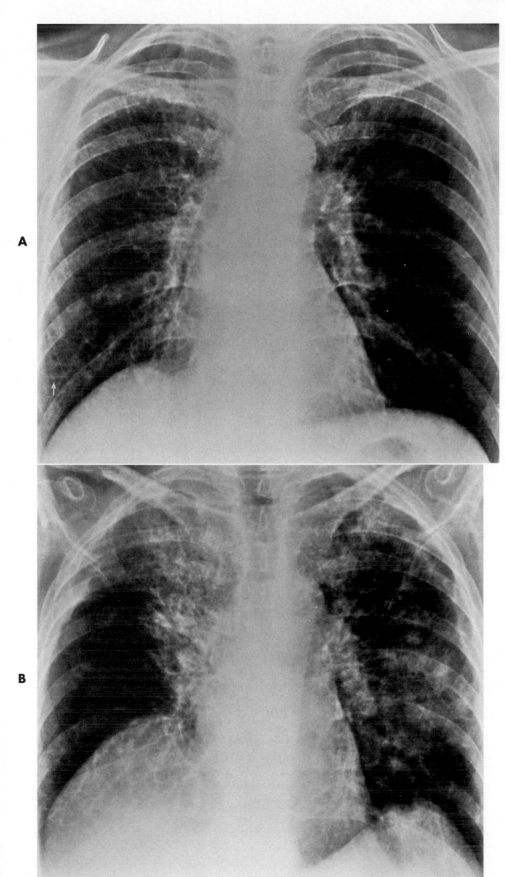

Fig. 7-19 Lymphangitic carcinomatosis. Patient who had bilateral mastectomies for breast cancer. **A,** PA radiograph shows fine linear opacities in both lungs. There are Kerley-B lines (*arrow*). **B,** Chest radiograph 3 months later shows more confluent opacities and bilateral pleural thickening.

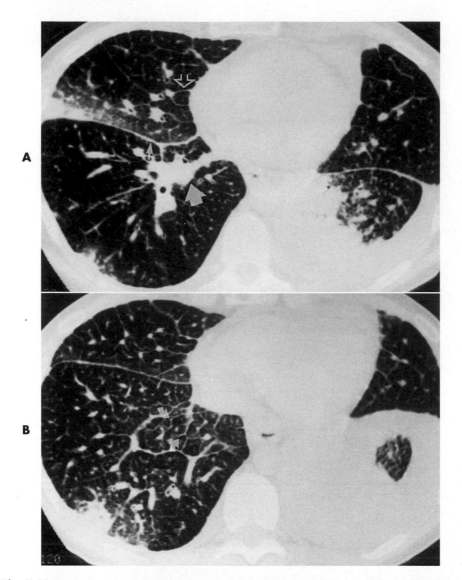

Fig. 7-20 Lymphangitic carcinomatosis. **A,** There is nodular thickening of the axial interstitium (*large white arrow*) as well as septal lines (*open white arrow*) and fissural thickening (*small arrow*). **B,** Note the prominent polygons with central dots (*arrows*).

Box 7-11   Idiopathic Pulmonary Fibrosis (IPF or UIP)

CHARACTERISTICS

Clinical
    40 to 60 years of age
    Dyspnea, dry cough

RADIOGRAPHIC FINDINGS

Linear opacities
Lower zones
Honeycombing
Small lungs

HIGH-RESOLUTION CT

Septal thickening
Intralobular thickening
Honeycombing
Bronchiolectasis
Traction bronchiectasis
Peripheral and subpleural

> ## Box 7-12 Desquamative Interstitial Pneumonia (DIP)
>
> ### CHARACTERISTICS
>
> Possible early inflammatory stage of idiopathic pulmonary fibrosis
> Active alveolitis
> Better prognosis—responds to steroids
>
> ### RADIOGRAPHIC FEATURES
>
> Lower zones
> Fine linear or ground-glass pattern
>
> ### HIGH-RESOLUTION CT FINDINGS
>
> Lower zones
> Ground-glass opacification

tendency to develop fibrosis. His classification included five types: usual interstitial pneumonia (UIP), desquamative interstitial pneumonia (DIP), lymphocytic interstitial pneumonia (LIP), giant cell interstitial pneumonia (GIP), and bronchiolitis with interstitial pneumonia (BIP). Although this terminology has been widely accepted, in the 1980s the more commonly used term of reference was idiopathic pulmonary fibrosis, which described the end-stage of these disorders. Fibrosis due to known causes was designated as such, for example, fibrosis associated with collagen vascular disease. In addition, the designation "fibrosing alveolitis," which encompasses both the inflammatory and the fibrotic aspects of this group of disorders, is used more commonly in Britain and the Commonwealth countries. All of these designations are in common usage in textbooks and references.

Types

The interstitial pneumonias described by Liebow do not represent individual diseases but rather characteristic ways in which the lung can respond to injury. More than one type of such interstitial pneumonias may be found in a single patient. The most common types are UIP and DIP (Boxes 7-11 and 7-12). DIP is felt by many pathologists to represent the very early or more inflammatory cellular phase of UIP or of idiopathic pulmonary fibrosis (IPF), and therefore the more potentially reversible phase (Box 7-12). LIP is uncommon and is seen in patients with a variety of immunologic disorders and in those with AIDS. LIP is now considered to be a prelymphomatous disorder. For more details, see Chapters 4 and 9. GIP is extremely rare. Although Liebow first described bronchiolitis with interstitial pneumonia, this entity is rather rare. More frequently, bronchiolitis may be associated with patchy air-space–organizing pneumonia, which is called bronchiolitis obliterans-organizing pneumonia or cryptogenic-organizing pneumonia. Despite the designation of bronchi-

olitis, this disease is not primarily a small airways disease but is often classified with the infiltrative lung disorders. IPF and the chronic interstitial pneumonias usually occur in patients between 40 and 60 years of age. The chief complaint in most patients with chronic interstitial pneumonia and idiopathic fibrosis is dyspnea and occasional dry cough. Pulmonary function tests show evidence of restriction and impairment of gas exchange with a lowered diffusing capacity.

Pathologic features

It is important to review some of the pathologic features of these entities. As mentioned above, UIP and DIP may not be distinct disease entities but represent different phases or stages of a single disease state. UIP is characterized histologically by alveolitis and mononuclear cell inflammatory changes in the alveolar wall. Eventually, fibrosis develops and this may lead to a drastic revision of pulmonary architecture in which the normal pattern of the distal air spaces is replaced by randomly communicating air spaces lined by thick fibrous walls. This end-stage is referred to as honeycomb lung. Such changes can also be identified in the collagen vascular diseases as well as in response to certain drugs such as bleomycin, cyclophosphamide, or busulfan. On the other hand, DIP is characterized by the presence of large numbers of cells filling the alveolar spaces. Most of these cells represent macrophages, although some may represent desquamated type II alveolar cells. In this disease the symptoms are usually milder, there is not necessarily progression to fibrosis, and patients have a much better prognosis and response to steroid therapy.

Radiologic findings

The characteristic radiologic findings on standard radiographs in IPF or UIP (Fig. 7-21) consist of a diffuse linear pattern obliterating normal vessels and often predominating at the bases. This may progress from fine reticulation to coarse irregular opacities. Small, well-formed cystic spaces less than 1 cm in diameter are designated as a "honeycomb" pattern. Identification of honeycombing indicates end-stage disease and severe architectural distortion and fibrosis. Severe reduction in lung volume is a frequent complication. In DIP, occasionally a "ground-glass" pattern of ill-defined opacities at the bases reflects an active alveolitis. More commonly, however, DIP is also characterized by a fine linear or reticular pattern that will eventually progress if untreated to findings consistent with IPF. HRCT is much superior to chest radiographs in the assessment of patients with IPF. The HRCT findings reflect the presence of fibrosis (Fig. 7-11). They include the following: smooth but irregular septal thickening, intralobular interstitial thickening, irregular interfaces between the lung and pleura, bronchiolectasis, honeycombing, and traction bronchiectasis. The findings are typically peripheral and subpleural in location and pre-

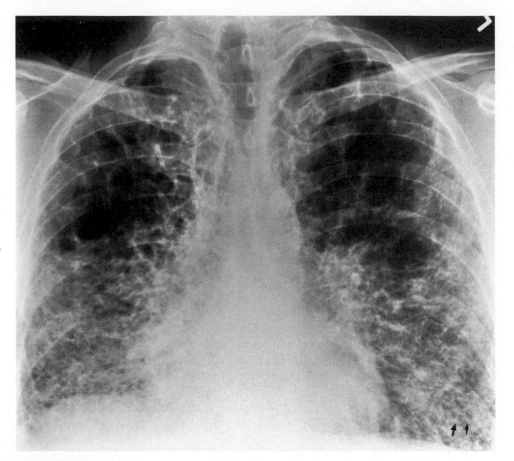

Fig. 7-21 Idiopathic pulmonary fibrosis or usual interstitial pneumonia. PA radiograph shows coarse reticular opacities predominating at the bases. There is also evidence of honeycombing (*arrows*).

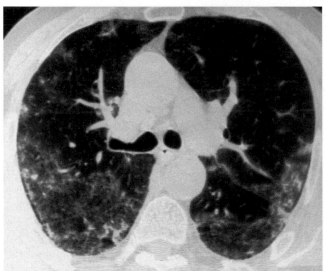

Fig. 7-22 Desquamative interstitial pneumonitis. High-resolution CT shows ground-glass opacities in the peripheral lung zones. There is no architectural distortion or honeycombing.

dominate at the bases. You may observe areas of ground-glass opacity; these most commonly represent active inflammatory change or alveolitis (DIP). In cases of IPF where honeycombing predominates there is often gross destruction of lung architecture. CT may have important clinical applications. It can be useful as a guide to the site

for lung biopsy. It is important to obtain diagnostic tissue by avoiding areas of extensive honeycombing. There are also recent studies showing that ground-glass opacification is more likely to correspond to active alveolitis and a DIP-like reaction (Fig. 7-22). Patients who have predominantly ground-glass opacification usually respond to therapy. You can also use CT for clinical follow-up.

Collagen Vascular Disease, Asbestosis, Drug Reactions

The collagen vascular diseases have features that are almost identical to IPF on both standard radiography and HRCT. The parenchymal fibrosis due to asbestos exposure ("asbestosis") both radiologically and pathologically resembles IPF. For more details about these entities, see Chapters 8 and 9. Similarly, reactions in the lung to drugs may be allergic in origin and occasionally may induce pulmonary fibrosis. (See Chapter 9).

CYSTIC PATTERN

Lymphangioleiomyomatosis

Lymphangioleiomyomatosis (LAM) (Box 7-13) is a rare disease occurring in young women. It is characterized pathologically by widespread proliferation of

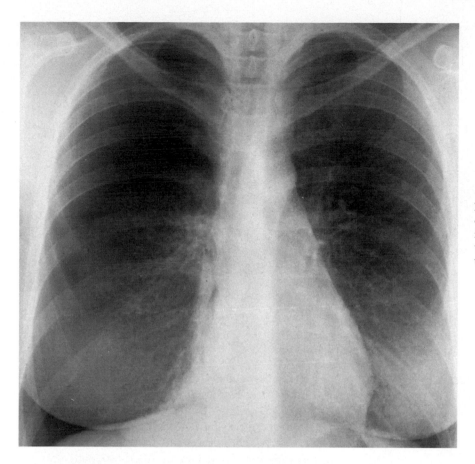

Fig. 7-23 Lymphangioleiomyomatosis. PA chest radiograph in a young woman shows a right pneumothorax and normal lung volumes. Cysts and linear opacities are difficult to appreciate on this standard film.

Box 7-13 Lymphangioleiomyomatosis

CHARACTERISTICS

Young women, reproductive age, tuberous sclerosis
Proliferation of immature smooth muscle
Chylothorax
Pneumothorax
Hemoptysis

RADIOGRAPHIC FEATURES

Linear pattern
Thin-walled cysts
Normal or increased lung volumes

HIGH-RESOLUTION CT FINDINGS

Thin-walled cysts
Diffuse
Otherwise normal parenchyma

---

immature smooth muscle, especially around bronchioles and in lymphatics. These changes may occur in both the chest and the abdomen. The process often leads to obstruction of the bronchioles with air trapping and the development of thin-walled lung cysts that may rupture and cause pneumothorax. Similarly, obstruction of the lymphatics can occur with subsequent development of chylous pleural effusions, and compression of venules may lead to hemoptysis. Most patients are in the reproductive age group, and symptoms include dyspnea. Tuberous sclerosis produces similar histologic findings.

Standard radiographic features include a diffuse linear pattern that may be associated with thin-walled cysts. The lung volumes are either normal or increased. The increase in lung volumes correlates with evidence of airway obstruction on function testing. Pneumothorax may be seen in 40% of patients, and 60% may develop chylous pleural effusions (Fig. 7-23). The HRCT findings are striking (Fig. 7-24) and show thin-walled cysts that may be difficult to recognize on standard radiography. On HRCT they are distributed diffusely throughout the lungs, unlike in honeycombing in which the cysts are thicker-walled and predominant in the subpleural zones. Usually the lung parenchyma between the cysts is normal and there is no evidence of lung distortion, although there may be occasional septal thickening and increased linear opacities or ground-glass opacity. Nodules are extremely unusual, but there is occasional adenopathy.

The prognosis for this disease has improved as a result of treatment with progesterone and oophorectomy.

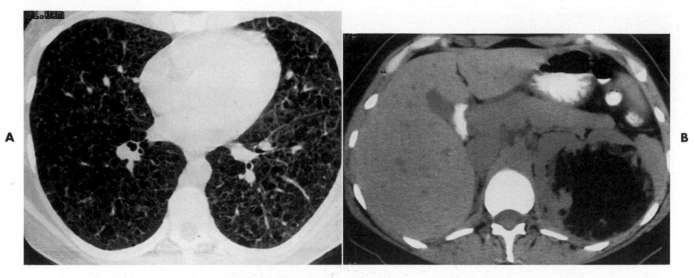

Fig. 7-24   Lymphangioleiomyomatosis in tuberous sclerosis. Young woman with recurrent pneumothoraces. **A,** HRCT demonstrates multiple thin-walled cysts distributed uniformly throughout the lungs without architectural distortion or small opacities. **B,** CT of the upper abdomen demonstrates a large angiomyolipoma (a tumor common in tuberous sclerosis) in the left kidney. There is abundant lipid in the lesion as demonstrated by the low-attenuation area.

Box 7-14   Histiocytosis

CHARACTERISTICS

Benign proliferation of histiocytes, granulomas
Young adults
Smokers

RADIOGRAPHIC FEATURES

Reticulonodular pattern
Upper-zone predominance
Pneumothorax
Cysts

HIGH-RESOLUTION CT FINDINGS

Thin-walled cysts
Nodules, ± cavitation
Upper-zone predominance

Histiocytosis X

Histiocytosis X (Box 7-14), more recently referred to as Langerhans' histiocystosis (eosinophilic granuloma), is an idiopathic disease characterized by benign proliferation of mature histiocytes. Early stages of the disease are characterized by multiple granulomas composed of histiocytes, Langerhans histiocytes, and varying numbers of eosinophils in the alveolar septa, bronchial walls, and perivascular areas. Eventually in the later stages some interstitial fibrosis and thin-walled cysts may develop.

It is an uncommon disease that occurs in young and middle-aged adults, and over 90% of the patients are smokers. Presenting symptoms usually consist of dyspnea and nonproductive cough. Radiographic features on standard radiographs (Fig. 7-25) include a reticulonodular pattern, that is, a combination of lines and nodules that are usually bilateral and symmetrical with the apical areas involved more than the bases. There is typical sparing of the costophrenic sulci. The lung volumes are characteristically normal or increased. Occasionally you can recognize thin-walled cysts. Pneumothorax is a frequent complication occurring in 20% to 30% of cases, and it may be recurrent. HRCT findings (Fig. 7-3) include thin-walled lung cysts usually less than 1 cm. Occasionally the cysts may have bizarre shapes. The other fairly constant feature of histiocytosis is the presence of nodules that are typically located in a centrilobular and peribronchiolar distribution (Fig. 7-26). They range in size from 1 mm to 1 cm. These nodules may cavitate, and there appears to be a progression from the purely nodular form through a phase of cavitation and subsequent development of thin-walled cysts. On CT you will note upper-lobe predominance with costophrenic angle sparing. Differential diagnosis includes primarily lymphangioleiomyomatosis, but the presence of nodules is a highly useful distinguishing feature. As in lymphangioleiomyomatosis, the cysts must be differentiated from honeycombing caused by IPF. Distinctive features are noted above. There is a large differential diagnosis of other diseases characterized by nodules, and if cysts are not present the differentiation may be difficult.

GROUND-GLASS ATTENUATION

Ground-glass opacity is a nonspecific finding that may occur in a number of disease processes. In most instances it represents an active and potentially

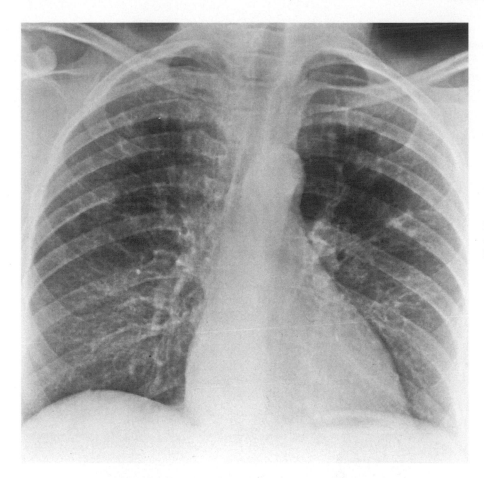

Fig. 7-25   Histiocytosis X. There is a reticular nodular pattern in the upper lobes. The lung volumes are preserved.

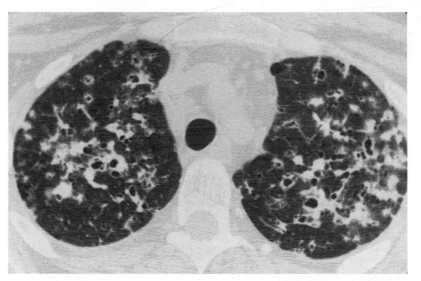

Fig. 7-26   Histiocytosis X. HRCT shows multiple irregular nodules, some of which are cavitating. There are also some thin-walled cysts.

reversible or treatable process, although in a minority of cases it may signify fibrosis. Many infiltrative lung diseases will demonstrate areas of ground-glass opacity interspersed with other patterns of disease that tend to be more predominant. These areas are likely to represent active alveolitis or active parenchymal disease. Hypersensitivity pneumonitis characteristically shows areas of ground-glass opacification on HRCT. (For more discussion, see Chapter 9).

Alveolar Proteinosis

Pulmonary alveolar proteinosis (Box 7-15) is a disease characterized pathologically by accumulation of large amounts of a proteinaceous material in the alveoli with little or no tissue reaction. The cause of the disease is unknown, although it has been suggested that excessive production or impaired removal of surfactant may be the mechanism underlying the alveolar filling process. The material in the alveoli stains positively with periodic acid-Schiff-positive (PAS-positive). Most cases are idiopathic, although some cases may result from overwhelming exposure to silica or immunologic disturbances due to hematologic and lymphatic malignancies

such as lymphoma or chemotherapy. The disease predominantly affects men between 30 and 50 years of age. Symptoms include nonproductive cough and dyspnea.

The chest radiographic findings are often dramatic (Fig. 7-27). The pattern is bilateral and symmetrical and is identical in both distribution and character to that of pulmonary edema. It consists of alveolar consolidation and ground-glass opacification in a typical butterfly or bat's-wing pattern. Occasionally there is a localized lobar consolidation or nodular pattern. You can differentiate this process from congestive heart failure by the absence of cardiomegaly and Kerley-B lines. Features on HRCT (Fig. 7-13) include primarily ground-glass opacity, although you can also see dense consolidation. Often the distribution is geographic with sharp demarcation of normal from abnormal areas. Thickening of the interlobular septa by edema may produce prominent septal lines. If smooth septal thickening is superimposed on the ground-glass opacification, it produces a pattern commonly referred to as crazy paving.

The prognosis in this disease has been improved by the use of bronchoalveolar lavage. However, relapse may occur after lavage, and repeated lavages may be necessary. Certain types of pulmonary infections may compli-

---

Box 7-15 Alveolar Proteinosis

CHARACTERISTICS

Cause unknown
Lipoproteinaceous material in alveoli
Male > Female, 30 to 50 years of age

RADIOGRAPHIC FEATURES

Consolidation or ground-glass opacities
Bilateral, symmetrical
Central

HIGH-RESOLUTION CT FINDINGS

Ground-glass opacity
Septal lines
Patchy distribution
"Crazy paving"

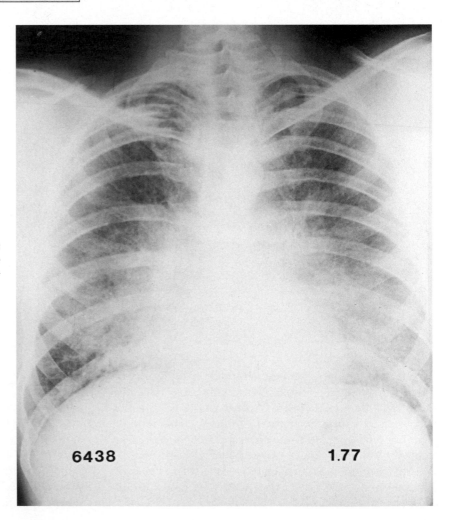

Fig. 7-27 Pulmonary alveolar proteinosis. There is ground-glass opacification and air space consolidation noted centrally in a pattern similar to pulmonary edema.

cate the course of alveolar proteinosis. These include particularly *Nocardiosis* and infection with *Aspergillus* and *Mucormycetes*.

PARENCHYMAL CONSOLIDATION

A number of diffuse infiltrative lung diseases may cause parenchymal consolidation or what has been previously referred to as "alveolar or air-space" disease. These may be chronic infiltrative disorders as well as acute diseases that are often infectious in etiology. (For discussion please see Chapters 3 and 11.)

Bronchiolitis Obliterans Organizing Pneumonia

Bronchiolitis obliterans organizing pneumonia (BOOP) (Box 7-16) is a typical example of a chronic infiltrative lung disease that produces parenchymal consolidation. It is characterized by the presence of granulation tissue and plugs within bronchioles that extend more peripherally into the alveolar ducts with patchy areas of organizing pneumonia. Despite the name of this disease, it is primarily an infiltrative lung disease rather than a true airway disease because the bronchiolitis tends to be a minor component. This disorder is referred to as cryptogenic organizing pneumonia in the United Kingdom.

The cause is unknown and most patients develop symptoms in middle age with a history of weeks to months of nonproductive cough. Dyspnea and a history of a flulike illness are common, but wheezing is rare. Many patients present with a history of antibiotic treatment for an atypical pneumonia. Most cases respond to steroid therapy, and the prognosis is good. On standard radiographs (Fig. 7-28) the characteristic

---

Box 7-16 Bronchiolitis Obliterans Organizing Pneumonia

CHARACTERISTICS

Patchy pneumonia and bronchiolitis
Middle age
Responds to steroids

RADIOGRAPHIC FEATURES

Patchy bilateral consolidation

HIGH-RESOLUTION CT FEATURES

May be peripheral
Bilateral patchy consolidation

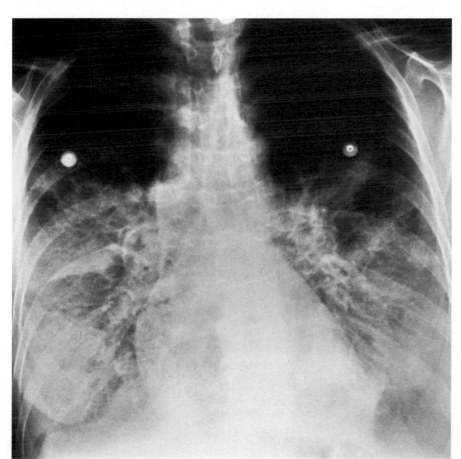

Fig. 7-28 Bronchiolitis obliterans-organizing pneumonia. PA radiograph shows areas of consolidation bilaterally in both lungs.

features of BOOP consist of patchy areas of air-space disease or consolidation, which are usually present bilaterally. This pattern occurs in close to 80% of patients. Small irregular or nodular opacities are uncommon. Pleural effusions, adenopathy, and cavitation are rare.

Relapse may occur after cessation of steroid therapy, and opacities may reappear in the same distribution.

On HRCT (Fig. 7-14) the typical feature is patchy air-space consolidation with air bronchograms. Approximately half of the cases may show a peripheral subpleural distribution. Often this distribution may not be readily evident on standard radiographs.

SUGGESTED READINGS

Carrington CB, Gaensler EA, Coutu RE et al: Natural history and treated course of usual and desquamative interstitial pneumonia, *N Engl J Med* 298:801-809, 1978.

Epler GR, Colby TV, McLoud TC et al: Idiopathic bronchiolitis obliterans with organizing pneumonia, *N Engl J Med* 312:152-159, 1985.

Epler GR, McLoud TC, Gaensler EA et al: Normal chest roentgenograms in chronic diffuse infiltrative lung disease, *N Engl J Med* 298:934-939, 1978.

Friedman PJ, Liebow AA, Sokoloff S: Eosinophilic granuloma of lung: clinical aspects of primary pulmonary histiocytosis in the adult, *Medicine* 60:385-396, 1981.

Godwin JD, Müller NL, Takasugi JE: Pulmonary alveolar proteinosis: CT findings, *Radiology* 169:609-613, 1988.

Heitzman ER: *Sarcoidosis,* St. Louis, 1984, Mosby–Year Book; pp 294-310.

Janower ML, Blennerhasset JB: Lymphangitic spread of metastatic tumor to lung, *Radiology* 101:267-273, 1971.

Lynch DA, Webb WR, Gamsu G: Computed tomography in pulmonary sarcoidosis, *J Comput Assist Tomogr* 13:405-410, 1989.

Mathisen JR, Mayo JR, Staples CA et al: Chronic diffuse infiltrative lung disease: comparison of diagnostic accuracy of CT and chest radiography, *Radiology* 171:111-116, 1989.

McLoud TC, Carrington CB, Gaensler EA: Diffuse infiltrative lung disease: a new scheme for description, *Radiology* 149:353-363, 1983.

McLoud TC: Diffuse infiltrative lung disease. In Putman CE, editor: *Pulmonary diagnosis: imaging and other techniques,* New York, 1991, Appleton Communications; pp 125-153.

Moore AD, Godwin JD, Müller NL et al: Pulmonary histiocytosis X: comparison of radiographic and CT findings, *Radiology* 172:249-254, 1989.

Müller NL, Chiles C, Kullnig P: Pulmonary lymphangioleiomyomatosis: correlation of CT with radiographic and functional findings, *Radiology* 175:335-339, 1990.

Müller NL, Miller RR, Webb WR et al: Fibrosing alveolitis: CT-pathologic correlation, *Radiology* 160:585-588, 1986.

Müller NL, Miller RR: Computed tomography of chronic diffuse infiltrative lung disease. Part II, *Am Rev Respir Dis* 142:1440-1448, 1990.

Müller NL, Miller RR: Computed tomography of chronic diffuse infiltrative lung disease. Part I, *Am Rev Respir Dis* 142:1206-1215, 1990.

Stein MG, May J, Müller N et al: Pulmonary lymphangitic spread of carcinoma. Appearances on CT scans, *Radiology* 162:371-375, 1987.

Webb WR, Müller NL, Naidich DP: *High resolution CT of the lung,* New York, 1992, Raven Press.

Webb WR: High resolution CT of the lung parenchyma, *Radiol Clin North Am* 27:1085-1097, 1989.

The Pneumoconioses

THERESA C. McLOUD

Many respiratory disorders can be occupationally induced. The most important of these are the pneumoconioses. A pneumoconiosis is a diagnosable disease produced by the inhalation of dust (particulate matter in the solid phase excluding living organisms). Mineral dust can be classified as fibrogenic, such as asbestos and silica; or inert, such as iron, tin, or barium. The metal dusts, beryllium and cobalt, are associated with granulomatous pneumonitis and giant cell pneumonitis, respectively (Table 8-1). Most pneumoconioses produce diffuse opacities on the chest radiograph that are similar to those seen in other infiltrative lung disorders.

INTERNATIONAL LABOUR ORGANIZATION CLASSIFICATION OF PNEUMOCONIOSES (BAR A)

The International Labour Organization (ILO) classification of the radiographic appearances of the pneumoconioses is a standardized internationally accepted system used to codify the radiographic changes in the pneu-

Table 8-1   Dust Diseases

Agent	Examples	Disorders
Mineral dusts	Asbestos	Pneumoconioses
	Silica	
	Coal	
Metal dusts	Iron	"Inert dust"
	Tin	pneumoconioses
	Barium	
Metal dusts	Beryllium	Granulomatous
		pneumonitis
	Cobalt	Giant cell pneumonitis
Biologic dusts	Spores	Hypersensitivity
	Mycelia	pneumonitis (allergic
	Bird droppings	alveolitis)

Box 8-1   International Labour Organization (ILO) Classification of Pneumoconioses

OPACITIES

Small
   Rounded (*p, q, r*)
   Irregular (*s, t, u*)
Large
   A (1–5 cm)
   B (cm^2 = RU)
   C (cm^2 > RU)

ZONES

RU LU
RM LM
RL LL

PROFUSION (SEVERITY)

0 (normal 0/–, 0/0, 0/1)
1 (slight 1/0, 1/1, 1/2)
2 (moderate 2/1, 2/2, 2/3)
3 (severe 3/2, 3/3, 3/+)

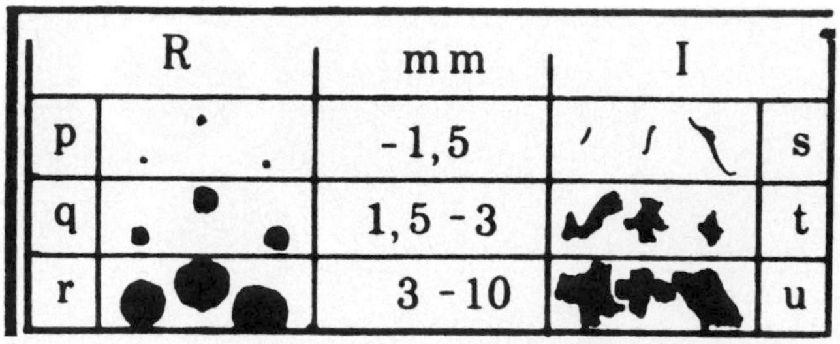

Figure 8-1. Diagrammatic representation of small opacities in the ILO classification. *R*, small rounded (nodules). *I*, small irregular (lines).

There are four basic categories: *0*, normal; *1*, slight; *2*, moderate; and *3*, advanced. The distribution and extent of opacities are recorded in six zones. In addition, there is a convention for large opacities that describes the conglomerate masses identified in some of the pneumoconioses.

The 1980 ILO classification also includes detailed categorization of pleural thickening that is quantified and classified as diffuse or circumscribed (plaque).

SILICOSIS

General Description

Silicosis (Box 8-2) is a fibrotic disease of the lungs caused by inhalation of dust containing free crystalline silica or silicon dioxide. It is the predominant constituent of the earth's crust. Silica dust may be encountered in almost any mining, quarrying, or tunneling operation. Occupations at risk, therefore, include the mining of heavy metals, such as gold, tin, copper, silver, nickel, and uranium and to a lesser extent coal; the pottery industry, sandblasting; foundry work; and stone masonry. Silicosis is usually a chronic slowly progressive disease that occurs with at least a latency period of 20 years.

Simple Silicosis

Simple silicosis (Box 8-3) has no symptoms or any significant changes in pulmonary function.

Pathologic findings

The pathologic findings consist of fibrotic nodules with a typical whorled appearance that have the greatest profusion in the apical and posterior regions of the upper and apical region of the lower lobes.

Radiographic findings

Classical radiographic findings consist of multiple nodules or "small rounded opacities" 1 to 10 mm in diameter (Fig. 8-2). Larger nodules often predominate, and the distribution is typically more in the upper lung zones. Occasionally the nodules calcify. Enlargement of lymph nodes is common and may precede the appearance of dif-

moconioses in a reproducible manner (Box 8-1). The advantage of the system is that it provides graphic and morphometric terms to describe diffuse lung patterns. The classification includes conventions of small rounded (nodules) and small irregular (linear and reticular) opacities (Fig. 8-1). The small rounded opacities are classified according to the approximate diameter of the predominant opacity: *p*, up to 1.5 mm in diameter; *q*, 1.5 to 3 mm in diameter; and *r*, 3 to 10 mm in diameter. Small irregular opacities are divided on the basis of thickness into: *s*, fine; *t*, medium; and *u*, coarse or blotchy irregular opacities.

The ILO scheme also provides for quantification of the radiographic severity or "profusion" on a 12-point scale.

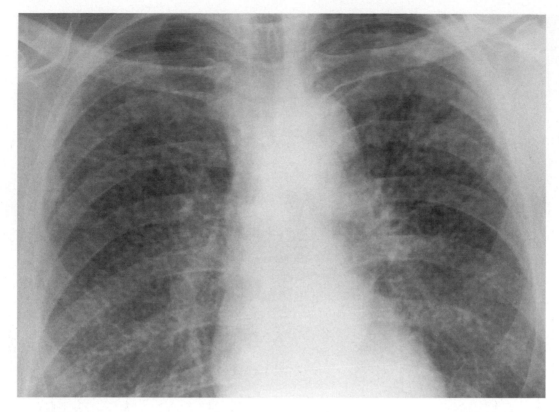

Figure 8-2. Simple silicosis. There are multiple small (2—4 mm) nodules distributed throughout the lungs with an upper lobe predominance.

Box 8-2 Silicosis

CHARACTERISTICS

Occupations
    Mining heavy metals
    Foundry work
    Pottery industry
    Sandblasting
20-year latency period

TYPES

Simple
Complicated
Acute or accelerated
Caplan's syndrome

Box 8-3 Simple Silicosis

CHARACTERISTICS

Pathology—fibrotic nodules
No changes pulmonary function

RADIOLOGIC FEATURES

Small nodules
Upper zones
Occasional calcification
Adenopathy, eggshell calcification

---

fuse nodularity. Calcification of the periphery of hilar and mediastinal nodes may occur. This is termed eggshell calcification and it has a characteristic appearance (Fig. 8-3).

Use of CT

Because both silicosis and coal worker's pneumoconiosis exhibit a nodular pattern, you should use both conventional CT and high-resolution CT (HRCT). CT clearly depicts the characteristic nodules in patients with simple silicosis, and it is more sensitive in the detection of such nodules than conventional radiographs. Conventional 10-mm CT is preferred because the thin sections in HRCT may cause you to underestimate the prevalence of nodules, and it is often difficult to differentiate small nodules from normal pulmonary vessels. However, you should supplement conventional scans with thin-section HRCT to depict fine parenchymal detail. You can limit these and perform them at preselected levels. Be sure to include at least three slices through the upper lung zones where nodules of silicosis predominate.

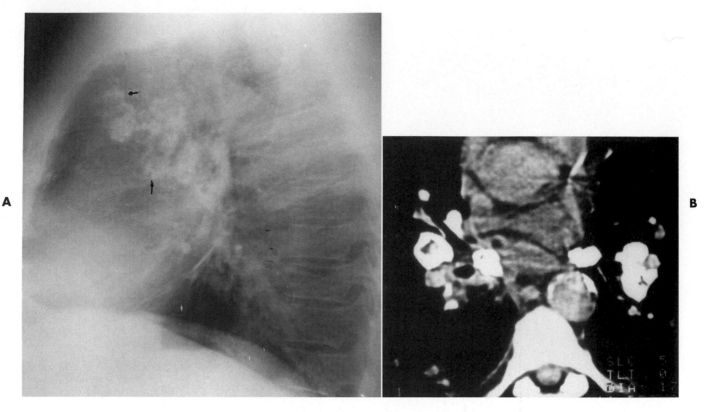

Figure 8-3. Eggshell calcification. **A,** Lateral chest radiograph shows multiple calcified nodes, some with peripheral calcification (*arrows*). **B,** CT of another patient with silicosis demonstrates densely calcified nodes; eggshell configuration can be seen in a right hilar node.

Complicated Silicosis

Characteristics

Complicated silicosis (Box 8-4) is characterized by the appearance of one or more areas in which the silicotic nodules have become confluent (>1 cm in size). These areas may contain obliterated blood vessels and bronchi. Complicated silicosis is associated with symptoms and often disability.

Radiographic findings

On the chest radiograph these opacities appear in the mid-zone or in the periphery of the lung in the upper lobes. (Fig. 8-4) They tend to migrate to the hilum, leaving overinflated emphysematous lung tissue in the surrounding lung, particularly at the bases. The more extensive the progressive massive fibrosis, the less the apparent nodularity in the remaining lungs.

As conglomeration develops the lungs gradually lose volume, and cavitation of the masses may occur secondary to ischemic necrosis. In this setting tuberculosis or infection with atypical mycobacteria may supervene. Superimposed tuberculosis may be difficult to detect radiographically; findings such as cavitation of conglomerate masses, pleural reaction at the apices, or other rapid radiographic changes are suggestive (Fig. 8-5). The

Box 8-4 Complicated Silicosis
CHARACTERISTICS
Confluent fibrosis
>1 cm
Associated with symptoms, dyspnea, cough
Complication: tuberculosis
RADIOLOGIC FEATURES
Upper or middle zones
Periphery migrating to hilum
Surrounding emphysema
Vertical orientation
Cavitation (ischemia or tuberculosis)
CT
Earlier detection of coalescence
Better detection of emphysema

diagnosis of supervening tuberculosis, however, is bacteriologic rather than radiologic.

CT findings

CT features are similar to those seen on standard radiographs, but coalescence of nodules and the develop-

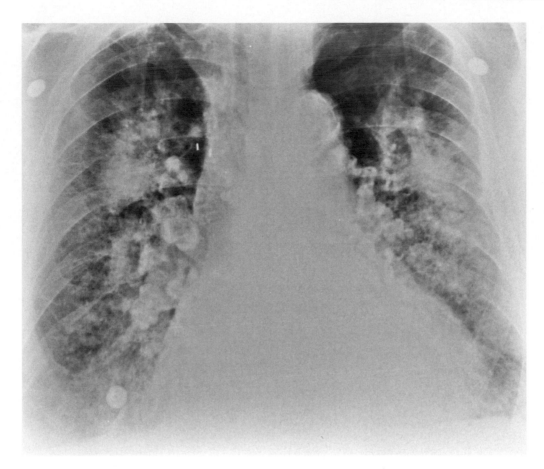

Figure 8-4. Complicated silicosis with progressive massive fibrosis. Large vertically oriented masses can be observed in the upper and middle lung zones midway between the hila and lateral pleura. Note eggshell calcification in nodes.

ment of conglomerate masses can often be detected at an earlier stage. Conglomerate masses of complicated silicosis can be seen to be associated with disruption of normal vessels and bulla formation (Fig 8-6). CT is also better at revealing gross disruption of the pulmonary parenchyma in the upper lung zones in complicated disease.

Accelerated Silicosis and Acute Silicosis

Accelerated silicosis

Accelerated silicosis (Box 8-5) often occurs after exposure to high concentrations of silica over a relatively short period, usually a few years. The radiographic and CT features are similar to those in simple silicosis.

Acute silicosis

Acute silicosis or silicoproteinosis (Box 8-5) generally occurs as a consequence of exposure to large quantities of fine particulate silica in enclosed spaces over a period of a few weeks. Pathologically the alveoli are filled with an eosinophilic and lipid-rich exudate, which is periodic-acid-Schiff (PAS) positive. The disease rapidly progresses, and death occurs due to respiratory failure.

Box 8-5   Accelerated and Acute Silicosis

ACCELERATED

High concentration of silica
Exposure over short period of time
Simple silicosis

ACUTE

Characteristics
    Few weeks' exposure
    Lipoproteinaceous fluid in alveoli (proteinosis)
    Rapidly progressive, high mortality
Radiologic features
    Air-space consolidation, perihilar
    Identical to pulmonary alveolar proteinosis

The radiographic appearance is quite different from classical simple silicosis. Acute silicosis has a pattern of diffuse consolidation or air-space disease with a perihilar distribution and air bronchograms. Radiographic and pathologic findings are similar to those in alveolar proteinosis. Mycobacterial infection is quite prevalent (25%), and half of the cases are due to atypical organisms.

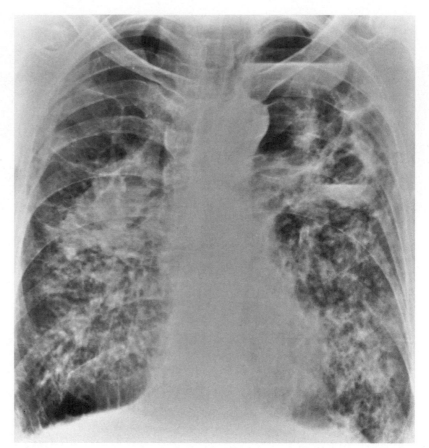

Figure 8-5. Silicotuberculosis. Areas of massive fibrosis are present in the right perihilar area and left upper lobe. There are cavities with air/fluid levels in the left upper lobe. Sputum culture positive for *Mycobacterium tuberculosis*.

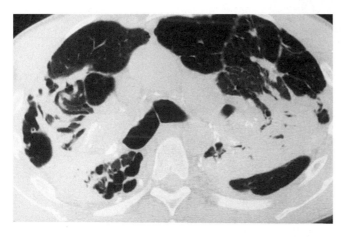

Figure 8-6. Complicated silicosis. Large masses are identified in the upper lobes associated with architectural distortion, bullae, and paracicatricial emphysema.

Caplan's Syndrome

A number of connective tissue diseases occur with increased prevalence in silicosis, including progressive systemic sclerosis, rheumatoid arthritis, Caplan's syndrome, and systemic lupus erythematosus. Caplan's syndrome (Box 8-6) consists of the presence of large necrobiotic nodules (rheumatoid nodules) superimposed on a background of simple silicosis or coal worker's pneumoconiosis (Fig. 8-7). It is a manifestation of rheumatoid

---

Box 8-6   Caplan's Syndrome

CHARACTERISTICS

Simple silicosis or coal worker's pneumoconiosis
Rheumatoid nodules

RADIOLOGIC FEATURES

Multiple nodules 0.5–5 cm
Cavitation
Calcification

---

lung disease and is seen more commonly in coal worker's pneumoconiosis than in silicosis. The nodules measure from 0.5 to 5 cm, and they may cavitate and calcify. Although they most often develop concomitantly with the joint disease, their formation may precede the onset of arthritis by months or years.

COAL WORKER'S PNEUMOCONIOSIS

Coal worker's pneumoconiosis (CWP) is a compensable occupational disease in the United States. This disease is common particularly in underground miners. In studies of CWP among this population prevalences varying from 9% to 27% have been reported.

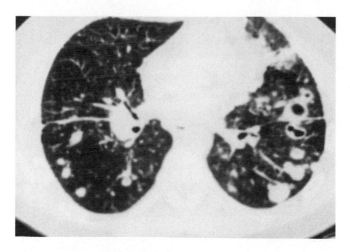

Figure 8-7. Caplan's syndrome. CT scan. Multiple nodules greater than 1 cm, several of which are calcified, can be identified. There is a background of smaller nodules due to simple CWP.

Box 8-7 Simple Coal Worker's Pneumoconiosis
CHARACTERISTICS Coal dust alone Pathology—coal macule Minimal fibrosis **RADIOLOGIC FEATURES** Small nodules Upper zones Lymphadenopathy Eggshell calcification **CT** Parenchymal and subpleural micronodules Pseudoplaques Centrilobular emphysema

---

Simple Coal Worker's Pneumoconiosis

Causes and pathology

Simple coal worker's pneumoconiosis (Box 8-7) results from the retention of coal dust alone. Pathologically, the hallmark of CWP is the coal macule. It consists of aggregations of dust around dilated respiratory bronchioles. There is minimal fibrosis. Simple coal worker's pneumoconiosis is not associated with any significant functional impairment, and workers are usually asymptomatic.

Radiographic findings

The findings on the chest radiograph consist of small nodules, which are predominant in the upper lobes. In contrast to silicosis, once the exposure to coal dust subsides or ceases, the nodules become stable without further evidence of progression.

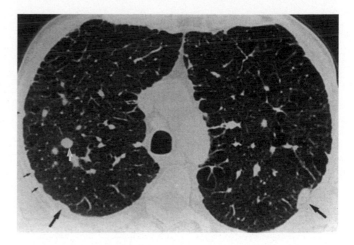

Figure 8-8. HRCT. Coal worker's pneumoconiosis. There are micronodules less than 7 mm in diameter subpleurally (*small black arrows*). In some areas they have become confluent, forming pseudoplaques (*large arrows*). Larger nodules can be seen deep in the lung parenchyma (*white arrow*). (Courtesy of Dr. Martine Remy-Jardin, Lille, France.)

CT findings

The CT findings in simple coal worker's pneumoconiosis include parenchymal and subpleural micronodules (nodules less than 7 mm in diameter) (Fig. 8-8). The nodules show an upper zone and right-sided predominance. When they occur in the subpleural zones they may become confluent, forming pseudoplaques. These consist of subpleural focal linear areas of increased attenuation that are less than 7 mm wide. Larger nodules between 7 and 20 mm in diameter can be seen scattered on a background of micronodules.

Hilar and Mediastinal Lymph Nodes

"Eggshell" calcification of hilar and mediastinal lymph nodes is a feature of CWP. Adenopathy may occur in any of the mediastinal lymph-node groups, but it seldom exceeds more than 2 cm in diameter.

Complicated Coal Worker's Pneumoconiosis

General description

Complicated coal worker's pneumoconiosis (Box 8-8) is also called progressive massive fibrosis (PMF). It occurs on a background of simple CWP. PMF may possibly result from additional exposure to silica. PMF may develop many years after exposure has ceased and it may progress in the absence of further exposure. It is associated with respiratory impairment, disability, and premature death.

Radiographic findings

The radiologic features consist of large opacities identical to those described above in silicosis. The ILO classification recognizes complicated CWP when a single opacity on the chest radiograph measures more than 1 cm in

Box 8-8 Complicated Coal Worker's Pneumoconiosis

CHARACTERISTICS

Progressive massive fibrosis (PMF)
>1 cm
Upper lobes and superior segments of lower lobes
Respiratory impairment

RADIOLOGIC FEATURES

Similar to complicated silicosis
Scar emphysema
Cavitation (tuberculosis)

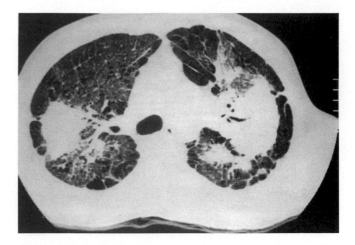

Figure 8-9. Complicated coal worker's pneumoconiosis. HRCT demonstrates large masses in the upper zones with irregular borders and associated paracicatricial emphysema.

diameter. Massive lesions tend to occur in the upper lobes or apical parts of the lower lobes and may cavitate.

CT findings

On CT you can identify two categories of lesions of PMF: (1) masses with irregular borders that are usually associated with gross disruption of the pulmonary parenchyma and scar emphysema occasionally with bulla formation (Fig. 8-9); (2) masses with regular borders and without emphysema. Aggregation and fusion of groups of smaller fibrotic nodules probably produce the first group. There is a typical predilection for the upper and posterior portions of the lung. Cavitation may occur and may be complicated by infections such as tuberculosis or intracavitary aspergilloma.

Emphysema

Coal miners have all types of emphysema, including panacinar, paraseptal, centrilobular, and scar. Centrilobular is the most common, and it is considered an integral part of the lesion of CWP. It is defined by a zone of enlarged air spaces within and around the coal dust macule. There are two major forms of emphysema in coal workers, and these are particularly visible on CT: (1) bullae and paracicatricial lesions, that is, scar emphysema around PMF lesions (Fig. 8-9); and (2) nonbullous emphysema, that is, centrilobular emphysema characterized by areas of low attenuation without definable walls. Centrilobular emphysema may occur in coal workers with nodular opacities independent of smoking history.

ASBESTOS-RELATED DISEASE

Public Health Interest

Exposure to asbestos is an important public health hazard in all industrial societies. The problem is of widespread public interest, in part because of the ubiquity of the material in daily life and also because of the asso-

ciation of pulmonary fibrosis and malignant disease with the inhalation of fibers. Asbestos is the generic term for several fibrous silicate minerals that share the property of heat resistance. There are two large groups: the serpentines and the amphiboles. Chrysotile is the only asbestos mineral in the serpentine group and accounts for more than 90% of asbestos used in the United States. The amphiboles include crocidolite (blue asbestos), amosite (brown asbestos), anthrophyllite, and tremolite. Although the use of asbestos has declined precipitously since the late 1970s, its use was widespread earlier in the century. The major sources of exposure to asbestos have included (1) primary occupations of asbestos mining and its processing in a mill; and (2) secondary occupations such as insulation manufacturing, textile manufacturing, construction, shipbuilding, and the manufacture and repair of gaskets and brake linings. High exposures in the United States ceased after the late 1970s because of federal regulations and strict industrial hygiene.

General Description

There is a 20-year latency period between initial exposure and the development of many asbestos-related diseases. Changes in the pleura are the most common finding. There may also be interstitial fibrosis (asbestosis) and benign masses in the lung that are usually associated with pleural thickening. A variety of malignancies can also occur.

Pleural Manifestations

Pleural plaques

Pleural plaques (Box 8-9) are the most common manifestation of asbestos exposure. They do not produce any symptoms and are incidentally discovered. You will see them as focal irregular areas of pleural thickening that involve the parietal pleura and occasionally the fissures. They are composed of dense bands of avascular collagen and are not considered premalignant.

On the chest radiograph, plaques are identifiable as localized, limited, plateaulike, smooth, and nodular areas of pleural thickening (Fig. 8-10). They may be seen in "profile" or "en face." A plaque seen in profile appears as a well-marginated dense band of soft tissue ranging from 1 to 10 mm in thickness paralleling the inner margin of the lateral thoracic wall. Plaques are usually bilateral, often symmetric, and more prominent in the lower half of the thorax between the sixth and ninth ribs. The apices and costophrenic angles are usually spared. When seen en face, a pleural plaque appears as a faint, ill-defined, veil-like opacity with irregular edges.

CT is more sensitive than standard radiographs in the detection of plaques and typically shows more pleural plaques and calcification (Fig. 8-11). It is also associated with fewer false positive readings of plaques than on standard films.

Diffuse pleural thickening

Diffuse pleural thickening (Box 8-10) is less frequently seen. It is characterized by a uniform homogeneous density, smooth contours (no nodularity), and frequently by obliteration of the costophrenic angle (Fig. 8-12). It is often a residual of a previous benign asbestos effusion or pleurisy. It may be associated with clinical symptoms and physiologic abnormalities that are comparable in severity to that resulting from fibrothorax from other causes.

Subcostal fat may mimic pleural thickening in obese individuals. Typically it appears as a symmetric, smooth, soft-tissue density that parallels the chest wall and is thickest over the lung apices. CT may be helpful in distinguishing fat from diffuse thickening, in the identification of localized fat, and in assessing patients with a combination of fat and plaques. CT easily shows subcostal fat because of its low attenuation (Fig. 8-13).

You can identify diffuse pleural thickening on CT when the pleural thickening extends greater than 8 cm craniocaudally, 5 cm wide, and 3 cm thick. Diffuse pleur-

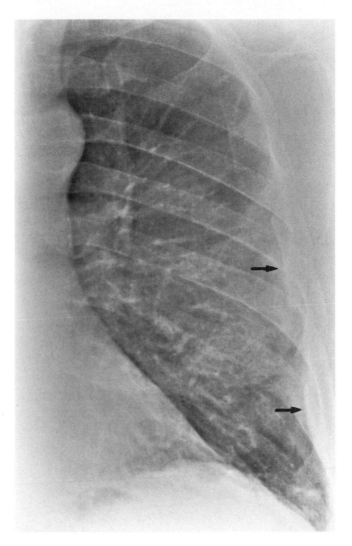

Figure 8-10. Pleural plaques. Multiple interrupted pleural plaques can be identified adjacent to the lateral chest wall (*arrows*). The apices and costophrenic angle are spared.

al thickening invariably involves the visceral pleura and the underlying lung parenchyma producing fibrous bands. There may be calcification.

Benign asbestos pleural effusion

A diffuse exudative pleural reaction following asbestos exposure (Box 8-11) may occur before other manifestations of asbestos-related disease (often within 10 years). The effusion may be unilateral, bilateral, or recurrent, and the diagnosis is made by exclusion of other diseases, particularly malignant mesothelioma. Occasionally the effusion may be bloody.

Most benign asbestos effusions are easily detected on standard PA and lateral chest radiographs. Decubitus films may be helpful in the demonstration of free-flowing fluid. Residual diffuse pleural thickening, usually with a blunted angle, occurs in roughly half of the patients with a benign asbestos pleurisy as the effusion resolves (Fig. 8-14).

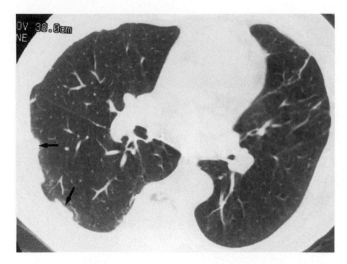

Figure 8-11. Pleural plaques. CT demonstrates multiple plaques on the right side (*arrows*).

Box 8-10   Diffuse Pleural Thickening

CHARACTERISTICS

Less common than plaques
Symptoms and respiratory impairment

RADIOLOGIC FEATURES

Smooth, extensive, involves costophrenic angle

CT

> 8 cm × 5 cm × 3 cm
Parenchymal bands

DIFFERENTIAL DIAGNOSIS

Subcostal fat
Malignant mesothelioma
Other causes of fibrothorax

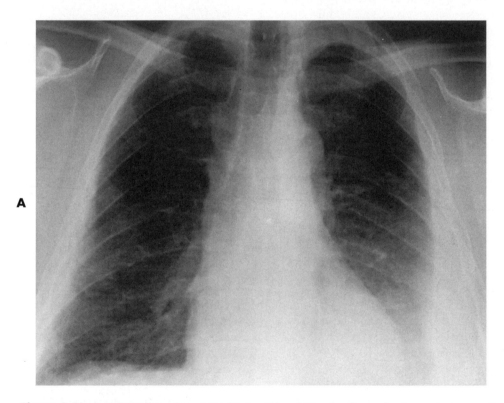

A

Figure 8-12. A & B, Diffuse pleural thickening. PA and lateral radiographs demonstrate smooth extensive thickening, which involves the lateral and posterior costophrenic angles on the left. Calcification may occur occasionally, as in this case (*arrow*).

Continued

B

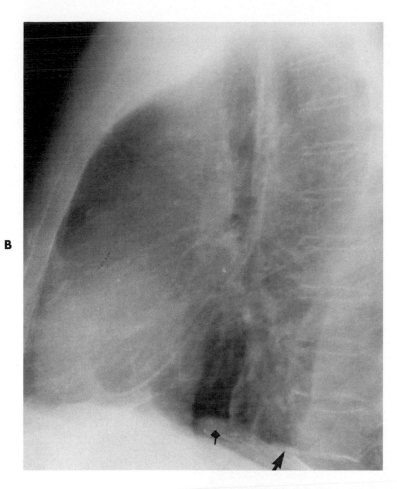

Figure 8-12, cont'd. For legend see opposite page.

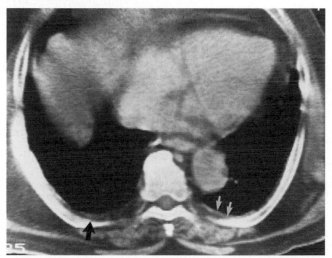

Figure 8-13. Extrapleural fat. CT scan demonstrates extrapleural fat (*black arrow*) deep to the posterior ribs bilaterally. There is also a pleural plaque on the left (*white arrows*). Note the prominent pericardial fat pad, which can often be seen in such patients. There may be associated mediastinal lipomatosis.

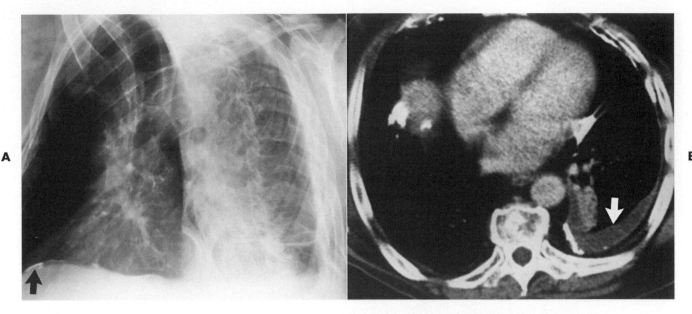

Figure 8-14. Benign asbestos pleurisy. Former shipyard worker with biopsy-proven, recurrent benign asbestos effusion. **A,** Right anterior oblique chest radiograph demonstrates diffuse pleural thickening on the left. There are also calcified plaques along the right hemidiaphragm (*arrow*). **B,** CT scan shows calcified pleural thickening on the left and a new left effusion (*arrow*).

Box 8-11   Benign Asbestos Effusion

CHARACTERISTICS

<10-year exposure
Exudate, may be bloody
Unilateral, bilateral, recurrent
Diagnosis of exclusion

RADIOLOGIC FEATURES

Effusion
Often leaves residual thickening

Box 8-12   Pleural Calcification

CHARACTERISTICS

Plaques or thickening
30 to 40 years after exposure

RADIOGRAPHIC FEATURES

Bilateral
Chest wall, diaphragm, cardiac border

Pleural calcification

Pleural calcification (Box 8-12) is a later manifestation of asbestos exposure, often seen 30 to 40 years after onset of exposure. It occurs within pleural plaques and occasionally within diffuse pleural thickening. Calcifications can be identified along the chest wall, diaphragm, or cardiac border. Viewed en face they show an irregular, unevenly dense pattern likened to the fringe of a holly leaf. PA and lateral chest radiographs best show pleural calcifications (Fig. 8-15). Oblique views and CT may be helpful in distinguishing calcified pleural plaques seen en face from underlying pulmonary parenchymal nodules.

Lung Manifestations

Diffuse interstitial fibrosis (also called asbestosis) is the most significant change that occurs in the lung secondary to asbestos exposure. You may also see several other benign radiographic changes in the lungs of these individuals.

Asbestosis

The term *asbestosis* (Box 8-13) should only refer to the pulmonary fibrosis that occurs in asbestos workers. Most workers in whom pulmonary fibrosis develops have been exposed to high dust concentrations for a prolonged period of time, and there is a definite dose—effect relationship. Symptoms include dyspnea and dry cough; functional abnormalities consist of progressive reduction of both vital capacity and diffusing capacity.

On pathologic examination pulmonary fibrosis is usually evident when there are 10 million asbestos fibers per gram of pulmonary tissue. The parenchymal fibrosis begins in and around the respiratory bronchioles in the lower lobes adjacent to the visceral pleura where asbestos fibers tend to accumulate. Progression of fibro-

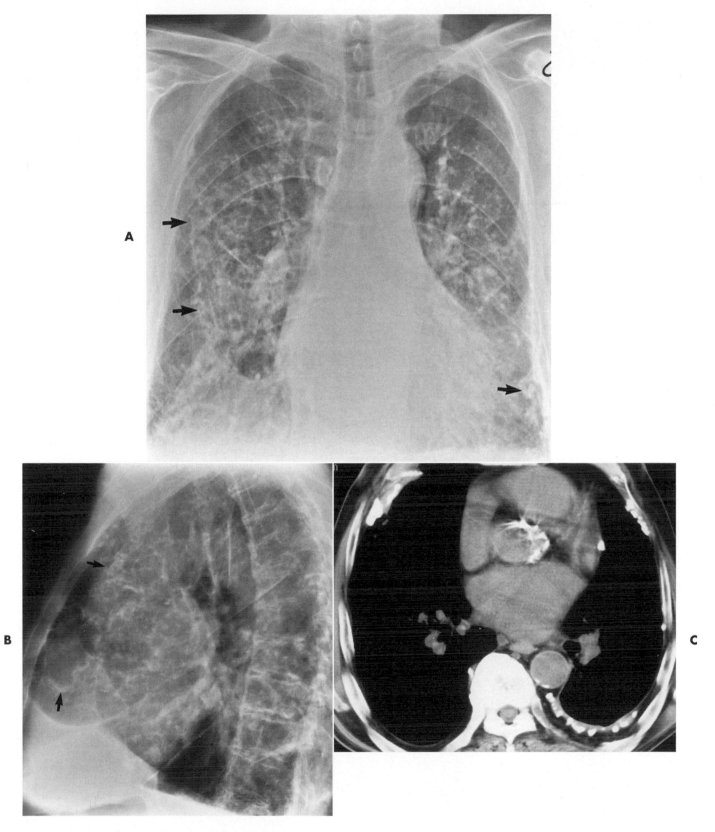

Figure 8-15. Pleural calcifications. **A & B,** Standard radiographs show extensive calcifications, many of which appear en face (*arrows*), reflecting calcified plaques along the anterior and posterior chest walls. **C,** CT scan confirms the presence of calcified plaques.

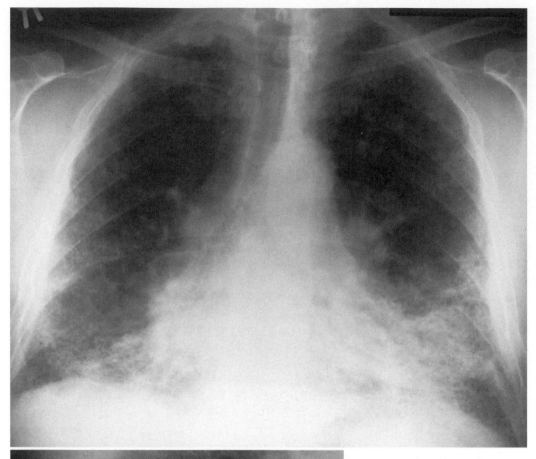

A

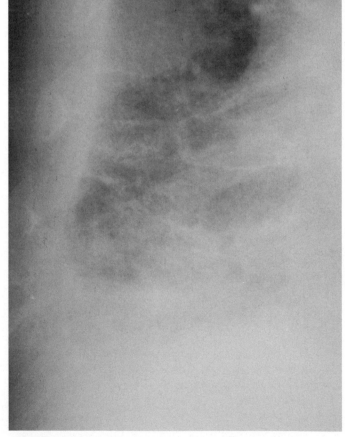

B

Figure 8-16. Asbestosis **A,** PA radiograph shows coarse linear opacities at both lung bases obscuring the cardiac borders. **B,** Cone-down view at the right base demonstrates associated pleural thickening.

Box 8-13   Asbestosis

CHARACTERISTICS

Pulmonary fibrosis
20-year latent period
Respiratory impairment

RADIOGRAPHIC FEATURES

Fine to coarse linear opacities
Bases
"Shaggy heart"
Plaques or diffuse thickening

CT

Early detection
Features
   Curvilinear subpleural lines
   Thickened interstitial short lines
   Subpleural dependent density
   Parenchymal bands
   Honeycombing

sis may lead to honeycombing with complete destruction of the alveolar architecture.

Standard radiographic findings include small linear or reticular opacities that predominate in the lung bases (Fig. 8-16). These may progress from a fine reticulation to a coarse linear pattern with honeycombing. A combination of parenchymal and pleural changes leads to partial obscuration of the heart border, the so-called shaggy heart. Radiographic findings are similar to those seen in idiopathic pulmonary fibrosis. The presence of pleural thickening or plaques lends support to the diagnosis of asbestosis, although plaques are not invariably present. Because lung biopsy is usually not warranted in individuals with asbestos exposure, the diagnosis of asbestosis rests on a combination of the history of exposure, restrictive pulmonary impairment including basilar crackles on physical examination, and radiographic evidence of small linear opacities. However, the standard radiograph may be normal in the presence of disease, and it may be further compromised by associated pleural disease, emphysema, and other parenchymal abnormalities.

CT is superior in characterizing and quantifying parenchymal abnormalities and in the detection of early asbestosis. It is currently the best noninvasive method to assess gross pathologic morphology. High-resolution CT with 1- to 2-mm collimation is preferred, and you should perform it through the bases of the lungs with the patient in both the prone and supine positions. All of the findings described on HRCT are nonspecific and may be seen in other interstitial lung disorders. Five major parenchymal abnormalities are identifiable on HRCT (Fig. 8-17): (1) curvilinear subpleural lines, (2) thickened interstitial short lines, (3) subpleural dependent density, (4) parenchymal bands, and (5) honeycombing. A subpleural curvilinear line is defined as a linear density of variable length within 1 cm and parallel to the chest wall. However, these lines may be observed in individuals without asbestos exposure; as a single finding they are certainly not diagnostic of asbestosis (Fig. 8-18). You may also see thickened interlobular septa that consist of lines 1 to 2 cm in length in the peripheral lung extending to the pleura. (For further discussion, see Chapters 1 and 7). These, the most common abnormalities in asbestosis, may be in combination with thickened core structures around the centrilobular bronchovascular bundles. Subpleural dependent density consists of a band of increased density 2 to 20 mm thick bordering the dependent pleura. Parenchymal bands (Fig. 8-19) or linear densities from 2 to 5 cm in length coursing through the lung are usually in contact with the pleura. These parenchymal bands are more likely secondary to pleural thickening and may represent atelectasis or fibrosis related to pleural disease rather than progressive interstitial fibrosis. Typical honeycombing occurs with advanced asbestosis.

In an asbestos-exposed individual with a normal chest radiograph, the presence of the above findings suggests the diagnosis of asbestosis but is not confirmatory. A combination of findings rather than isolated features is more likely to be conclusive.

Benign parenchymal lesions

In addition to asbestosis, other parenchymal abnormalities may occur in the lung parenchyma in individuals exposed to asbestos. These include rounded atelectasis, benign fibrotic masses, and transpulmonary bands.

Rounded atelectasis The most common of these is rounded atelectasis (Box 8-14), a form of peripheral lobar collapse that develops in patients with pleural disease. On a standard chest radiograph (Fig. 8-20), rounded atelectasis appears as a rounded, sharply marginated mass abutting the pleura. The mass, which has an intrapulmonary location as manifested by an acute angle between it and the pleura, usually occurs at the base of the lung. There is always pleural thickening and it often has greatest dimensions near the mass. The mass often has a curvilinear tail frequently referred to as comet tail sign. This is produced by the crowding together of bronchi and blood vessels that extend from the lower border of the mass to the hilum, creating a whorled appearance of the bronchovascular bundle. Occasionally, findings of volume loss may be associated with rounded atelectasis, although they are usually minimal. You should differentiate this mass from bronchogenic carcinoma, which occurs commonly in individuals exposed to asbestos. You can often appreciate these features on standard PA and lateral radiographs, but oblique views may be useful to demonstrate the rela-

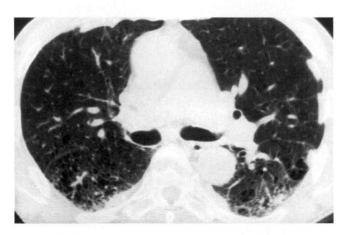

Figure 8-17. HRCT in asbestosis. There is evidence of subpleural-dependent density, interstitial lines, and honeycombing.

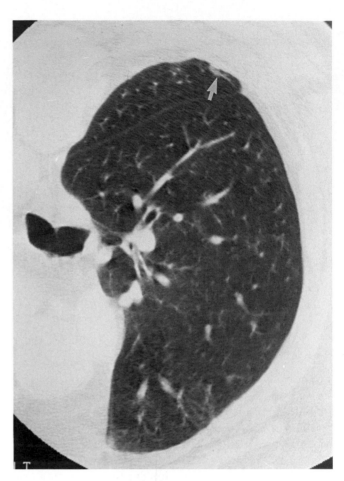

Figure 8-18. Subpleural curvilinear opacity. Prone HRCT shows a single short line paralleling the chest wall (*arrow*). As an isolated finding it is not diagnostic of asbestosis.

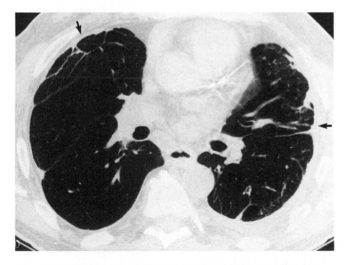

Figure 8-19. Parenchymal bands. HRCT demonstrates long linear bands bilaterally extending into the lung parenchyma. There is underlying pleural thickening on both sides (*arrows*).

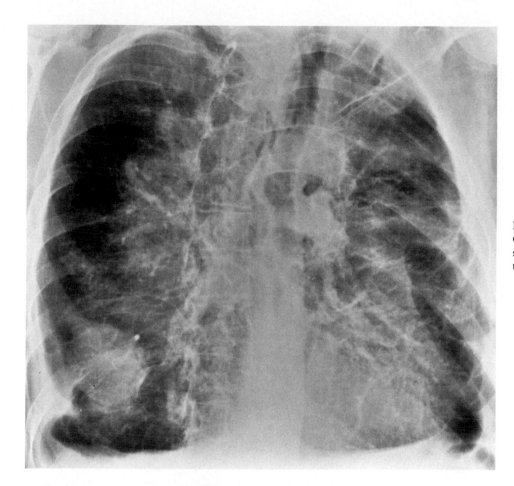

Figure 8-20. Rounded atelectasis. Oblique view of the chest demonstrates a right lower-lobe mass abutting pleural thickening.

Box 8-14   Rounded Atelectasis

CHARACTERISTICS

Peripheral location
Pleural disease

RADIOGRAPHIC AND CT FEATURES

Well-marginated mass
Occurs at base of lung
Pleural thickening
"Comet tail" sign

---

tionship of the peripheral mass to a thickened pleura. CT, however, is often required to make a definitive diagnosis (Fig. 8-21).

Other benign fibrotic masses   Other focal benign fibrotic masses may also occur in asbestos-exposed individuals. These are usually in a subpleural or occasionally a more central intraparenchymal location (Fig. 8-22). They may be wedge-shaped, lentiform, or rounded and may be associated with parenchymal bands that radiate into the surrounding lung. You must exclude bronchogenic carcinoma in patients with a parenchymal mass or nodules and known exposure to asbestos. You

should do a needle biopsy rather than radiographic follow-up because of the very high association between bronchogenic carcinoma and asbestos exposure.

Transpulmonary bands   Parenchymal or transpulmonary bands consist of linear opacities crossing the lungs that are generally found in the lower lobes (Figs. 8-19 and 8-22). They may be identified on standard radiographs, although they were originally described on CT. Frequently associated with visceral or parietal pleural thickening, they are thought to represent fibrotic projections that have merged with the pleura. Such bands may be involved with the development of rounded atelectasis because they serve as tethers to the atelectatic lung and the pleural-based mass. When the bands are multiple and radiate from a single point on the pleura they may produce a "crow's feet" appearance.

Malignant Neoplasms

Bronchogenic carcinoma

Bronchogenic carcinoma is estimated to develop in 20% to 25% of heavily exposed asbestos workers; it is a major cause of death in that group. Asbestos workers who smoke are at greater risk, perhaps as much as 80 to 100 times that in the nonsmoking, nonexposed population. The clinical presentation and radiographic features

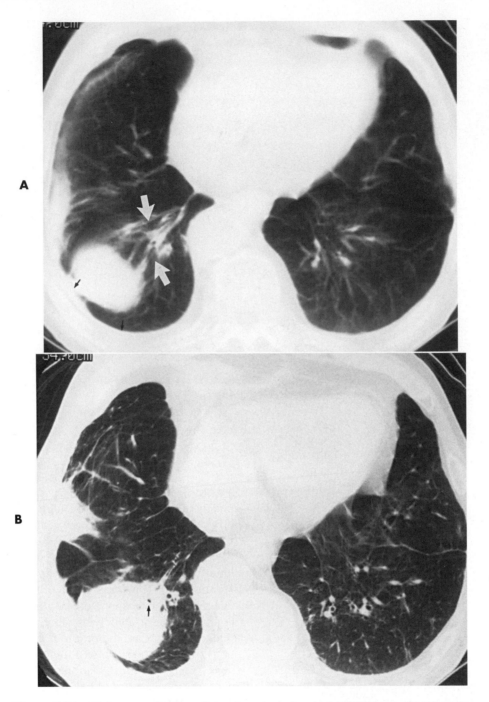

Figure 8-21. CT demonstrating rounded atelectasis. **A,** Standard CT (10-mm collimation) demonstrates a peripheral mass associated with pleural thickening (*black arrows*). Vessels and bronchi medial to the mass are crowded together forming a "comet tail" (*white arrows*). **B,** HRCT demonstrates loculations of air in the mass (pseudocavitation) (*arrow*).

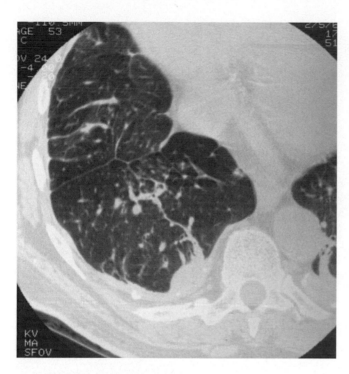

Figure 8-22. Benign fibrotic mass. CT shows a lentiform mass in the right lower lobe. There is associated pleural thickening, calcification, and parenchymal bands.

in asbestos workers with lung cancer are no different from other patients with this tumor. (For further discussion, see Chapter 11.)

Malignant mesothelioma

Malignant mesothelioma is an uncommon and fatal neoplasm of the pleural cavity, peritoneum, or both. It is highly associated with asbestos exposure, and the risk of mesothelioma in an asbestos worker is approximately 10% over his or her lifetime.

CHRONIC BERYLLIUM DISEASE

General Description

Chronic beryllium disease (Box 8-15) is a multisystem disorder caused by exposure to dust, fumes, or aerosols of beryllium metal or its salts. The major portal of entry is through the respiratory tract. Beryllium disease occurs in two forms: (1) an acute toxic chemical pneumonitis occurring after brief exposure to extremely high levels of airborne beryllium; and (2) chronic granulomatous pulmonary disease representing an immunologic response to long-term exposure. The acute form is a disease of the past and is rarely if ever identified.

Beryllium is used in a number of industries. It may be used as an alloy with copper in the manufacture of air-

---

Box 8-15   Chronic Beryllium Disease

CHARACTERISTICS

Multisystem disorder
Chronic granulomatous pulmonary disease
10- to 20-year latency
Pathology—Noncaseating granulomas

RADIOGRAPHIC FEATURES

Small nodules
All lung zones
Hilar adenopathy
Late disease
    Linear opacities
    Conglomerate masses
    Upper-lobe fibrosis

---

plane landing gear, electronics, undersea communication cables, and a wide variety of household appliances, including air conditioners and electric ranges. It is also used in aerospace applications and in glass windows of x-ray tubes.

Chronic beryllium disease is a granulomatous process involving primarily the lungs, but occasionally also the liver, spleen, lymph nodes, and bone marrow. You will sometimes see skin lesions. Chronic beryllium disease represents a cell-mediated hypersensitivity reaction to beryllium bound to tissue proteins. The characteristic pathologic finding is the epithelioid cell granuloma, which cannot be distinguished from the noncaseating granuloma of sarcoidosis. The disease usually presents 10 to 20 years after last exposure, and the most common presenting symptom is exertional dyspnea. Pulmonary function tests show a typical restrictive defect. Treatment of choice is corticosteroids, which usually prevent further progression and associated death and mortality.

Radiographic findings

The radiographic findings in chronic beryllium disease closely resemble those of sarcoidosis (Fig. 8-23). The most common finding is a nodular pattern or small rounded opacities, or occasionally, reticulonodular opacities involving all lung zones. Very small nodules up to 2 mm in diameter are most common and can produce a granular or sandpaper appearance. The small opacities may show gradual decrease over time, and following treatment with steroids the chest radiograph may show dramatic clearing.

In addition to small opacities, conglomerate masses occasionally develop. Radiographically they are similar in appearance to the conglomerate masses in patients with

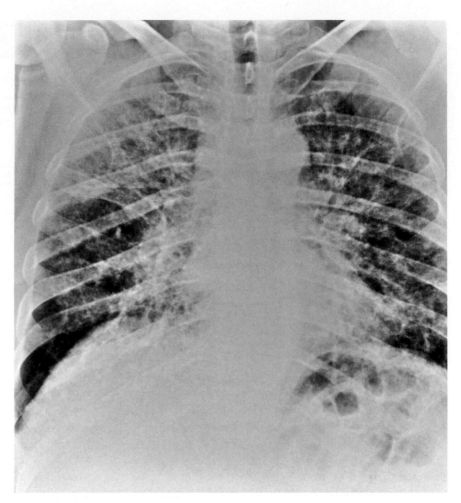

Figure 8-23. Chronic berylliosis. There are diffuse reticular-nodular opacities associated with right hilar and right paratracheal adenopathy.

silicosis. Hilar lymphadenopathy is also common with chronic beryllium disease. In long-standing disease, pulmonary fibrosis and contraction of the upper lobes may occur associated with emphysematous bullae. The opacities in the lung are usually linear at this stage. Pleural thickening may also develop, usually in the upper and middle zones of the thorax.

CT findings

There are few reports on the CT findings in berylliosis, but they are classically said to resemble those of sarcoidosis. You may find prominent thickening of the bronchovascular bundles and in the end stage, thin- and thick-walled cysts with traction bronchiectasis and lung distortion, particularly in the upper lobes.

NONFIBROGENIC DUSTS AND THEIR EFFECTS

Iron

Workers who inhale dust containing a high content of iron usually in the form of iron oxide may develop siderosis, a condition that is not associated with fibrosis or functional impairment. Workers at risk include those involved in the mining and processing of iron ore and metallic pigment and welding.

The radiographic pattern is a combination of lines and nodules creating a reticulonodular appearance involving all lung zones. The opacities may disappear partly or completely when patients are removed from dust exposure.

Tin

Pneumoconiosis caused by inhalation of tin is referred to as stannosis. Workers at risk include those who are employed in the handling of tin after it has been mined, especially in industries in which tin oxide fumes are created. The condition is not of any functional significance.

The radiographic findings are striking because of the high density of tin. Typically small nodules of high density, about 1 mm in diameter, are distributed evenly throughout the lungs.

Barium

Pulmonary disease secondary to exposure to barium and its salts, particularly barium sulfate, is known as barytosis. Because of the high density of barium (atomic number 56), the discrete opacities are extremely opaque. The apices and bases are usually spared, and large opacities do not occur. The lesions are usually nodular and characteristically regress after the patient is removed from the dust-filled environment.

SUGGESTED READINGS

Aronchick JM, Rossman MD, Miller WT: Chronic beryllium disease: diagnosis, radiographic findings, and correlation with pulmonary function tests, *Radiology* 163:677-682, 1987.

International Labour Office: Guidelines for the use of the ILO international classification of radiographs of pneumoconioses, 1980, Geneva, International Labour Office.

McLoud TC: Conventional radiography in the diagnosis of asbestos-related disease, *Radiol Clin North Am* 30:1177-1189, 1992.

Morgan WRC, Seaton A: *Occupational lung disease,* Philadelphia, 1984, WB Saunders.

Remy-Jardin M, Degreef JM, Beuscart R et al: Coal worker's pneumoconiosis: CT assessment in exposed workers and correlation with radiographic findings, *Radiology* 177:363-371, 1990.

Shipley RT: The 1980 ILO classification of radiographs of the pneumoconioses, *Radiol Clin North Am* 30:1135-1145, 1992.

Staples CA: Computed tomography in the evaluation of benign asbestos-related disorders, *Radiol Clin North Am* 30:1191-1207, 1992.

Staples CA, Gamsu G, Ray CS et al: High resolution computed tomography and lung function in asbestos-exposed workers with normal chest radiographs, *Am Rev Respir Dis* 139:1502-1508, 1989.

Stark P, Jacobsen F, Shaffer K: Standard imaging in silicosis and coal worker's pneumoconiosis, *Radiol Clin North Am* 30:1147-1154, 1992.

CHAPTER 9

Diseases of Altered Immunologic Activity

THERESA C. McLOUD, BEATRICE TROTMAN-DICKENSON

Radiologic Features
   Hydrochlorothiazide
   Interleukin-2 (IL-2)
   Amiodarone
   Nitrofurantoin
   Methotrexate
   Busulfan
   Bleomycin
   Cyclosporine
   Oily substances (lipoid pneumonia)
Pulmonary Lymphoproliferative Disorders
   General description
   Plasma-cell granuloma
   Psuedolymphoma
   Lymphocytic interstitial pneumonitis (LIP)
   Lymphomatoid granulomatosis
   Posttransplant lymphoproliferative disorders
Suggested Readings

A number of pulmonary disorders are associated with systemic or local bronchopulmonary immunologic alterations. Some of these disorders primarily involve the lung, and in others the pulmonary manifestations are secondary to disease arising elsewhere. The choice of diseases included in this chapter is somewhat arbitrary. For example, asthma is addressed elsewhere with other types of chronic obstructive pulmonary disease. Some of the infiltrative lung diseases such as sarcoidosis and occupational lung diseases such as silicosis and asbestosis are associated with multiple immunologic aberrations, but these are also discussed elsewhere.

IMMUNE REACTIONS

There are four basic types of immunologic reaction, all of which may be responsible for diseases in the lung. These reactions are not mutually exclusive, and the development of one type may be accompanied by the simultaneous or subsequent development of another (Box 9-1).

Type I

- Involves immediate hypersensitivity mediated by nonprecipitating antibody IgE or reagin
- Takes place on the surface of the mast cells
- Leads to the release of histamine and other mediators
- May be manifested by allergic asthma, the classic prototype in the lung

---

Box 9-1 Immune Reactions

TYPE
I   Immediate hypersensitivity
II   Cytotoxic
III   Immune complexes
IV   Delayed or tuberculin

- Is immediate and causes local infiltration with eosinophils

Type II

- Depends on cytotoxic tissue–specific antibodies
- Usually has complement that reacts with cells or other tissue elements
- Causes pathologic changes or death of cells
- Includes Goodpasture's syndrome involving the lung, the hemolytic anemias, and thrombocytopenic purpura

Type III

- Involves the formation of circulating immune complexes composed of antigen and antibody of the IgG or IgM type
- Activates complement
- Results in tissue damage of various types such as vasculitis, pneumonitis, and granulomatosis
- Results in a vasculitis if the complexes are precipitated within the endothelium of small vessels
- Is identifiable in collagen vascular disorders such as systemic lupus erythematosus, rheumatoid arthritis, and polyarteritis nodosa
- Has a reaction time of usually 2 to 4 hours
- Referred to as the Arthus reaction
- Includes allergic bronchopulmonary aspergillosis (sometimes associated with Type I reaction), hypersensitivity pneumonitis, and possibly interstitial fibrosis

Type IV

- Referred to as the delayed (or tuberculin) hypersensitivity
- Typically develops 24 to 48 hours after contact with the antigen
- Is mediated by sensitized T-lymphocytes
- Involves neither circulating antibodies nor complement

Box 9-2 Goodpasture's Syndrome

CHARACTERISTICS

Pulmonary hemorrhage
Iron-deficiency anemia
Glomerulonephritis

PATHOLOGY

Autoimmune
Antiglomerular basement membrane (anti-GBM)
   antibody

CLINICAL FEATURES

Young adult males
Hemoptysis
Anemia
Anti-GBM in serum

RADIOGRAPHIC FEATURES

Diffuse homogeneous consolidation
All lung zones
Irregular linear opacities during resolution

anti-GBM, antiglomerular basement membrane.

- Usually features granulation formation
- Includes the infectious and noninfectious granulomatous disease (tuberculosis and hypersensitivity pneumonitis)

GOODPASTURE'S SYNDROME

Characteristics

Goodpasture's syndrome (Box 9-2) is a disorder of unknown etiology characterized by repeated episodes of pulmonary hemorrhage, iron deficiency anemia, and glomerulonephritis. It is often rapidly progressive. The immunopathologic nature of the disease is apparent because of the linear deposits of immunoglobulins, which can be demonstrated in both the glomerular basement membrane and alveolar septa.

Pathology

The disorder is an autoimmune disease in which the renal and pulmonary lesions are mediated by an antiglomerular basement membrane (anti-GBM) antibody that cross-reacts with lung basement membrane. The majority of patients with Goodpasture's syndrome have circulating anti-GBM antibodies.

Clinical Features

The syndrome is classically a disease of young adult males. The initial and most frequent symptom is hemoptysis. Iron deficiency anemia is invariably present. Pulmonary hemorrhage commonly antedates the clinical manifestations of renal disease. Anti-GBM antibodies can be identified in the sera of patients with the disease.

Radiographic Features

The classic radiographic appearance of Goodpasture's syndrome consists of diffuse homogeneous consolidation or alveolar opacities distributed fairly uniformly throughout all lung zones (Fig. 9-1). These changes are characteristic of both the early stages of the disease and the development of acute pulmonary hemorrhage. Although the radiographic pattern is similar to that of cardiogenic pulmonary edema, conspicuosly absent features are cardiomegaly, Kerley-B lines, and pleural effusions. In the later stages the changes are dependent on the time sequence and the number of hemorrhages that have occured in the past. The alveolar consolidation seen during the acute episode may resolve in 2 to 3 days. Irregular or linear opacities often persist for an extended period. If bleeding is continuous or repetitive, these linear and occasionally nodular opacities become permanent as increasing amounts of hemosiderin are deposited within the interstitial tissue. You must distinguish Goodpasture's syndrome from pulmonary hemorrhage due to other causes such as idiopathic pulmonary hemorrhage (hemosiderosis) and numerous causes of vasculitis. Hemorrhage may occur rarely in patients receiving systemic anticoagulants.

Therapy

Current treatment consists of a combination of immunosuppressive therapy with cyclophosphamide, prednisone, and plasmaphoresis, which reduces the level of circulating anti-GBM antibody. Prognosis, however, still remains guarded.

CONNECTIVE TISSUE DISEASES

The connective tissue or collagen vascular diseases are a group of immunologically mediated disorders characterized by inflammation of joints, serosal membranes, connective tissue, and blood vessels in various organs. Pathologically, alterations occur in the connective tissue ground substance, which contains elastin, collagen, and reticulin. Edema, fibrinoid degeneration, and vascular lesions are characteristic.

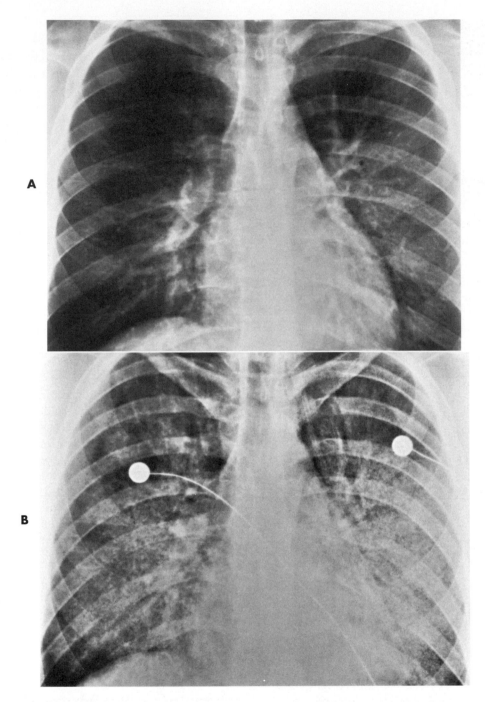

Figure 9-1. Goodpasture's syndrome. PA chest radiographs several days apart demonstrate consolidation in the left lung, **A,** which progressed to diffuse alveolar disease (consolidation), **B.**

Rheumatoid Disease

General description

Rheumatoid arthritis is a subacute or chronic disease that primarily affects the joints with a symmetrical inflammatory arthritis. Constitutional symptoms are frequent, and laboratory abnormalities include an elevated erythrocyte sedimentation rate and a high rheumatoid factor. Occasionally, rheumatoid arthritis may involve other organs and tissues including the lungs and pleura.

There are five pleuropulmonary abnormalities associated with rheumatoid disease. These include (1) pleurisy with or without effusion, (2) diffuse interstitial pneumonitis or fibrosis, (3) pulmonary (necrobiotic) nodules, (4) Caplan's syndrome (pneumoconiotic nodules), and (5) pulmonary hypertension secondary to rheumatoid vasculitis.

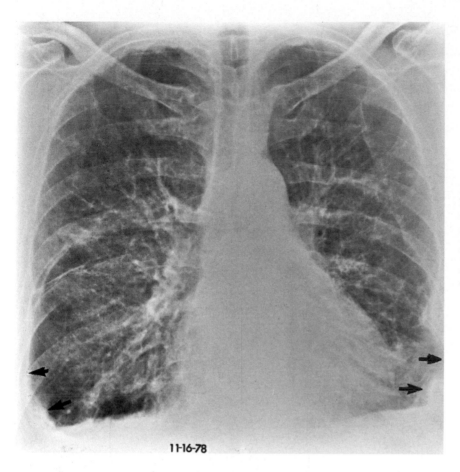

Figure 9-2. Rheumatoid lung—pleuropulmonary disease. PA chest radiograph shows linear opacities diffusely in both lungs indicating interstitial fibrosis. There is also bilateral pleural thickening (*arrows*) with blunting of both costophrenic angles. The patient had had recurrent bilateral rheumatoid pleurisy with effusions.

Box 9-3 Rheumatoid Pleurisy

Characteristics
  5% of cases
  Men > women
  Pleural fluid (low pH, low glucose, + Rheumatoid factor)
Radiographic features
  Small to moderate effusion
  Unilateral
  Often chronic

Rheumatoid pleurisy

Pleural involvement is the most common thoracic manifestation of rheumatoid disease (Box 9-3). Clinical evidence of rheumatoid pleurisy appears in about 5% of patients, but pleural involvement may be found in 50% of autopsy series. Pleural disease occurs much more frequently in men than in women with rheumatoid disease. Rheumatoid pleurisy usually occurs in the sixth decade of life and is associated with moderate to severe arthritis. Rheumatoid factor is present in both the serum and the pleural fluid in high titers. The pleural fluid is exudative and characterized by a low glucose concentration and low pH.

The chest radiograph usually shows a small- to moderate-sized pleural effusion. It is typically unilateral with a slight predominance on the right. Rheumatoid effusions tend to remain unchanged for many months or even years. Other manifestations of rheumatoid lung disease such as interstitial fibrosis are usually absent. The effusions may be recurrent and occasionally result in a diffusely thickened pleura or fibrothorax (Fig. 9-2).

Interstitial fibrosis and pneumonitis

Usual interstitial pneumonitis (UIP) and interstitial fibrosis (Box 9-4) may be seen in a variety of collagen vascular diseases. Pathologic changes are identical to idiopathic pulmonary fibrosis, although often the disease is less severe and more slowly progressive. The prevalence may be as high as 30%. Immunologically mediated injury most likely plays a central role in this interstitial pneumonitis, and immune complexes (Type III reaction) containing rheumatoid factor have been identified in alveolar walls and pulmonary capillaries by immunofluorescence.

The interstitial lung disease may occur before, after, or with the onset of arthritis. Symptoms classically consist of progressive dyspnea, and pulmonary function tests show evidence of restrictive ventilatory impairment.

The radiologic features of rheumatoid interstitial disease are identical to those seen in idiopathic pulmonary

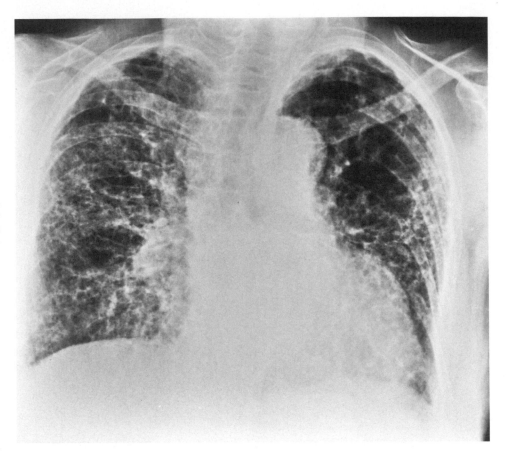

Figure 9-3. Rheumatoid interstitial fibrosis. There is advanced disease with a coarse linear pattern, which is diffuse and shows evidence of honeycombing.

Box 9-4 **Rheumatoid Interstitial Fibrosis and Pneumonitis**

CHARACTERISTICS

Type III reaction
Dyspnea and restrictive impairment

RADIOGRAPHIC FEATURES

Linear opacities
Bases
Honeycombing

CT FINDINGS

Reticular opacities
Subpleural zones
Thickened interlobular septa
Honeycombing

---

fibrosis (Fig. 9-3). In the early stages a pattern of fine linear or irregular opacities can be identified predominantly in the bases. This may progress to coarse reticulation with end-stage cystic changes and honeycombing. CT findings include reticular opacities located predominantly in the subpleural regions in the lung bases; irregular pleural and mediastinal interfaces; thickened interlobular septa; and honeycomb cysts. Progressive loss of volume or "shrinking lungs" may be observed on serial studies. Pleural effusion or thickening may be present. Occasionally other features of rheumatoid disease may be observed in the bony thorax, including typical arthritic changes in the shoulder, joints, and tapering of the distal clavicles.

Necrobiotic nodules

The intrapulmonary rheumatoid or necrobiotic nodule is pathologically identical to the subcutaneous nodule in rheumatoid arthritis. It may occur in the pleura and pericardium in addition to the lung parenchyma. It is a relatively rare manifestation of pulmonary rheumatoid disease, and it is usually associated with the presence of advanced arthritis and subcutaneous nodules.

Radiographically these lesions appear as multiple well-circumscribed pulmonary nodules usually located in the periphery of the lungs (Fig. 9-4). Cavitation is common, and the walls are usually thick and smooth. Changes in the size of nodules may be observed; these correlate with the activity and treatment status of the disease.

On pathologic examination these lesions are identical to the subcutaneous rheumatoid nodule, and they contain a central zone of fibrinoid necrosis surrounded by a zone of palisading fibroblasts oriented at right angles to the zone of necrosis. External to the palisade is a zone of cellular granulation tissue.

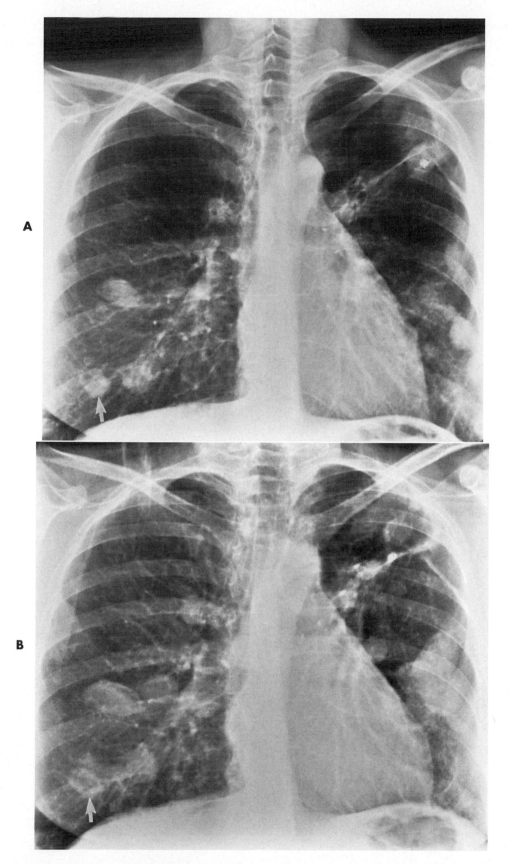

Figure 9-4. Rheumatoid necrobiotic nodules. **A** and **B,** Radiographs obtained 4 years apart show multiple nodules that are slowly increasing in size. There is cavitation in some of the nodules (*arrows*). An open-lung biopsy was performed of a nodule in the left upper lobe.

Caplan's syndrome

Please see Chapter 8 on the Pneumoconioses.

Pulmonary vasculitis and hypertension

In rare cases pulmonary vasculitis may cause pulmonary hypertension in rheumatoid arthritis; more commonly, pulmonary hypertension is secondary to end-stage fibrosis. The radiographic features consist of enlargement of the right side of the heart and dilation of central pulmonary arteries with rapid tapering of peripheral branches.

Scleroderma (Progressive Systemic Sclerosis)

Characteristics

Progressive systemic sclerosis or scleroderma (Box 9-5) is a connective tissue disease characterized by fibrosis and atrophy of the skin, lungs, gastrointestinal tract, heart, and kidneys. Patients are usually affected in the fourth to sixth decade of life, and the disease is three times more common in women than in men.

Following the esophagus, the lung is the second most frequently involved visceral organ. Chest radiographic abnormalities have been reported in up to 25% of cases. The pulmonary manifestations of scleroderma may take one of three forms: interstitial fibrosis is the most common, but pulmonary vascular disease and pleural changes may also occur. Although the pathogenesis of interstitial lung disease is unknown, an immunologic mechanism is likely. Vascular disease involving the arterioles and capillary bed frequently occurs in the lungs of scleroderma patients. These changes appear to be unrelated to the interstitial fibrosis and may occur independently. Pulmonary hypertension may develop as a consequence of these lesions.

Clinical features

Clinical symptoms include dyspnea and nonproductive cough. Pulmonary function abnormalities consist of restrictive pattern with a diminished diffusing capacity. Signs of cor pulmonale may occur at a later stage. Pulmonary hypertension is a frequent complication of sclerodema, and it appears to be independent of the duration of the disease or the severity of the interstitial fibrosis. It results from primary lesions in the small- and medium-sized pulmonary arteries that are characterized by intimal proliferation with myxomatous changes. Severe pulmonary hypertension is also found in CREST syndrome (calcinosis cutis, Raynaud's phenomenon, esophageal dysfunction, sclerodactyly, and telangectasia). It is a benign variant of scleroderma.

Pulmonary symptoms may also occur as a result of recurrent aspiration pneumonia secondary to disturbances of esophageal motility and distal esophageal strictures.

Radiographic features

The radiographic pattern is usually identical to that seen in idiopathic pulmonary fibrosis or rheumatoid lung. A fine linear pattern of small irregular opacities can be identified with predominant involvement at the bases. As the disease progresses, the pattern becomes coarser and eventually honeycomb cysts develop. Progressive loss of volume occurs over several years. Pleural involvement, however, is uncommon. On high-resolution CT (Fig. 9-5), findings are similar to those described in rheumatoid lung disease.

Box 9-5   Scleroderma (Progressive Systemic Sclerosis)

CHARACTERISTICS

Fibrosis and atrophy
    Skin
    Lung—second most common site
    Gastrointestinal tract (esophagus most common)

CLINICAL FEATURES

Females > males
Age 40 to 70 years
Dyspnea, cough, restrictive disease
Pulmonary hypertension
Recurrent aspiration

RADIOGRAPHIC FEATURES

Fibrosis
    Linear opacities
    Bases
    Calcinosis—soft tissues
    "Air esophagram"
Pulmonary arterial hypertension
    Dilated central arteries
    Rapid tapering
Chronic aspiration
    Basilar opacities
    Bronchiectasis

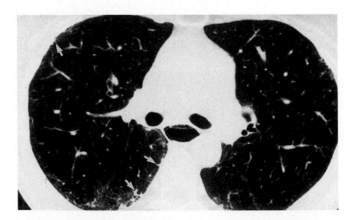

Figure 9-5. Progressive systemic sclerosis. HRCT. There are fine linear subpleural opacities (*arrows*) as well as a dilated esophagus.

Other nonpulmonary manifestations of scleroderma may be identified on the chest radiograph. Calcinosis may be present in the skin and subcutaneous tissue of the thorax, particularly about the shoulders. Atrophy and atony of the esophagus that results in absent peristalsis may also lead to dilation of the esophagus. On the chest radiograph and CT this is manifested by the presence of gas without an air/fluid level in a distended esophagus, the so-called air esophagram (Fig. 9-5). Dilation of the central pulmonary arteries with rapid tapering of peripheral vessels is characteristic of pulmonary arterial hypertension (Fig. 9-6).

Systemic Lupus Erythematosus

Systemic lupus erythematosus (SLE) is a chronic disease of unknown etiology that affects the components of connective tissue of multiple organs including the lungs. The vascular system, the epidermis, and serous and synovial membranes are the most commonly involved sites. The diagnosis of SLE is established by clinical and laboratory phenomena including a positive antinuclear antibody test and the lupus cell (LE cell phenomenon). SLE is the prototype of disease caused by a Type III immunologic reaction.

Young women are affected four times as often as men. Renal and central nervous system involvement and various infections are common determinants of survival. The lungs and pleura are involved more frequently in SLE than in any other collagen vascular disease, the prevalence ranging from 30% to 70% in several series.

The clinical manifestations of pleural pulmonary lupus are variable. Symptoms include cough with or without dyspnea, and pleuritis. Pleuritis occurs in 35% to 40% of patients and is often painful and accompanied by fever. Occasionally hemoptysis associated with pulmonary hemorrhage may be noted. The radiographic manifestations may be classified into the six categories (Box 9-6). More than one of these entities may be present in an individual patient.

Pleuritis and/or effusion

Pleuritis, effusion, or both are the most common pleuropulmonary abnormalities in SLE. Pleuritis is often an early manifestation of disease and is associated with exacerbations. The effusions are frequently bilateral and small, although they may be massive. Pericardial effusions may also be present (Fig. 9-7). The fluid is an exudate with a high protein content and normal glucose concentration.

Atelectasis

Atelectasis usually of the subsegmental variety can be identified on chest radiographs in patients with SLE.

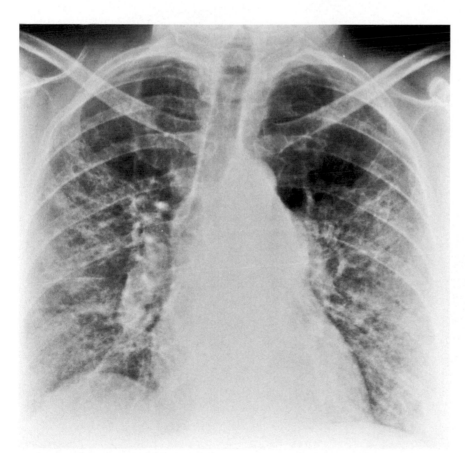

Figure 9-6. Scleroderma with pulmonary arterial hypertension. There is enlargement of the central pulmonary arteries as well as diffuse linear opacities in both lungs, indicative of interstitial fibrosis.

Figure 9-7. Lupus pleurisy and pericarditis. **A,** PA film shows enlargement of the cardiac silhouette suggestive of a pericardial effusion. There is also a small left pleural effusion. **B,** Four days later after steroid therapy, both the pericardial and pleural effusion have resolved.

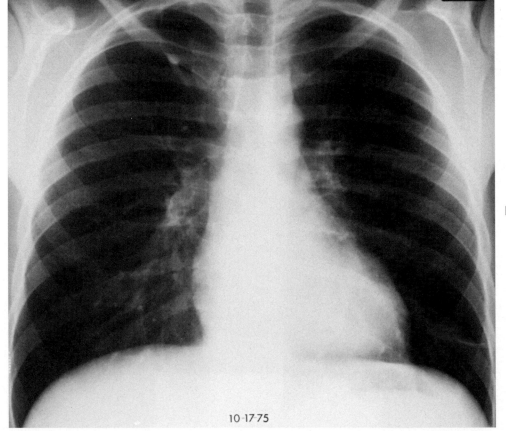

Box 9-6   Systemic Lupus Erythematosus

CHARACTERISTICS

Type III reaction
Positive antinuclear antibodies
Vascular system, epidermis, serous and synovial membranes
Young women more than men
Lungs and pleura
    30% to 70% cases
    Pleuritis

RADIOGRAPHIC FEATURES
Pleuritis and/or Effusion

Most common
Early
Bilateral, small
Pericardial effusion

Atelectasis

Subsegmental
Bases

Uremic Pulmonary Edema

Central alveolar opacities
Cardiac enlargement

Acute Lupus Pneumonitis

Uncommon
Vasculitis, hemorrhage
Widespread consolidation
Focal opacities at bases

Diffuse Interstitial Disease

Uncommon
Appearance identical to idiopathic pulmonary fusion

Diaphragmatic Dysfunction

Low lung volumes
Elevated hemidiaphragms

Box 9-7   Polymyositis/Dermatomyositis

CHARACTERISTICS

Autoimmune
Weakness, pain, atrophy of proximal muscle
Violaceous skin rash in about 50% of cases
Women:men = 2:1, first, fifth, and sixth decades
Types of lung disease
    Chronic interstitial pneumonia (<5%)
    Aspiration pneumonia
    Hypostatic pneumonia

RADIOGRAPHIC FEATURES

Basilar linear opacities
Small lung volumes
Unilateral or bilateral aspiration pneumonia
Soft-tissue calcification

These areas appear as horizontal line shadows generally at the bases. They may be migratory and fleeting. Such areas are often associated with pleural effusion or diaphragmatic dysfunction.

Uremic pulmonary edema

Uremic pulmonary edema is seen in the presence of severe renal failure in patients with SLE. The chest radiograph reveals evidence of cardiac enlargement and central alveolar opacities in a classic "butterfly" or "bat's wing" distribution.

Acute lupus pneumonitis

Acute lupus pneumonitis is an uncommon but well-recognized manifestation of SLE. It is characterized by severe dyspnea, nonproductive cough, fever, and hypoxia. The radiographic features (Fig. 9-8) consist of either poorly defined focal areas of increased opacity at the bases or widespread extensive unilateral or bilateral consolidation. These pulmonary opacities usually respond to steroids or cytotoxic drugs. The pathogenesis of this disorder is unclear, but histologic alterations include vasculitis and hemorrhage.

Diffuse interstitial lung disease

In contrast to other collagen vascular diseases, chronic interstitial lung disease in SLE is distinctly uncommon. Estimates of prevalence vary from 1% to 6%. Clinical symptoms and pulmonary function tests are identical to those found in other collagen vascular diseases with interstitial fibrosis. The radiographic changes are identical to idiophatic pulmonary fibrosis.

Diaphragmatic dysfunction

Diaphragmatic dysfunction with loss of lung volume is a fairly recently described abnormality in SLE. The etiology of this disorder is related to a diffuse myopathy affecting the diaphragmatic muscles. A chest radiograph will show evidence of elevated hemidiaphragms and loss of lung volume. On fluoroscopic examination diaphragmatic movement is sluggish.

Pleural effusions and pulmonary disease may be seen in cases of drug-induced lupuslike syndromes. Unlike cases of idiopathic SLE, the prognosis is excellent once the offending agent is discontinued.

Polymyositis/Dermatomyositis

General description

Polymyositis and dermatomyositis (Box 9-7) include a group of autoimmune disorders characterized by diffuse

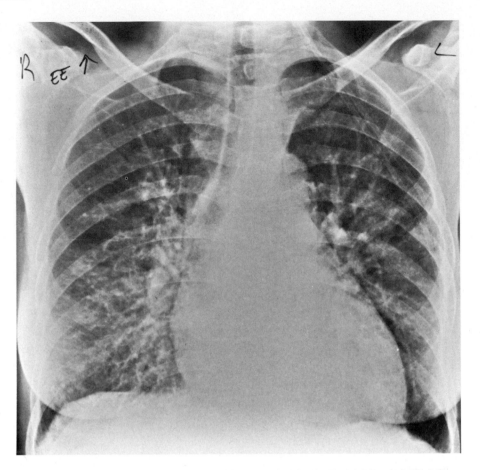

Figure 9-8. Acute lupus pneumonitis. Patchy consolidation is present in the right lung. Biopsy showed vasculitis and hemorrhage.

inflammatory and degenerative changes in striated muscle. A minority are associated with underlying malignancy. Symptoms include dyspnea on exertion and nonproductive cough. There is evidence of restriction on pulmonary function testing, and there may be a profound weakness of the muscles of respiration. The cause is unknown, and unlike other collagen vascular diseases, there are no circulating immune complexes.

Three types of pulmonary disease can be identified in this disorder: (1) chronic interstitial pneumonitis, (2) aspiration pneumonia due to a hypotonic esophagus, and (3) hypostatic pneumonia secondary to chest-wall involvement with resultant hypoventilation. The prevalence of interstitial pneumonitis is low, estimated to be around 5%.

Dermatomyositis/polymyositis is twice as common in women as in men and shows a peak incidence in the first decade and the fifth and sixth decades.

Radiologic features

The radiologic features consist of diffuse linear opacities of varied coarseness that predominate at the bases similar to other collagen vascular diseases. However, many patients may have a normal chest radiograph. When polymyositis involves the muscles of respiration, then diaphragmatic elevation with small lung volumes and areas of subsegmental atelectasis are apparent. Unilateral or bilateral aspiration pneumonia may result

when pharyngeal muscle paralysis is a feature. You may identify diffuse soft-tissue calcification on the chest film, a finding more often seen in children than in adults.

Mixed Connective Tissue Disease

Mixed connective tissue disease is a rheumatic disease syndrome that overlaps features of SLE, polymyositis, and scleroderma. It is distinguished from other collagen vascular diseases by the presence of a specific antibody to an extractable nuclear antigen (ENA) in the serum. Many patients with this disorder have been reported to have interstitial lung disease. The pulmonary involvement may be mild and responsive to steroids, but occasionally rapidly progressive fibrosis and pulmonary hypertension develop.

Ankylosing Spondylitis

Involvement of the thoracic spine is common in ankylosing spondylitis. In addition, 1% to 2% of patients may develop pleuropulmonary manifestations most commonly in the form of upper-lobe fibrotic and bullous disease (Fig. 9-9). Although it is rare, you should consider ankylosing spondylitis in the differential diagnosis of chronic infiltrative lung disorders that cause upper-lobe scarring and fibrosis.

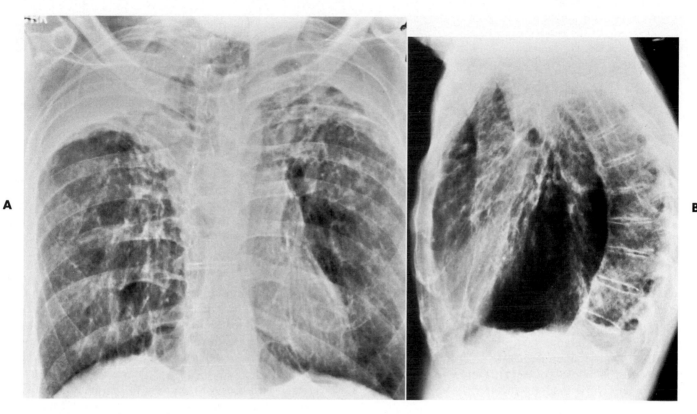

Figure 9-9. Ankylosing spondylitis. **A,** PA radiograph demonstrates marked upper lobe fibrosis and retraction with bullae and pleural thickening. **B,** Lateral chest radiograph shows the typical features of ankylosing spondylitis of the thoracic spine. Note the calcification of the anterior longitudinal ligament.

Box 9-8 Classification of the Pulmonary Vasculidities

CATEGORY—GRANULOMATOUS VASCULITIS

Classic Wegener's granulomatosis
"Limited" Wegener's granulomatosis
Lymphomatoid granulomatosis
Allergic granulomatosis and angiitis
Necrotizing sarcoidal angiitis and granulomatosis
Bronchocentric granulomatosis

CATEGORY—HYPERSENSITIVITY VASCULITIS

Anaphylactoid purpura
Essential mixed cryoglobulinemia with leukocytoclastic
    vasculitis
Vasculitis associated with malignancy, infection, or drugs
Extrinsic allergic alveolitis

CATEGORY—PULMONARY VASCULITIS ASSOCIATED WITH CONNECTIVE TISSUE DISEASES

Rheumatoid disease
Systemic lupus erythematosus
Progressive systemic sclerosis
Dermatomyositis/polymyositis
Mixed connective tissue disease

CATEGORY—VASCULITIS ASSOCIATED WITH PULMONARY ARTERY ANEURYSM

Behçet's disease
Hughes-Stovin syndrome

From Dreisin RB: Pulmonary vasculitis, *Clin Chest Med* 3(3): 608, 1982.

VASCULIDITIES AND GRANULOMATOSES

General Description

Any disease characterized pathologically by an inflammatory response within blood vessels may be considered a vasculitis. If the inflammation produces destruction of vessel walls, the process is termed a *necrotizing vasculitis.* Most vascular diseases are systemic, although frequently there is a target organ. The lungs are often involved by a number of different types of vasculitis. Box 9-8 provides a classification that divides these disorders into four groups. This section deals with diseases in Category 1, those that histopathologically have a granu-

---

Box 9-9 Wegener's Granulomatosis

CHARACTERISTICS

Upper respiratory tract, lungs, kidneys
Women > men, middle age
Cough, hemoptysis
Positive antineutrophilic cytoplasmic antibody

RADIOGRAPHIC FEATURES

Multiple nodules or masses
    Cavitation
    Peripheral
Focal or diffuse consolidation

Box 9-10 Lymphomatoid Granulomatosis

CHARACTERISTICS

Granulomatous vasculitis
Now considered a B-cell lymphoma
Middle age, men > women

RADIOGRAPHIC FEATURES

Multiple nodules or masses
    Numerous
    Cavitation

---

lomatous appearance and have been characterized by Liebow as pulmonary angiitis and granulomatosis. In all these diseases, the lung is the major site of involvement. These granulomatous vasculidities include classic and limited Wegener's granulomatosis, lymphomatoid granulomatosis, allergic granulomatosis (Churg-Strauss syndrome), necrotizing sarcoid angiitis and granulomatosis, and bronchocentric granulomatosis.

Wegener's Granulomatosis

General description

Wegener's granulomatosis (Box 9-9) usually consists of a disease triad of necrotizing vasculitis that involves the upper respiratory tract, lungs, and glomeruli of the kidneys. However, there is also a limited form of Wegener's that is confined to the lungs.

In Wegener's granulomatosis the mean onset of age is 40 years, and there is a female to male ratio of 2:1. Symptoms are usually related to the upper respiratory tract such as sinus pain and rhinorrhea. Pulmonary symptoms include cough with mild sputum production and occasionally hemoptysis. Renal involvement in classic Wegener's granulomatosis is usually asymptomatic and revealed only on subsequent evaluation. There is no single laboratory test that is diagnostic of Wegener's granulomatosis. However, elevated levels of antineutrophilic cytoplasmic antibody (ANCA) in the serum are suggestive. There is also striking elevation of the erythrocyte sedimentation rate. Wegener's granulomatosis can often be successfully treated with a combination of steroids and cyclophosphamide.

Radiologic findings

The radiologic features of Wegener's granulomatosis are varied. The most frequent and characteristic pattern is that of multiple rounded nodules or masses generally well defined and ranging in size from a few millimeters

to 9 cm in diameter. They may cavitate (Fig. 9-10), and they are commonly bilateral and multiple. The cavities have thick and irregular walls. The nodules may be peripheral in location and may simulate pulmonary infarcts. CT may demonstrate a peripheral distribution of pulmonary opacities that are wedge-shaped and associated with a feeding vessel, suggesting an angiocentric process. It is also not uncommon to see focal or diffuse areas of consolidation that are transient and fleeting in nature, these are most likely due to associated pulmonary hemorrhage (Fig. 9-11). This type of involvement is usually more fulminating and more severe. Hilar and mediastinal adenopathy as well as pleural effusions are rare. However, CT may demonstrate slightly enlarged nodes in a minority of patients.

Lymphomatoid Granulomatosis

Characteristics

Lymphomatoid granulomatosis (Box 9-10) is a systemic disease characterized by an angiocentric, angiodestructive lymphoreticular granulomatous vasculitis primarily involving the lungs but frequently involving the kidneys, skin, and central nervous system. For many years lymphomatoid granulomatosis was considered to represent a continuum from a more benign lymphocytic angiitis to frank lymphoma. Now there is general agreement that this disease entity is a frank lymphoma of the B-cell variety with rich T-cell components.

Presentation and diagnosis

Lymphomatoid granulomatosis generally occurs in patients at early middle age. There is a male predominance of 2:1. Symptoms such as cough and dyspnea may be present and may be accompanied by neurologic or systemic symptoms or cutaneous lesions. The radiographic features are similar to those of Wegener's. The most common radiographic presentation consists of multiple pulmonary nodules that range in size from 1 to 10

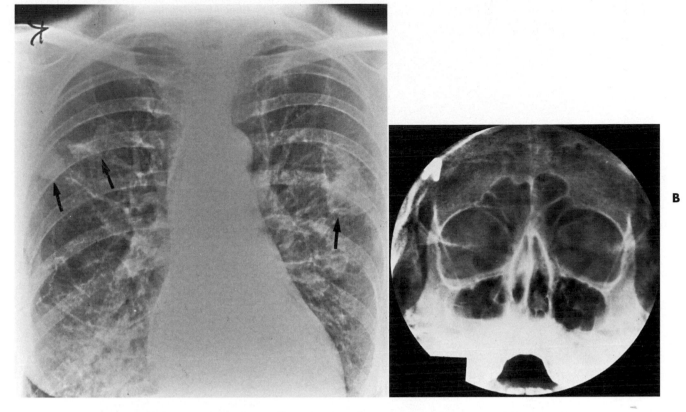

Figure 9-10. Wegener's granulomatosis. **A,** PA chest shows multiple pulmonary nodules (*arrows*). The one on the left is cavitated. There is also consolidation at the right base **B,** Sinus films show disease in both maxillary antra with an air/fluid level on the right.

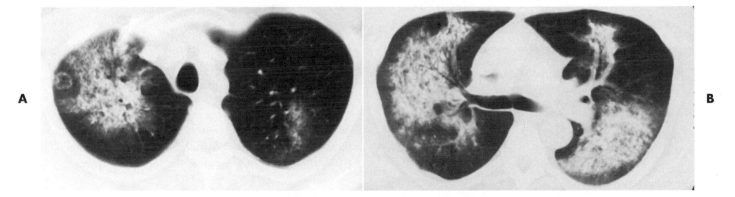

Figure 9-11. Wegener's granulomatosis. CT shows **A,** A peripheral cavitary nodule abutting the pleura in the right upper lobe. **B,** There is also bilateral air-space consolidation with air bronchograms due to pulmonary hemorrhage.

cm (Fig. 9-12). The nodules are often much more numerous than in Wegener's granulomatosis and may simulate advanced metastatic disease. The lower lung zones are more frequently involved, and initially the nodules may be ill-defined. Occasionally they coalesce, producing a more pneumonic appearance. Cavitation is common, and hilar adenopathy is rare.

The diagnosis is usually made by open-lung biopsy. Treatment consists of a combination of steroids and

cyclophosphamide, and the prognosis is very poor with rapid morbidity in the absence of treatment.

Allergic Angiitis and Granulomatosis (Churg-Strauss Syndrome)

General description

Allergic angiitis and granulomatosis (Box 9-11) is a disease characterized by inflammation and vascular necro-

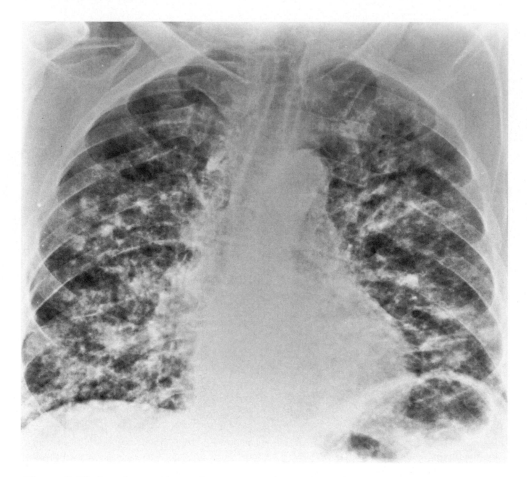

Figure 9-12. Lymphomatoid granulomatosis. PA chest radiograph shows multiple ill-defined nodules, some of which are cavitated. The nodules are smaller and much more numerous than in Wegener's.

Box 9-11 Allergic Angiitis and Granulomatosis (Churg-Strauss Syndrome)

CHARACTERISTICS

Organs: heart, lungs, skin, nervous system, kidneys
Asthma history
Pronounced eosinophilia
Any age

RADIOGRAPHIC FEATURES

Patchy areas of consolidation
Multiple nodules
Fleeting opacities

---

sis of many organs, including the heart, lungs, skin, nervous system, and kidneys. It occurs almost exclusively in patients with a history of asthma, and it is accompanied by pronounced peripheral eosinophilia. Many patients have signs of a systemic necrotizing vasculitis that may be indistinguishable from periarteritis nodosa. The disease is very similar to periarteritis nodosa, but its distinguishing characteristics include the presence of pulmonary disease and eosinophilia.

Patients may develop symptoms at any age with extreme manifestations of atopy. They always have asthma or a history of asthma. Systemic symptoms are common and include fever, anemia, and weight loss accompanied by pronounced peripheral eosinophilia. The patient's asthma may clear as the vasculitis develops.

Radiologic findings

The radiographic features are varied (Fig. 9-13). The appearances range from patchy areas of ground glass or alveolar disease to multiple bilateral nodules without cavitation. The former appearance is more common. However, there may also be a pattern of diffuse interstitial disease. The opacities may be fleeting, and new lesions may appear while older lesions are resolving. Complete regression of pulmonary lesions with corticosteroid therapy may occur. The diagnosis is often made by a biopsy of skin lesions if present, or a lung biopsy may be required. Histologic examination shows fibrinoid, necrotizing, and eosinophilic granulomatous lesions with frequent involvement of the pulmonary arteries.

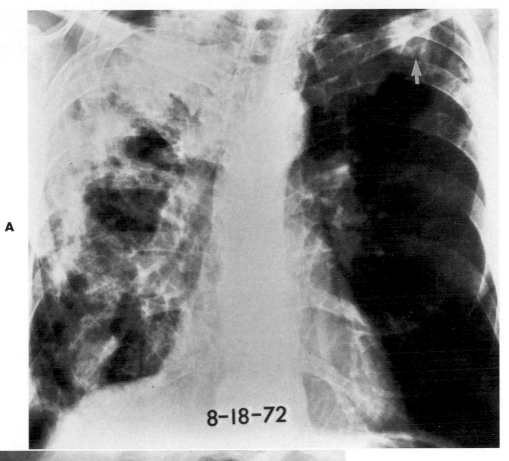

8-18-72

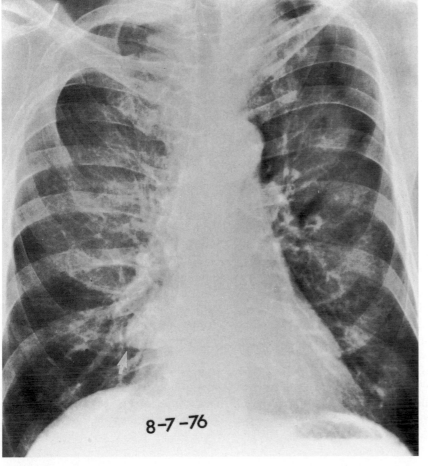

8-7-76

Figure 9-13. Allergic angiitis and granulomatosis. **A,** Original PA chest radiograph demonstrates peripheral air-space consolidation in the right lung and a nodule (*arrow*) in the left upper lobe in this asthmatic patient. **B,** A recurrent episode occurred 4 years later. There is a nodule in the right middle lobe (*arrow*).

Necrotizing Sarcoid Granulomatosis

Necrotizing sarcoid granulomatosis probably represents a vascular manifestation of disseminated or localized sarcoidosis. Patients are often asymptomatic and the disease is discovered on an incidental chest radiograph. The radiographic findings consists of multiple bilateral and often confluent nodules. Hilar and mediastinal adenopathy is usually not present, although nodes are often involved pathologically. The diagnosis is made by lung biopsy, and the prognosis is excellent with marked response to corticosteroid therapy.

Bronchocentric Granulomatosis

Although this lesion is classified as a vasculitis, the predominant pathologic feature is a necrotizing granulomatous reaction of the bronchial wall that only secondarily invades accompanying vessels. It is seen characteristically in atopic and asthmatic patients who have bronchopulmonary aspergillosis and mucoid impaction. In and of itself, it causes few symptoms and is usually diagnosed by biopsy of a lung mass discovered radiographically. The radiologic features, similar to those of bronchopulmonary aspergillosis, consist of lobar and segmental consolidation, atelectasis, and branching central "gloved finger" opacities due to mucoid impaction in abnormal bronchi.

EOSINOPHILIC LUNG DISEASE

General Description

The term pulmonary eosinophilia was originally used to describe a group of diseases in which radiographic abnormalities were seen in association with blood eosinophilia. The descriptive term pulmonary infiltration with eosinophilia—"PIE syndrome" is sometimes used to identify these disorders. However, eosinophilic infiltration of the lung can exist in the absence of blood eosinophilia. The following are the classifications of such disorders.

Löeffler's Syndrome (Simple Pulmonary Eosinophilia)

General description

Löeffler's syndrome (Box 9-12) consists of fleeting radiographic opacities associated with blood eosinophilia. Most patients have a background of atopy. Löeffler's syndrome may occur without an exciting extrinsic agent or allergen, but it may occur secondary to infestations with parasites or drug therapy. Indeed, in the original cases *Ascaris lumbricoides* was a common finding. Drug-related eosinophilia is described later in this chapter.

Box 9-12 Löeffler's Syndrome (Simple Pulmonary Eosinophilia)

CHARACTERISTICS

Atopy
Causes
   Idiophatic
   Parasites
   Drug-induced
Mild symptoms and eosinophilia

RADIOGRAPHIC FEATURES

Peripheral consolidation
Fleeting opacities
Photographic negative of pulmonary edema

Patients may be asymptomatic, and the syndrome is discovered incidentally on a chest radiograph. Symptoms when present are usually mild and consist of cough, slight fever, and chest pain. A low-level eosinophilia is present in the peripheral blood.

Radiologic findings

Radiographic features are highly characteristic in Löeffler's syndrome (Fig. 9-14). These consist of single or multiple areas of opacity that are usually ill-defined but homogeneous, typically occurring in the peripheral or axillary portions of the lungs. The areas of consolidation are transient and frequently shift from one area to another, although stability may be noted over several days. Cavitation, pleural effusion, and lymphadenopathy do not occur.

The prognosis is excellent, and both the opacities and blood eosinophilia usually resolve spontaneously. Careful search for a parasitic or drug reaction should be undertaken and the underlying disease treated.

Chronic Eosinophilic Pneumonia

General description

Chronic eosinophilic pneumonia (Box 9-13) is a more serious disease that requires treatment. Most patients are middle-aged women. Prominent symptoms include dyspnea, fever, chills, night sweats, and weight loss. Asthma is present in only 50% of cases. The disease is often insidious. Peripheral blood eosinophilia (greater than 6% of total white cell count) is present in the majority of patients, but is often mild or moderate.

Radiographic patterns

The typical radiographic pattern is said to be virtually diagnostic of this disorder (Fig. 9-15). There are typically dense opacities with ill-defined margins and with-

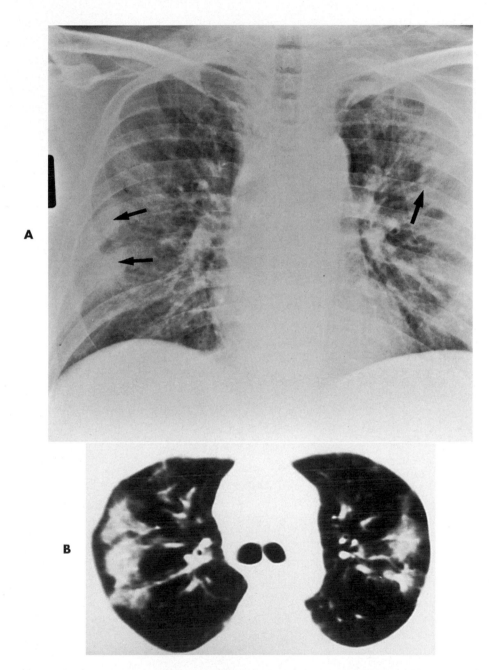

Figure 9-14. Löeffler's syndrome. **A,** PA chest radiograph shows multiple ill-defined radiographic opacities (*arrows*). **B,** CT confirms the peripheral location of the patchy consolidation.

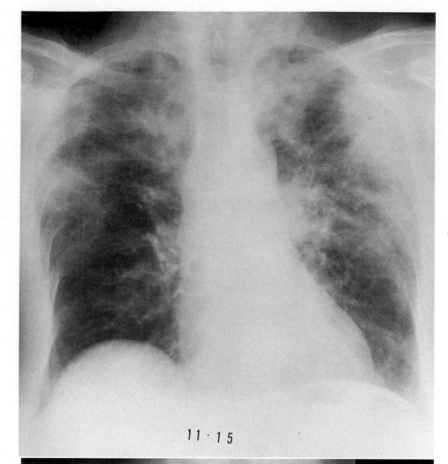

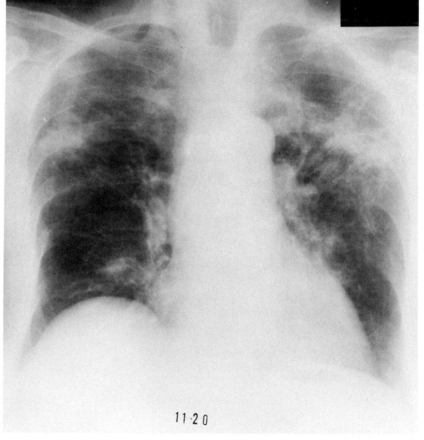

Figure 9-15. Chronic eosinophilic pneumonia. **A,** PA chest radiograph demonstrates peripheral consolidation in the upper axillary zones of both lungs (photographic negative of pulmonary edema). **B,** Five days later following steroid therapy there is significant improvement.

Box 9-13   Chronic Eosinophilic Pneumonia

CHARACTERISTICS

Middle-aged women
Mild or moderate eosinophilia
More severe disease than Löeffler's, insidious onset
Rapid response to steroids

RADIOGRAPHIC FEATURES

Peripheral consolidation
Upper zones
Photographic negative of pulmonary edema
Differential diagnosis: tuberculosis

Box 9-14   Acute Eosinophilic Pneumonia

CHARACTERISTICS

Acute febrile illness
Respiratory failure
Complete response to steroids
Absence of atopic history

RADIOGRAPHIC FEATURES

Diffuse consolidation
Not peripheral
CT
   Diffuse parenchymal consolidation
   Effusion
   No lymphadenopathy

out lobar or segmental distribution peripherally apposed to the pleura. The opacities are usually in an apical or axillary location, but occasionally they may be basal. When the opacities surround the lung, the appearance is that of a photographic negative or reversal of opacities usually seen in pulmonary edema. The opacities sometimes disappear and recur in exactly the same location. Oblique or vertical lines with no anatomic reference occasionally appear during resolution. CT will show peripheral consolidation even when the chest radiograph fails to show the peripheral location of the opacities. One half of patients have mediastinal adenopathy on CT that is also not apparent on the standard radiograph. You should consider tuberculosis in the differential diagnosis because of the apical or upper-lobe location.

Histologic examination will demonstrate eosinophil and leukocyte accumulation in the alveoli and in the interstitium with thickened alveolar walls.

Outcome

The prognosis in this disease is excellent, although if untreated it is likely to be protracted and may be fatal. One of the characteristic features of chronic eosinophilic pneumonia is a dramatic response to corticosteroid treatment with clinical improvement in hours and radiographic resolution within a few days. A trial of corticosteroids may be used as a diagnostic tool.

Acute Eosinophilic Pneumonia

General description

Idiopathic acute eosinophilic pneumonia (Box 9-14) was first described in 1989 and represents a clinical entity distinct from other idiopathic eosinophilic lung disease, such as chronic eosinophilic pneumonia. Diagnostic criteria include an acute febrile illness of less than 5 days duration; respiratory failure; eosinophils greater

than 25% on bronchoalveolar lavage; absence of parasitic, fungal, or other infection; prompt and complete response to corticosteroids; and failure to relapse after discontinuation of corticosteroids. Patients do not usually have a history of atopy or asthma.

Radiologic findings

Radiographic findings usually include subtle linear opacities, which progress to a consolidative pattern that is usually bilateral, extensive, and involving all lobes. Unlike chronic eosinophilic pneumonia and many of the other eosinophilic syndromes, the opacities are usually not peripheral in location. CT shows diffuse parenchymal consolidation, pleural effusions, pronounced thickening of the interlobular septa, and normal-size lymph nodes.

Diagnosis and treatment

The cause of this disease is unknown, but it may represent an acute hypersensitivity phenomenon to an unidentified inhaled antigen. In the differential diagnosis, you must exclude infectious disease. Patients respond rapidly to high doses of corticosteroids usually within 24 to 48 hours. If untreated they may progress rapidly to acute respiratory failure.

Idiopathic Hypereosinophilic Syndrome

General description

Idiopathic hypereosinophilic syndrome (Box 9-15) is a rare fatal disorder characterized by blood eosinophilia of greater than 1500/ml for more than 6 months with absence of parasitic or other causes of secondary eosinophilia. Initially this disease was termed eosinophilic leukemia.

The disease usually occurs in the third or fourth decades, and there is marked 7:1 male predominance. Symptoms include night sweats, anorexia, weight loss,

---

Box 9-15 Idiopathic Hypereosinophilic Syndrome

CHARACTERISTICS

High chronic eosinophilia (30%—70%) ("eosinophilic leukemia")
Third and fourth decades
Marked male predominance

RADIOGRAPHIC FEATURES

Reticular nodular opacities

---

cough, and fever. There is a profound peripheral eosinophilia of 30% to 70% with a total white count greater than 10,000. Cardiac involvement may occur and is a cause of morbidity and mortality. Pulmonary involvement occurs in up to 40% of patients and typically presents with cough.

Radiologic Findings

The chest radiograph shows interstitial linear or nodular opacities that are nonlobar in distribution, and approximately half of patients will have pleural effusions. Thromboembolic disease occurs in two thirds of patients. About half of the patients will have a good clinical response to steroids alone, but others may require cytotoxic therapy.

Asthma

Please see Chapter 10.

Allergic Bronchopulmonary Aspergillosis

Please see Chapter 13.

Bronchocentric Granulomatosis

Please see previous discussion in this chapter.

Allergic Angiitis and Granulomatosis

Please see previous discussion in this chapter.

Parasitic Infections

Many parasites can cause pulmonary consolidation with blood and/or alveolar eosinophilia. Among those causing infection in the United States include *Strongyloides, Ascaris, Toxocara,* and *Ancylostoma*. Radiographic features in most of the parasitic infections are typically those of fleeting migratory peripheral areas of consolidation. Tropical pulmonary eosinophilia is caused by filarial worms.

Box 9-16 Hypersensitivity Pneumonitis

CHARACTERISTICS
Cause: Inhaled Organic Dust, Occupational Antigens

Animal proteins
Saprophytic fungi
Dairy and grain products
Water vaporizers

Stages

Acute (4-6 hours)
Subacute—after resolution of acute stage, between episodes
Chronic—fibrosis, months or years after exposure

Diagnosis

History related to exposure
Precipitating antibodies
Positive inhalational challenge

RADIOGRAPHIC CHANGES
Acute

Air-space consolidation—diffuse
Rapid clearing

Subacute

Nodular or reticular nodular opacities
Upper zones
CT
    Centrilobular nodules
    Ground-glass opacity

Chronic

Medium to coarse linear opacities
Honeycombing
Upper zones

HYPERSENSITIVITY PNEUMONITIS

Background

Hypersensitivity pneumonitis (Box 9-16), also known as extrinsic allergic alveolitis, describes a spectrum of granulomatous and interstitial pulmonary disorders associated with intense and often prolonged exposure to a wide range of inhaled organic dust and related occupational antigens. The site of inflammatory host response in these disorders is located primarily in the alveolar air exchange portion of the lung and not in the large conducting airways that are involved in asthmatic diseases.

A variety of organic antigens may cause hypersensitivity pneumonitis. These antigens, usually disseminated as aerosol dust, can be derived from animal dander and proteins; saprophytic fungi (spores) in contaminated vegetables, wood, bark or water reservoir vaporizers; and

Table 9-1 Some Etiologic Agents in Hypersensitivity Pneumonitis

Major Antigens	Exposure or Source	Disease
THERMOPHILIC BACTERIA		
Micropolyspora faeni	Moldy hay	Farmer's lung
Thermoactinomyces vulgaris	Moldy grain	Grain handler's lung
M. faeni, T. vulgaris	Mushroom compost	Mushroom worker's lung
Thermoactinomyces sacchari	Moldy sugar cane (bagasse)	Bagassosis
T. vulgaris, Streptomyces candidus, M. faeni	Heated water reservoirs	Humidifier or air conditioner lung
OTHER BACTERIA		
Bacillus subtilis	Water	Detergent worker's lung
Bacillus cereus	Water reservoir	Humidifier lung
TRUE FUNGI		
Cryptostroma corticale	Moldy bark	Maple bark stripper's lung
Aspergillus clavatus	Moldy malt, barley	Malt worker's lung
Aureobasidium pullulans and *graphium* sp.	Moldy redwood dust	Sequoiosis
Mucor stolonifer	Moldy paprika pods	Paprika splitter's lung
Sitophilus granarius	Infested wheat flour	Wheat weevil's disease
Penicillium caseii	Cheese mold	Cheese worker's lung
Penicillium frequentans	Moldy cork dust	Suberosis
Aspergillus spores	Water reservoir	Aspergillosis
ANIMAL PROTEINS		
Avian proteins (serum and excreta)	Pigeons, parakeets	Bird breeder's lung
Chicken feathers, serum	Chickens	Chicken handler's lung
Turkey feathers, serum	Turkeys	Turkey handler's lung
Duck feathers	Ducks	Duck fever
Rat urine, serum	Rats	Rodent handler's disease
Porcine and bovine pituitary protein	Pituitary snuff	Pituitary snuff-taker's lung
AMEBA		
Acanthamoeba	Water	Humidifier lung
BACTERIAL PRODUCTS		
Endotoxin (?)	Cotton brac	Byssinosis
Streptomyces verticillus glycopeptides	Bleomycin	Bleomycin hypersensitivity lung (in contrast to fibrosis)

From Reynold HY: Hypersensitivity pneumonitis, *Clin Chest Med* 3:503, 1982.

dairy and grain products. These diseases and the major inciting antigens are listed in Table 9-1.

The exposure is often occupational. The organic antigen may be a microbial organism, and the most commonly incriminated is thermophilic actinomyces, a ubiquitous bacterium that has the morphologic features of a fungus. This is the offending antigen in one of the most common types of hypersensitivity pneumonitis, farmer's lung.

Stages of Disease

Three stages of the disease can be identified: acute, subacute, and chronic. Acute disease usually results from heavy exposure to the inciting antigen and occurs 4 to 6 hours after exposure. The subacute stage is seen after resolution of acute abnormalities or between episodes of acute exposure, and the chronic stage is characterized by the presence of fibrosis, which may develop months or years after initial exposure.

Presentation and Diagnosis

The first clue to the diagnosis of hypersensitivity pneumonitis is a good clinical history that suggests the temporal relationship between the patient's symptoms and certain activities including hobbies and occupations. The acute form of the disease is characterized by cough, dyspnea, and fever, which usually begins 4 to 6 hours after exposure to large quantities of the causative agent. There is often a leukocytosis, and pulmonary function studies reveal restrictive dysfunction. Usually characterized by dyspnea and chronic cough, subacute and chronic disease associated with low-grade exposure to the offending antigen may be confused with other forms of interstitial lung disease. Laboratory studies consistent with the diagnosis include precipitating antibodies reactive to the offending dust antigen as well as a positive inhalational challenge that will reproduce the symptoms.

Radiologic Findings

The radiographic features vary with the stage of the disease. In the acute form, the chest radiograph may be normal, but after heavy exposure to the appropriate antigen you may observe alveolar consolidation especially in the lower lung zones. This reflects pathologic findings of alveolar filling by polymorphonuclear leukocytes, eosinophils, lymphocytes, and large mononuclear cells. This air-space consolidation may be quite extensive, simulating pulmonary edema, but it is transitory and usually clears within hours or days. The subacute form is characterized by a fine nodular or reticulonodular pattern that tends to predominate in the upper-lung zones (Fig. 9-16). This nodular appearance corresponds pathologically with alveolitis, interstitial infiltration, small granulomas, and some degree of bronchiolitis. Histologic abnormalities are usually most severe in a peribronchiolar distribution. CT may be helpful in the diagnosis of the subacute form (Fig. 9-17). The findings usually consist of small nodular opacities often distributed in a centrilobular location as well as areas of ground-glass opacity.

In the chronic stage of hypersensitivity pneumonitis where there is continued exposure to the antigen, the diffuse reticulonodular pattern is replaced by changes characteristic of diffuse interstitial fibrosis, that is, medium to coarse linear opacities, with loss of lung volume and honeycombing. The fibrosis tends to be more pronounced in the upper zones. Similar reticular opacities can be identified on CT scans.

Treatment

If the environmental source of the inhaled antigen is identified, simple avoidance is sufficient treatment: the acute form of the disease will abate without specific therapy. With chronic forms of disease a trial of corticosteroids can be given.

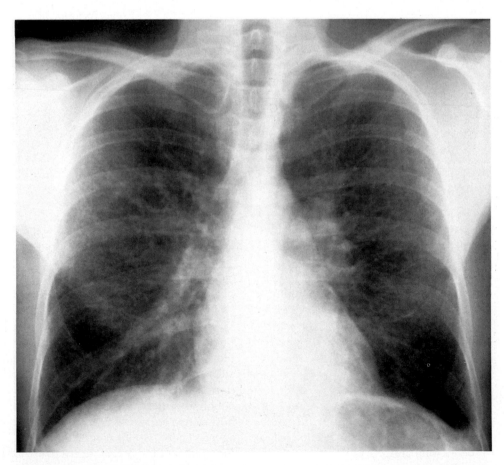

Figure 9-16. Hypersensitivity pneumonitis. Subacute stage. Humidifier lung. There are small nodular opacities more predominant in the upper lung zones.

Specific Diseases

Farmer's lung

This was the first occupationally related form of hypersensitivity pneumonitis to be clearly described and understood. *Thermophilic actinomyces vulgaris* is the most important antigen in farmer's lung. It is found in moldy hay that has been improperly dried for storage.

Farmer's lung typically affects men between 40 and 50 years of age. The disease occurs in late winter or early spring when the lower levels of hay, which have had the longest time to compost, are reached. A classic acute onset occurs in a third of cases, but a more common clinical presentation is insidious and is characterized by gradual progression of cough and dyspnea, weight loss, and fever. Prevalence of the syndrome among farmers is estimated to be between 1% and 10%.

Humidifier lung

Equipment used to heat, humidify, or cool air may harbor microorganisms responsible for hypersensitivity pneumonitis. This entity can develop in unsuspecting people who do not have obvious known exposure, and it may affect large numbers of people in an epidemic form. The diagnosis may be obvious when exposure occurs at home. However, contamination of heating and air conditioning or humidifying equipment with microorganisms in an office or commercial establishment is difficult to prove. The causative agents are usually thermophilic *Actinomyces.* An accurate diagnosis requires a thorough history and detailed environmental probing, including a visit to suspicious areas and cultures from contaminated appliances.

Pigeon breeder's lung (Bird Fancier's Disease)

This disease differs from farmer's lung or humidifier lung in that it is caused by inhaled proteins rather than microbial antigens and spores. Exposure to excreta and proteinaceous material from pigeons and other fowl and birds provokes the disease. It may produce either an acute or chronic reaction.

DRUG-INDUCED LUNG DISEASE

Drug-induced lung toxicity is common and may result from either complex chemotherapeutic regimens or the abuse of elicit drugs. Many drugs may produce a similar clinical syndrome, and individual drugs may cause a variety of reactions. Many drug reactions are immunologically mediated, although some may occur as a result of direct toxicity. Direct toxicity is usually dose-related. The pathologic reaction consists of permeability pulmonary edema, which may progress to diffuse alveolar damage and pulmonary fibrosis. The injury may be mediated by the generation of reactive oxygen species. On the other hand, hypersensitivity reactions are not dose-related and require prior sensitization to

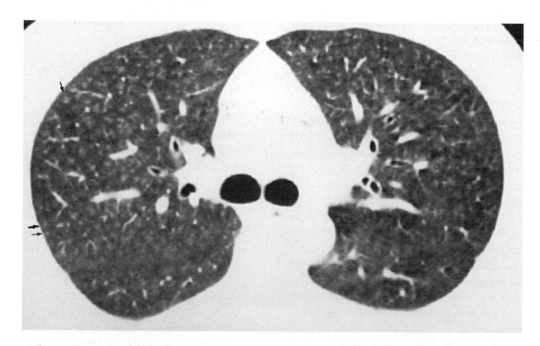

Figure 9-17. Hypersensitivity pneumonitis. Fish-plant worker. HRCT shows multiple ill-defined, low-attenuation nodules. In the subpleural zones the nodules occupy a centrilobular location 2 to 3 mm deep to the pleural surface (*arrows*). (Courtesy of Victoria General Hospital, Halifax, Nova Scotia.)

the drug. This reaction is the result of the interaction between the drug and humeral antibodies or sensitized lymphocytes. Idiosyncratic toxicity is not dose-related and does not require prior sensitization. Such reactions are usually acute, presenting with noncardiogenic pulmonary edema.

Patterns of Injury

Noncardiogenic pulmonary edema

Noncardiogenic pulmonary edema is a common complication of a variety of drugs, particularly cytotoxic agents—for example, interleukin, methotrexate, cytosine, and arabinoside. The pulmonary edema typically occurs within hours of administration. It is a well-recognized complication of opiate (heroin) and salicylate overdose.

Pulmonary hemorrhage

Pulmonary hemorrhage is most commonly a complication of anticoagulant therapy or drug-induced thrombocytopenia. Penicillamine may rarely cause a pulmonary renal syndrome similar to Goodpasture's syndrome. Acute and even fatal pulmonary hemorrhage has been reported with nitrofurantoin therapy, but more commonly this drug is associated with hypersensitivity pneumonitis or pulmonary fibrosis. Cocaine abuse is increasingly recognized as a cause of intraalveolar hemorrhage.

Pulmonary fibrosis

Pulmonary fibrosis usually develops as a chronic insidious process and is typically seen with a wide variety of cytotoxic and noncytotoxic drugs such as busulfan and bleomycin.

Eosinophilic pneumonia

Drug reactions are one of the most commonly reported causes of pulmonary opacities associated with blood or alveolar eosinophilia (Box 9-17). Among the most commonly reported are sulfasalazine, which is used for inflammatory bowel disease. Eosinophilia-myalgia syndrome is an interesting multiorgan disorder caused by contaminants found in batches of L-tryptophan that were manufactured in the late 1980s. The disease involved approximately half of the persons ingesting the contaminated drug who developed acute peripheral blood eosinophilia accompanied by severe myalgias. Approximately half of the patients had respiratory symptoms. Typical peripheral pulmonary consolidation was identified on chest radiographs.

Drug-induced eosinophilia may be mild or present as a fulminant acute eosinophilic pneumonia-like syndrome. Most patients respond to withdrawal of the drug, although steroid therapy may be necessary.

Box 9-17 Drugs Causing Eosinophilic Lung Disease

Ampicillin
Beclomethasone dipropionate (inhaled)
Bleomycin
Carbamazepine
Chlorpromazine
Clofibrate
Cocaine (inhaled)
Cromolyn (inhaled)
Desipramine
Diclofenac
Fenbufen
Glafenine
Ibuprofen
Interleukin-2
Interleukin-3
Iodinated contrast dye
L-tryptophan
Mephenesin carbamate
Methotrexate
Methylphenidate
Minocycline
Naproxen
Nickel
Nitrofurantoin
Paraaminosalicylic acid
Penicillin
Pentamidine (inhaled)
Phenytoin
Pyrimethamine
Rapeseed oil
Sulfadimethoxine
Sulfadoxine
Sulfasalazine
Sulindac
Tamoxifen
Tetracycline
Tolazamide
Tolfenamic acid
Vaginal sulfonamide cream

Exogenous lipoid pneumonia

Exogenous lipoid pneumonia has been described as a complication of accidental aspiration of mineral oil. Endogenous phospholipoidosis induced by amiodarone is an important cause of pulmonary toxicity.

Drug-induced lupus syndrome

Drug-induced lupus syndrome is more common than the idiopathic form of systemic lupus erythematosus. It has however a more benign course and is usually reversible. Common manifestations include pleural and pericardial effusions. Subsegmental atelectasis and basilar consolidation are typical radiographic findings. Drugs implicated include hydralazine, procainamide, and phenytoin. The majority of patients have a positive antinuclear antibody (ANA).

Bronchiolitis obliterans

Bronchiolitis obliterans is characterized pathologically by the proliferation of granulation tissue in the small airways with obliteration of their lumens. It is an uncommon drug-induced complication, most frequently associated with penicillamine therapy prescribed for rheumatoid arthritis.

Illicit drug use

The pulmonary manifestations of drug abuse include a wide variety of infectious and inflammatory complications. The adverse effects are related to the route of administration as well as the type of drug. Talcosis results from intravenous injection of aqueous solutions of oral preparations contaminated by talc. Talc is a filler used in the manufacture of tablets to prevent them from sticking to the mouth. When injected, the talc particles become lodged in peripheral pulmonary arterioles and capillaries, producing pulmonary hypertension and vasculitis.

Radiologic Features

Clinical and radiologic features of drug-induced lung disease are summarized in Box 9-18.

Hydrochlorothiazide

Hydrochlorothiazide produces noncardiogenic pulmonary edema due to a hypersensitivity reaction. Reported cases have occurred in women, and the radiographic features consist of bilateral diffuse air-space opacities.

Interleukin-2 (IL-2)

Interleukin-2 is used to treat advanced malignant disease. Pulmonary edema has been reported in up to 70% of patients and usually occurs within a week of commencing therapy. The radiographic findings consist of mild interstitial or frank alveolar pulmonary edema often associated with pleural effusions and ascites.

Amiodarone

Amiodarone is a triiodinated compound used in the treatment of cardiac arrhythmias. Pulmonary toxicity is a common complication occurring in up to 18% of patients. Toxicity appears to be dose-related. The onset is usually subacute. Radiographic findings consist of patchy alveolar and diffuse linear opacification often with an upper-lobe and peripheral distribution. Pleural reaction may occur, but effusions are uncommon. CT may demonstrate the characteristic high density of the pleuropulmonary lesions as a result of the iodine content of the amiodarone (Fig. 9-18).

Box 9-18   Clinical and Radiologic Features of Drug-Induced Lung Disease

HYDROCHLORTHIAZIDE

Noncardiogenic pulmonary edema

INTERLEUKIN-2 (IL-2)

Noncardiogenic edema
Pleural effusions and ascites

AMIODARONE

Treatment of cardiac arrhythmias
Patchy alveolar and diffuse linear opacities
Upper lobe and peripheral distribution
CT: high attenuation (iodine)

NITROFURANTOIN

Urinary tract infections
Eosinophilia
Patchy and peripheral air-space consolidation
Fibrosis (with chronic use)

METHOTREXATE

Treatment of inflammatory diseases and malignancy
Allergic response
Diffuse reticular nodular opacities or widespread consolidation
Adenopathy
Lung-base and middle-zone distribution

BUSULFAN

Rx of chronic granulocytic leukemia
Diffuse reticulonodular opacities

BLEOMYCIN

Treatment of lymphoma, solid tumors
Dose-related
Pulmonary fibrosis
Linear subpleural basilar opacities

CYCLOSPORINE

Prevention of transplant rejection
Lymphoproliferative disorder (3%—5%)
Lungs, nodes, gastrointestinal tract distribution
Solitary mass, multiple nodules, with or without adenopathy

LIPOID PNEUMONIA

Aspiration of oily substances
Chronic multifocal basal areas of consolidation
Air bronchograms
CT: attenuation of fat

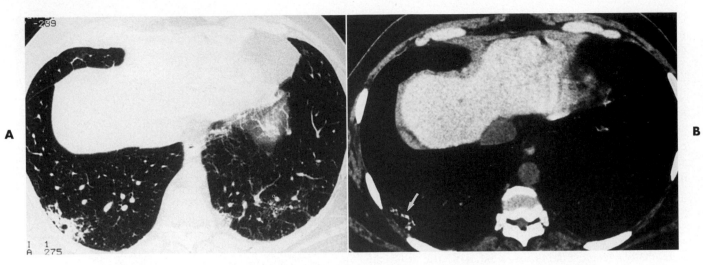

Figure 9-18. Amiodarone toxicity. CT. **A,** Lung windows demonstrate fine reticular and some confluent opacities in both lower lobes subpleurally. **B,** Mediastinal windows reveal high attenuation of the pulmonary opacities (*arrow*) and a high-attenuation liver.

Nitrofurantoin

Nitrofurantoin is a drug widely used in the treatment of urinary tract infections. It is an important cause of pulmonary eosinophilia, which occurs in the majority of patients. It may cause both acute onset of pneumonitis and chronic interstitial pneumonia. The chest radiograph will demonstrate bilateral patchy and occasional peripheral air-space consolidation (Fig 9-19). Pleural effusions may occur. Pulmonary fibrosis develops with prolonged use of nitrofurantoin, and the fibrosis is likely secondary to chronic drug toxicity rather than a hypersensitivity reaction.

Methotrexate

This drug is used to treat a variety of inflammatory diseases such as rheumatoid arthritis and psoriasis as well as malignant disorders. Methotrexate toxicity is unique is several respects. Discontinuation of the drug is not always required for recovery, and reintroduction of the drug is not necessarily associated with recurrent symptoms. Toxicity may occur with low-dose therapy, and it appears to be related to the frequency of administration. The features are usually that of an allergic response with a subacute illness associated with pulmonary eosinophilia. A typical radiographic appearance is that of diffuse reticulonodular opacities, but there may be widespread consolidation with hilar and mediastinal lymphadenopathy (Fig. 9-20). A predilection for the lung bases and middle zones has been described. Most patients recover completely even if the drug is continued, and residual pulmonary fibrosis is uncommon.

Busulfan

Busulfan is used almost exclusively in the treatment of chronic granulocytic leukemia. Pulmonary toxicity is usually related to the duration of therapy and is increased with combination chemotherapy. The chest radiograph usually shows a diffuse reticulonodular appearance. The prognosis is poor, with a mortality of roughly 50%.

Bleomycin

Bleomycin is used in the treatment of lymphomas, squamous cell cancer, and testicular tumors. Pulmonary toxicity occurs in about 4% of patients and is an important factor limiting dosage. The incidence of toxicity is related to the cumulative dose. Pulmonary fibrosis is the most serious complication, although acute hypersensitivity reaction has been described. The chest radiograph may be normal or may show typical basal subpleural reticular opacities similar to those seen in idiopathic pulmonary fibrosis (Fig. 9-21). CT may demonstrate abnormalities even when the chest radiograph is normal. In the early stages of the disease, regression may occur after stopping therapy, but fibrosis may progress resulting in death.

Cyclosporine

Cyclosporine inhibits cytotoxic T-cells and is used to control rejection in transplant patients. Approximately 3% to 5% of patients treated with cyclosporine will develop a drug-induced lymphoproliferative disorder typically within 4 to 6 months of commencing therapy. The lungs, lymph nodes, and gastrointestinal tract may be involved. All reported patients have evidence of Epstein-Barr virus infection. This virus selectively affects B-cells, causing B-cell proliferation that is normally controlled by cytotoxic T-cells. Pulmonary radiologic manifestations include a solitary mass, multiple pulmonary nodules, and hilar adenopathy (Fig. 9-22).

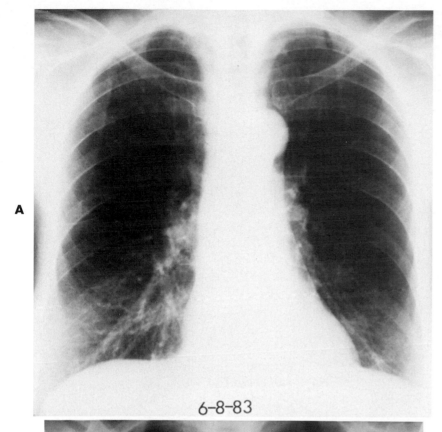

6-8-83

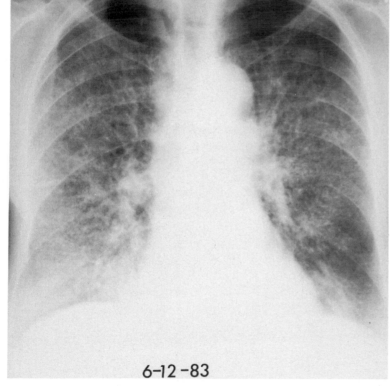

6-12-83

Figure 9-19. Nitrofurantoin reaction. **A,** Baseline radiograph is normal. **B,** Several days after administration of the drug for a urinary tract infection there are diffuse bilateral reticular opacities and areas of consolidation. There is no evidence of a peripheral distribution.

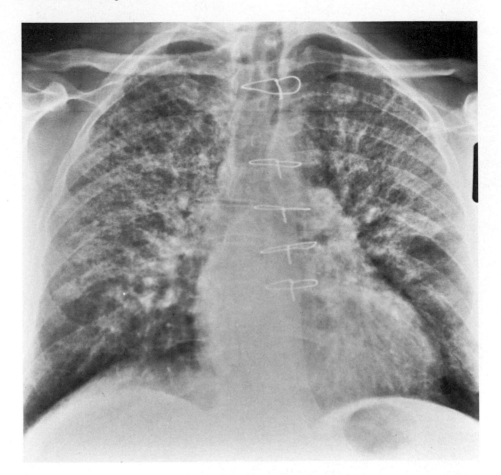

Figure 9-20. Methotrexate pulmonary disease. PA radiograph shows diffuse reticulonodular and patchy opacities.

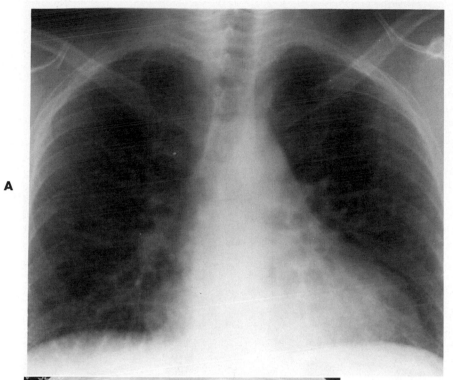

A

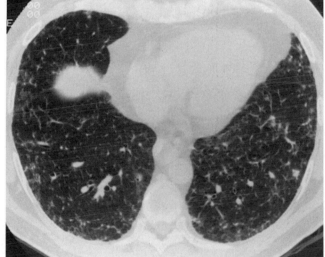

B

Figure 9-21. Bleomycin lung. **A,** PA radiograph shows fine reticular opacities at the lung bases. **B,** HRCT. There are linear opacities with intralobular lines and septal thickening most pronounced in the subpleural basal lung.

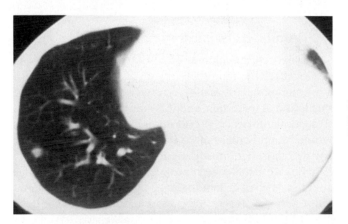

Figure 9-22. Lymphoproliferative disorder following cardiac transplant and cyclosporine therapy. CT scan shows a solitary nodule in the right lower lobe.

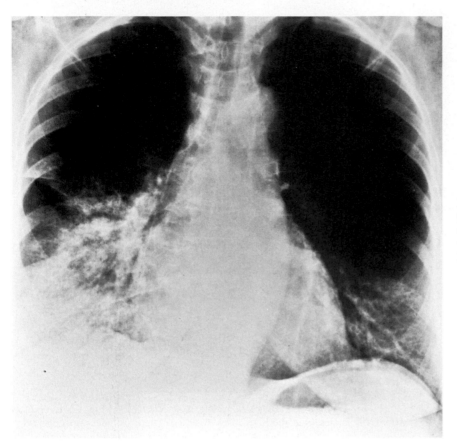

Figure 9-23. Lipoid pneumonia. Elderly patient who had taken mineral oil regularly for chronic constipation. There is consolidation with air bronchograms at the base of the right lung.

Oily substances (lipoid pneumonia)

Lipoid pneumonia usually occurs as the result of inadvertent aspiration of oily substances such as mineral oil. This usually results in multifocal areas of consolidation typically at the bases of the lungs. Such areas of consolidation tend to be chronic with prominent air bronchograms (Fig. 9-23). The diagnosis can be made on CT. CT density numbers of the areas of consolidation will be in the range of fatty tissue and are therefore pathognomonic of lipoid pneumonia (Fig. 9-24).

PULMONARY LYMPHOPROLIFERATIVE DISORDERS

General Description

There are a number of nonlymphomatous lymphoproliferative disorders that may occur in the lung. There is considerable overlap between these disorders and lymphoma. The normal lung contains abundant lymphoid tissue. Lymph nodes are present within the hila and along the tracheobronchial branches, and there is submucosal lymphoid tissue along the respiratory tract at the level of the pulmonary acinus. Lymphoid clusters can be found at the level of the distal respiratory bronchiole. There is also a chain of subpleural lymphatics abutting the visceral pleura. The benign lymphoid disorders of the lung are felt to represent hyperplasia of the pulmonary lymphoid system in response to chronic antigenic stimulation. They are associated with an abnormality of immune response. These pulmonary extranodal and lymphoid disorders include plasma cell granuloma, pseudolymphoma, lymphocytic interstitial pneumonitis, lymphomatoid granulomatosis, and lymphoproliferative disorders associated with cyclosporine use following transplant. The lymph-node disorders include giant lymph-node hyperplasia (Castleman's disease) and angioblastic lymphadenopathy.

Plasma-Cell Granuloma

Plasma-cell granuloma (Box 9-19) of the lung consists of a localized benign proliferation of a variety of cells with a predominance of mature plasma cells. Pathogenesis of this lesion is uncertain, and it is sometimes referred to as a postinflammatory pseudotumor. The disease affects women slightly more often than men, and it may occur at any age, although most patients are under the age of 30. Patients are usually asymptomatic, and the lesion is discovered as a solitary pulmonary nodule on an incidental chest radiograph (Fig. 9-25). The nodule may range from 1 to 12 cm in diameter and occasionally may cavitate or

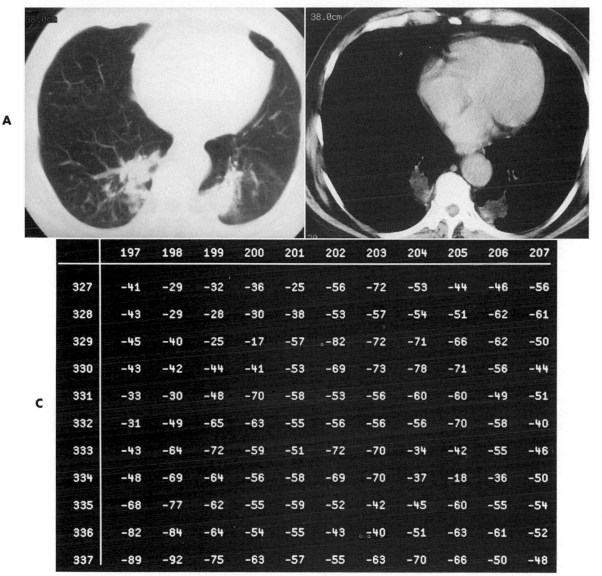

	197	198	199	200	201	202	203	204	205	206	207
327	−41	−29	−32	−36	−25	−56	−72	−53	−44	−46	−56
328	−43	−29	−28	−30	−38	−53	−57	−54	−51	−62	−61
329	−45	−40	−25	−17	−57	−82	−72	−71	−66	−62	−50
330	−43	−42	−44	−41	−53	−69	−73	−78	−71	−56	−44
331	−33	−30	−48	−70	−58	−53	−56	−60	−60	−49	−51
332	−31	−49	−65	−63	−55	−56	−56	−56	−70	−58	−40
333	−43	−64	−72	−59	−51	−72	−70	−34	−42	−55	−46
334	−48	−69	−64	−56	−58	−69	−70	−37	−18	−36	−50
335	−68	−77	−62	−55	−59	−52	−42	−45	−60	−55	−54
336	−82	−84	−64	−54	−55	−43	−40	−51	−63	−61	−52
337	−89	−92	−75	−63	−57	−55	−63	−70	−66	−50	−48

Figure 9-24. Lipoid pneumonia. Patient had been a regular user of oily nose drops. CT. **A,** Lung windows demonstrate focal patchy areas of consolidation in the basal segments of both lower lobes. **B,** Mediastinal windows show areas of low attenuation within the opacities. **C,** Printout of CT numbers of pixels through the abnormal area in the right lower lobe show values equal to fat attenuation (−50 to −150 HU).

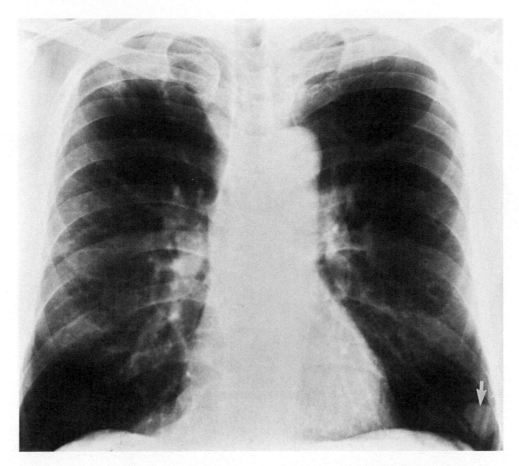

Figure 9-25. Plasma cell granuloma. PA chest radiograph shows a well-defined, approximately 2-cm nodule near the left costophrenic angle (*arrow*).

Box 9-19 Plasma Cell Granuloma

CHARACTERISTICS

Postinflammatory pseudotumor
Women > men
Young, under 30
Asymptomatic

RADIOGRAPHIC FEATURES

Solitary nodule
1-12 cm
Slow growth, ± Ca++ and cavitation

Box 9-20 Pseudolymphoma

CHARACTERISTICS

Asymptomatic
Autoimmune diseases (Sjögren's syndrome), dysgamma-globulinemias

RADIOGRAPHIC FEATURES

Chronic consolidation
Single or multiple focal areas
Air bronchograms

---

calcify. It usually grows slowly in a matter of months to years. Complete surgical resection with as little removal of adjacent lung as possible is the treatment of choice.

Pseudolymphoma

Although most patients are asymptomatic, pseudolymphoma (Box 9-20) may be seen in patients with a variety of autoimmune diseases (Sjögren's syndrome) or dysgammaglobulinemias. Patients are reusually of middle age.

Pseudolymphoma usually presents as a localized area of parenchymal consolidation (Fig. 9-26). It is caused by lymphoid interstitial proliferation, which compresses the air spaces and creates air bronchograms. The consolidation is usually between 2 and 5 cm in size, and it may be scattered randomly throughout the lung. Lymphadenopathy and pleural effusions are absent. Differentiation from lymphocytic lymphoma is difficult, and malignant transformation is reported in 15% to 80% of cases.

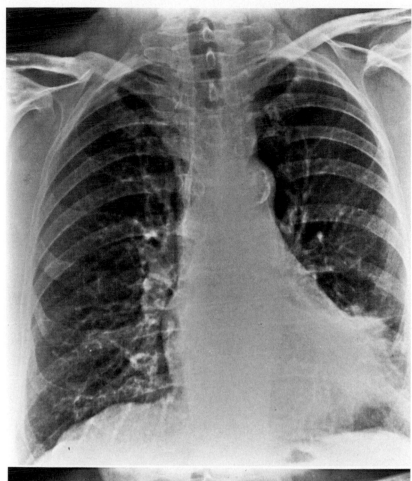

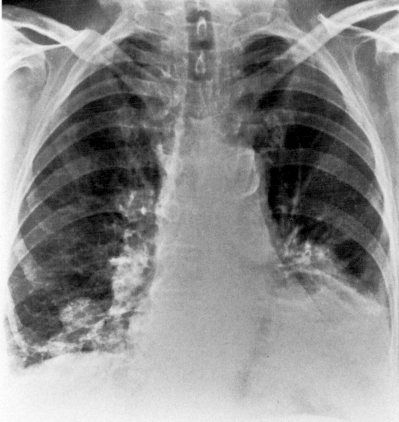

Figure 9-26. Pseudolymphoma. Patient with Sjögren's syndrome. **A,** PA radiograph shows an ill-defined opacity with faint air bronchograms in the lingula obliterating the left heart border. **B,** Two years later the area of opacification on the left has increased in size and there are new nodules at the right base.

Lymphocytic Interstitial Pneumonitis (LIP)

Lymphocytic interstitial pneumonitis (Box 9-21) is a diffuse interstitial infiltration of the lung characterized predominantly by lymphocytes with varying admixtures of plasma cells and other elements. In pseudolymphoma the lymphocytic infiltration is localized. In LIP the involvement is diffuse. Although the cause is unknown, it may be associated with abnormalities in the immune system such as Sjögren's syndrome, pernicious anemia, chronic active hepatitis, and myasthenia gravis, or it may be secondary to viral infection. The disease may occur with some frequency in children with AIDS.

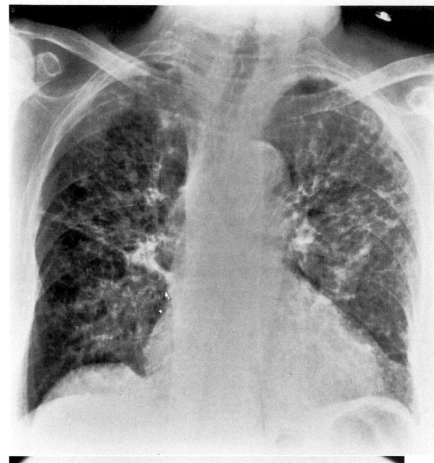

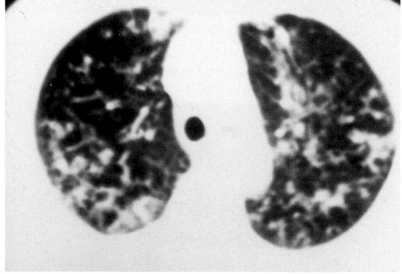

Figure 9-27. Lymphocytic interstitial pneumonitis. **A,** PA chest radiograph shows a coarse reticulonodular pattern diffusely in both lungs. **B,** CT scan demonstrates a predominately nodular pattern with a lymphatic distribution both along the bronchovascular bundles and in the subpleural zones.

Box 9-21 Lymphocytic Interstitial Pneumonitis

CHARACTERISTICS

Diffuse lymphocytic infiltration of the lung
Associated autoimmune diseases, children with AIDS
Progression to lymphoma in some non-AIDS

RADIOGRAPHIC FEATURES

Bilateral linear or reticular nodular opacities
Basilar
Coarse, flamelike opacities
Late honeycombing
Adenopathy rare

The radiographic appearance is variable, but it often consists of a bilateral linear or reticulonodular pattern with basilar predominance (Fig. 9-27). Coarse flamelike opacities or diffuse confluent lesions have been described. If a nodular pattern is present, the nodules tend to be smaller than those seen in lymphoma. In later stages, honeycombing may be seen. Pleural effusion occasionally occurs, but hilar and mediastinal adenopathy is rare. Neoplastic transformation may occur, and the reported incidence varies from a small percentage to 50% of cases.

Lymphomatoid Granulomatosis

Please see previous discussion in this chapter.

Posttransplant Lymphoproliferative Disorders

Posttransplant lymphoproliferative infiltration of the lung is usually seen in association with cyclosporine and can occur in 3% of post transplant patients. It usually occurs 4 to 6 months after transplantation. The radiographic features include solitary masses, multiple nodules, and occasionally hilar adenopathy (Fig. 9-22). There may also be involvement of gastrointestinal tract. The disorder usually regresses with decrease of immunosuppression.

SUGGESTED READINGS

Aberle DR, Gamsu G, Lynch D: Thoracic manifestations of Wegener's granulomatosis, *Radiology* 174:703-706, 1990.

Allen JN, Davis WB: Eosinophilic lung diseases, *Am J Respir Crit Care Med* 150:1423-1438, 1994.

Allen JN, Pacht ER, Gadek JE, Davis WB: Acute eosinophilic pneumonia as a reversible cause of noninfectious respiratory failure, *N Engl J Med* 321:569-574, 1989.

Ansell G: *Radiology of adverse reactions to drugs and toxic hazards,* ed 2, London, 1987, Chapman & Hall.

Badesch DB, King TE, Schwarz MI: Acute eosinophilic pneumonia: a hypersensitivity reaction? *Am Rev Respir Dis* 139:249-252, 1989.

Buchheit J, Eid N, Rodgers F Jr, Feger T, Yakoub O: Acute eosinophilic pneumonia with respiratory failure: a new syndrome? *Am Rev Respir Dis* 145:716-718, 1992.

Carrington CB, Addington WW, Goff AM et al: Chronic eosinophilic pneumonia, *N Engl J Med* 280:787-790, 1969.

Churg J, Strauss L: Allergic granulomatosis, allergic angiitis, and periarteritis nodosa, *Am J Pathol* 27:277-283, 1951.

Cooper JA, editor: Drug induced pulmonary disease, *Clin Chest Med* 11:1-194, 1990.

Cooper JA, White DA, Matthay RA: Drug induced pulmonary disease. Part I: cytotoxic drugs, *Am Rev Respir Dis* 133:321-340, 1986.

Cooper JA, White DA, Matthay RA: Drug induced pulmonary disease. Part II: noncytotoxic drugs, *Am Rev Respir Dis* 133:488-505, 1986.

Dreisin RB: Pulmonary vasculitis, *Clin Chest Med* 3(3):607-618, 1982.

Fauci AS, Haynes BF, Katz P: The spectrum of vasculitis: clinical, pathologic, immunologic, and therapeutic considerations, *Ann Intern Med* 89:660-664, 1978.

Fraser RG, Paré JAP: *Diagnosis of diseases of the chest,* ed 2, vol 2, Philadelphia, 1978, WB Saunders.

Gaensler EA, Carrington CB: Peripheral opacities in chronic eosinophilic pneumonia: the photographic negative of pulmonary edema, *AJR* 128:1-5, 1977.

Gefter WB: Drug induced disorders in the chest. In Taveras JM, Ferrucci JT, editors: *Radiology-diagnosis-imaging-intervention,* Philadelphia, 1984, JB Lippincott.

Kuhlman JE, Hruban RH, Fishman EK: Wegener's granulomatosis: CT features of parenchymal lung disease, *J Comput Assist Tomogr* 15:948-952, 1991.

Liebow AA, Carrington CB, Friedman PJ: Lymphomatoid granulomatosis, *Hum Pathol* 3:457-461, 1972.

Liebow AA: The J Burns Amberson Lecture: Pulmonary angiitis and granulomatosis, *Am Rev Respir Dis* 108:1-5, 1973.

Malo J, Pepys J, Simon G: Studies in chronic allergic bronchopulmonary aspergillosis. 2. Radiological findings, *Thorax* 32:262-265, 1977.

Matthay RA, Putman CE: Pulmonary-renal syndromes. In Putman CE, editor: *Pulmonary diagnosis: imaging and other techniques,* New York, 1981, Appleton Communications.

Matthay RA, Schwartz M, Petty TL: Pleuro-pulmonary manifestations of connective tissue diseases, *Clin Notes Respir Dis* 16:3-6, 1977.

Matthay RA, Schwartz MI, Petty TL et al: Pulmonary manifestations of systemic lupus erythematosus: review of 12 cases of acute lupus pneumonitis, *Medicine* 54:397-401, 1975.

McCarthy DS, Pepys J: Allergic bronchopulmonary aspergillosis: clinical immunology. I. Clinical features, *Clin Allergy* 1:261-264, 1971.

McLoud TC, Carrington CB, Gaensler EA: A new scheme for description of diffuse infiltrative lung disease, *Radiology* 149:353-357, 1983.

Müller NL, Miller R: Computed tomography of chronic diffuse infiltrative lung disease. Part I, *Am Rev Respir Dis* 142:1206-1210, 1990.

Müller NL, Miller R: Computed tomography of chronic diffuse infiltrative lung disease. Part II, *Am Rev Respir Dis* 142:1440-1445, 1990.

Pepys J: Hypersensitivity disease of the lungs due to fungi and organic dusts. In *Monographs in allergy,* Basel, 1969, Starger.

Pepys J: Pulmonary hypersentivity disease due to inhaled organic antigens, *Ann Intern Med* 64:943-946, 1966.

Schwartz MI, Matthay RA, Lahn SA et al: Interstitial lung disease in polymyositis, dermatomyositis. Analysis of six cases and a review of the literature, *Medicine* 55:89-95, 1976.

Symposium: Lung and heart disease associated with drug therapy and abuse, *J Thorac Imag* 6(1):1-84, 1991.

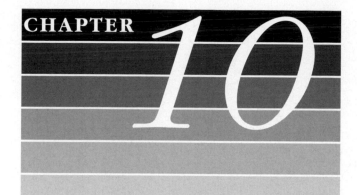

CHAPTER 10

Chronic Obstructive Pulmonary Disease

THERESA C. McLOUD

CHRONIC OBSTRUCTIVE PULMONARY DISEASE

Chronic obstructive pulmonary disease (COPD) consists of a group of disorders characterized by airway obstruction leading to decreased expiratory flow rates, and increased airways resistance with decrease in intrapulmonary diameters. COPD (Box 10-1) includes chronic bronchitis, which is defined in clinical terms, and emphysema, which is defined anatomically. Other disease entities sometimes classified as COPD include asthma and diffuse bronchiectasis (e.g., cystic fibrosis) and bronchiolitis obliterans. The latter two entities are discussed in Chapter 13. COPD is predominantly a disease of smokers, although only about 15% of smokers develop disabling air-flow obstruction.

The chest radiograph is an important imaging modality in the assessment of patients with COPD. However, it has limitations both in the detection and differential diagnosis of obstructive airways disease. It is relatively insensitive in the detection of early emphysema, and it is frequently normal in patients with pure chronic bronchitis and asthma. However, the recent development of high-resolution CT has significantly improved our ability to image morphologic abnormalities associated with chronic air-flow obstruction, particularly in emphysema, bronchiectasis, and bronchiolitis. In addition, CT permits the delineation of functional abnormalities such as air trapping and decreased perfusion.

EMPHYSEMA

Emphysema is defined as a condition of the lung characterized by abnormal permanent enlargement of the air spaces distal to the terminal bronchiole, accompanied by destruction of their walls without obvious fibrosis (Box 10-2).

Pathology

There are four major types of emphysema defined anatomically. These are: (1) centrilobular or centriacinar; (2) panlobular or panacinar; (3) paraseptal (distal acinar) emphysema; and (4) paracicatricial (irregular). The acinus is the air-exchanging unit of the lung located distal to the terminal bronchiole. It includes the respiratory bronchioles, alveolar ducts, alveolar sacs, and alveoli (Fig. 10-1). Although this classification relies on the relationship of emphysema to the acinus, acini cannot be resolved on high-resolution CT, and it may be more useful for the radiologist to consider the types of emphysema relative to their location at the lobular level (i.e., centrilobular, panlobular, and paraseptal).

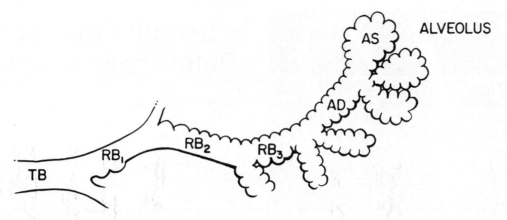

Figure 10-1. The acinus. The acinus is that part of the lung distal to the terminal bronchiole. *RB* = respiratory bronchiole, *AD* = alveolar duct, *AS* = alveolar sac. (From Thurlbeck WM: *Chronic airflow obstruction in lung disease,* Philadelphia, 1976, WB Saunders.)

Box 10-1   Chronic Obstructive Pulmonary Disease

Emphysema
Chronic bronchitis
Asthma
Cystic fibrosis and other causes of diffuse bronchiectasis
Bronchiolitis obliterans

Centrilobular emphysema (proximal acinar emphysema, centriacinar emphysema) affects predominately the respiratory bronchioles in the central portion of the secondary pulmonary lobule (Fig. 10-2). It is usually identified in the upper-lung zones, and it is associated with cigarette smoking. Panlobular (panacinar) emphysema involves all of the components of the acinus and therefore involves the entire lobule (Fig. 10-3). It is classically associated with alpha-1 protease inhibitor (alpha-1 antitrypsin) deficiency, although it may also be seen without protease deficiency in smokers, in the elderly, and distal to bronchial and bronchiolar obstruction. Thurlbeck has described this entity as a "diffuse simplification of the lung structure with progressive loss of tissue until little remains but the supporting framework of vessels, septa, and bronchi." Paraseptal emphysema (distal acinar emphysema) is characterized by involvement of the distal part of the secondary lobule, that is, the alveolar ducts and sacs, and therefore it occurs in a subpleural location (Fig. 10-4). It can be seen in the periphery of the lung adjacent to the chest wall but also along the interlobular septa and the fissures. Paraseptal emphysema, which can be an isolated phenomenon in young adults, is associated with spontaneous pneumothorax without other evidence of restriction in lung function. However, it can also be seen in older patients with centrilobular emphysema. These three

---

Box 10-2   Emphysema

PATHOLOGY

Centrilobular (central lobule)
Panlobular (entire lobule)
Paraseptal (distal lobule, subpleural)
Paracicatricial (around scars)

CLINICAL FEATURES

Cigarette smoking
Dyspnea
Chronic air-flow obstruction ($\downarrow$ FEV$_1$, $\uparrow$ TLC, $\uparrow$RV, $\downarrow$ DL$_{CO}$)

RADIOLOGY—STANDARD RADIOGRAPHS

Overinflation
Low, flat diaphragm
Increased retrosternal clear space

VASCULAR DEFICIENCY

Areas of irregular lucency
Bullae

DL_{CO}, diffusing capacity for carbon monoxide; FEV_1, forced expiratory volume in one second; RV, residual volume; TLC, total lung capacity.

forms of emphysema often can be distinguished morphologically, but as emphysema becomes severe, distinction among the three types becomes more difficult.

Paracicatricial or irregular emphysema refers to abnormal air-space enlargement associated with pulmonary fibrosis. This is most frequently a localized phenomenon.

Clinical Features

Emphysema is defined anatomically and pathologically. Emphysema may occur without detectable chronic airway obstruction. Mild degrees of emphysema are fre-

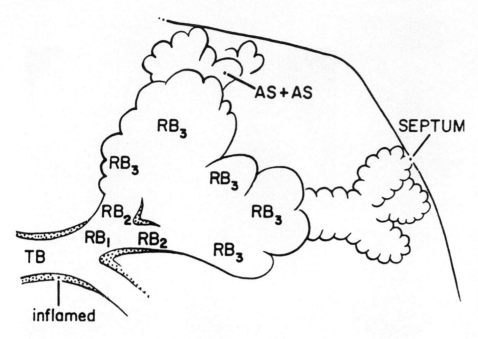

Figure 10-2. Centrilobular emphysema. The respiratory bronchioles are selectively and dominantly involved. (From Thurlbeck WM: *Chronic airflow obstruction in lung disease,* Philadelphia, 1976, WB Saunders.)

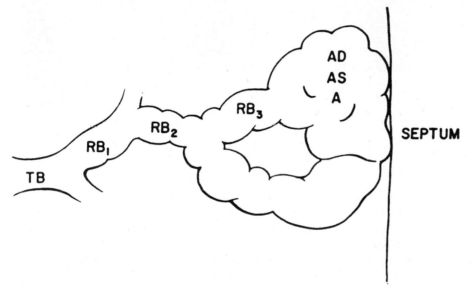

Figure 10-3. Panlobular emphysema. The enlargement and destruction of air spaces involve the acinus more or less uniformly. (From Thurlbeck WM: *Chronic airflow obstruction in lung disease,* Philadelphia, 1976, WB Saunders.)

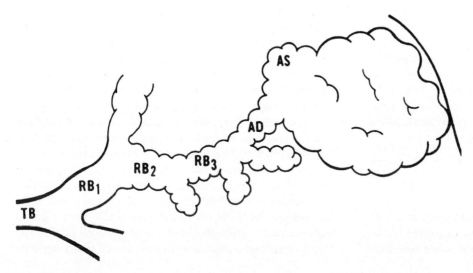

Figure 10-4. Paraseptal emphysema. The peripheral part of the acinus (alveolar ducts and sacs) is dominantly and selectively involved. (From Thurlbeck WM: *Chronic airflow obstruction in lung disease,* Philadelphia, 1976, WB Saunders.)

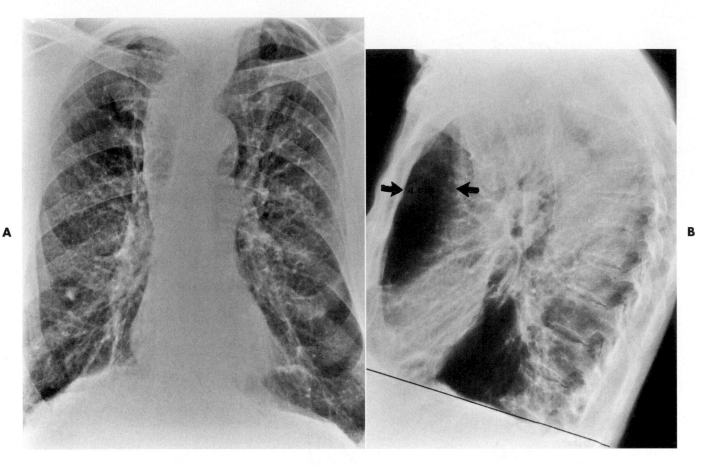

Figure 10-5. Emphysema. PA, **A,** and lateral, **B,** views of standard radiographs demonstrate low, flat hemidiaphragms and a retrosternal clear space *(arrows)* that measure 4 cm. The highest level of the dome of the diaphragm abuts a line drawn between the costophrenic junction and the vertebral phrenic junction. The heart is long and narrow.

quently found in smokers at autopsy. Widespread and severe emphysema is usually associated with a history of cigarette smoking, chronic air-flow obstruction, and dyspnea. The air-flow obstruction can be measured with pulmonary function tests by a diminution of the forced expiratory volume in one second (FEV_1) or the ratio of the FEV_1 to the forced vital capacity (FVC). Lung volumes increase in emphysema as a result of hyperinflation with increases in the total lung capacity, functional residual capacity, and residual volume with a concomitant decrease in vital capacity as the emphysema becomes more severe. The loss of the internal surface area of the lung and of the alveolar capillary bed, two components of emphysema, is reflected in a decrease in the diffusing capacity of carbon monoxide.

Radiographic Features

The standard radiograph

Emphysema can be diagnosed by standard radiography when the disease is severe. If the lungs are mildly affected by emphysema, the chest radiograph is usually normal. In addition, only about half of the cases of moderately severe emphysema are diagnosed radiologically. The standard radiograph is generally not considered a reliable tool for diagnosing and quantitating emphysema. However, there are certain radiographic signs that, when present, are accurate in the diagnosis of emphysema (Fig. 10-5). These include: (1) overinflation of the lungs. Hyperinflation is characterized by a low, flat diaphragm particularly on the lateral view. The diaphragm is considered flattened when the highest level of the dome is less than 1.5 cm above a straight line drawn between the costophrenic junction and the vertebral phrenic junction. The angle formed by the diaphragm and the anterior chest wall is often 90° or greater, compared with the acute angle seen with a normal upwardly curved diaphragm. Another criterion of overinflation is a widened retrosternal air space greater than 2.5 cm in diameter. The cardiac silhouette tends to be long and narrow. Similar radiographic findings are seen in severe asthma, but the signs of overexpansion abate with clinical improvement. In emphysema, however, they persist. (2) The second major sign of emphysema is a rapid tapering

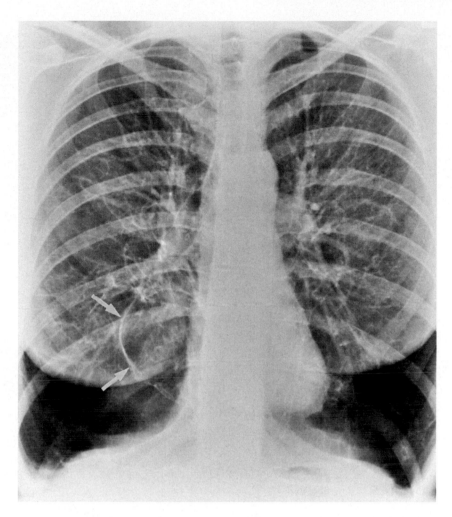

Figure 10-6. Emphysema. Patient with alpha-1 antitrypsin deficiency. This disorder is characterized by panlobular emphysema that is most marked at the bases. Note the attenuation of pulmonary vessels and increased lucency at the lung bases. There is a bulla in the right lower lobe *(arrows)*.

and attenuation of pulmonary vessels accompanied by irregular radiolucency of affected areas (Fig. 10-6). Although this is an important radiographic finding, it is subjective and difficult to detect before the disease is severe. Localized lucent areas, particularly if they are surrounded by consolidation, may be apparent in the periphery of the lungs.

Bullae may occur in emphysema (Fig. 10-6). A bulla is defined as a sharply demarcated area of emphysema measuring 1 cm or more in diameter and having a wall less than 1 mm in thickness. You should look carefully for evidence of bullae on the standard radiograph as supporting evidence for the presence of emphysema. Bullae reflect only locally severe involvement and do not necessarily mean that the disease is widespread.

High-resolution computed tomography

Computed tomography (CT) is superior to chest radiography in showing the presence, extent, and severity of emphysema. High-resolution CT (HRCT) has been shown to have elevated sensitivity and high specificity for emphysema. It is also possible with HRCT to distinguish among the anatomic types of emphysema (Box 10-3).

Centrilobular emphysema is characterized on HRCT by the presence of multiple small round areas of abnormally low attenuation, several millimeters to a centimeter in diameter and distributed throughout the lung but usually with an upper-lobe predominance (Fig. 10-7). The centrilobular location of these lucencies can sometimes be recognized. The lucencies tend to be multiple, small, and "spotty." Classically the areas of low attenuation of centrilobular emphysema lack visible walls. As the disease becomes more severe, the areas of lung destruction become more confluent and the centrilobular distribution may no longer be recognizable (Fig. 10-8). The HRCT appearance can then closely simulate panlobular emphysema.

Panlobular emphysema is characterized on HRCT by the presence of fewer and smaller-than-normal pul-

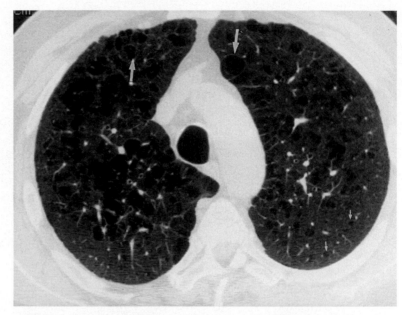

Figure 10-7. Centrilobular emphysema. There are multiple round areas of low attenuation without visible walls. Some measure only a few millimeters *(small white arrows)* while others are larger and qualify as bullae (>1 cm well-defined thin walls) *(large white arrows)*. The emphysema predominates in the upper lobes.

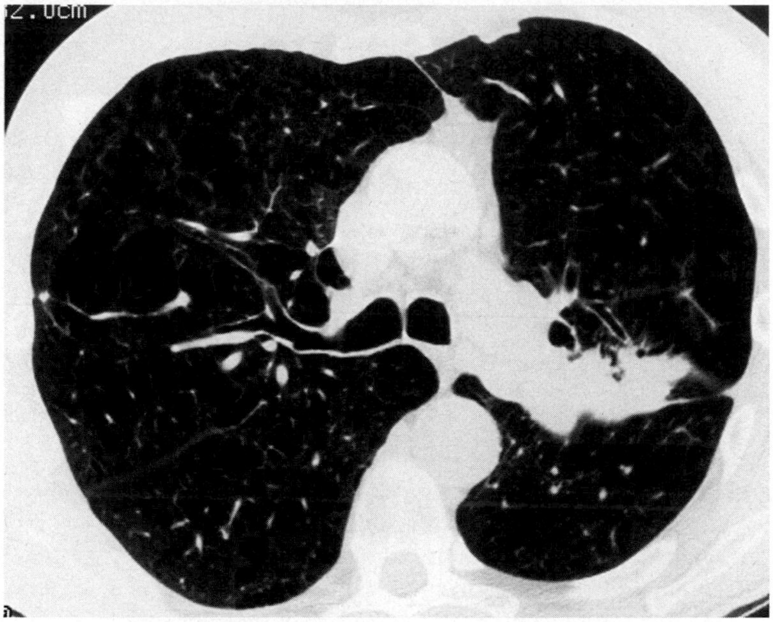

Figure 10-8. Severe centrilobular emphysema in a heavy smoker. There are confluent areas of lung destruction with marked attenuation of the pulmonary vasculature. The centrilobular distribution is not apparent.

Box 10-3 Emphysema as Seen on HRCT

TYPES

Centrilobular
    Multiple small areas of low attenuation
    No walls
    Upper lobes
Panlobular
    Fewer and smaller vessels
    Lower lobes
Paraseptal
    Subpleural and along fissures
    Thin walls
    Single row

Paracicatricial
    Usually focal
    Associated with scars

DIFFERENTIAL DIAGNOSIS

Honeycombing
Pneumatoceles
Cystic lung disease
Bronchiolitis obliterans

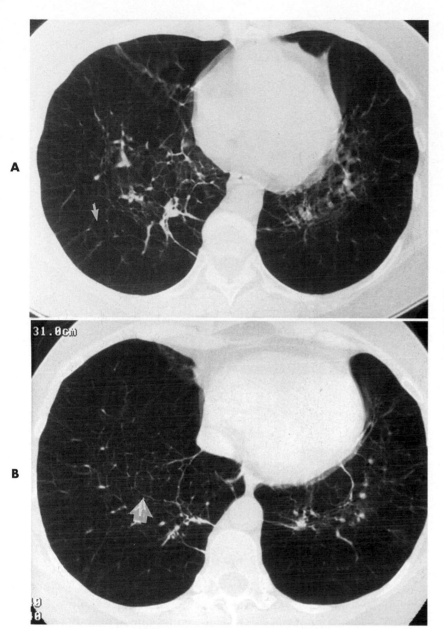

Figure 10-9. A and **B,** Panlobular emphysema. Patient with alpha-1 antitrypsin deficiency. There is pronounced paucity of vessels in both lower lobes. "Empty" secondary pulmonary lobules nearly devoid of vessels can be identified *(arrows).*

monary vessels (Fig. 10-9). It is almost always more severe in the lower lobes but may appear diffuse. When it is advanced, extensive lung destruction can be identified and the associated paucity of vessels is readily detectable. However, in moderate disease, increased lucency of the lung parenchyma and limited slight decrease in the caliber of the pulmonary vessels may be more difficult to recognize.

Mild paraseptal emphysema (Fig. 10-10) is easily detected by HRCT. The appearance is that of multiple areas of subpleural emphysema often with visible thin walls that correspond to interlobular septa. The emphysema is localized in the subpleural zones and along the interlobar fissures. When larger than a centimeter, areas of paraseptal emphysema are most appropriately termed

"bullae." Subpleural bullae are manifestations of paraseptal emphysema, although they may be seen in all types of emphysema. They are often associated with spontaneous pneumothorax in young adults.

Paracicatricial or irregular emphysema (Fig. 10-11) is focal emphysema usually found adjacent to parenchymal scars, in diffuse pulmonary fibrosis, and in the pneumoconioses particularly when progressive massive fibrosis is present. It is usually recognized on CT when the associated fibrosis is identified.

Clinical indications   HRCT is infrequently used as a diagnostic tool in emphysema. The diagnosis is usually made on a combination of clinical features, a smoking history, and compatible pulmonary function abnormalities. However, HRCT may be useful in patients whose

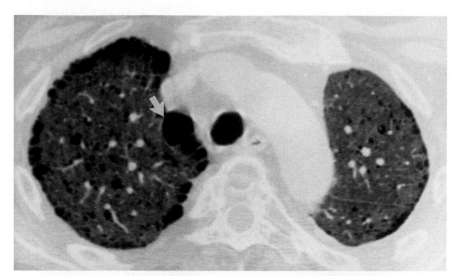

Figure 10-10. Paraseptal emphysema. Multiple areas of emphysema localized to the subpleural zones bilaterally. A bulla is noted on the right medially *(arrow).*

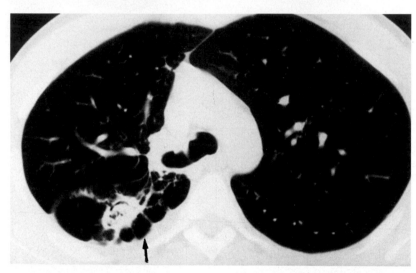

Figure 10-11. Paracicatricial emphysema. Focal emphysema *(arrow)* is seen surrounding an old tuberculous cavity with an intracavitary fungus ball.

clinical findings suggest another disease process such as interstitial lung disease or pulmonary vascular disease, namely shortness of breath and a low diffusing capacity without evidence of airway obstruction on pulmonary function tests. In such patients HRCT can be valuable in detecting the presence of emphysema and in excluding other abnormalities in the chest. There are a number of HRCT methodologies available to quantitate the degree and severity of emphysema.

Differential diagnosis Several entities should be considered in the differential diagnosis of emphysema on HRCT. These include: (1) *Honeycombing.* This occurs in pulmonary fibrosis and is characterized by areas of subpleural cystic lesions somewhat mimicking the appearance of paraseptal emphysema. However, honeycomb cysts are usually smaller; they occur in several layers along the pleural surface, are localized in the lung bases, and are associated with other findings of fibrosis. Paraseptal emphysema, on the other hand, is often associated with bullae, and the areas of emphysema are larger and occur in a single layer. They predom-

inate in the upper lobes without evidence of fibrosis. (2) *Pneumatoceles.* A pneumatocele is defined as a thin-walled, gas-filled space within the lung, usually occurring in association with acute pneumonia or more chronic infections such as *Pneumocystis carinii* pneumonia. They are usually transient and can be identical to bullae on HRCT. However, the association with current or previous infection should suggest the diagnosis. (3) *Cystic lung disease.* Multiple thin-walled lung cysts can be seen in a variety of disorders, particularly the infiltrative lung diseases such as lymphangioleiomyomatosis and histiocytosis. These cysts usually can be differentiated from centrilobular emphysema because the walls are more distinct and lung cysts appear larger. When the lucency can be clearly identified as within the center of the pulmonary lobule, it is diagnostic of centrilobular emphysema. (4) *Bronchiolitis obliterans.* Bronchiolitis obliterans, a disease of the small airways, can result in increased lung volume and oligemia similar to panlobular emphysema. It is usually, however, patchy in distribution, an important distinguishing fea-

BULLAE

Features
    Paraseptal and centrilobular emphysema
    >1 cm in diameter
    Well-defined wall, <1mm thick
"Vanishing lung" syndrome
    Young men
    Upper-lobe giant bullae
    Preoperative assessment CT

LUNG-REDUCTION SURGERY

Resection of selected areas of emphysema
Evaluation with CT

Box 10-5 Chronic Bronchitis

CLINICAL AND PATHOLOGIC FEATURES

Clinical definition
Pathology—mucous-gland hyperplasia

RADIOGRAPHIC FEATURES

Normal
Thickened bronchial walls
    End-on ring shadows
    Tram lines (in profile)
Overinflation

ture. Some dilation of the central airways with mild bronchiectasis is also more common in patients with bronchiolitis obliterans than in patients with panlobular emphysema.

Other features

Box 10-4 summarizes other features of emphysema.

Bullous emphysema does not represent a specific pathologic entity but refers to the presence of emphysema associated with large bullae. Bullae can develop in association with any type of emphysema, but they are most common in paraseptal and centrilobular emphysema. A bulla is defined as a sharply demarcated area of emphysema measuring more than 1 cm in diameter and possessing a well-defined wall less than 1 mm in thickness. Bullae occasionally can become quite large and may be rather focal; occasionally, they are not associated with diffuse emphysema. Large bullae may result in compromised respiratory function. This syndrome has been referred to variously as bullous emphysema, vanishing lung syndrome, and primary bullous disease of the lung (Fig. 10-12). This entity may occur in young men and is characterized by large progressive upper-lobe bullae. Most are smokers, but the entity may occur in nonsmokers. CT, particularly HRCT, may be helpful in delineating the volume, location, and number of bullae as well as the degree of compression of the underlying lung and the severity of emphysema in the remainder of the lung parenchyma (Fig. 10-12). Such an assessment is often helpful because such bullae can be resected with marked improvement in pulmonary function. CT is of value in the preoperative assessment of such patients.

HRCT may also be useful in the preoperative evaluation of patients with severe emphysema who are selected for lung volume-reduction surgery. This surgery involves the resection of target areas of emphy-

sema in both lungs that can be excised to reduce lung volume without significant sacrifice of lung tissue. In selected patients this procedure has been shown to improve respiratory mechanics, diminish oxygen requirement, reduce dyspnea, and improve the quality of life.

CHRONIC BRONCHITIS

Clinical and Pathologic Features

Chronic bronchitis (Box 10-5), unlike emphysema, is defined in clinical rather than pathologic terms. It is defined as a productive cough occurring on most days for at least 3 consecutive months and for not less than 2 consecutive years. Other causes of chronic productive cough including bronchiectasis, tuberculosis, and other chronic infections must be excluded before the diagnosis of chronic bronchitis can be made. Most patients with chronic bronchitis are smokers, and frequently emphysema is present.

Pathologically, the hallmark of chronic bronchitis is mucous-gland hyperplasia. There is an increased volume of the mucous glands; this can be assessed by the bronchial gland:bronchial-wall ratio, termed the Reid index.

Radiographic Features

The radiographic features are nonspecific, and the chest radiograph is most frequently normal. Described features include thickened bronchial walls seen either end-on in cross-section or in "profile" (tram lines), as well as hyperinflation of the lungs (Fig. 10-13). Bronchial-wall thickening is a nonspecific finding that may be seen in patients with interstitial pulmonary edema as well as other interstitial diseases, asthma, and bronchiectasis, and occasionally in healthy subjects. On HRCT the most prominent finding is usually that of emphysema, although some bronchial-wall thickening and mild dila-

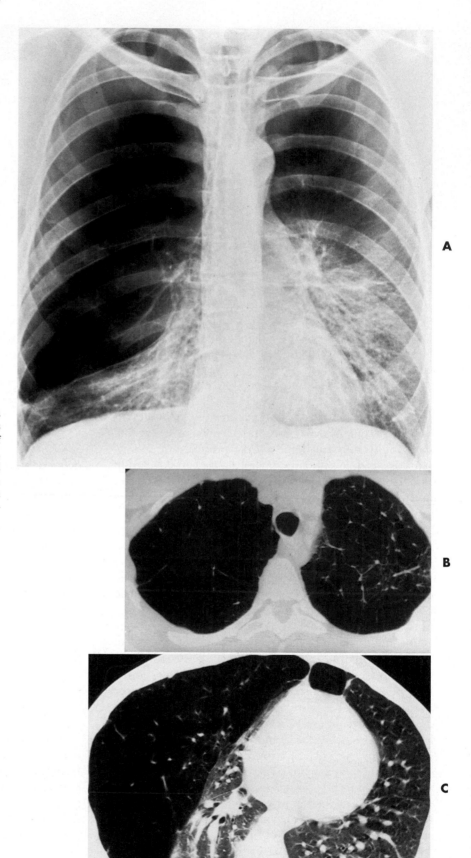

Figure 10-12. "Vanishing lung" syndrome in a 30-year-old man. **A,** PA chest radiograph shows bilateral upper lobe bullae with compression of the basilar lung. The minor fissure is depressed. **B,** HRCT through the upper lobes shows bilateral bullae with the right side more severely affected. **C,** HRCT at the bases demonstrates compression of the middle and lower lobes, which are relatively free of emphysema.

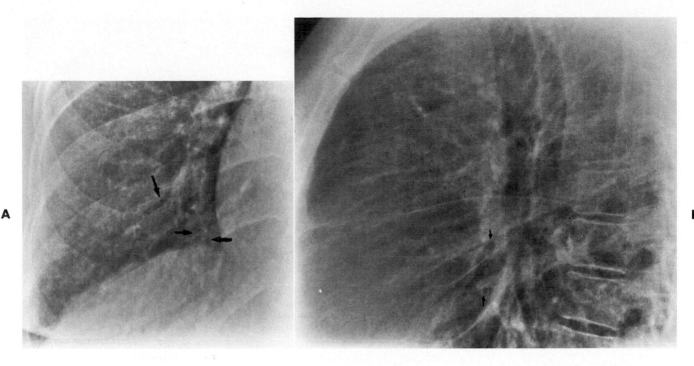

A   **B**

Figure 10-13. Chronic bronchitis. **A,** PA radiograph demonstrates bronchial-wall thickening in profile ("tram tracking") *(arrows)* Bronchi are seen more peripherally in the lung than is normally the case. **B,** The lateral radiograph shows thickened end on bronchi peripheral to the hilar areas.

tion can be observed. The diagnosis of chronic bronchitis is based on clinical rather than radiographic findings.

ASTHMA

Clinical Features

Asthma (Box 10-6) is a chronic illness that causes widespread narrowing of the tracheobronchial tree. It is characterized by reversible bronchospasm that may be provoked by a variety of stimuli. There are often acute exacerbations that resolve spontaneously or with therapy. It is a common disease, estimated to affect 3% to 5% of the population of the United States. At least two thirds of patients are atopic, and the pathogenesis of asthma in these individuals is related to a reaction to different types of allergens. Mortality, though rare, has been increasing for several years. Pathologically, the disease is characterized by an active inflammatory process in the airways, even when patients are asymptomatic. Further features include edema of the bronchial mucosa and excessive mucus production.

Radiographic Features

Uncomplicated asthma

There is some controversy regarding the indications for a chest radiograph in asthma. In adults it is generally agreed that a chest radiograph should be obtained when

---

Box 10-6 Asthma

CLINICAL AND PATHOLOGIC FEATURES

Reversible bronchospasm
Two thirds atopic
Active inflammation of the airways

RADIOGRAPHIC FEATURES

Uncomplicated
  Normal in majority
  Signs of hyperinflation
  Bronchial-wall thickening
  HRCT—bronchial-wall thickening and mild dilation
  of bronchi
Complicated
  Pneumonia
  Lobar or segmental atelectasis
  Allergic bronchopulmonary aspergillosis (ABPA)—
  mucoid impaction
  Pneumomediastinum
  Pneumothorax

---

asthma is first suspected and when conventional treatment is ineffective in order to exclude other causes of wheezing, such as neoplasm, congestive heart failure, bronchiectasis, and foreign bodies. In pediatric patients, chest radiographs are seldom abnormal and should be obtained only when (1) there is no improvement or

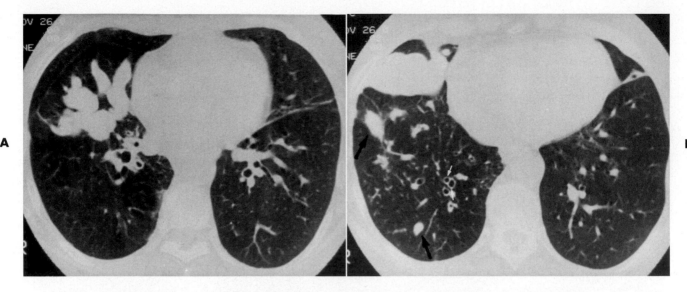

Figure 10-14. Mucoid impaction with allergic bronchopulmonary aspergillosis (ABPA) in an asthmatic patient. **A,** Branching V-shaped, mucus-filled, dilated bronchi are identified in the right lung anteriorly. **B,** There are mucous plugs in the lower lobes, which are more oval or round in shape *(black arrows)*. Bronchi are slightly dilated with wall-thickening *(small white arrows)*.

when there is worsening of symptoms despite conventional therapy; (2) when there is fever in association with ausculatory findings that persist after treatment; and (3) when there is a clinical suspicion of a complication such as pneumothorax.

In most patients with asthma the chest radiograph is normal. Radiographic changes, more common in children than in adults, usually consist of signs of hyperinflation, flattening of the hemidiaphragms best identified on the lateral radiograph, and increase in the retrosternal air space. Another radiographic feature of asthma is that of bronchial-wall thickening. In children the walls of secondary bronchi are normally not discernible beyond the mediastinum and hila; when visualized more peripherally in the lung, they are considered abnormal. In both adults and children, the thickening of the bronchial walls can best be detected in bronchi seen in cross-section most commonly in the perihilar areas. Bronchi seen in the longitudinal plane often appear as "tram lines," paired parallel lines separated by lucency. Occasionally the thickening of the bronchial walls may produce a perihilar haze or stringy linear opacities in the perihilar areas. Transient pulmonary hypertension during severe attacks of asthma will increase the size of the central pulmonary arteries on standard radiographs. This is probably secondary to alveolar hypoxia.

On HRCT, mild bronchial dilation has been reported in 15% to 77% of asthmatic patients, and over 90% may have bronchial-wall thickening.

Complicated asthma

The most frequent complication in asthma is pneumonia. In the pediatric age group, the majority of exacerbations are viral and are particularly due to respiratory syncytial virus in infants and parainfluenza and rhinoviruses in older children. The radiographic appearance is similar to viral pneumonias in the nonasthmatic population. Lobar or segmental atelectasis can occur in asthma, but it is unusual. It is seen more commonly in children and most frequently involves the right middle lobe secondary to the retention of mucus in the large airways.

Allergic bronchopulmonary aspergillosis is discussed in more detail in the chapter dealing with the airways. The most characteristic finding is the presence of central bronchiectasis frequently involving or predominating in the upper lobes. The ectatic bronchi are often filled with mucoid material that contains aspergillus. Radiographic findings of mucoid impaction include a bandlike opacity that appears like fingers of a glove; this can also be V-shaped, Y-shaped, or round (Fig. 10-14). Mucous plugs are typically located centrally in the perihilar areas and upper lobes. (See Chapter 13.)

Pneumomediastinum is a complication of asthma that is said to occur in approximately 1% to 5% of asthma cases and has a bimodal distribution peaking at ages 4 to 6 and 13 to 18. The postulated mechanism is a mucus plug or infection that causes a check-valve obstruction that increases intraalveolar pressure. With deep inspiration or cough the alveolar wall may rupture with tracking of interstitial air towards the hilum and eventual extension into the mediastinum along the perivascular sheaths. Patients usually have symptoms of chest or neck pain. Radiographic findings are described in detail in Chapter 5. The findings are often subtle (Fig. 10-15). Air encircling major bronchi and hilar vessels and outlining

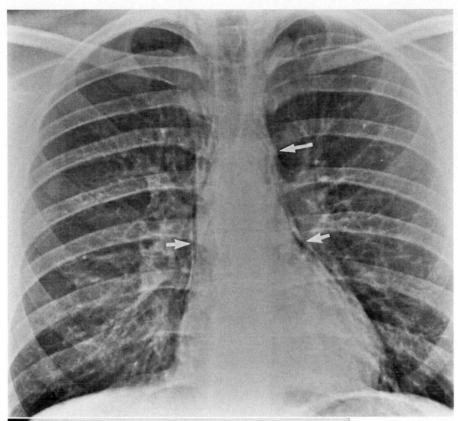

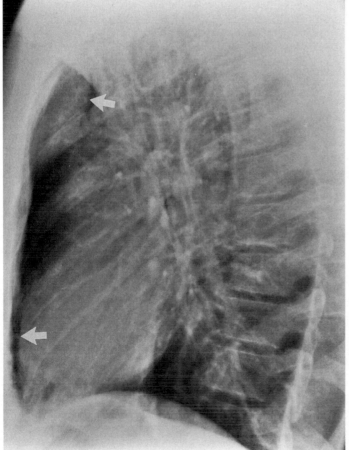

Figure 10-15. Pneumomediastinum in 19-year-old man with asthma. **A,** Streaks of air can be seen outlining the heart, aorta, and superior vena cava *(arrows)*. **B,** On the lateral view air is seen behind the sternum and outlining the thymus *(arrows)*.

the trachea and the esophagus, the aorta, and the heart is characteristic. It may be observed more easily on the lateral view. Air will eventually dissect into the neck, and you should carefully search the soft tissues of the neck for evidence of air, which can often be more easily detected than air in the mediastinum. Occasionally, inferior dissection of air may result in either pneumoperitoneum or an extraperitoneal air collection.

Pneumothorax may occur in conjunction with pneumomediastinum and, although rare, may be fatal. It may be secondary to barotrauma in intubated asthmatic patients. It usually occurs with long-standing disease. A small pneumothorax may be important in patients who are intubated and maintained on intermittent positive-pressure breathing. The chest radiograph will be diagnostic, and expiratory films may increase the visibility of a small pneumothorax.

SUGGESTED READINGS

Bergin CJ, Müller NL, Nichols DM et al: The diagnosis of emphysema: a computed tomographic-pathologic correlation, *Am Rev Respir Dis* 133:541-546, 1986.

Blair DN, Coppage L, Shaw C: Medical imaging in asthma, *J Thorac Imag* 1:23-35, 1986.

Burrows B: Airways obstructive diseases: pathogenetic mechanisms and natural history of the disorders, *Med Clin North Am* 74:547-559, 1990.

Cardoso WV, Thurlbeck WM: Pathogenesis and terminology of emphysema, *Am J Respir Crit Care Med* 149:1383, 1994.

Carr DH, Pride NB: Computed tomography in pre-operative assessment of bullous emphysema, *Clin Radiol* 35:43-45, 1984.

Foster WL Jr, Gimenez EI, Roubidoux MA, Sherrier RH et al: The emphysemas: radiologic—pathologic correlations, *Radio-Graphics* 13:311-328, 1993.

Foster WL Jr, Pratt PC, Roggli VL, Godwin JD, Halvorsen RA, Putman: Centrilobular emphysema: CT-pathologic correlation, *Radiology* 159:27-32, 1986.

Fraser RG, Fraser RS, Renner JW, Bernard C, Fitzgerald PJ: The roentgenologic diagnosis of chronic bronchitis: a reassessment with emphasis on parahilar bronchi seen end-on, *Radiology* 120:1-9, 1976.

Fraser RG, Paré JAP, Paré PD, Fraser RS, Genereux GP: *Diagnosis of diseases of the chest,* ed 3, Philadelphia, 1990, WB Saunders; pp 1969-2221.

Heitzman RB: Chronic obstructive pulmonary disease. In Heitzman RB, ed 2, St. Louis, 1984, Mosby–Year Book; pp 429-456.

Hodson ME, Simon G, Batten JC: Radiology of uncomplicated asthma, *Thorax* 29:296-303, 1974.

Kim JS, Müller NL: Obstructive lung disease. In Freundlich IM, Bragg DG, editors: *A radiologic approach to diseases of the chest,* ed 2, Baltimore, 1997, Williams & Wilkins; pp 709-722.

Kinsella M, Müller NL, Abboud RT, Morrison NJ, Bybuncio A: Quantitation of emphysema by computed tomography using a "density mask" program and correlation with pulmonary function test, *Chest* 97:315-321, 1990.

Klein J, Gamsu G, Webb WR, Golden JA, Müller NL: High-resolution CT diagnosis of emphysema in symptomatic patients with normal chest radiographs and isolated low diffusing capacity, *Radiology* 182:817-821, 1992.

Lynch DA, Newell JD, Tschomper BA, Cink TM, Newman LS, Bethel R: Uncomplicated asthma in adults: comparison of CT appearance of the lungs in asthmatic and healthy subjects, *Radiology* 188:829-833, 1993.

McFadden ER, Gilbert IA: Asthma, *New Engl J Med* 327(27):1928-1937, 1992.

Miller RR, Müller NL, Vedal S, Morrison NJ, Staples CA: Limitations of computed tomography in the assessment of emphysema, *Am Rev Respir Dis* 139:980-983, 1989.

Miniati M, Filippi E, Falaschi F, Carrozzi L, Milne ENC, Sostman HD, Pistolesi M: Radiographic evaluation of emphysema in patients with chronic obstructive pulmonary disease, *Am J Respir Crit Care Med* 151:1359-1367, 1995.

Müller NL, Staples CA, Miller RR, Abboud RT: "Density mask": an objective method to quantitate emphysema using computed tomography, *Chest* 94:782-787, 1988.

Neeld DA, Goodman LR, Gurney JW, Greenberger PA, Fink JN: Computerized tomography in the evaluation of allergic bronchopulmonary aspergillosis, *Am Rev Respir Dis* 142:1200-1206, 1990.

Pratt PG: Role of conventional chest radiography in diagnosis and exclusion of emphysema, *Am J Med* 82:998-1006, 1987.

Snider GL: Emphysema: the first two centuries—and beyond. Part I & II, *Am Rev Respir Dis* 146:1334-1344; 1615-1622, 1992.

Snider GL, Kleinerman J, Thurlbeck WM, Bengali ZH: The definition of emphysema. Report of a National Heart, Lung, and Blood Institute, Division of Lung Diseases Workshop, *Am Rev Respir Dis* 132:182-185, 1985.

Spouge D, Mayo JR, Cardoso W, Müller NL: Panacinar emphysema: CT and pathologic correlation, *J Comput Assist Tomogr* 17:710-713, 1993.

Stern EJ, Webb WR, Weinacker A, Müller NL: Idiopathic giant bullous emphysema (vanishing lung syndrome): imaging findings in nine patients, *AJR* 162:279-282, 1994.

Thurlbeck WM: *Chronic airflow obstruction in lung disease,* Philadelphia, 1976, WB Saunders; pp 12-30.

Thurlbeck WM, Henderson JA, Fraser RG, Bates DV: Chronic obstructive lung disease: comparison between clinical, roentgenologic, functional and morphologic criteria in chronic bronchitis, emphysema, asthma, and bronchiectasis, *Medicine* 48:82-145, 1970.

Thurlbeck WM, Müller NL: Emphysema: definition, imaging, and quantification, *AJR* 163:1017-1025, 1994.

Thurlbeck WM, Simon G: Radiographic appearance of the chest in emphysema, *AJR* 130:429-440, 1978.

Webb WR: High-resolution computed tomography of obstructive lung disease, *Radiol Clin North Am* 32:745-755, 1994.

Webb WR, Müller NL, Naidich DP: *High resolution CT of the lung,* ed 2, Philadelphia, 1996, Lippincott-Raven; pp 227-265.

Pulmonary Neoplasms

THERESA C. McLOUD

The most important neoplasm involving the lung is lung cancer (bronchogenic carcinoma), the leading cause of cancer mortality in the United States. It accounts for over 150,000 deaths each year. In addition to lung cancer, there are a number of other primary malignant neoplasms as well as benign neoplasms and other tumoral processes that originate in the lung. The lungs are a frequent site of metastases from extrathoracic malignancies.

BENIGN NEOPLASMS AND OTHER TUMORS OF NONNEOPLASTIC NATURE

A wide variety of benign tumoral lesions can occur in the lung. Some of these are true neoplasms and others are of uncertain nature or origin. Benign neoplasms may arise in the tracheobronchial glands, soft tissue, bone, and cartilage, or they may be from mixed mesenchymal origin. Nonneoplastic tumors include hamartomas and inflammatory pseudotumors.

Hamartoma

Characteristics
Hamartomas (Box 11-1) are acquired lesions composed of tissues normally found within the organ but demonstrating disorganized growth. Hamartomas, the most common benign tumors of the lung, account for 5% to 8% of solitary pulmonary nodules.

Clinical features
The peak incidence occurs in the sixth decade of life, with an age range of 30 to 70. The lesions are slightly more predominant in women. Most patients are asymptomatic, and the hamartoma is discovered on a routine chest radiograph as a solitary pulmonary nodule. Occasionally, however, hamartomas can occur endobronchially and may produce obstructive symptoms.

Pathologic features
These tumors contain nests of cartilage surrounded by fibrous tissue and mature fat cells. Other mesenchymal components such as bone, vessels, and smooth muscle may be present.

Radiographic features
Characteristically, hamartomas appear as well-defined, solitary, spherical nodules or masses. They are usually less than 4 cm in diameter, and they have well-defined margins (Fig. 11-1). Calcification is reported to be present in 10% to 15% of cases on standard radiographs, although it is more frequently identified on CT. The calcification has a characteristic morphology that produces

---

Box 11-1   Hamartomas

CHARACTERISTICS

Acquired
Tissues normal to organ
Disorganized growth
5% to 8% solitary pulmonary nodules

CLINICAL

30 to 70 years
Asymptomatic

PATHOLOGY

Cartilage
Fat
Fibrous tissue

RADIOLOGY

Solitary, well-defined pulmonary nodule
Ca^{++} 10% to 15%
CT—fat and calcium (25%)

---

a "popcorn" appearance (Fig. 11-1). Hamartomas typically grow slowly, and in rare cases they can be multiple.

Thin collimation CT can be valuable in diagnosing pulmonary hamartomas. The presence of focal deposits of fat (-50 to -150 HU) is most helpful in making this diagnosis (Fig. 11-2). In approximately 25% of cases, calcification can also be identified.

Amyloid

Characteristics
Amyloid, (Box 11-2) a waxy pink material that stains with Congo red, has a typical birefringence with polarization microscopy. It occurs in two major forms, primary and secondary. Lung involvement in primary amyloidosis is estimated to occur in 30% to 90% of cases. Secondary amyloidosis is usually associated with rheumatoid arthritis, suppurative disease such as osteomyelitis, and malignant neoplasms. Amyloidosis may also be seen in association with multiple myeloma. In the thorax, amyloid occurs in two locations. The first is the tracheobronchial tree. Airway amyloidosis is discussed in Chapter 12. Amyloidosis may also involve the lung parenchyma in either a nodular form or as a diffuse infiltrative process.

Clinical features
The nodular disease usually occurs late in life, in the seventh decade, with an equal sex prevalence. Patients are usually asymptomatic, and the prognosis is excellent. The diffuse infiltrative form is less common and usually

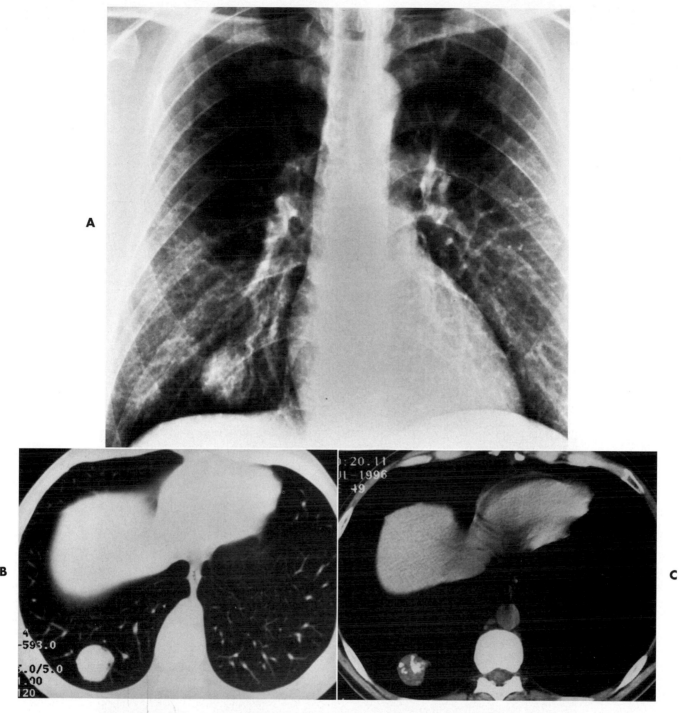

Figure 11-1. Hamartoma. **A** and **B,** Frontal radiograph and CT scan show a well-defined 3-cm spherical nodule in the right lower lobe. **C,** The nodule has classic "popcorn" calcification.

occurs in the sixth decade. Patients with the diffuse form are symptomatic. Diffuse infiltration of amyloid material associated with giant cells and plasma cells involves both vascular walls and the interstitial compartments of the lung. The disease is accompanied by symptoms of progressive dyspnea and leads to eventual death from respiratory insufficiency.

Radiographic features

The radiologic appearance of the nodular form consists of solitary or multiple nodules and masses (Fig. 11-3). Calcification is common, occurring in 30% to 50%, of patients but cavitation is rare. The lower lobes are more frequently involved, often in a subpleural distribution. These nodules may exhibit slow growth.

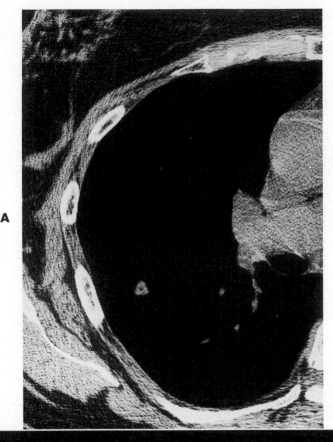

	209	210	211	212	213	214	215	216	217	218	219
313	-577	-217	-47	-44	-25	25	14	24	-37	-289	-613
314	-473	-105	14	25	20	21	35	25	5	-76	-370
315	-294	-26	28	-5	11	37	25	17	17	-38	-328
316	-107	1	36	33	6	15	10	4	-33	-34	-289
317	-58	-9	-20	14	22	-46	-18	13	-1	9	-138
318	-8	24	-7	-66	-42	-45	-20	39	40	50	34
319	0	0	-12	-14	-85	-101	-35	-20	28	35	-25
320	-41	-2	48	1	-14	-87	5	35	19	32	-14
321	18	9	28	-5	26	3	37	36	15	23	21
322	42	12	70	22	46	21	1	-30	2	25	43
323	4	33	48	44	31	-2	-2	-32	37	5	-35

Figure 11-2. Hamartoma. **A,** Thin collimation CT scan (1.5 mm) demonstrates a solitary nodule with a low-attenuation center in the right lung. **B,** A printout of CT numbers through each pixel in the lesion shows a cluster of values equal to fat attenuation.

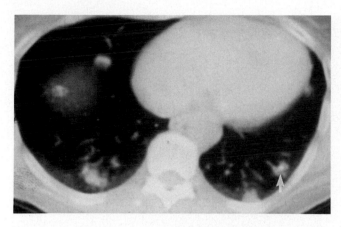

Figure 11-3. Amyloidosis, nodular form. CT scan in an asymptomatic elderly man shows multiple pulmonary nodules. One in the left lower lobe is calcified *(arrow)*.

Box 11-2   Amyloid

CHARACTERISTICS

Waxy pink material stains with Congo red
Forms
    Primary
    Secondary
Thoracic involvement
    Airway
    Parenchyma
        Nodules
        Diffuse infiltration

CLINICAL FEATURES

Nodular
    Seventh decade of life
    Asymptomatic
Infiltrative
    Sixth decade of life
    Symptomatic

RADIOGRAPHIC FEATURES

Nodular
    Solitary or multiple masses
        Ca^{++} in 30% to 50%
        Slow growth
Infiltrative
    Fine bilateral linear or nodular pattern

In the diffuse infiltrative form, bilateral fine linear, nodular, or reticulonodular patterns may be present (Fig. 11-4). There is no specific distribution in the lung parenchyma. There may be associated nodal calcification.

Laryngotracheal Papillomatosis

This is discussed in Chapter 12.

Box 11-3   Pulmonary Pseudotumors

CHARACTERISTICS

Types
    Plasma cell granuloma
    Inflammatory pseudotumor
    Histiocytoma
    Xanthoma
    Mast cell granuloma
Etiology
    May be sequela of organized pneumonia

CLINICAL FEATURES

Wide age range
Asymptomatic

RADIOGRAPHIC FEATURES

Solitary, well-defined nodules
20% Ca^{++}

Leiomyoma

Neoplasms of smooth muscle are among the most common primary soft-tissue tumors of the lung. A leiomyoma usually presents as a solitary, well-circumscribed nodule; it is peripheral and occasionally may calcify.

Other Benign Soft Tissue Tumors of the Lung

Lipomas, chondromas, and fibromas may represent a one-dimensional histologic expression of hamartoma. These typically represent as solitary, peripheral, pulmonary nodules. The chondromas are frequently calcified.

Pulmonary Pseudotumor

Characteristics

Pulmonary pseudotumors (Box 11-3) include a number of histologic entities such as plasma-cell granuloma, inflammatory pseudotumor, histiocytoma, xanthoma, and mast-cell granuloma. The etiology of pulmonary pseudotumors is unknown, though they have been thought to represent a localized form of organizing pneumonia in patients with subclinical infection. Plasma cell granuloma is discussed more extensively in Chapter 9. Pulmonary pseudotumors occur slightly more frequently in males than in females over a wide age range. Patients are often asymptomatic, and antecedent infection can be documented in less than a fifth of cases.

Pathologic features

These tumors usually consist of a mixture of spindle cells, plasma cells, lymphocytes, and histiocytes with plasma cells predominating in the plasma cell granuloma form.

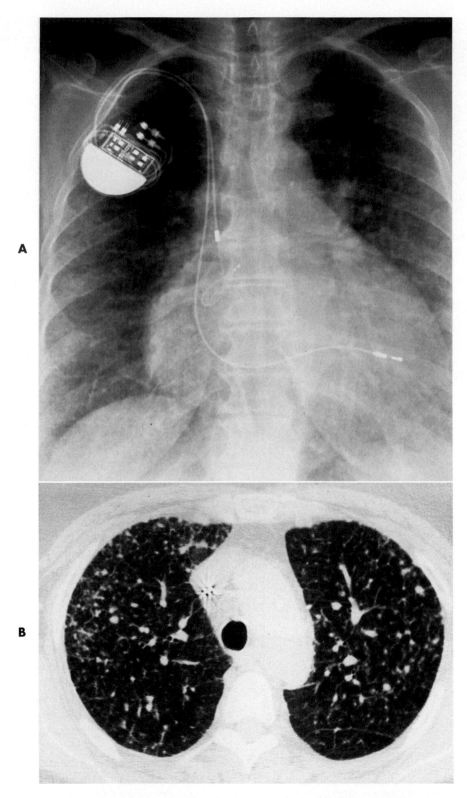

Figure 11-4. Amyloidosis, diffuse infiltrative form. Patient with known cardiac and pulmonary amyloid. **A,** Frontal radiograph shows a diffuse reticulonodular pattern. **B,** On HRCT there are linear and nodular opacities with septal thickening.

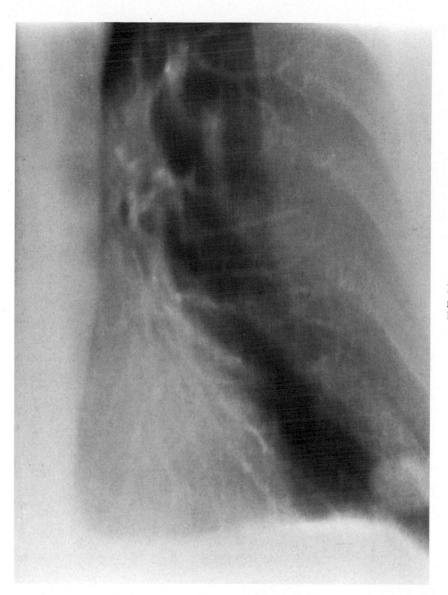

Figure 11-5. Plasma cell granuloma. AP tomogram shows a smooth, well-defined peripheral lung nodule.

Radiographic features

Pulmonary pseudotumors present as solitary, peripheral, pulmonary nodules that are well marginated (Fig. 11-5). Calcification occurs in about a fifth of cases, and airway involvement is uncommon. Rarely, particularly in children, these tumors may invade adjacent structures. Airway involvement is unusual.

LUNG CANCER

Lung cancer (bronchogenic carcinoma) is the leading cause of cancer mortality in the United States, with over 160,000 individuals diagnosed each year and over 140,000 succumbing to the disease. It is the most common cancer in men worldwide and it has now surpassed breast cancer as the leading cause of cancer death in women. Indeed, lung cancer one of the most common lung diseases that radiologists in practice encounter. Both computed tomography (CT) and magnetic resonance imaging (MRI), in addition to standard radiography, play an important role in the diagnosis and staging of patients with lung cancer.

Clinical features

Eighty-five percent to 90% of lung cancer deaths are directly attributable to cigarette smoking. The risk is related to the number of cigarettes smoked, the duration of smoking years, the age at which smoking began, and the depth of inhalation. The risk decreases with cessation of smoking but never completely disappears. Other etiologic factors may play a role in the development of bronchogenic carcinoma. These factors include genetic, occupational, and the presence of concomitant disease in the lungs.

It is well known that certain occupational agents may increase the risk of lung cancer. These are listed in Box 11-4. The most important of these is asbestos. A combi-

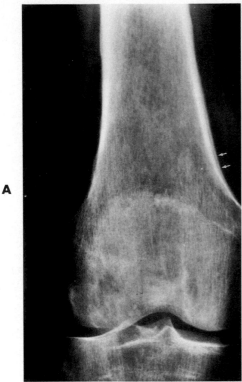

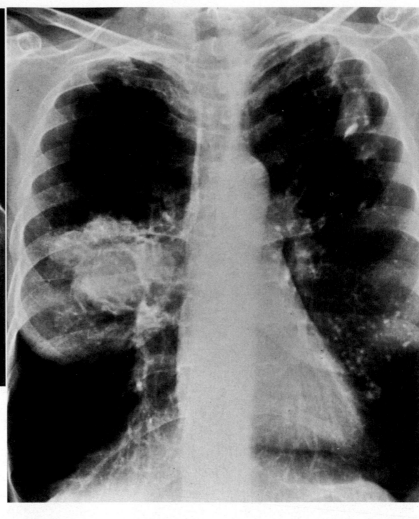

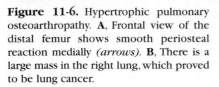

Figure 11-6. Hypertrophic pulmonary osteoarthropathy. **A**, Frontal view of the distal femur shows smooth periosteal reaction medially *(arrows)*. **B**, There is a large mass in the right lung, which proved to be lung cancer.

Box 11-4 Occupational and Environmental Agents Associated with Lung Cancer

Asbestos
Coke
Arsenic
Chromium
Chloromethyl ether
Mustard gas

Box 11-5 Diseases Associated with Lung Cancer

Tuberculosis
Asbestosis
Idiopathic pulmonary fibrosis
Scleroderma

---

nation of asbestos exposure and cigarette smoking is multiplicative and results in a marked increased risk of lung cancer, particularly if asbestosis is present in the parenchyma of the lungs. Most of the concomitant lung diseases associated with bronchogenic carcinoma reflect the presence of fibrosis in the lungs (Box 11-5). These include any cause of end-stage lung disease such as idiopathic pulmonary fibrosis and localized fibrosing disease such as tuberculosis.

Only 10% of patients with lung carcinoma are asymptomatic (Box 11-6). Most often symptoms are due to central tumors that result in obstruction of a major bronchus. This leads to cough, wheezing, hemoptysis, and postobstructive pneumonia. Local intrathoracic spread may result in related symptoms such as pleuritic or chest-wall pain, Pancoast syndrome, and symptoms related to obstruction of the superior vena cava. Occasionally, patients may have symptoms that result from distant metastases (i.e., a seizure related to metastases to the brain).

There are a number of paraneoplastic syndromes associated with lung carcinoma. These include clubbing as well as hypertrophic pulmonary osteoarthropathy, which consists of periosteal new bone formation usually involving the bones of the lower arms and legs (Fig. 11-6). It is usually associated with pain. Other paraneoplastic syndromes include migratory thrombophlebitis and ectopic hormone production including Cushing's syndrome from adrenocorticotropic hormone (ACTH) production, hyponatremia associated with inappropriate antidiuretic hormone (ADH) syndrome, and hypercalcemia due to excessive parahormone production. There are also a variety of neurologic paraneoplastic syndromes.

Radiologic-Pathologic Correlation

The common cell types of lung cancer include adenocarcinoma, squamous cell carcinoma, small-cell carcinoma, and large-cell undifferentiated carcinoma. Multidifferentiated tumors may also occur, although uncommonly. Adenocarcinoma includes the subset of bronchioloalveolar carcinoma.

Adenocarcinoma

Clinical features Adenocarcinoma (Box 11-7) has been increasing in incidence; it is now the most common cell type, accounting for approximately 50% of cases. It is the most common cell type in women and in nonsmokers. Because these lesions are typically peripheral in the lung, they may not produce symptoms and hence they are found incidentally on a routine chest radiograph.

Pathologic features Adenocarcinomas typically grow slowly. However, they tend to metastasize early. An association has been noted with focal and diffuse pulmonary fibrosis. Pathologically, adenocarcinomas are characterized by the formation of glands or papillary structures, and typically they have either intracellular or extracellular mucin. They are most frequently peripheral and subpleural in location, and they show evidence of expansile growth. Occasionally they may occur endobronchially.

Radiographic features These neoplasms are typically peripheral in location and present as a solitary nodule or mass often with lobulated, spiculated, and ill-defined borders (Fig. 11-7).

Bronchioloalveolar carcinoma

Bronchioloalveolar carcinoma (Box 11-8) is generally considered a subtype of adenocarcinoma. It may present with one of three distinct radiologic patterns. The most common is a solitary nodule. Such nodules share the same appearance as adenocarcinoma, although they are often rather hazy and ill-defined (Fig. 11-8). They are peripheral in location and exhibit lipidic growth, that is, growth along the alveolar walls that probably accounts for the relatively low density on standard radiographs. On CT they may exhibit "ground-glass" opacification, particularly around the periphery of the nodule. The solitary nodule is associated with an excellent prognosis when it is resected at this stage. An air bronchogram may be identified on both standard films and on CT (Fig. 11-8). The second appearance is that of a pneumonia-like consolidation, which occurs in approximately 20% of cases (Fig. 11-9). This consolidation may be asso-

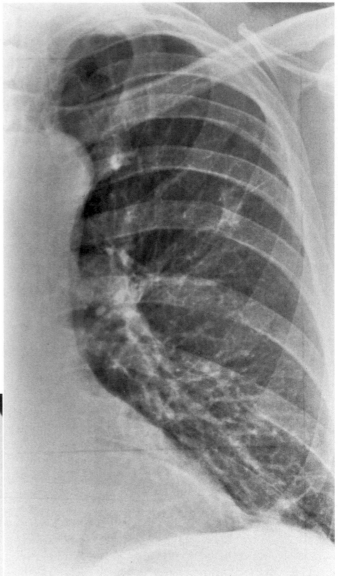

Figure 11-7. Adenocarcinoma. **A,** Frontal radiograph shows a small irregular and spiculated lesion in the periphery of the left upper lobe. **B,** Thin collimation CT of the lesion better illustrates the irregular margins. There is a "tail" (arrow) extending to the major fissure. This may represent either a fibrous strand or local tumor extension.

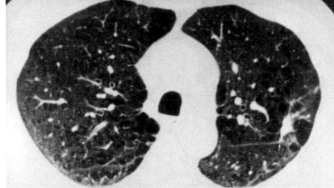

Box 11-8   Bronchioloalveolar Carcinoma

SUBTYPE OF ADENOCARCINOMA

CLINICAL FEATURES
Severe bronchorrhea

RADIOGRAPHIC FEATURES
Solitary nodule
  Most common
  Hazy, ill-defined
  "Ground-glass" on CT
  Air bronchogram
Consolidation
Multiple nodules

ciated with nodules either in the same lobe or in other lobes of either lung. This appearance reflects the presumed mode of dissemination of this tumor through the tracheobronchial tree. The final appearance is that of multiple nodules scattered throughout both lungs (Fig. 11-10). These nodules are typically 5 to 6 mm in diameter and tend to have very irregular borders. This presentation is found in a small minority of patients.

One of the classic clinical features of bronchioloalveolar carcinoma is the presence of bronchorrhea, which may be extreme and may lead to the expectoration of a large amount of mucus with severe morbidity.

Squamous-cell carcinoma

Clinical features Squamous-cell carcinoma (Box 11-9) represents about a third of all lung cancers. It is associated with the best prognosis. Although it grows rapid-

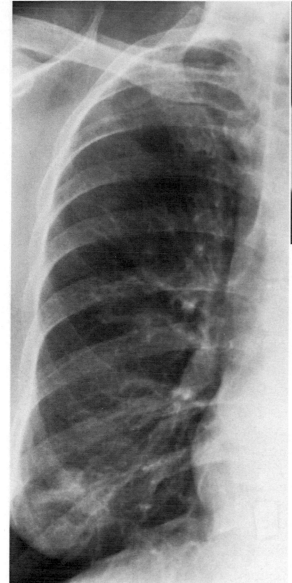

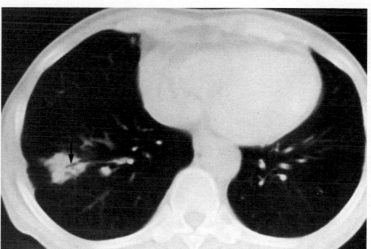

Figure 11-8. Bronchioloalveolar carcinoma. Solitary nodule. **A,** Frontal radiograph shows an irregular focal opacity at the base of the right lung. **B,** On CT an air bronchogram can be identified *(arrow).*

ly, distant metastases occur at a later phase than in adenocarcinoma. There is an extremely strong association with cigarette smoking. Squamous-cell carcinoma is the most common cause of Pancoast syndrome, and the cell type is most commonly associated with hypercalcemia due to ectopic parathormone production.

Superior sulcus tumors (Pancoast tumors) (Box 11-10) are tumors that occur at the very apex of the lung in the superior sulcus. They are typically characterized by pain, Horner's syndrome, destruction of bone, and atrophy of hand muscles. Such tumors typically invade the chest wall and extend into the neck. Such local extension may result in involvement of the brachial plexus, spread to the spinal canal and vertebral bodies, involvement of the sympathetic ganglion, and anterior extension with invasion of the subclavian artery. If the local tumor is not extensive, such lesions can be treated

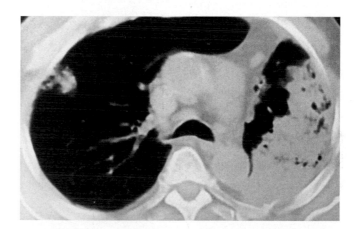

Figure 11-9. Bronchioloalveolar carcinoma. Pneumonic form. CT scan shows consolidation due to tumor in the left lung that contains air bubbles and air bronchograms. There is spread to the opposite lung, and this has produced a nodule in the right upper lobe.

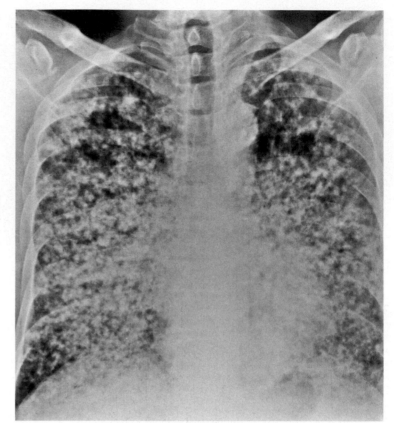

Figure 11-10. Bronchioloalveolar carcinoma. Diffuse nodular form. There are multiple nodules of varying sizes in both lungs. The nodules have fuzzy irregular borders.

Box 11-9   Squamous-Cell Carcinoma

CLINICAL FEATURES

Best prognosis
One third of all lung cancers
Pancoast syndrome
Ectopic parathormone production

PATHOLOGIC FEATURES

Central, endobronchial
Local metastases to lymph nodes
Central necrosis

RADIOGRAPHIC FEATURES

Two thirds central
    Endobronchial lesion best seen on CT
    Atelectasis of lung or lobe
    Postobstructive pneumonitis
One third peripheral
    Thick-walled, cavitary mass
    Solitary nodule

Box 11-10   Superior Sulcus Carcinoma

CLINICAL FEATURES

Pain
Horner's syndrome
Bone destruction
Atrophy of hand muscles

PATHOLOGIC FEATURES

Most common: squamous cell
Invasion
    Chest wall
    Base of neck
    Brachial plexus
    Vertebral bodies and spinal canal
    Sympathetic ganglion
    Subclavian artery

RADIOGRAPHIC FEATURES

Apical mass or asymmetric thickening
Bone destruction
MRI
    Multiplanar imaging
    Local extension

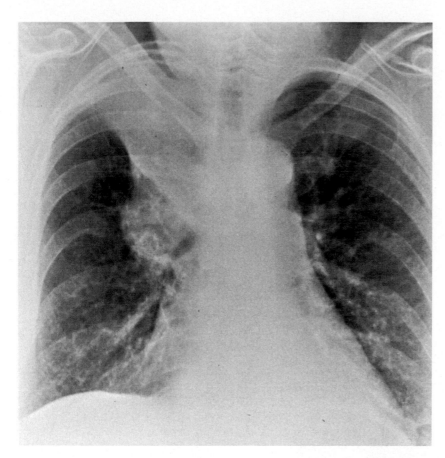

Figure 11-11. Squamous cell carcinoma. Frontal radiograph shows a large right hilar mass with atelectasis of the right upper lobe.

successfully with a combination of preoperative radiation and chemotherapy followed by lobectomy and chest-wall resection.

Pathologic features Squamous-cell carcinomas often arise in areas of squamous metaplasia, and there appears to be an orderly progression of alterations in bronchial mucosa in cigarette smokers from squamous metaplasia to invasive carcinoma. Typically these tumors occur in main, segmental, or subsegmental bronchi, and they grow endobronchially. Eventually bronchial wall invasion occurs with proximal growth along the bronchial mucosa. Metastases to regional lymph nodes are common, and these may occur by direct extension. Central necrosis is a frequent feature. Histologic features typical for squamous-cell carcinomas include the formation of keratin pearls and intracellular bridges.

Radiographic features The radiologic presentation depends on the location of the carcinoma. The most common finding is that of a central endobronchial obstructing lesion, which produces a hilar or perihilar mass (Fig. 11-11). Involvement of the central bronchus may range from focal thickening to complete occlusion. When the lesion is small, the tumor may not be evident on the standard radiograph, but the bronchial-wall abnormalities will be well depicted on CT scanning (Fig. 11-12). Atelectasis or obstructive pneumonitis is usually present distal to the obstructed bronchus.

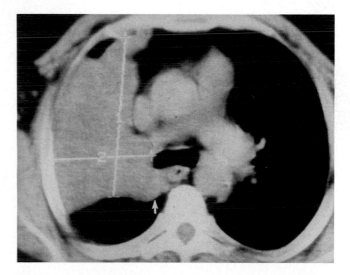

Figure 11-12. Squamous cell carcinoma. CT scan shows tumor surrounding the posterior wall of the right main bronchus *(arrow)*. The origin of the right upper lobe bronchus cannot be identified and is occluded. There is distal obstructive pneumonitis in the right upper lobe.

Any patient presenting with atelectasis and signs of infection should be followed radiographically to complete resolution and reexpansion of the involved lobe. Failure of resolution is highly suggestive of a central lung carcinoma.

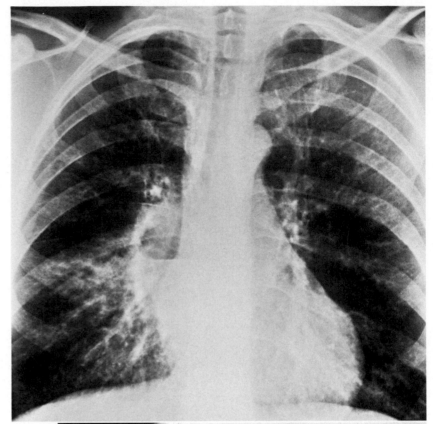

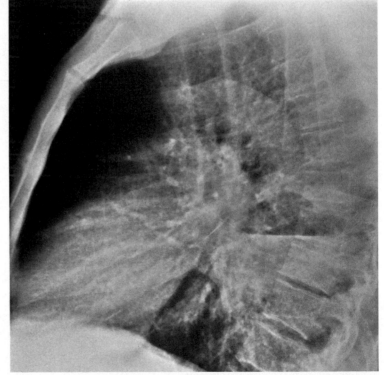

Figure 11-13. Cavitary squamous cell carcinoma. **A** and **B**, Frontal and lateral radiographs demonstrate a thick-walled cavity with an air/fluid level in the superior segment of the right lower lobe.

Approximately one third of squamous-cell carcinomas occur in the lung periphery. The most characteristic appearance is a thick-walled, cavitary mass usually without an air/fluid level. The size ranges from 2 to 10 cm (Fig. 11-13). Such a cavity may be indistinguishable radio-graphically from a primary lung abscess. A solitary nodule or mass without cavitation can also occur in the periphery of the lung parenchyma.

On standard radiographs, a superior sulcus tumor usually appears as an apical mass or an asymmetric pleural thickening with irregularity occasionally associated with rib destruction. Apical thickening alone may be a normal finding; usually its prevalence is related to age. Much more commonly seen in older individuals, it is usually bilateral but it may be asymmetric. However, any irregular apical thickening that is 5 mm or greater than that on the opposite side should be considered with suspicion. However, most patients with superior sulcus tumors do have clinical symptoms of chest pain. MRI is the preferred modality for evaluating superior sulcus tumors because of its ability to visualize structures at the apex of the thorax in multiple planes. Features of superior sulcus tumors on MRI are discussed below in the section on staging.

Small-cell carcinoma

Clinical features Small-cell carcinoma (Box 11-11), the most aggressive form of lung cancer, is characterized by rapid growth and early metastases, which are present in two thirds of patients at the time of presentation. It is associated with the poorest survival, and it has the strongest and most irrefutable association with cigarette smoking. It accounts for approximately 15% to 20% of all lung cancers. Small-cell carcinoma does not respond to surgical treatment, but it is often managed successfully with chemotherapy. However, long-term survival is extremely poor, and when treated the median survival is 9 to 18 months. Patients with limited stage disease, that is, disease confined to the thorax, have approximately a 25% 2-year survival.

Small-cell carcinoma is the most common cause of superior vena cava (SVC) syndrome. It is also associated with both Cushing's syndrome and inappropriate secretion of ADH.

Pathologic features Small-cell carcinoma most often occurs as a large central mass associated with stenosis of a bronchial lumen, although an endobronchial lesion is seldom identified. It is characterized by extensive tumor necrosis and hemorrhage.

Radiographic features The radiographic features usually consist of a hilar or perihilar mass associated with massive bilateral mediastinal adenopathy (Fig. 11-14). There may be associated lobar collapse. The primary tumor may not be readily evident because it is obscured by the extensive adenopathy. However, CT may show the primary tumor to better advantage. Occasionally a small-cell carcinoma presents as a peripheral nodule that can be resected, and in these relatively uncommon cases the prognosis is better.

Large-cell undifferentiated carcinoma

Clinical features Large-cell carcinomas (Box 11-12) account for 2% to 5% of lung cancers, and they have a strong association with cigarette smoking. They are characterized by rapid growth, early metastases, and a poor prognosis.

Pathologic features Typically these tumors are peripheral in location, although they may involve segmental or subsegmental bronchi by bronchial extension. They are characterized by large cells with large nuclei, and on gross inspection they are large and bulky, often greater than 4 cm in diameter with areas of necrosis. Giant-cell carcinoma, a subtype of large-cell carcinoma, is characterized by the presence of multiple giant cells with bizarre shapes. It has a highly aggressive behavior with poor prognosis.

Box 11-11 Small-Cell Carcinoma

CLINICAL FEATURES

Most aggressive
Strongest association with smoking
Poorest survival
15% to 20% of cancers
Treated with chemotherapy
Inappropriate ADH production, ectopic ACTH

PATHOLOGIC FEATURES

Large central mass
Tumor necrosis

RADIOGRAPHIC FEATURES

Hilar or perihilar mass
Massive adenopathy, often bilateral
Lobar collapse
Rare—peripheral nodule

ACTH, adrenocorticotropic hormone; *ADH,* antidiuretic hormone.

Box 11-12 Large-Cell Undifferentiated Carcinoma

CHARACTERISTICS

2% to 5% of lung cancers
Strong association with cigarette smoking
Rapid growth
Early metastases
Poor prognosis

PATHOLOGIC FEATURES

Peripheral
Large, >4 cm

RADIOLOGIC FEATURES

Peripheral
>4 cm

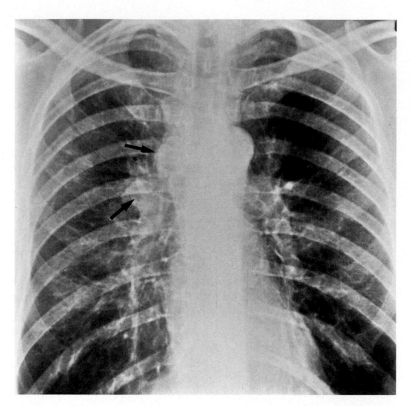

Figure 11-14.   Small-cell carcinoma. Frontal radiograph shows right paratracheal and right hilar adenopathy *(arrow)*. The primary tumor is not identified.

Radiographic features   The lesions are usually peripheral and quite large, with greater than 70% of the tumors being more than 4 cm on presentation (Fig. 11-15).

Multidifferentiated tumors

Adenosquamous carcinoma is a type of tumor that consists of malignant squamous and glandular components. It is typically peripheral and is associated with early metastases and poor prognosis.

Staging of Lung Cancer

TNM classification

Staging of any tumor consists of the determination of the extent of the disease. The only strong rationale for staging is to select patients who will benefit from surgical resection. Staging also determines prognosis.

The TNM system is widely used to classify lung tumors. In the TNM classification, *T* indicates the features of the primary tumor, *N* indicates metastasis to regional lymph nodes, and *M* refers to the presence or absence of distant metastasis (Tables 11-1 and 11-2). In 1986 the staging system was revised based on epidemiologic evidence of improved survival following surgical resection in patients who had previously been classified as having unresectable disease.

In the old lung cancer classification, stages I and II were considered amenable to surgical management, and stage III tumors were considered unresectable. The current system consists of four stages; stage IV includes only those patients with evidence of distant metastasis (M1).

Stage III has been redefined and divided into two stages, stages IIIa and IIIb. Of these two categories, stage IIIb is considered unresectable disease. Tumors with limited invasion of the chest wall and mediastinum are included in the operable category in this classification (IIIa). The designation T4 is used to describe lesions with extensive invasion of the mediastinum or diaphragm, that is, involvement of vital mediastinal structures such as the great vessels, heart, and aerodigestive tract. N1 disease refers to ipsilateral metastases to hilar nodes. The presence of ipsilateral hilar adenopathy alters the overall survival rate, but it does not alter the decision regarding surgery, and such patients are considered resectable. Patients with N2 disease (metastases to ipsilateral mediastinal nodes) are considered potentially resectable. However, most patients with N2 disease are usually entered into protocols that may consist of neoadjuvant chemotherapy sometimes combined with radiation therapy before operation. The category N3 refers to contralateral mediastinal and hilar lymph node involvement or supraclavicular lymph-node metastasis; it is considered unresectable disease.

Although the TNM system is used for the classification of both non–small-cell and small-cell carcinoma, a more useful classification for small-cell carcinoma includes two categories: (1) limited (involving the thorax only), and (2) extensive (metastatic disease outside the thorax).

Computed tomography & magnetic resonance imaging

A number of different imaging modalities have historically been used in staging lung cancer. These have

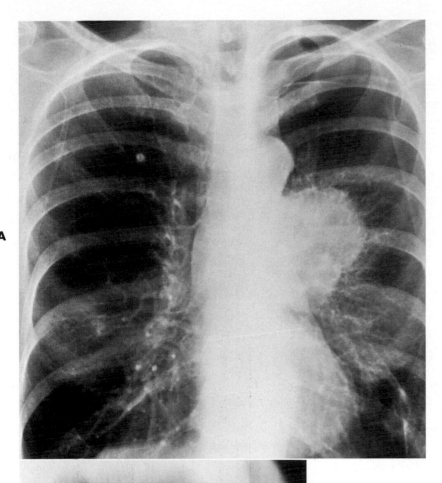

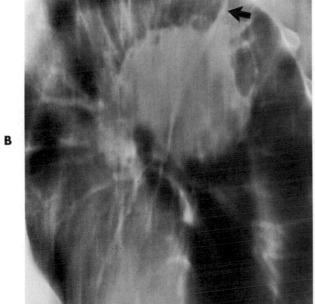

Figure 11-15. Giant cell (large cell) carcinoma. Frontal view, **A,** and lateral tomogram, **B,** demonstrate a 5-cm mass in both the left upper lobe and left lower lobe that is crossing the major fissure *(arrow).*

Table 11-1   TNM classification of lung cancer

Stage	Description
PRIMARY TUMOR (T)	
TX	Tumor proved by the presence of malignant cells in bronchoscopy secretions, but not visualized by radiography or bronchoscopy. Or, any tumor that cannot be assessed, as in a retreatment staging.
T0	No evidence of primary tumor.
T1S	Carcinoma in situ.
T1	A tumor 3 cm or less in greatest diameter, surrounded by lung or visceral pleura and without evidence of invasion proximal to a lobar bronchus at bronchoscopy (except superficial endobronchial tumors, which may extend proximal to the main bronchus and still be called T1).
T2	A tumor more than 3 cm in greatest diameter. Or, a tumor of any size that either invades the visceral pleura or has associated atelectasis or obstructive pneumonitis extending to the hilar region. At bronchoscopy, the proximal extent of demonstrable tumor must be within a lobar bronchus or at least 2 cm distal to the carina. Any associated atelectasis or obstructive pneumonitis must involve less than an entire lung.
T3	A tumor of any size with direct extension into the chest wall (including superior sulcus tumors), diaphragm, or the mediastinal pleura or pericardium, without involving the heart, great vessels, trachea, esophagus, or vertebral body. Or, a tumor in the main bronchus within 2 cm of the carina without involving the carina.
T4	A tumor of any size with invasion of the mediastinum involving heart, great vessels, trachea, esophagus, vertebral body, or carina. Or, presence of malignant pleural effusian (cytologically positive).
NODAL INVOLVEMENT (N)	
N0	No demonstrable metastasis to regional lymph nodes.
N1	Metastasis to lymph nodes in the peribronchial region, the ipsilateral hilar region, or both, including direct extension.
N2	Metastasis to ipsilateral mediastinal lymph nodes and subcarinal lymph nodes.
N3	Metastasis to contralateral mediastinal or hilar lymph nodes, ipsilateral or contralateral scalene, or supraclavicular nodes.
DISTANT METASTASIS (M)	
M0	No (known) distant metastasis.
M1	Distant metastasis present—specify site(s).

Derived from Mountain CF: Value of the new TNM staging system for lung cancer, *Chest* 96:47-49, 1989, and from Friedman PJ: Lung cancer: Update on staging classification, *AJR Am J Roentgenol* 150:261-264, 1988.

Table 11-2   TNM classification of lung carcinoma

Stage grouping		Description
Occult carcinoma	TX N0 M0	An occult carcinoma with bronchopulmonary secretions containing malignant cells, but without other evidence of the primary tumor or evidence of metastasis.
Stage 0	T1S N0 M0	Carcinoma in situ.
Stage I	T1 N0 M0	A tumor that can be classified T1 or T2, without any nodal or distant metastasis.
	T2 N0 M0	
Stage II	T1 N1 M0	A tumor classified as T1 or T2, with metastasis to the lymph nodes in the peribronchial region and/or ipsilateral hilar region only.
	T2 N1 M0	
Stage IIIa	T3 N0 M0	A tumor more extensive than T2, but without invasion of a vital structure, or any tumor up to T3, with metastasis to ipsilateral mediastinal or subcarinal lymph nodes.
	T3 N1 M0	
	T1-3 N2 M0	
Stage IIIb	Any T N3 M0	Any tumor with invasion of vital mediastinal structures or metastasis to nonresectable nodes, but without spread beyond the thorax.
	T4 Any N M0	
Stage IV	Any T Any N M1	A tumor with metastatic spread beyond the thorax and its regional lymph nodes (i.e., beyond scalene or superclavicular nodes).

Derived from Mountain CF: Value of the new TNM staging system for lung cancer, *Chest* 96:47-49, 1989, and from Friedman PJ: Lung cancer: Update on staging classification, *AJR Am J Roentgenol* 150:261-264, 1988.

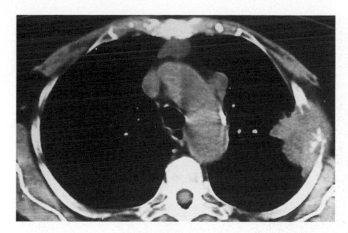

Figure 11-16. Lung cancer with definite chest wall invasion. CT shows rib destruction and extension of the mass into the soft tissues of the chest wall. There is also anterior mediastinal and prevascular adenopathy.

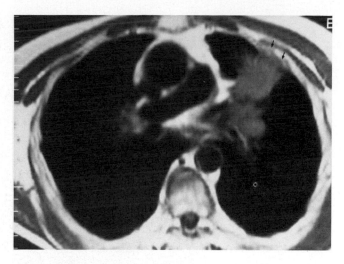

Figure 11-17. Chest wall invasion. MRI T_1-weighted sequence shows tongues of tumor *(arrows)* extending into the subcostal fat.

included standard and conventional tomography as well as computed tomography (CT) and magnetic resonance imaging (MRI). In some instances, accurate staging and the determination of appropriate treatment for patients with lung cancer can be made noninvasively with imaging modalities alone, although in most instances some degree of surgical staging is also necessary.

Computed tomography has now become the major imaging modality of choice for the evaluation of patients with lung carcinoma. CT is not only useful for staging but also as a guide to surgical management and in the determination of appropriate methods for surgical staging.

Evaluation of the primary tumor (the T factor) T3 tumors include tumors of any size with direct extension into the chest wall, diaphragm, the mediastinal pleura, or pericardium without involvement of vital mediastinal structures. T4 tumors are tumors of any size with invasion of the mediastinum (heart, great vessels, trachea, esophagus), vertebral body, carina, or with associated malignant pleural effusion.

It is not always possible to distinguish T3 from T4 lesions with imaging studies. Lesions with chest wall invasion are classified as T3 lesions and are potentially resectable. Surgical treatment, however, requires en bloc resection of the pulmonary malignancy and the contiguous chest wall, it is associated with an operative mortality in the range of 8% to 15%. In selecting patients as operative candidates it is sometimes desirable, therefore, to determine preoperatively if chest-wall invasion is present.

The value of CT in the determination of chest-wall invasion is somewhat limited. Although CT certainly provides incremental information over standard films, many of the findings described in the literature that are said to be associated with chest-wall invasion have been shown to be neither sensitive nor specific. These include pleural thickening adjacent to the tumor, encroachment on

or increased density of extrapleural fat, or an obtuse angle between the pulmonary mass and the pleural surface. Only the presence of a mass in the chest wall or definite rib destruction are helpful indicators of chest-wall invasion (Fig. 11-16). MRI has a slight advantage over CT in the evaluation of chest-wall invasion. Both T1- and T2-weighted spin-echo sequences may show direct tumor extension into the chest wall, and the yield is improved with the use of gadolinium contrast (Fig. 11-17).

Superior sulcus carcinomas are defined as bronchogenic carcinomas occurring at the extreme apex of the lung. Such tumors, which may be considered resectable, are usually managed with radiation therapy followed by surgery with chest-wall resection if there is no evidence of mediastinal or distant metastases. However, accurate assessment of the local extent of disease is an important aspect in the staging of these lesions. MRI is useful in determining certain parameters of unresectability such as invasion of the vertebral body and involvement of the subclavian artery and brachial plexus (Fig. 11-18). Sagittal and coronal images are particularly useful in imaging such lesions. T2-weighted images help to differentiate apical tumor from surrounding muscle and to define the extension of the tumor into the base of the neck.

CT may be useful when extensive mediastinal invasion is present. Contrast-enhanced images may show vascular encasement and involvement of major mediastinal organs (Fig. 11-19). However, CT in some instances is unable to distinguish contiguity of tumor with the mediastinum from actual invasion of the walls of vital mediastinal structures. Again, MRI has been shown to be more accurate than CT in delineating the extent of malignant invasion. Findings consistent with invasion include encasement or distortion of major mediastinal organs (Fig. 11-20). However, often the decision regarding

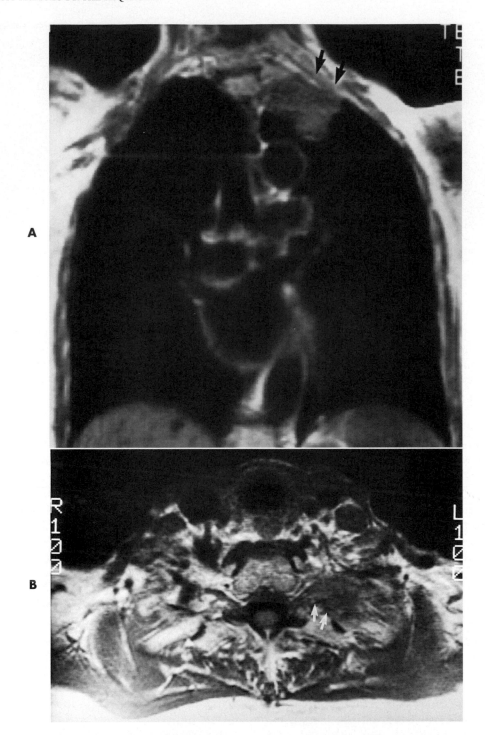

Figure 11-18.   Superior sulcus (Pancoast) tumor. **A,** Coronal MRI demonstrates a mass impinging on the lowest branch of the brachial plexus *(arrows).* **B,** Surface coil axial T1-weighted image shows tumor extending into the intervertebral foramen *(arrows).* Compare with bright signal intensity of epidural fat on the opposite side. (From Choplin RH, MacMahon H, McLoud TC, Müller NL, Reed JC: ACR professional self-evaluation program. In Siegel BA, Proto AC, editors: *Chest disease* (fifth series). *Test and syllabus.* Reston, Va, 1996, American College of Radiology.

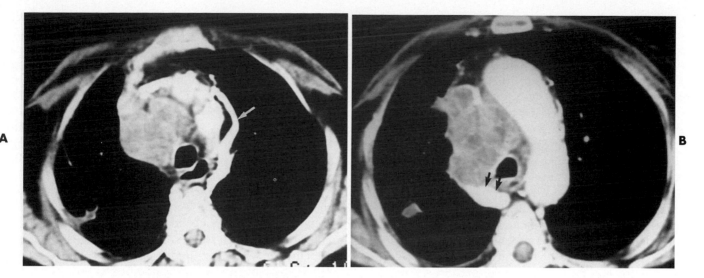

Figure 11-19. Superior vena caval obstruction, lung cancer. CT performed with contrast material. **A** and **B**, There are enlarged metastatic nodes in the right paratracheal area. The superior vena cava is occluded and not opacified. Multiple collaterals can be identified in the mediastinum (superior intercostal vein—*white arrow*) and the azygos vein is dilated *(black arrow).*

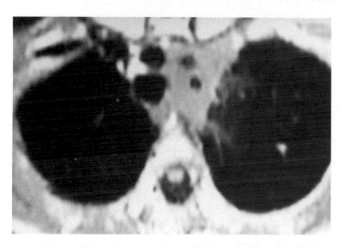

Figure 11-20. MRI—mediastinal invasion by lung carcinoma. Axial T1-weighted image shows tumor replacing mediastinal fat and encasing the left common carotid and subclavian arteries.

resectability of lung cancers with suspected mediastinal invasion is made at the operating table.

Evaluation of nodal metastases (the N factor) Computed tomography has become the method of choice for the assessment of mediastinal nodes in bronchogenic carcinoma. Previously, patients with mediastinal nodal metastases from bronchogenic carcinoma were not considered to benefit from surgical therapy. However, several studies have consistently documented improved survival of selected patients after resection of limited mediastinal nodal disease combined with adjuvant radiation therapy. The new American Joint Committee on Cancer Staging now considers patients with ipsilateral mediastinal lymph-node metastases (N2) as potentially surgically resectable stage IIIa disease. Included in this group are patients with (1) intracapsular rather than extracapsular

involvement, and (2) positive nodes identified at thoracotomy after negative mediastinoscopy. In addition, current reports indicate that even patients with gross and bulky ipsilateral nodal metastases (N2) may benefit from surgery if this treatment is combined with neoadjuvant chemotherapy and radiation therapy. However, patients with contralateral mediastinal nodal involvement (N3) are considered to have nonoperable stage IIIb disease.

Several studies have addressed the accuracy of CT in the staging of mediastinal nodal metastases in lung cancer. In most studies nodes greater than 1 cm in the short axis are considered abnormal and should cause suspicion concerning nodal metastases. Some early investigations reported a high sensitivity in the range of 88% to 94%, values that are equivalent to the sensitivity of mediastinoscopy. Opinions based on such data suggested that mediastinoscopy was unnecessary in cases in which the CT scan showed no evidence of enlarged nodes. More recent studies that have employed total nodal sampling and the American Thoracic Society (ATS) lymph node classification have shown a lower sensitivity for CT in the detection of nodal metastases, in the range of 60% to 79% with specificities of 60% to 80%. The limitations of CT in the identification of N2 and N3 disease are now well accepted. MRI is constrained by similar limitations, and there appears to be no clear advantage to MRI over CT in identifying lymph-node involvement by tumor.

Despite the limitations of CT in staging mediastinal lymph nodes, this imaging modality does provide important information concerning the nodal status of patients with lung cancer. Identification and localization of enlarged lymph nodes aid in the selection of the appropriate invasive procedure for surgical staging. Mediastinoscopy, performed in the pretracheal plane, allows an adequate approach to paratracheal and anterior subcarinal lymph nodes. However, nodes in the aorticopulmonary window and anterior mediastinal nodes cannot be biopsied with this procedure (Fig. 11-16). Such nodes may require a small anterior thoracotomy (Chamberlain procedure), percutaneous transthoracic needle biopsy, or video-assisted thoracoscopic biopsy. Evidence of extensive lymphadenopathy with secondary signs such as obstruction of the SVC or destruction of the vertebral bodies may preclude further need for staging procedures if the histologic characteristics of the primary lesion are known.

A negative CT scan for mediastinal adenopathy is a more controversial issue. It is the opinion of this author that such patients still merit mediastinoscopy because of the limitations of CT. However, in some institutions mediastinoscopy may not be available or preferred. If patients are selected immediately for thoracotomy without precedent mediastinoscopy, careful nodal sampling must be done at the time of surgery. Because of the low specificity of CT, enlarged lymph nodes require biopsy before surgery. Enlarged hyperplastic nodes occur frequently in the setting of central tumors associated with obstructive pneumonitis (Fig. 11-21). Various procedures are available for such sampling, including mediastinoscopy, Wang needle biopsy, and percutaneous needle biopsy.

The issue of CT staging of the mediastinum in T1 lesions is controversial. T1 tumors are defined as lesions 3 cm or less in greatest diameter, surrounded by lung or visceral pleura without evidence of invasion proximal to the lobar bronchus. Several studies have suggested a low prevalence of mediastinal nodal metastatic disease with T1 cancers (5% to 15%). Because of such a low prevalence, it has been suggested that CT may not be necessary in such patients and that the preoperative staging should be limited to plain chest radiographs. However, Seely and others, in a study of 104 patients with T1 lesions, found a higher prevalence of nodal metastases (21%). The sensitivity of CT in this study was 77%. The high prevalence of metastases to the mediastinum suggests the need for further careful preoperative staging in such patients, to include CT scanning.

Evaluation of distant metastases (the M factor) The role of imaging in the determination of extrathoracic metastases from bronchogenic carcinoma is somewhat controversial. Most studies indicate that it is not cost-effective to search for distant metastases with imaging unless the patient is symptomatic or has positive physical signs or chemical abnormalities (e.g., abnormal liver function tests).

Because the adrenal glands are one of the most common sites for extrathoracic metastases, CT scans used in staging lung cancer should include the upper abdomen. The prevalence of adrenal metastases at time of presentation ranges from 5% to 10%. Examination of the adrenal glands and in fact the liver can be done easily at the time of the CT examination of the chest. However, two thirds of adrenal masses identified by CT in patients with lung carcinoma are not malignant. Adrenal adenomas are quite common. CT characteristics of adrenal adenomas include size less than 3 cm in diameter and low attenuation (less than 10 HU) due to fat content (Fig. 11-22). However, in lesions not meeting these criteria, chemical shift MRI may be helpful in distinguishing adenomas from metastatic disease. With the advent of helical CT it

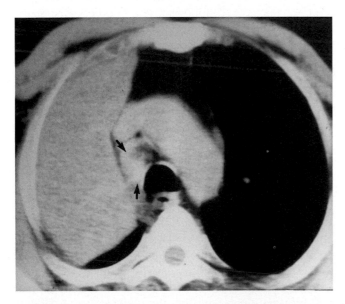

Figure 11-21. Enlarged hyperplastic nodes. CT shows an enlarged, 2-cm right paratracheal lymph node *(arrow)*. There is obstructive pneumonitis involving the right upper lobe. Histology of the node showed only reactive changes with no evidence of metastatic cancer.

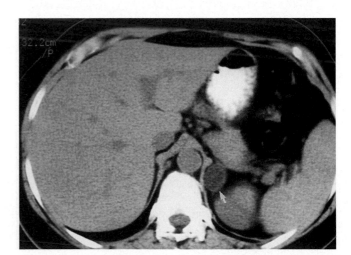

Figure 11-22. Adrenal adenoma. CT scan of the abdomen. There is a well-defined, 2-cm low-attenuation mass in the left adrenal (-5 HU) *(arrow)*

is possible to image the liver with contrast material in an expeditious fashion as part of the thoracic CT scan. Though its efficacy has not been proven, the approach provides a convenient method of imaging the liver as well as the chest at no extra cost and only with slightly extra time required.

OTHER PRIMARY MALIGNANT NEOPLASMS

Other primary malignant neoplasms of the lungs are listed in Box 11-13. Most of these tumors are uncommon. The most frequently encountered is the carcinoid tumor. Carcinoid tumors were previously classified with adenoid cystic carcinomas and mucoid epidermoid carcinomas as types of "bronchial adenoma," a term no longer in use. These tumors are not adenomas but are actually low-grade malignancies. Adenoid cystic carcinomas and mucoepidermoid carcinomas, which occur almost exclusively in the trachea and central bronchi, are discussed in Chapters 12 and 13.

Carcinoid Tumors

Carcinoid tumors (Box 11-14) are among a group of neoplasms that arise from pulmonary neuroendocrine cells. Such neuroendocrine tumors are classified into three types: *type 1,* typical carcinoid tumor; *type 2,* atypical carcinoid tumor; and *type 3,* small-cell lung cancer. Carcinoid tumors are low-grade malignant neoplasms that represent between 0.6% and 2.5% of all primary pulmonary neoplasms. They generally have a good prognosis with approximately 90% 5-year survival, and there is no association with cigarette smoking.

Clinical features

Males and females are equally affected over a wide age range, with the median age being 50 years. Presenting symptoms include cough and hemoptysis.

Box 11-13 Other Malignant Neoplasms of the Lung

PULMONARY NEUROENDOCRINE CELL ORIGIN

Carcinoid tumor

TRACHEOBRONCHIAL GLANDS ORIGIN

Adenoid cystic carcinoma
Mucoepidermoid carcinoma

LYMPHORETICULAR NEOPLASMS AND LEUKEMIA

Hodgkin's disease
Non-Hodgkin's lymphoma
Leukemia

NEOPLASMS OF SOFT TISSUE, BONE, AND CARTILAGE

Muscle
   Leiomyosarcoma
Vascular tissue
   Kaposi's sarcoma
   Intravascular bronchioloalveolar tumor
   Angiosarcoma
Bone and cartilage
   Chondrosarcoma
   Osteosarcoma
Adipose tissue
   Liposarcoma
Fibrous tissue
   Malignant fibrous histiocytoma

MISCELLANEOUS

Pulmonary blastoma
Carcinosarcoma

Box 11-14 Carcinoid Tumors

CHARACTERISTICS

Arise from neuroendocrine cells
Type 1, typical carcinoid
Type 2, atypical carcinoid
Low-grade malignancy in type 1
Good prognosis

CLINICAL FEATURES

Median age—50
Males and females equally affected
Cough, hemoptysis
Rarely, Cushing's syndrome

PATHOLOGIC FEATURES

Small cells
Neurosecretory granules
Atypical carcinoids
   Peripheral
   10% of cases
   Metastasize in 40% to 50% of cases

RADIOGRAPHIC FEATURES

Central
   80% of cases
   Lobar, segmental, subsegmental bronchi
   Hilar mass
   Obstructive pneumonia and atelectasis
Peripheral
   20% of cases
   Slow growth if typical
   Large and faster growth if atypical
   Calcification seen on CT

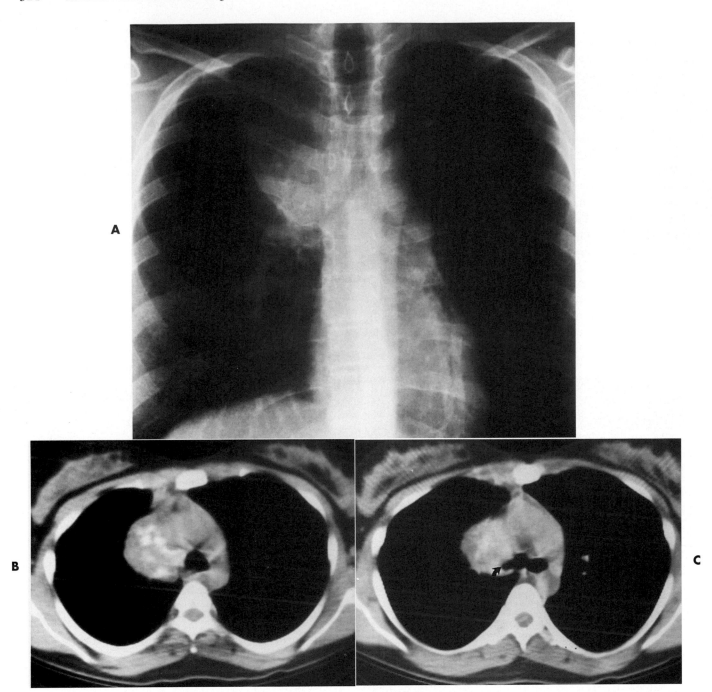

Figure 11-23. Central carcinoid tumor. **A,** Frontal radiograph of the chest shows a hilar mass with partial atelectasis of the right upper lobe. **B,** CT scan demonstrates a calcified central mass. **C,** This obstructs the origin of the right upper lobe bronchus *(arrow).*

Carcinoid tumors may be associated with ectopic hormone production, specifically ACTH. However, these tumors do not produce the clinical carcinoid syndrome unless liver metastases are present.

Pathologic features

Carcinoid tumors are composed of small cells that are arranged in nests or trabeculae with a vascular stroma. Electron microscopy studies show an ultrastructure consisting of neurosecretory granules. Typical carcinoid tu-

mors rarely metastasize. However, atypical carcinoid tumors exhibit metastases in 40% to 50% of patients. Atypical carcinoids account for 10% of cases, and they tend to be peripheral in location. They may be associated with early metastases, particularly osteoblastic bone metastases.

Radiographic features

Carcinoid tumors may be either central or peripheral. The central tumors account for the majority of cases in

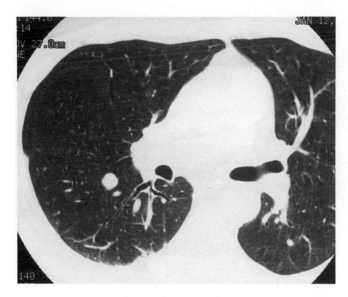

Figure 11-24. Carcinoid tumor. CT scan shows a well-defined nodule in the right lower lobe.

80% of patients and are discussed in more detail in Chapter 13. They originate in the lobar, segmental, or subsegmental bronchi (Fig. 11-23). They may appear as a small endobronchial nodule or a hilar or perihilar mass with associated postobstructive pneumonia and atelectasis. Because they are slow-growing they may produce low-grade infection with bronchiectasis in the involved lobe. Approximately 20% of cases will occur as a solitary pulmonary nodule in the periphery of the lung (Fig. 11-24). Typical carcinoids in the periphery will grow at a slow rate, and carcinoid tumors should be considered in the differential diagnosis of slow-growing solitary pulmonary nodules. Atypical carcinoids also occur in the periphery and are usually large. In pathologic studies, up to 30% of carcinoid tumors contain calcification or ossification. Although such calcification is usually not identified on standard radiographs, it can be identified on CT scans. The majority of carcinoid tumors will also show vigorous enhancement after contrast administration because of their vascular nature .

Intravascular Bronchoalveolar Tumor

This is an uncommon multifocal pulmonary neoplasm that arises from endothelial cells and is characterized by extensive intravascular spread. The radiographic features consist of multiple well-defined or ill-defined nodules measuring up to 2 cm in diameter; these show little or no growth on serial studies.

Carcinosarcoma

Carcinosarcomas are rare tumors that occur mainly in middle-aged and elderly men. They carry a poor progno-

sis because of their aggressive nature characterized by local invasion of surrounding structures and widespread metastases. These tumors consist of an epithelial component of either squamous-cell carcinoma or adenocarcinoma and a mesenchymal component most commonly of the spindle cell type. These tumors may occur centrally with endobronchial growth or peripherally as a large mass.

The radiographic features correspond to the location and may consist of a large, peripheral, sharply circumscribed mass or a central lesion with atelectasis and obstructive pneumonitis. There is an upper-lobe predominance. Extension to the pleura, chest wall, and mediastinum may occur.

Pulmonary Blastoma

Pulmonary blastoma is an uncommon primary lung tumor with a mixture of immature epithelial and mesenchymal components. It morphologically mimics embryonal lung. The tumor occurs predominantly in men in the first and seventh decades of life, with a biphasic age distribution. It is associated with a generally poor prognosis. The radiologic findings usually consist of a well-circumscribed, large peripheral mass (Fig. 11-25) with occasional pleural invasion and metastases.

Other Malignant Mesenchymal Tumors

Malignant tumors of mesenchymal origin are rare in the lung. They include neoplasms arising from muscle, vascular tissue, bone and cartilage, and neural and adipose tissue, as well as from fibrohistiocytic tissue. Examples include fibrosarcoma, leiomyosarcoma, and osteogenic sarcoma.

Lymphoma

Both Hodgkin's and non-Hodgkin's lymphoma frequently involve the thorax. Although the most common sites are the mediastinal and hilar lymph nodes, the chest wall, lung parenchyma, and pleura may also be involved.

Hodgkin's disease

Pathologic classification The pathologic classification for Hodgkin's disease is listed in Tables 11-3 and 11-4. The pathologic diagnosis is based on the recognition of typical Reed-Sternberg cells. The nodular sclerosing form is associated with abundant fibrous tissue stroma.

Clinical features In Hodgkin's disease (Box 11-15) there is a bimodal age peak of presentation. It is most commonly seen in young adults in the late teens and twenties. A second peak occurs later, in elderly men. The

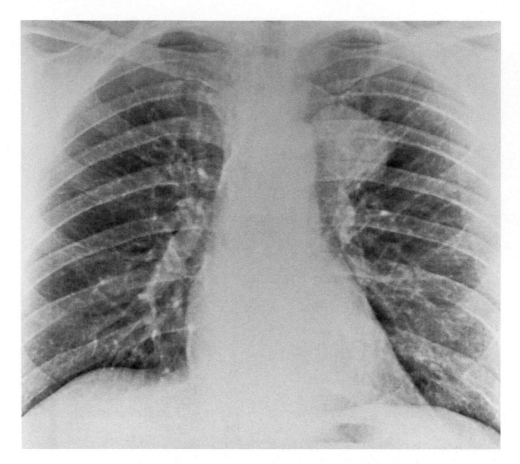

Figure 11-25.   Pulmonary blastoma. Frontal view demonstrates a well-defined 3-cm mass in the left upper lobe.

Table 11-3   Hodgkin disease classification (Rye modification of Lukes and Butler System)

Subtype	Frequency	Prognosis	Involvement	Comment
Lymphocyte predominance (LP)	Less than 5% (young patients)	Most favorable	Early stage disease	Nodular and diffuse forms
Nodular sclerosis (NS)	Most common (less than 75%)	Less favorable than LP	Mediastinum usually involved	Large fibrotic component, few cells (infrequent Reed-Sternberg cell)
Mixed cellularity	Second most frequent (older patients)	Less favorable than NS	More advanced stage presentation than NS	Frequent Reed-Sternberg cells
Lymphocytic depletion	Uncommon (less than 5%)	Worst prognosis	Advanced disease, older patient, systemic symptoms	Frequent Reed-Sternberg cells

From Bragg DG: Hodgkin disease and non Hodgkin lymphoma of the thorax. In Freundlich IM, Bragg DG, editors: *A radiologic approach to diseases of the chest*, Baltimore, 1997, Williams & Wilkins.

Table 11-4 Cotswold's staging classification of Hodgkin's disease

Classification	Description
Stage I	Involvement of a single lymph-node region or lymphoid structure.
Stage II	Involvement of two or more lymph-node regions on the same side of the diaphragm (the mediastinum is considered as a single site, whereas hilar lymph nodes are considered bilaterally); the number of anatomic sites should be indicated by a subscript (e.g., II_3).
Stage III	Involvement of lymph-node regions or structures on both sides of the diaphragm.
III_1	With or without involvement of splenic, hilar, celiac, or portal nodes.
III_2	With involvement of paraaortic, iliac, and mesenteric nodes.
Stage IV	Involvement of one or more extranodal sites in addition to a site for which the designation "E" has been used (see below).

DESIGNATIONS APPLICABLE TO ANY DISEASE STAGE

A	No symptoms.
B	Fever (temperature, >38° C), drenching night sweats, unexplained loss of >10% of body weight within the preceding 6 months.
X	Bulky disease (a widening of the mediastinum by more than one third, or the presence of a nodal mass with a maximum dimension greater than 10 cm).
E	Involvement of a single extranodal site that is contiguous or proximal to the known nodal site.
CS	Clinical stage.
PS	Pathologic stage (as determined by laparotomy).

Derived from Urba WJ, Longo DL: Hodgkin disease in adults, *Invest Radiol* 28:737-752, 1993.

Box 11-15 Hodgkin's Disease

CLINICAL FEATURES

Bimodal age distribution
    Young adults
    Elderly men
Mass in neck or groin
Systemic symptoms—"B" classification
Survival of 75%—Stage I and II radiotherapy alone

RADIOGRAPHIC FEATURES

CT for staging
85%—thoracic involvement
Hilar and mediastinal adenopathy
Multiple lymph-node groups
Anterior mediastinum most common
Lung involvement
    Primary-lung Hodgkin's rare
    Nodules, masses
        Perihilar
        Cavitation
        Air bronchograms
Follow-up
    Recurrence adjacent to radiation portal
    Pericardial nodes
MRI
    Differentiates residual from recurrent tumor from fibrosis
    T2-weighted
        Fibrosis—low SI
        Tumor—bright SI
Eggshell calcification in nodes

SI, signal intensity.

original Ann Arbor Staging System has been expanded to the currently accepted system, called Cotswold's Staging Classification (Table 11-4). Patients may seek treatment because of an enlarging painless mass in the neck or groin. The presence of systemic symptoms such as fever, weight loss, or pruritis is classified by the modifier "B" in the staging system, and such symptoms are often associated with extensive intraabdominal disease. The majority of Hodgkin's patients have localized stage I or stage II disease at presentation. Long-term survival approximating 75% can be achieved with radiotherapy alone. The addition of chemotherapy reduces the rate of recurrence. Combination treatment with chemotherapy and radiation is usually reserved for the patient who has massive mediastinal involvement and advanced-stage disease.

Radiographic features Computed tomography is usually required for the staging evaluation of patients with Hodgkin's disease. Approximately 85% of cases will have intrathoracic involvement. The most common location in the thorax is mediastinal and hilar nodes (Fig. 11-26). Hodgkin's disease usually produces involvement of multiple lymph-node groups, but the anterior mediastinal compartment is the most frequently involved. Mediastinal involvement is seen most frequently in the nodular sclerosing type. Bulky and massive mediastinal adenopathy may produce superior vena caval syndrome or life-threatening compression of the trachea. Patients with Hodgkin's disease will exhibit mediastinal lymph-node involvement in the majority of cases (approximately 80% to 85%). CT is necessary to define the extent of Hodgkin's disease within the thorax. MRI has no advantage over CT in staging, but it may be useful in patient follow-up.

The lung parenchyma may be involved with Hodgkin's disease. Primary pulmonary Hodgkin's disease is extremely uncommon. More frequently, the lung is involved when the disease is widespread, and there is abundant bulky mediastinal and hilar adenopathy. The pattern is

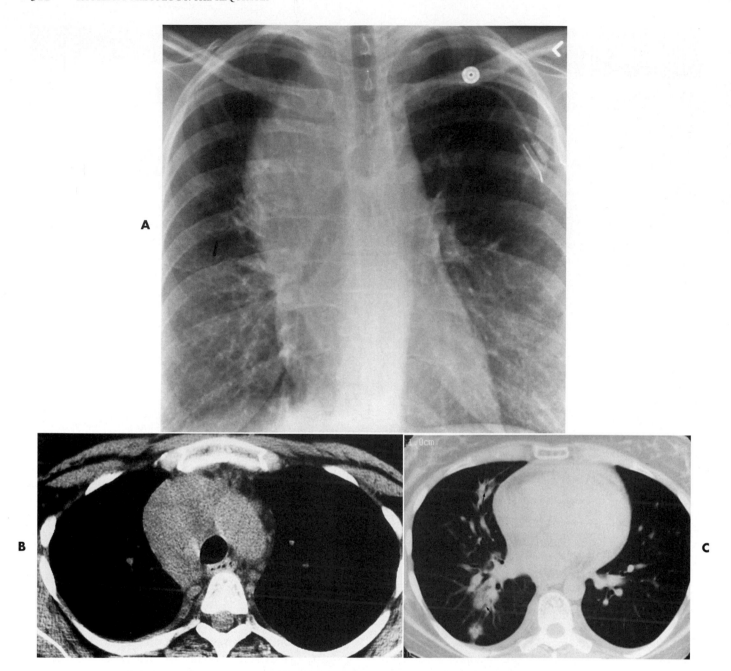

Figure 11-26.   Hodgkin's disease. **A,** Frontal view demonstrates a large mediastinal mass. **B,** CT scan. There is a large anterior and paratracheal mass caused by enlarged lymph nodes. **C,** Lung windows demonstrate pulmonary parenchymal involvement. There are ill-defined nodules distributed axially along the bronchovascular bundles. Air bronchograms can be identified in the nodules *(arrows).*

usually that of ill-defined masses and nodules that spread out from the hila in an axial distribution along the bronchovascular bundles (Fig. 11-26). The appearance may simulate that seen in sarcoidosis or Kaposi's sarcoma, particularly on high-resolution CT. Cavitation may occur, and air bronchograms are a conspicuous feature of parenchymal Hodgkin's disease.

If Hodgkin's disease recurs, it is often within the thorax. Recurrence is typically seen close to the radiation treatment port margins in the adjacent untreated areas of the lung. Such recurrences may appear as nodular or mass lesions in the lung or as perihilar, ill-defined opacities. Involvement of pericardial or diaphragmatic nodes that are not included in the mantle radiation treatment portal may be noted; these appear initially as a mass in the cardiophrenic angle (Fig. 11-27). Such patients should be evaluated with CT, which will demonstrate the nature of the cardiophrenic angle mass.

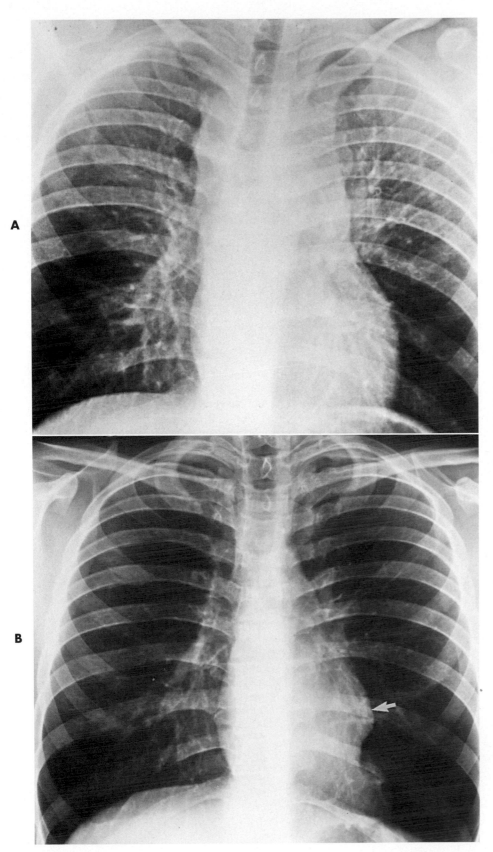

Figure 11-27. Recurrent Hodgkin's disease involving pericardial nodes. **A,** On the initial pretreatment radiograph there is marked widening of the superior mediastinum due to enlarged lymph nodes. Following treatment, the adenopathy resolved. **B,** Subsequent follow-up frontal radiograph several months later shows a bulge along the left heart border produced by an enlarged pericardial lymph node *(arrow)* secondary to recurrent tumor.

In some patients with Hodgkin's disease, particularly those with a nodular sclerosing histologic subtype, a mediastinal mass may persist after treatment. It is difficult using CT alone to differentiate residual masses due to fibrosis from active or recurrent disease. MRI may make the differentiation more accurately. On T2-weighted images, a node replaced by fibrosis will have low signal intensity in contrast to a node that contains active tumor; the latter will be of bright signal intensity. Gadolinium may demonstrate enhancing lymph nodes if active tumor is present.

Calcification may occur in mediastinal lymph node sites following treatment with radiation or chemotherapy (Fig. 11-28). Typically these nodes are calcified in an eggshell distribution.

Non-Hodgkin's lymphoma

Pathologic classification   The histologic classification of non-Hodgkin's lymphoma (Box 11-16) has undergone many changes over the past 25 years. Table 11-5 shows both the Rappaport and Working Formulation for Clinical Usage classifications. The Working Formulation subdivides non-Hodgkin's lymphomas into low, intermediate, and high grade. The low-grade lymphomas are typically found in older men with widespread disease, whereas the high-grade lymphomas occur in younger patients with localized disease.

Clinical features   Older patients with fairly generalized lymphadenopathy and low-grade non-Hodgkin's lymphoma may not complain of any symptoms. Such patients may not undergo treatment unless they develop symptoms of a more aggressive high-grade lymphoma. However, younger patients with intermediate or high-grade non-Hodgkin's lymphoma are treated with aggressive chemotherapy.

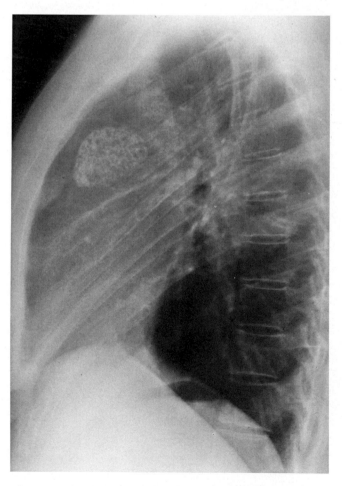

Figure 11-28. Hodgkin's disease, calcified nodules posttreatment. Lateral view shows a large area of calcification in the area of a treated anterior mediastinal mass.

Box 11-16   Non-Hodgkin's Lymphoma

CLINICAL FEATURES

Low grade
  Older patients
  Generalized lymphadenopathy
  Asymptomatic
Intermediate and high grade
  Younger patients
  Treatment with aggressive chemotherapy
Immunocompromised hosts
  AIDS
  Transplant recipients
<50% intrathoracic involvement

RADIOGRAPHIC FEATURES

Similar to Hodgkin's disease
Chest-wall involvement
  More common
  Direct extension or primary site
Pleura
  Direct extension
  Localized plaque-like seeding
  Pleural effusions—lymphatic obstruction
Lung parenchyma
  Primary extranodal site
  Mass with air bronchogram
  Multiple masses or consolidation
Follow-up
  Localized recurrence
  Within 2 years

RADIATION PNEUMONITIS AND FIBROSIS

  6 to 8 weeks posttreatment
  Conforms to portal
  Consolidation with air bronchograms
  Fibrosis
    Loss of volume
    Linear opacities
    Traction bronchiectasis

Table 11-5 Working Formulation/Rappaport Comparison

Working Formulation Type	Rappaport	5-year survival	Comments
LOW			
Small lymphocytic	Lymphocytic, well differentiated	59%	Uncommon
Follicular, small cleaved cell	Nodular, poorly differentiated	70%	Most frequent type
Follicular, mixed cell	Nodular, mixed	50%	
INTERMEDIATE			
Follicular, large cell	Nodular, histiocytic	45%	
Diffuse, small cleaved cell	Diffuse, lymphocytic, poorly differentiated	33%	
Diffuse, mixed cell	Diffuse, mixed	38%	
Diffuse, large cell	Diffuse, histiocytic	35%	GI involvement 25%
HIGH			
Immunoblastic	Diffuse, histiocytic	32%	GI involvement 35%
Lymphoblastic	Lymphoblastic	26%	Usually T-cell origin; mediastinal mass in young males.
Small, noncleaved cell	Diffuse, undifferentiated (Burkitt and non-Burkitt)	23%	Usually B-cell origin; abdomen involvement—North America. Craniofacial form—Africa.

The Working Formulation is described by prognostic grade and cell type and is compared with the Rappaport classification. The 5-year survival percentages are estimated from the Working Formulation report. The classification does not include the miscellaneous category, which includes tumors such as myocosis fungoides. *GI*, gastrointestinal.

From Bragg DG: Hodgkin disease and non Hodgkin lymphoma of the thorax. In Freundlich IM, Bragg DG, editors: *A radiologic approach to diseases of the chest*, Baltimore, 1997, Williams & Wilkins.

Non-Hodgkin's lymphomas may occur in immuno-compromised patients, particularly transplant recipients and patients with AIDS. These lymphomas tend to be aggressive and typically involve the central nervous system.

The majority of low-grade lymphomas will be defined as either stage III or stage IV on initial presentation, whereas the intermediate and high-grade lymphomas will usually be localized stage I tumors. Intrathoracic disease is found with non-Hodgkin's lymphoma at presentation in less than 50% of adult cases.

Radiographic features Less than 50% of non-Hodgkin's lymphoma patients will have thoracic involvement on initial presentation. The appearance is generally similar to that of Hodgkin's disease.

Chest-wall involvement is much more common in non-Hodgkin's lymphoma as a result of direct extension of disease from the mediastinum. Occasionally the chest wall will be involved as a primary site of extranodal lymphoma. It usually appears as a destructive lesion of a rib with a surrounding soft tissue mass.

The pleura may be involved by a direct extension from a contiguous chest wall mass or parenchymal lung disease. Occasionally, localized plaque-like opacities may be observed on the pleural surface, and these represent direct seeding of the pleura from known lymphoma (Fig. 11-29). Pleural involvement is best evaluated with CT.

The majority of patients with lymphoma who have pleural effusions have no direct involvement of the pleura by the lymphomatous process. The effusion most likely occurs secondary to lymphatic obstruction from enlarged hilar and mediastinal nodes.

The lung parenchyma is a common site of involvement by extranodal non-Hodgkin's lymphoma. This is sometimes referred to as primary pulmonary lymphoma. It usually appears as a mass lesion frequently with an air bronchogram (Fig. 11-30). Multiple masses or areas simulating air space consolidation can also be noted. Other patterns are identical to that described above in Hodgkin's disease.

Follow-up As in Hodgkin's disease, most patients with high-grade, non-Hodgkin's lymphomas usually experience recurrences within 2 years after completion of treatment. With the intermediate and high-grade tumors of non-Hodgkin's lymphoma, tumor recurrences tend to occur at the initial localized disease site.

Radiation pneumonitis and fibrosis can be observed in the majority of patients who have received mantle radiation therapy for either Hodgkin's or non-Hodgkin's lymphoma. Classically, radiation pneumonitis can be identified within 6 to 8 weeks after the completion of treatment on standard radiographs, but it often becomes demonstrable on CT at an earlier point in time (Fig. 11-31). The consolidative process is limited by the radiation

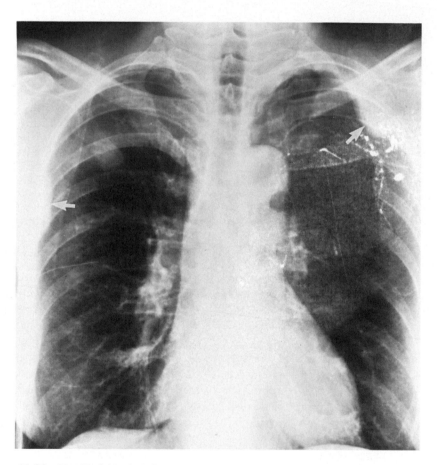

Figure 11-29   Non-Hodgkin lymphoma, pleural involvement. There are plaque-like and more rounded areas of pleural involvement bilaterally *(arrows)*.

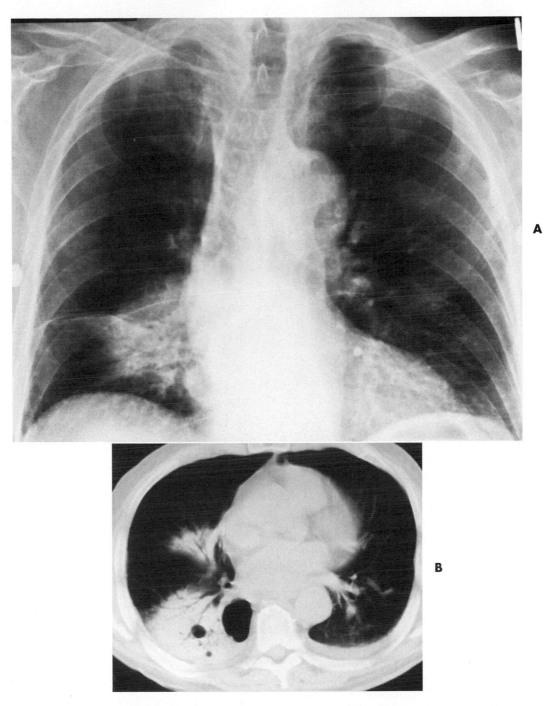

Figure 11-30. Primary pulmonary lymphoma (non-Hodgkin). **A,** Frontal view shows a masslike consolidation at the base of the right lung. **B,** CT scan demonstrates air space consolidation with air bronchograms and cavitation in the right middle and lower lobes.

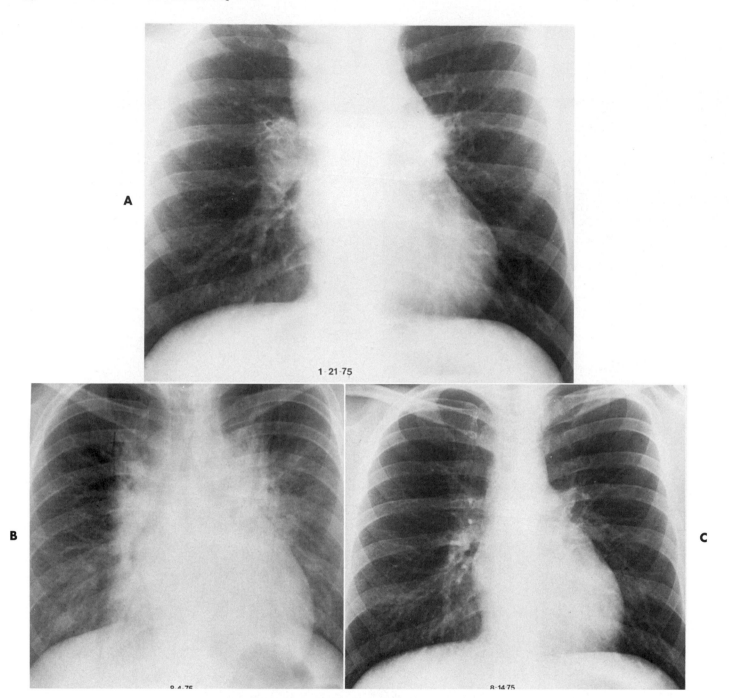

Figure 11-31 Radiation pneumonitis. Hodgkin's disease. **A,** Frontal view shows a widened mediastinum and bilateral hilar adenopathy. **B,** Eight weeks following radiation therapy to the mediastinum there is paramediastinal opacity bilaterally with air bronchograms and a sharp lateral margin especially on the right side. **C,** After steroid treatment the chest radiograph is normal.

portals, and it usually has a sharp lateral margin. Air bronchograms are frequent. Fibrosis usually develops within 6 to 12 months following radiation therapy. Volume loss can be identified in the paramediastinal lung; this involves the upper lobes with dilated air bronchograms as a result of traction bronchiectasis.

METASTATIC DISEASE

Pulmonary metastases, which represent the most common lung neoplasms, occur in 30% to 50% of patients diagnosed with malignancy. The most common

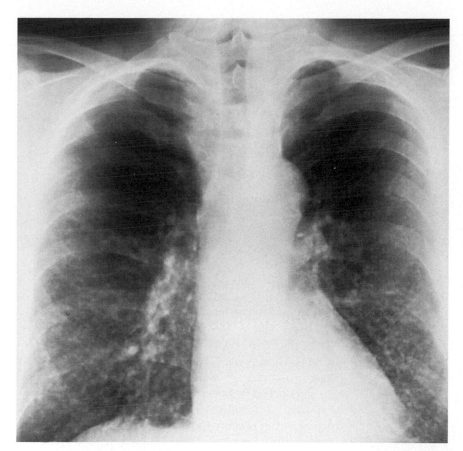

Figure 11-32. Metastases from thyroid cancer. On the frontal view there are multiple small nodules at the bases that represent hematogenous metastases. This pattern is typical for thyroid cancer.

sites of primary malignancies metastatic to the lung include breast, colon, pancreas, stomach, skin (melanoma), head and neck, and kidney.

Mechanisms of Spread

Tumors may spread by direct extension or seeding of body cavities such as the pleura. However, true metastatic disease to the lungs occurs by one of three mechanisms and through one or more of three pathways: hematogenous, lymphatic, and endobronchial. Hematogenous spread is the most common, and endobronchial spread occurs rarely in bronchioloalveolar carcinoma and in malignancies that involve the upper airways or paranasal sinuses. Lymphangitic spread of carcinoma may result initially from bloodborne metastases with extension into the lymphatics from the capillaries. Retrograde lymphatic spread from the upper abdomen may also occur.

Radiographic Features

Hematogenous metastases

Usually both lungs are affected by metastases (Box 11-17). The bases of the lungs are more frequently involved than the apices (Fig. 11-32). Eighty percent to 90% of metastases occur in the periphery, and most lie in close proximity to the pleura (Fig. 11-33). CT is the most sen-

Box 11-17   Metastatic Disease— Hematogenous Spread

CT

High sensitivity, low specificity, false positives owing to intraparenchymal lymph nodes, granulomas

BOTH LUNGS, LOWER LOBES

Periphery
Round, well marginated
Variable doubling times
Ca^{++}
   Primary bone and cartilage tumors
   Mucinous adenocarcinomas
Cavitation
   Metastatic squamous cell
Solitary pulmonary nodule
   <10% of cases
   If squamous cell, likely a lung primary

sitive modality for the detection of metastatic disease. However, CT findings are often nonspecific. Granulomas and subpleural intraparenchymal lymph nodes, both of which tend to measure less than 5 mm in diameter, can be indistinguishable from metastases.

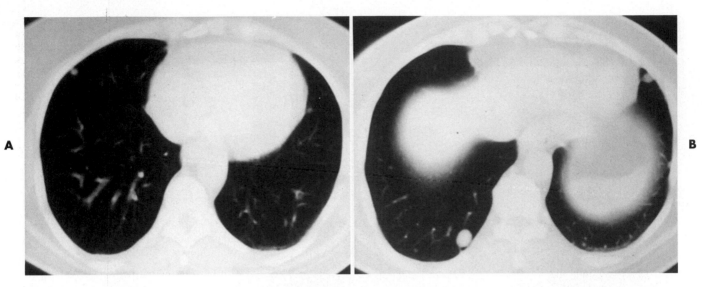

Figure 11-33 Multiple hematogenous metastases from colon carcinoma. CT demonstrates typical peripheral subpleural location of metastases. They are smooth and well defined.

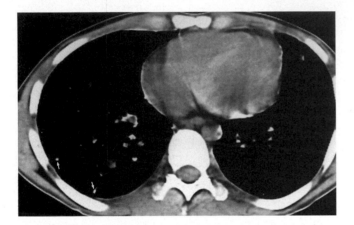

Figure 11-34 Metastases from osteogenic sarcoma. There are multiple small ossified metastases *(arrows)*.

Most metastases tend to be round and very sharply marginated, and they can vary from between 1 and 2 mm to 5 cm or larger. Irregular margins are usually attributable to hemorrhage around the periphery of the metastatic nodule. Choriocarcinoma is cited as the classic example of such an appearance, but hemorrhage and irregularity can occur in other types of metastases after therapy. There is great variability in the growth rates of hematogenous metastases. The tumor doubling time is the time required for a nodule to double in volume or increase 25% in diameter. Carcinoma of the thyroid is an example of an extremely slow-growing tumor that may take months to double in volume. On the other hand, most sarcomas, melanomas, and germ-cell tumors have rapid doubling times. They may even approach 1 to 2 weeks.

Calcification may occur in a number of metastatic lesions (Fig. 11-34). These include primary bone and cartilage tumors such as osteogenic sarcoma and chondrosarcoma as well as papillary and mucinous adenocarcinomas. Dystrophic calcification occurs in areas of necrosis after therapy. Cavitation is infrequent and is most common in squamous-cell carcinomas that are metastatic from the head and neck in men and from the cervix in women. However, such cavities are typically thick-walled. Occasionally, pneumothorax may be associated with cavitation of a subpleural metastatic focus, particularly in sarcomas. The incidence of pulmonary metastases presenting as a solitary nodule is low, less than 10%. However, solitary metastasis can occur in a number of primary tumors, including carcinoma of the colon; sarcoma; and carcinomas of the breast, bladder, kidney, and testicle. A solitary nodule in an adult with an extrathoracic primary squamous cell carcinoma is more likely to represent a primary lung cancer than a metastatic tumor. If the primary tumor is an adenocarcinoma, the likelihood of the nodule in the lung representing a solitary metastasis is equal to the incidence of a second primary tumor. However, with melanoma or sarcoma, solitary metastasis is more likely.

Following chemotherapy, many metastatic lesions will either decrease in size or completely resolve. However, some metastatic lesions will initially respond to therapy and then become stable in size. Such nodules may only contain necrotic or fibrous tissue without viable tumor. Occasionally, biologic markers may distinguish viable tumor from residual fibrotic disease.

Lymphangitic metastases

As mentioned above, most lymphangitic metastases are believed to result from hematogenous spread (Box

---

Box 11-18   Metastatic Disease— Lymphangitic Spread

CHARACTERISTICS

May result from hematogenous spread
Primary sites
   Lung
   Breast
   Upper-abdominal malignancy
More commonly bilateral

RADIOGRAPHIC FEATURES

Standard radiograph
   Reticulonodular pattern
   Kerley B lines
   Pleural effusion (60%)
   Adenopathy (25%)
High-resolution CT
   Nodular thickening of bronchovascular bundles
   Polygonal arcades
   Beaded septal thickening

Box 11-19   Metastatic Disease— Endobronchial Metastases

SITE OF PRIMARY MALIGNANCY

Kidney
Melanoma
Thyroid
Breast
Colon

RADIOGRAPHIC FEATURES

Atelectasis
Hilar mass

Box 11-20   Metastatic Disease— Intrathoracic Adenopathy

SITES OF PRIMARY MALIGNANCY

Genitourinary
Head and neck
Breast
Skin (melanoma)

RADIOGRAPHIC FEATURES

Adenopathy
± Parenchymal metastases

11-18). Primary sites of origin of lymphangitic spread of tumor include carcinomas of the lung, breast, and upper abdominal malignancies such as stomach and pancreas. The spread may be unilateral or bilateral, although unilateral involvement is less common. Lymphangitic spread of primary lung cancer can occur to other areas of the same lung or to the opposite side.

The standard radiograph may be normal, but there is often a mixed reticulonodular pattern (Fig. 11-35). This may be associated with prominent thickening of the interlobular septa (Kerley B and Kerley A lines). The pattern is usually bilateral; it is associated with pleural effusion in 60% of cases and with hilar adenopathy in less than 25% of cases. CT is more sensitive than conventional chest radiographs in the diagnosis of lymphangitic carcinomatosis. Such CT should be performed using high-resolution technique as described in Chapter 7. The typical findings include nodular thickening of the bronchovascular bundles centrally and the interlobular septa (Fig. 11-36). The septal thickening is usually beaded, and it produces a pattern of polygonal arcades. These arcades represent secondary pulmonary lobules. In the center of the arcade is a prominent dot that represents the centrilobular core consisting of the pulmonary artery surrounded by infiltrating tumor. The pattern is usually diffuse, though it may be focal in fewer than half the cases. In addition, small isolated nodules and pleural effusions may be identified. Lymphadenopathy is more commonly identified on CT than on standard radiographs.

Endobronchial metastases

Metastases to major bronchi are uncommon and occur in fewer than 5% of patients at autopsy (Box 11-19). Common sites of primary tumors include the kidney, skin (melanoma), thyroid, breast, and colon. Patients often present with cough and hemoptysis. The radiographic findings consist of lobar, segmental, or subsegmental atelectasis sometimes associated with postobstructive pneumonitis (Fig. 11-37). A hilar or central mass may be present. You must distinguish this appearance from a primary bronchogenic carcinoma.

Intrathoracic adenopathy

Extrathoracic primary tumors may metastasize to mediastinal and hilar lymph nodes either alone or in combination with parenchymal metastases (Fig. 11-38) (Box 11-20). The most common sites of origin include genitourinary neoplasms, those arising in the head and neck, breast carcinoma, and skin (melanoma). Concomitant parenchymal metastases are present in 40% of cases.

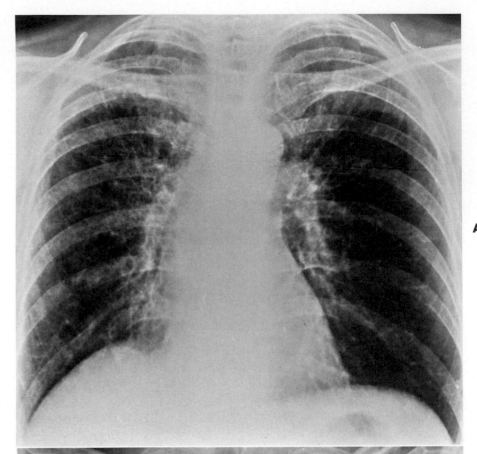

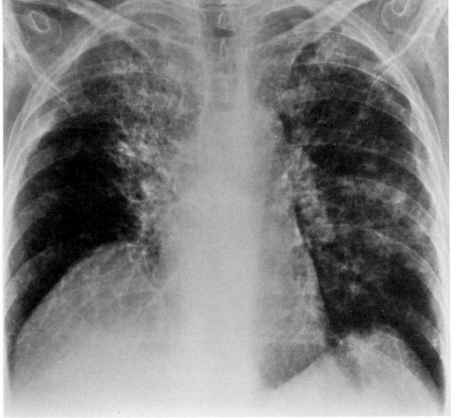

Figure 11-35 Lymphangitic metastases in a woman who had bilateral mastectomies for breast carcinoma. Frontal views (**A** and **B**) several weeks apart show a reticulonodular pattern, which becomes more confluent over time. There is bilateral hilar adenopathy, **B.**

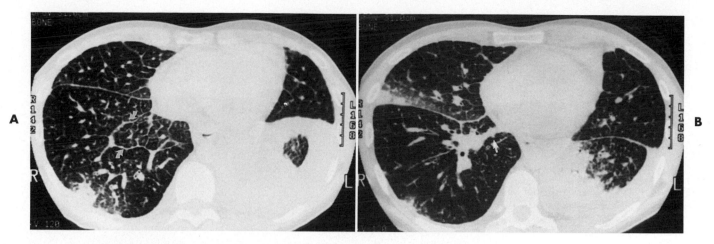

Figure 11-36 Lymphangitic spread of tumor from a lung primary in the left lower lobe. **A,** There is nodular septal thickening creating polygonal arcades *(arrows).* **B,** There is also nodular thickening along bronchovascular bundles *(arrow).*

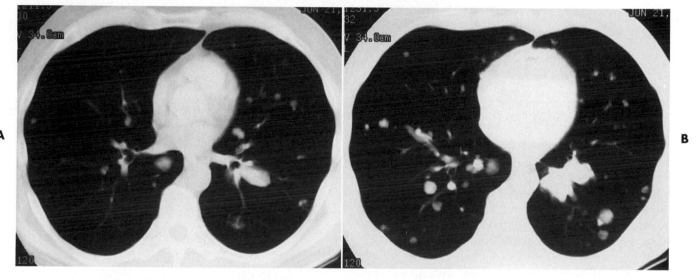

Figure 11-37 Endobronchial metastases from thyroid carcinoma. **A** and **B,** There is a tubular branching structure in the basal segments of the left lower lobe produced by an endobronchial metastases with some associated mucoid impaction.

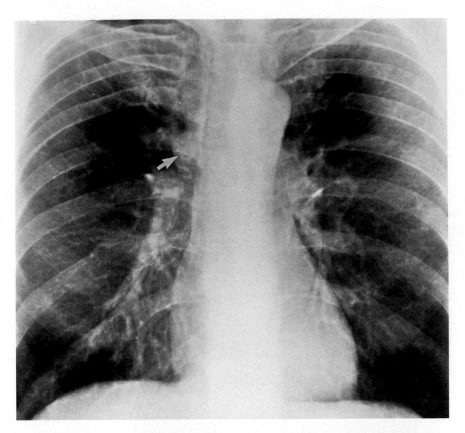

Figure 11-38. Metastasis from malignant melanoma to right paratracheal area. There is an enlarged node in the azygos area on the frontal view *(arrow)*.

Diagnostic Workup

The diagnosis of pulmonary metastases can often be made on standard chest radiographs, and comparison with previous examinations is important. Computed tomography has markedly higher sensitivity as compared with standard radiographs, but it has lower specificity because of the inability to differentiate granulomas and intraparenchymal lymph nodes from small metastases.

Approximately 3% to 4% of all cancers will present with metastatic carcinoma to the lung without a known primary. These are typically adenocarcinomas. The average survival from diagnosis is 3 to 7 months. An extensive imaging search for a primary tumor in such situations is somewhat controversial. Needle aspiration biopsy of a lung metastasis may establish the diagnosis and identify the types of adenocarcinoma that may be likely to respond to specific treatments (i.e., hormone therapy in prostate and breast carcinoma).

SOLITARY PULMONARY NODULE

The solitary pulmonary nodule represents a common clinical problem. In series in which such "coin" lesions have been resected, approximately half are found to be benign, about 40% represent primary lung cancer, and 10% are solitary metastases. A solitary pulmonary nodule

Table 11-6 Clinical indicators of benign vs. malignant solitary pulmonary nodule

Clinical	Benign	Malignant
Age	<35 years of age	>35 years of age
Sex	Female	Male
History	Endemic granuloma area	Primary lesion elsewhere
	Exposure to tuberculosis	

can be defined as a well-circumscribed round or oval lesion measuring less than 3 cm in diameter.

There are a number of clinical indicators that may be helpful in distinguishing benign from malignant solitary nodules (Table 11-6). Unfortunately these are only indicators and they are not sufficiently specific to be helpful in individual cases. However, solitary pulmonary nodules in patients under the age of 35 who with no history of an extrathoracic malignancy are generally considered to be benign and may not require a further diagnostic workup.

Standard Radiographs

A number of criteria have been described to help separate benign from malignant solitary nodules, such as: size, shape, contour, location, edge definition, the presence of satellite lesions, and cavitation. However, none of

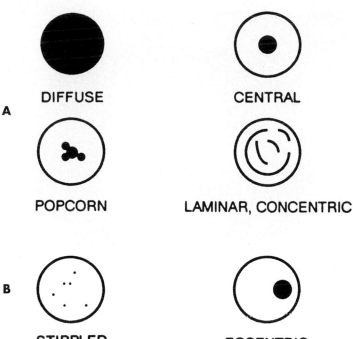

Figure 11-39 Patterns of calcification in benign, **A**, and malignant, **B**, nodules. Benign nodule must be less than 3 cm in diameter and have smooth borders. (From Webb WR: Radiologic evaluation of the solitary pulmonary nodule, *AJR Am J Roentgenol* 154:701-708, 1990.)

these findings is very specific. The only specific and reliable signs of the benign nature of a solitary nodule include the identification of certain "benign" types of calcification and the absolute absence of growth over a 2-year period. "Benign" types of calcification (Figs. 11-1 & 11-39) include those with a central nidus, "popcorn" and laminated. Stippled or eccentric calcification may be identified in 7% to 15% of malignant lung carcinomas. The growth rate or doubling time is an indicator, but this is not a useful discriminant between benign and malignant lesions. Generally speaking, benign lesions have a doubling time of less than 1 month or greater than 16 months. However, there is significant overlap of growth rates among rapidly growing nodules. Only nodules that are stable over a 2-year period can be considered benign. Occasionally, certain acute processes such as infarcts or focal pneumonias may produce a solitary nodule. However, frequently there are important clinical clues such as fever and chest pain. It is important in such a clinical context to follow such lesions for a 2- to 6-week period to ensure that they resolve and do not represent coincidental carcinoma.

Computed Tomography

Computed tomography (CT) is helpful and often diagnostic in the workup of solitary pulmonary nodules. In some cases the morphologic characteristics of a solitary lesion on CT can establish a specific diagnosis, and CT densitometry may allow the identification of benign lesions such as hamartomas and granulomas. You should perform CT either with a conventional scanner obtaining 1- to 2-mm–thick sections (HRCT) or on a helical scanner with a single breathhold and 1-mm sections through the nodule.

Certain lesions in the lung may produce the appearance of a nonspecific solitary pulmonary nodule or lesion on standard studies. However, CT may identify specific diagnostic features. Such entities include arteriovenous (AV) fistulas, rounded atelectasis, fungus balls, mucoid impaction, and infarcts. AV fistulas can be diagnosed because of the presence of a feeding artery and draining vein as well as intense enhancement after the administration of contrast material (Fig. 11-40). The features of rounded atelectasis include a peripheral rounded lesion in the lung abutting pleural thickening associated with a classic "comet tail" sign consisting of a crowding of pulmonary vessels and bronchi leading to the mass (see Chapter 1). A fungus ball within a preexisting cavity may appear as a solitary pulmonary nodule on standard films. However, CT will clearly identify the presence of a nodule within a cavity (see Chapters 3 and 4). Mucoid impaction on CT can be diagnosed because of the classic features of branching opacities located endobronchially that are often associated with bronchiectasis (Fig. 11-41). Finally, infarcts on CT may have a classic appearance. They abut the pleura and are round or wedge-shaped in appearance, and they often contain pseudocavities or air bronchograms.

CT densitometry is useful in detecting both the presence and distribution of calcification and fat within solitary nodules. CT is more sensitive than standard studies in the detection of calcification. Between 22% and 38% of uncalcified nodules on standard studies appear calcified on CT. The presence of calcification can often be

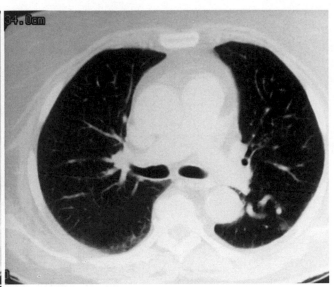

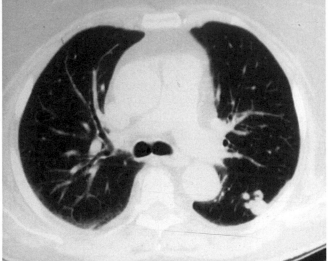

Figure 11-40   Arteriovenous malformation. CT scan, **A, B, C,** through a nodular lesion shows feeding and draining vessels.

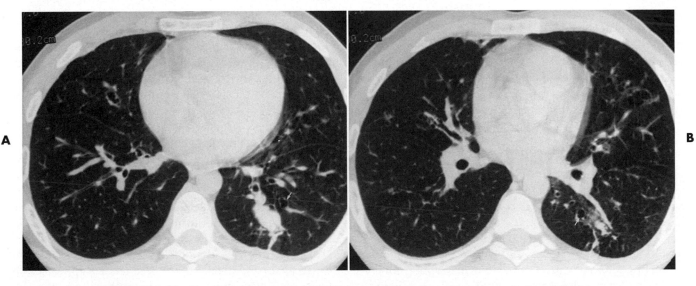

Figure 11-41   Mucoid impaction. **A** and **B,** CT shows a tubular branching opacity in the left lower lobe with areas of surrounding bronchiectasis *(arrows)*.

Box 11-21   Solitary Noncalcified Nodule (Over Age 35)

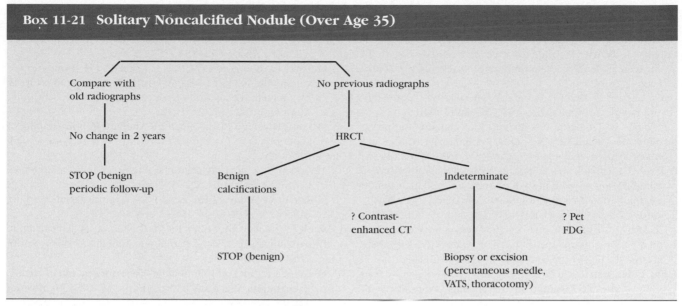

HRCT, high resolution CT; *PET FDG*, positron emission tomography with flurodesoxyglucose; *VATS*, video assisted thorasoscopy

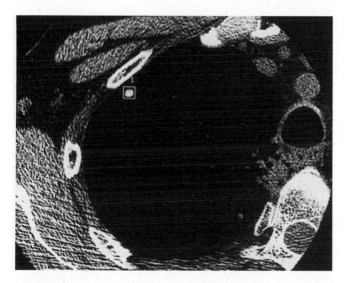

Figure 11-42   Calcified granuloma. CT densitometry. Thin collimation image of a solitary nodule in the right lung shows dense calcification. CT numbers throughout the lesion showed values greater than + 1200.

confirmed visually by direct examination of the image, or a pixelogram can be obtained by placing a cursor over the lesion (Fig. 11-42). A printout of each of the CT numbers in every pixel through the lesion is required. Values greater than + 200 are indicative of the presence of calcification.

Fat may be present in hamartomas. Fat will appear of low attenuation and measure between approximately –50 to –150 HU (Fig. 11-2). In a study of 47 hamartomas, 30 were correctly diagnosed on CT by the presence of fat alone, either focal or diffuse; by a combination of fat and calcification; or by the presence of "popcorn" calcification alone.

Newer Imaging Techniques

There are some promising newer imaging techniques for the evaluation of solitary pulmonary nodules. It has been shown that malignant pulmonary nodules enhance to a greater degree than benign lesions after the administration of contrast material. Enhancement of greater than 20 HU is highly sensitive for the presence of malignancy, although the specificity is slightly lower because occasionally active inflammatory lesions may also enhance. Positron emission tomography with fluorodeoxyglucose (PET FDG) may also be used to distinguish benign from malignant lesions. High sensitivities for malignancy have been reported. FDG is an analog of glucose and is taken up avidly by malignant tumors because of increased metabolism.

Diagnostic Workup

A scheme for the proposed diagnostic workup of a solitary pulmonary nodule is presented in Box 11-21.

SUGGESTED READINGS

Balakrishnan J, Meziane MA, Siegelman SS, Fishman EK: Pulmonary infarction: CT appearance with pathologic correlation, *J Comput Assist Tomogr* 13:941-945, 1989.

Bragg D: Hodgkin disease and non-Hodgkin lymphoma of the thorax. In Freundlich IM, Bragg DG, editors: *A radiologic approach to diseases of the chest,* Baltimore, 1997, Williams & Wilkins, pp 597-608.

Braman SS, Whitcomb ME: Endobronchial metastasis, *Arch Intern Med* 135:543-547, 1975.

Chalmers N, Best JJK: The significance of pulmonary nodules detected by CT but not by chest radiography in tumor staging, *Clin Radiol* 44:410-412, 1991.

Chang AE, Schaner EG, Conkle DM et al: Evaluation of computed tomography in detection of pulmonary metastases: A prospective study, *Cancer* 43:913-916, 1979.

Coppage L, Shaw C, McBride-Curtis A: Metastatic disease to the chest in patients with extrathoracic malignancy, *J Thorac Imag* 2:24-37, 1987.

Crow J, Slavin G, Kreel L: Pulmonary metastases: A pathologic and radiologic study, *Cancer* 47:2595-2602, 1981.

Cummings SR, Lillington GA, Richard RJ: Estimating the probability of malignancy in solitary pulmonary nodules: A Bayesian approach, *Am Rev Respir Dis* 134:449-452, 1986.

D'Angio GJ, Iannaccone G: Spontaneous pneumothorax as a complication of pulmonary metastases in malignant tumors of childhood, *AJR Am J Roentgenol* 86:1092-1102, 1961.

Edwards WM, Cox RS Jr, Garland LH: The solitary nodule (coin lesion) of the lung: An analysis of 52 consecutive cases treated by thoracotomy and a study of prospective diagnostic accuracy, *AJR Am J Roentgenol* 88:1020-1042, 1962.

Faling LJ, Pugatch RD, Jung-Legg Y: Computed tomography scanning of the mediastinum in the staging of bronchogenic carcinoma, *Am Rev Respir Dis* 124:690-695, 1981.

Filderman AE, Shaw C, Matthay RA: Lung cancer. Part I: Etiology, pathology, natural history, manifestations, and diagnostic techniques, *Invest Radiol* 21:80-90, 1986.

Forster BB, Müller NL, Miller RR, Nelems B, Evans KG: Neuroendocrine carcinomas of the lung: Clinical, radiologic, and pathologic correlation, *Radiology* 170:441-445, 1989.

Fraser RG, Paré JAP: *Diagnosis of diseases of the chest,* ed 3, vol 2, Philadelphia, 1989, WB Saunders; pp 1327-1699.

Friedman PJ: Lung cancer: Update on staging classifications, *AJR Am J Roentgenol* 150:261-264, 1988.

Glazer GM, Orringer MB, Gross BH, Quint LE: The mediastinum in non-small cell cancer: CT-surgical correlation, *AJR Am J Roentgenol* 142:1101-1105, 1984.

Gurney JW, Lyddon DM, McKay JA: Determining the likelihood of malignancy in solitary pulmonary nodules with Bayesian analysis. Part II: Application, *Radiology* 186:415-422, 1993.

Gurney JW: Determining the likelihood of malignancy in solitary pulmonary nodules with Bayesian analysis. Part I: Theory, *Radiology* 186:405-413, 1993.

Haggar AM, Perlberg JL, Froelich JW et al: Chest wall invasion by carcinoma of the lung: Detection by MR imaging, *AJR Am J Roentgenol* 148:1075-1078, 1987.

Hill CA: Bronchioloalveolar carcinoma: A review, *Radiology* 150:15-20, 1984.

Janower ML, Blennerhassett JB: Lymphangitic spread of metastatic cancer to the lung, *Radiology* 101:267-273, 1971.

Kuriyama K, Tateishi R, Doi O et al: CT-pathologic correlation in small peripheral lung cancers, *AJR Am J Roentgenol* 149:1139-1143, 1987.

Libshitz HI, Jing BS, Wallace S et al: Sterilized metastases: A diagnostic and therapeutic dilemma, *AJR Am J Roentgenol* 140:15-19, 1983.

Libshitz HI, McKenna RJ Jr, Haynie TP, McMurtney MJ, Mountain C: Mediastinal evaluation in lung cancer, *Radiology* 151:295-299, 1984.

Libshitz HI, McKenna RJ: Mediastinal lymph node size in lung cancer, *AJR Am J Roentgenol* 143:715-718, 1984.

Libshitz HI: Pulmonary metastatic disease. In Freundlich IM, Bragg DG, editors: *A radiologic approach to diseases of the chest,* Baltimore, 1997, Williams & Wilkins; pp 561-576.

Mayo JR, Webb WR, Gould R et al: High-resolution CT of the lungs: An optimal approach, *Radiology* 163:507-510, 1987.

McHugh K, Blaquiere RM: CT features of rounded atelectasis, *AJR Am J Roentgenol* 153:257-260, 1989.

McLoud TC, Bourgouin PM, Greenberg RW et al: Bronchogenic carcinoma: Analysis of staging in the mediastinum with CT by correlative lymph node mapping and sampling, *Radiology* 182:319-323, 1992.

McLoud TC, Filion RB, Edelman RR, Shepard JO: MR imaging of superior sulcus carcinoma, *J Comput Assist Tomogr* 13:233-239, 1989.

Mountain C: A new international staging system for lung cancer, *Chest* 89(Suppl):225-233, 1986.

Mountain CF: Value of the new TNM staging system for lung cancer, *Chest* 96:47-49, 1989.

Munk PL, Müller NL, Miller RR et al: Pulmonary lymphangitic carcinomatosis: CT and pathologic findings, *Radiology* 166:705-709, 1988.

O'Connell RS, McLoud TC, Wilkins EW: Superior sulcus tumor: Radiographic diagnosis and workup, *AJR Am J Roentgenol* 140:25-30, 1983.

Pancoast HK: Superior pulmonary sulcus tumor; tumor characterized by pain, Horner's syndrome, destruction of bone and atrophy of hand muscles, *JAMA* 99:1391-1396, 1932.

Patz EF, Lowe VJ, Hoffman JM et al: Focal pulmonary abnormalities: Evaluation with F-18 fluorodeoxyglucose PET scanning, *Radiology* 188:487-290, 1993.

Pennes DR, Glazer GM, Wimbish KJ, Gross BH, Long RW, Orringer MB: Chest wall invasion by lung cancer: Limitations by CT evaluation, *AJR Am J Roentgenol* 144:507-511, 1985.

Pugatch RD, Munden RF: Primary pulmonary neoplasm. In Freundlich IM, Bragg DG, editors: *A radiologic approach to diseases of the chest,* Baltimore, 1997, Williams & Wilkins; pp 543-560.

Remy J, Remy-Jardin M, Wattinne L et al: Pulmonary arteriovenous malformations: Evaluation with CT of the chest before and after treatment, *Radiology* 182:809-816, 1992.

Remy-Jardin M, Remy J, Giraud F et al: Pulmonary nodules: Detection with thick-section spiral CT versus conventional CT, *Radiology* 187:513-520, 1993.

Schaner EG, Chang AE, Doppman JL et al: Comparison of computed and conventional whole lung tomography in detecting pulmonary nodules: A prospective radiology-pathology study, *AJR Am J Roentgenol* 131:51-54, 1978.

Seely J, Mayo JR, Miller RR, M;auuller NL: T1 lung cancer: Prevalence of mediastinal nodal metastases (diagnostic accuracy of CT), *Radiology* 186:129-132, 1993.

Shuman LS, Libshitz HI: Solid pleural manifestations of lymphoma, *AJR Am J Roentgenol* 142:269-273, 1984.

Siegelman SS, Khouri NF, Leo FP, Fishman EK, Braverman RM, Zerhouni EA: Solitary pulmonary nodules: CT assessment, *Radiology* 160:307-312, 1986.

Siegelman SS, Khouri NF, Scott WW Jr et al: Pulmonary hamartoma: CT findings, *Radiology* 160:313-317, 1986.

Skarin A, Jochelson M, Sheldon F et al: Neoadjuvant chemotherapy in marginally resectable stage III MO non-small cell lung cancer: Long-term follow-up in 41 patients, *J Surg Oncol* 40:266-274, 1989.

Staples CA, Müller NL, Miller RR, Evans KG, Nelems B: Mediastinal nodes in bronchogenic carcinoma: Comparison between CT and mediastinoscopy, *Radiology* 167:367-372, 1988.

Swensen SJ et al: Pulmonary nodules: CT evaluation of enhancement with iodinated contrast material, *Radiology* 194:393-398, 1995.

Swensen SJ, Morin RL, Schueler BA et al: Solitary pulmonary nodule: CT evaluation of enhancement with iodinated contrast material—A preliminary report, *Radiology* 182:343-347, 1992.

Theros EG: 1976 Caldwell lecture. Varying manifestations of peripheral pulmonary neoplasms: A radiologic-pathologic correlative study, *AJR Am J Roentgenol* 128:893-914, 1977.

Tisi GM, Friedman PH, Peters RM et al: American Thoracic Society: Clinical staging of primary lung cancer, *Am Rev Respir Dis* 127:659-664, 1983.

Webb WR, Gatsonis C, Zerhouni E et al: CT and MR imaging in staging non-small cell bronchogenic carcinoma: Report of the Radiology Diagnostic Oncology Group, *Radiology* 178:705-713, 1991.

Webb WR: Radiologic evaluation of the solitary pulmonary nodule, *AJR Am J Roentgenol* 154:701-708, 1990.

Webb WR: The solitary pulmonary nodule. In Freundlich IM, Bragg DG, editors: *A radiologic approach to diseases of the chest,* Baltimore, 1997, Williams & Wilkins; pp 101-108.

Zerhouni EA, Stitik FP, Siegelman SS et al: CT of the pulmonary nodule: A cooperative study, *Radiology* 160:319-327, 1986.

Zwiebel BR, Austin JHM, Grines MM: Bronchial carcinoid tumors: Assessment with CT of location and intratumoral calcification in 31 patients, *Radiology* 179:483-486, 1991.

Zwirewich CV, Vedal S, Miller RR et al: M;auuller NL: Solitary pulmonary nodule: High-resolution CT and radiologic-pathologic correlation, *Radiology* 179:469-476, 1991.

The Trachea

JO-ANNE O. SHEPARD

ANATOMY

The trachea is a cartilaginous and membranous tube that extends from the larynx to the carina, measuring approximately 11 cm in length. The trachea is nearly cylindrical with slight flattening posteriorly. Its diameter from side-to-side is approximately 2 to 2.5 cm. The trachea and extrapulmonary bronchi are comprised of incomplete rings of hyaline cartilage, fibrous tissue, muscular fibers, mucous membrane, and glands. The tracheal cartilages form an imperfect ring that occupies the anterior two thirds of the trachea. The bronchial cartilages are shorter and narrower than those of the trachea, but they have the same shape and arrangement. Posteriorly, the membranous wall of the trachea and main bronchi is completed by fibrous tissue and nonstriated muscular fibers.

RADIOGRAPHIC EVALUATION

Plain Films

There are several radiographic studies used to evaluate the trachea and main bronchi (Table 12-1). The plain chest radiograph in the posteroanterior (PA) and lateral projections is the most frequently used screening study. A high-kilovoltage (140 kVp) technique is preferred because it reduces the visibility of the bony thorax and improves imaging of the various mediastinal interfaces. However, it is easy to miss a tracheal or main bronchial lesion on standard PA and lateral chest radiographs because there is considerable overlap of the trachea with the mediastinum and bony thorax. Bilateral oblique chest radiographs improve visibility of the trachea and main bronchi by rotating the spine so that it is not superimposed on the central airways (Fig. 12-1). In the majority of cases, additional imaging is usually indicated.

Computed Tomography

Computed tomography (CT) has become the imaging modality of choice for most tracheobronchial lesions. Because of the clarity of anatomic detail on cross-sectional imaging there is a direct display of tracheobronchial anatomy. The superior contrast resolution, compared with conventional radiography, permits evaluation of adjacent mediastinal soft tissues. This is of particular importance in cases of tracheal neoplasms, which may invade the adjacent mediastinum,

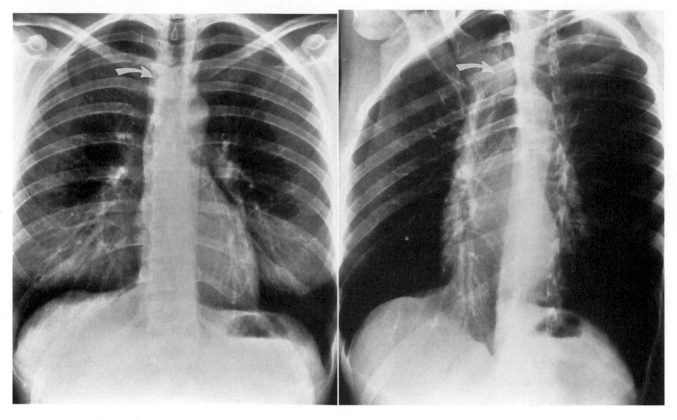

Fig. 12-1 Tracheal tumor. **A,** Posteroanterior view of the chest reveals a focal area of increased opacity in the mid trachea projected over the spine. (*arrow*). **B,** A left anterior oblique projection projects the trachea to the right of the spine. A focal well-defined intraluminal mass (*arrow*) is better characterized in the midtrachea, representing an adenoid cystic carcinoma.

Table 12-1 Approach to diagnostic imaging of the trachea

Study	Clinical indication
Chest radiographs (posteroanterior, lateral, oblique projections)	Screening study
Conventional tomography (anteroposterior, lateral, 55-degree posterior oblique projections)	Postintubation tracheal stenosis
	Preoperative assessment of length of lesion
	Postoperative assessment of bronchial anastomosis
Computed tomography	Tracheobronchial tumor location and extent
	Density determination
	Vascularity of tumor
	Airway diameter
	Wall thickness
	Tracheomalacia (inspiration/expiration CT)
	Compression of airway by mediastinal mass or vessel
	Tracheobronchial rupture
	Tracheobronchial dehiscence
Magnetic resonance imaging	Multiplanar imaging
	Mediastinal invasion by airway, neoplasm
	Airway obstruction by vascular rings
Fluoroscopy	Tracheomalacia
	Air trapping due to bronchial obstruction

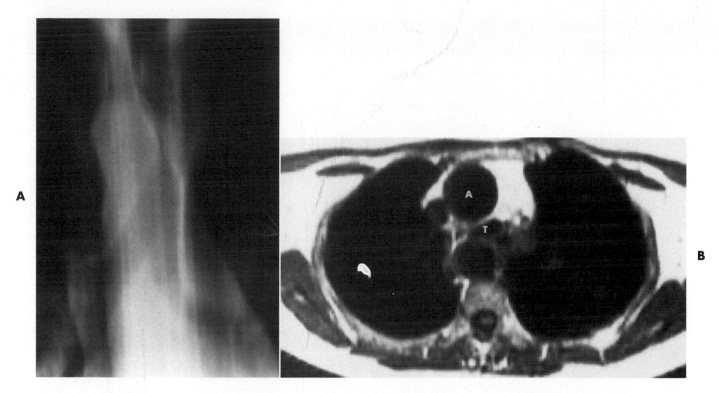

Fig. 12-2 Tracheal compression by a right aortic arch. **A,** Anteroposterior tomogram demonstrates extrinsic compression and smooth narrowing of the midtrachea by a right paratracheal mass. **B,** MRI with T1-weighted axial image demonstrates a slightly dilated ascending aorta *(A)*, which extrinsically compresses and narrows the tracheal lumen *(T)*.

or in cases of mediastinal masses such as goiters or vascular rings, which may compress the trachea. CT has the ability to identify calcific and fatty densities as well as vascular enhancement of tumors and aneurysms following intravenous contrast administration. Paired inspiratory/expiratory CT scans can identify abnormal collapsibility of the trachea and main bronchi in cases of tracheobronchomalacia. High-resolution computed tomography (HRCT) can be obtained with the use of thin (1 to 1.5 mm) sections and bone reconstruction algorithm. The major disadvantage of conventional CT is that craniocaudally oriented trachea and bronchi are not imaged in the long axis. Although images may be reconstructed in sagittal and coronal planes, the resolution is limited by the inherent scan thickness on conventional CT scans. Fortunately, volumetric scanning on newer spiral scanners has overcome this problem. Thin-section multiplanar reconstructions may be obtained in any plane, as well as three-dimensional images.

Historically, conventional tomography in the anteroposterior (AP), lateral, and oblique projections was routinely used to evaluate the trachea and central bronchi. With refinements in CT scanning, conventional airway tomography is no longer routinely employed. However, it does permit an accurate assessment of patency or the degree of obstruction in the central airways and provides

a direct image of the airways in the long axis. Conventional tomograms have the ability to determine accurately the length of tracheal lesions relative to the larynx or carina. Of course, the major disadvantage of conventional tomography is the inability to visualize adjacent mediastinal structures.

Magnetic Resonance Imaging

The role of magnetic resonance imaging (MRI) in the evaluation of the trachea and bronchi is limited. The trachea, main bronchi, and lobar bronchi are well demonstrated on spin echo images, but the spatial resolution of MRI permits observation of only an occasional segmental bronchus. MRI offers the advantages of multiplanar imaging, high-contrast resolution without the use of intravenous contrast agents, and absence of ionizing radiation. MRI is particularly useful in patients with vascular rings or tracheal compression by vascular anomalies and other mediastinal masses (Fig. 12-2).

TRACHEAL STENOSIS

Diffuse tracheal narrowing is seen in a number of conditions including chronic obstructive pulmonary disease (COPD); following tracheal trauma; as the result of viral,

Table 12-2 Diffuse tracheal stenosis

Disease	Tracheobronchial findings	Other findings
Idiopathic	• Smooth, tapered, irregular, lobulated or eccentric • 2-4 cm in length	• ± Laryngeal involvement
Postintubation cuff injury	Smooth narrowing with hourglass configuration	——
Posttraumatic	Smooth narrowing with hourglass configuration	• ± Upper rib and sternal fractures
Saber Sheath Trachea	• Smooth narrowing of intrathoracic trachea • Coronal diameter ≤ half sagittal diameter	Hyperinflated lungs
Tracheopathia Osteochondroplastica	• Submucosal nodularity of anterolateral walls of trachea and main bronchi with ossification • Membranous wall is spared	——
Relapsing Polychondritis	• Diffusely thickened tracheobronchial walls with diffuse narrowing of trachea and main bronchi • ± Calcification of wall • ± Tracheobronchomalacia	• Auricular and nasal chondritis, arthritis
Wegener's Granulomatosis	• Focal or diffuse tracheobronchial wall-thickening and narrowing • ± Enlarged calcified cartilages	• Renal involvement
Amyloidosis	• Diffuse tracheobronchial wall-thickening and narrowing • Focal nodular masses • ± Calcification • Contrast enhancement of masses on CT or MRI • Slowly progressive	• ± Lymphadenopathy, may calcify
Sarcoidosis	• Smooth, irregular, or nodular stenosis • Tracheobronchial wall thickening • Bronchial compression by lymph node	• ± Lymphadenoapathy, ± calcification • ± Reticular/nodular interstitial lung disease
Infectious		
Tracheobronchial papillomatosis	Diffuse nodules or masses in trachea and bronchi	• Laryngeal involvement • ± Multiple pulmonary nodules, may cavitate • Complicated by squamous cell carcinoma
Rhinosclerosis	• Nodular masses or diffuse symmetric narrowing of trchea and bronchi • Slowly progressive	
Tuberculous		
Hyperplastic stage	Irregular trachobronchial wall thickening and narrowing	• Hilar and/or mediastinal lymphadenopathy
Fibrostenotic stage	Smooth tracheobronchial narrowing	• Parenchymal cavitation and consolidation • Atelectasis and scarring • Bronchiectasis • Calcified lymph nodes

fungal, tuberculous, or bacterial infections; and in other diseases such as sarcoidosis, Wegener's granulomatosis, relapsing polychondritis, amyloidosis, and tracheobronchopathia osteochondroplastica. Such narrowing may be idiopathic and may involve the larynx (Table 12-2).

Idiopathic Laryngotracheal Stenosis

Idiopathic laryngotracheal stenosis is an uncommon cause of narrowing in the larynx and subglottic trachea. It typically affects middle-aged women who have no history of intubation, trauma, infection, or other underlying systemic disease. Clinically, patients experience progressive shortness of breath accompanied by wheezing, stridor, and/or hoarseness. The average duration of symptoms is approximately 2 years.

The radiologic appearance of idiopathic laryngotracheal stenosis is variable including lesions that may be smooth and tapered (Fig. 12-3), or irregular, lobulated, and eccentric (Fig. 12-4). The length of the stenosis varies from 2 to 4 cm, with severe compromise of the lumen measuring no more than 5 mm at the narrowest point.

Histologically, the stenotic areas show dense keloid fibrosis involving the adventitia and the lamina propria, sparing the mucosa, muscularis propria, and the cartilage. Small areas of spindle-cell proliferation similar to fibrosing mediastinitis or retroperitoneal fibrosis occur. The mucosa may show squamous metaplasia without

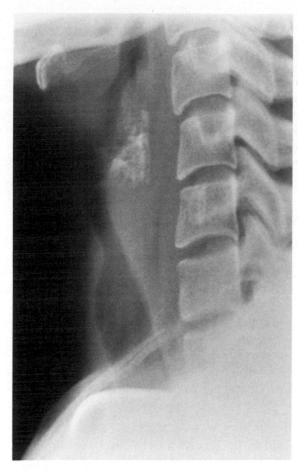

Fig. 12-3 Idiopathic laryngotracheal stenosis. A lateral soft-tissue view of the neck reveals a smooth and tapered stenosis of the subglottic larynx and proximal trachea.

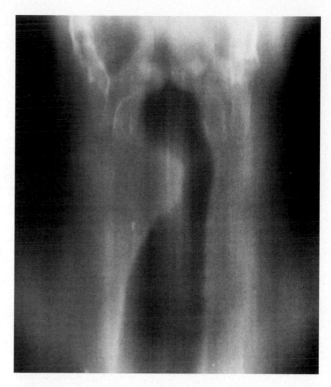

Fig. 12-4 Idiopathic tracheal stenosis. An anteroposterior tomogram of the larynx and proximal trachea reveals a focal eccentric and lobulated stenosis of the proximal trachea.

dysplastic changes. The lesions may be treated surgically or conservatively with dilation, intubation, stenting, steroid injection, cryotherapy, or electrocoagulation.

Box 12-1 Postintubation Injury

Tracheal stenosis
    At stomal level
    At cuff site (most frequent)
    At tube tip
Tracheoesophageal fistula
Tracheoarterial fistula

Postintubation Injuries

Most long-term complications of intubation relate to cuff injury. Cuffed endotracheal tubes became commonplace only after the introduction of intermittent positive pressure breathing for the treatment of respiratory failure during the poliomyelitis epidemic of 1952. As patients survived longer periods with respiratory assistance, new long-term complications arose including tracheal stenosis, tracheoesophageal fistula, and tracheoinnominate artery fistula (Box 12-1).

A *stenosis* may occur at the level of the tracheostomy stoma or rarely where the tip of the tube impinges on the tracheal mucosa. However, pressure necrosis at the cuff site is responsible for most long-term postintubation complications. If the cuff pressure exceeds capillary pressure, blood supply to the mucosa is compromised, leading to ischemic necrosis. Initially the mucosa

becomes inflamed, followed by ulceration in the mucosa overlying the cartilaginous rings. As the ulcers enlarge there is increasing exposure of the cartilage, which becomes colonized with bacteria. With further pressure on the wall there is the development of necrosis, softening and dissolution of the cartilage leading to tracheomalacia or to scarring and stenosis formation. Radiographically such a stenosis will have a smooth gradual narrowing with an hourglass configuration (Fig. 12-5). Typically, symptoms of stenosis will develop in 2 to 6 weeks postextubation and, in some patients, months later. The majority of stenoses are appropriately treated with resection of the damaged segment and end-to-end anastomosis. In the past 20 years, most tracheostomy and endotracheal tubes have been designed with large-volume, low-pressure cuffs, which has dramatically reduced

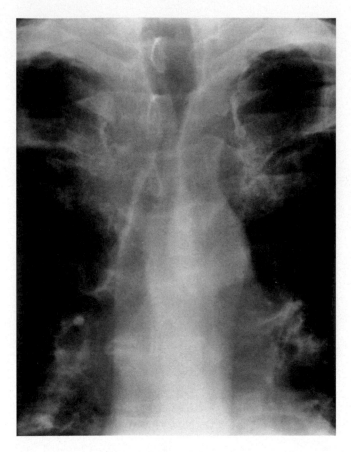

Fig. 12-5 Postintubation tracheal stenosis. An anteroposterior view of the proximal trachea reveals the typical hourglass configuration of tracheal stenosis related to cuff injury.

the incidence of tracheal stricture. Postintubation tracheal strictures do continue to occur but at a much reduced rate.

Tracheoesophageal fistula may occur from ventilation with a cuffed tube, most often when an indwelling esophageal tube is also being used in neurologically impaired patients who are ventilated for a long time. The mechanism of injury is pressure necrosis resulting from pressure exerted by the cuff on the tracheal wall against a foreign body in the esophagus. The injury occurs most often from the cuff on a tracheostomy tube rather than that on an endotracheal tube. The marked inflammatory reaction that ensues causes fusion of the tissue planes. As a result, the fistula enters the esophagus directly without communication with the mediastinum. Such a fistula often results in recurrent aspiration pneumonias manifest as patchy parenchymal consolidations (Fig. 12-6) (See Chapter 13 for further discussion.)

Most *tracheoarterial fistulas* will occur from erosion by the angle of the tube itself. Rarely will the cuff erode the vessel directly.

Posttraumatic Tracheal Stenosis

If a tracheal tear is incomplete and there is preservation of the peritracheal connective tissue, or if the tear is occluded by a cuff or fibrin deposition, pneumothorax or pneumomediastinum may not be present. Tears that present in this fashion may be missed initially and have a delayed presentation. If healing ensues, an untreated partial laceration will develop a stenosis with the typical hourglass configuration (Fig. 12-7 on page 354).

Saber-Sheath Trachea

Saber-sheath trachea is an abnormality of the intrathoracic trachea that affects men who smoke and have COPD. Typically, there is an abrupt change in the tracheal caliber beginning at the thoracic inlet that may extend the entire intrathoracic length of the trachea. The trachea is narrowed in the coronal diameter such that the coronal diameter is no more than half of the corresponding sagittal diameter (Fig. 12-8 on page 355). Changes in the configuration of the trachea in this entity result from abnormal intrathoracic transmural pressures.

Tracheopathia Osteochondroplastica

Tracheopathia osteochondroplastica is a condition of unknown etiology in which there are multiple submucosal osteocartilaginous nodules along the anterolateral walls of the trachea and cartilage bearing bronchi. The posterior membranous wall is typically spared because of the absence of cartilage in this area, a distinguishing feature from many other diffuse tracheal diseases. The submucosal deposits may cause distortion and narrowing of the airways. Radiographically, the tracheobronchial cartilages are thickened and nodular in appearance, with resultant narrowing of the lumen. Ossification within the nodules can be detected by CT. The membranous wall maintains a normal thin appearance (Fig. 12-9 on page 356).

Relapsing Polychondritis

Relapsing polychondritis is a rare inflammatory disease of unknown cause that affects the cartilages of the ears, nose, upper respiratory tract, and joints. Recurrent episodes of cartilaginous inflammation result in fragmentation of the cartilages, which are replaced by fibrosis. Auricular chondritis is the most common manifestation. The respiratory tract is affected in approximately 50% of patients and airway obstruction is the major cause of death.

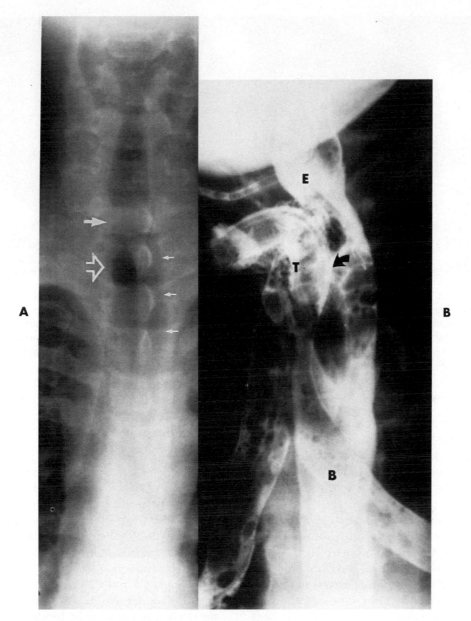

Fig. 12-6   Tracheoesophageal fistula in a neurologically impaired patient following prolonged mechanical intubation and indwelling nasogastric tube. **A,** An anteroposterior radiograph of the trachea reveals a tracheal stenosis *(arrow)* proximal to a tracheostomy stoma *(open arrow).* The proximal esophagus is distended with air *(arrows)* in proximity to the tracheoesophageal fistula. **B,** A contrast esophagram demonstrates filling of the tracheoesophageal fistula *(arrow)* and aspiration of contrast medium from the esophagus *(E)* into the trachea *(T)* and main bronchi *(B).*

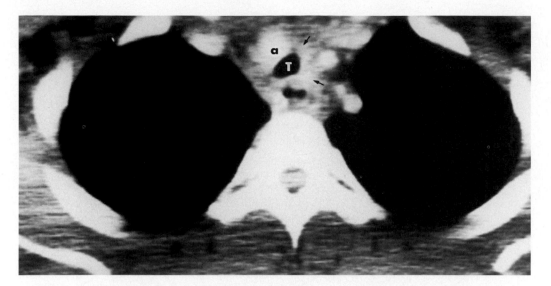

Fig. 12-7   Posttraumatic tracheal stenosis with delayed presentation following tracheal laceration. A contrast-enhanced CT examination through the superior mediastinum just cephalad to the aortic arch reveals a narrowed and misshapen tracheal lumen *(T)*. The wall of the trachea is thickened and irregular in its interface with the mediastinum, representing fibrous tissue at the site of laceration *(arrows)*. The innominate artery *(a)* is closely applied to the tracheal lumen and was found to occlude part of the anterior wall of the trachea at the time of tracheal repair.

A spectrum of changes affects the airways. Early in the disease when mucosal edema is present, the airways become narrowed. As the cartilage dissolves, the airways become more collapsible and as the destroyed cartilages are replaced by fibrous tissue, fixed stenosis of the airway develops.

The radiographic appearance is that of a diffusely thickened tracheobronchial wall with diffuse smooth narrowing of the trachea and main bronchi (Fig. 12-10 on page 357). In addition to the tracheal and main bronchial narrowing, CT demonstrates stenoses involving the segmental and subsegmental bronchi in some cases, and the tracheobronchial walls are thickened (Fig. 12-11 on page 357). There is occasionally calcification within the tracheobronchial wall.

Wegener's Granulomatosis

Wegener's granulomatosis, a granulomatous vasculitis, may involve the upper and lower respiratory tract most often in conjunction with renal and other organ involvement. Diffuse tracheobronchial involvement is rare and usually presents late in the disease process. Radiographic findings include tracheobronchial narrowing and thickening as well as an irregularity of the wall that may be diffuse or focal (Fig. 12-12 on page 358). Granulomatous tissue may obstruct a bronchus and cause atelectasis. You can often detect mediastinal adenopathy by CT. Enlarged calcified tracheal cartilages have also been reported.

Amyloidosis

Amyloidosis is manifested by the extracellular deposition of an insoluble protein that stains with Congo red. Involvement of the respiratory tract is more commonly seen in the primary form of the disease. Amyloidosis may involve any portion of the respiratory tract in a focal or diffuse fashion. Any level of airway can be involved, but distal tracheal and central bronchial involvement is the most common.

Radiographs and CT demonstrate focal (Fig. 12-13 on page 359) or diffuse (Fig. 12-14 on page 359) narrowing of the trachea and bronchi by the amyloid deposits that protrude into and narrow the lumen. The tracheobronchial walls appear thickened and you may see calcification in some lesions. Typically, amyloid lesions are slowly growing over many years. Associated adenopathy is sometimes present. Focal lesions may enhance with intravenous iodin-ated contrast on CT or with gadolinium on MRI.

Sarcoidosis

Sarcoidosis is a systemic granulomatous disease of unknown cause in which noncaseous epithelioid granulomas are present on biopsy specimens. Airway abnormalities include tracheobronchial mural thickening, which may be smooth, irregular, or nodular; luminal narrowing (Fig. 12-15 on page 360); and airway compression by lymphadenopathy. Tracheobronchial-wall thickening represents the presence of granulomas in the

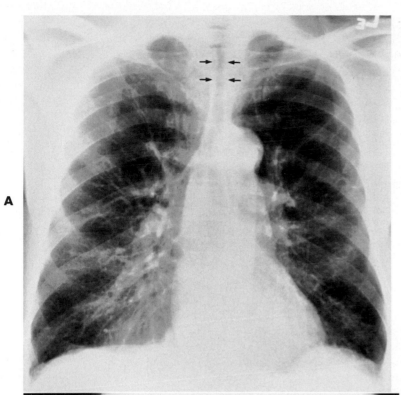

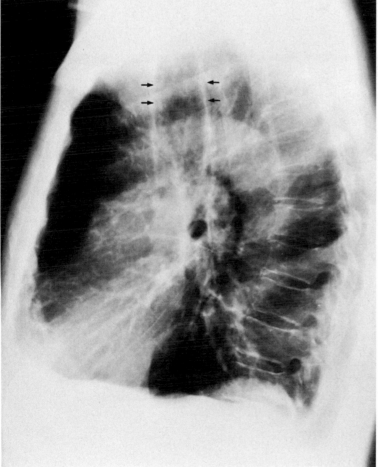

Fig. 12-8   Saber-sheath trachea. Posteroanterior, **A,** and lateral, **B,** view of the chest reveal hyperinflated lungs. The trachea is narrowed in the coronal plane but increased in diameter in the sagittal plane *(arrows)*. Note the point of transition from normal cervical trachea to narrowed intrathoracic trachea at the thoracic inlet.

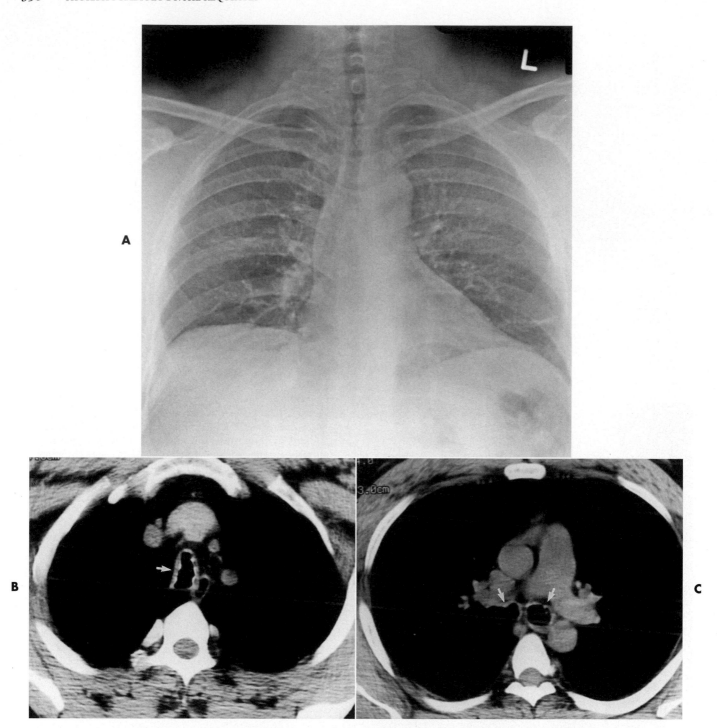

Fig. 12-9   Tracheopathia osteochondroplastica. Posteroanterior radiograph reveals diffuse irregular narrowing of the cervical and thoracic trachea. CT scan through the trachea, **B,** and main bronchi, **C,** demonstrates nodularity of the anterior and lateral cartilaginous walls of the trachea and main bronchi *(arrows)*. Note the smooth, normal-appearing posterior membranous wall.

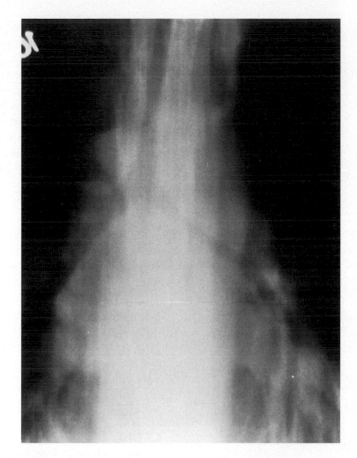

Fig. 12-10   Relapsing polychondritis. An anteroposterior tomogram of the trachea and main bronchi reveals diffuse smooth stenosis of the trachea and bronchi.

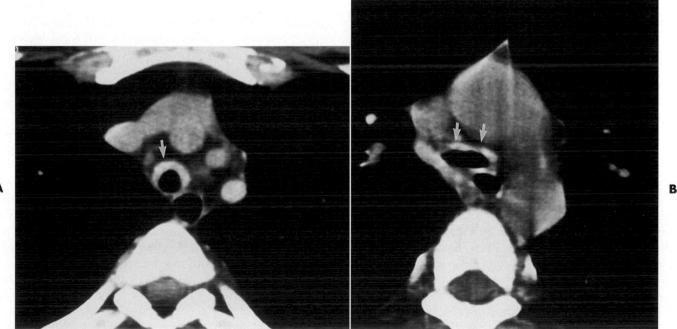

A   B

Fig. 12-11   Relapsing poychondritis. CT at the level of the trachea, **A,** and carina, **B,** demonstrates slight stenosis of the airway lumen in addition to thickening of the wall *(arrows)*.

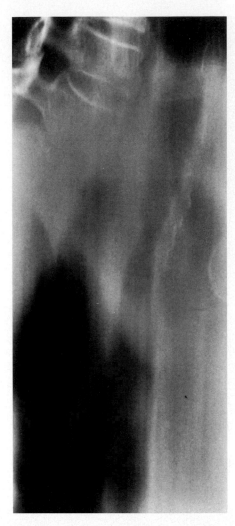

Fig. 12-12 Wegener's granulomatosis. An oblique tomogram of the trachea reveals an hourglass stenosis of the mid trachea, representing changes of Wegener's granulomatosis.

bronchial mucosa and along the peribronchovascular interstitium (Fig. 12-16 on page 360). This accounts for the high diagnostic success of transbronchial biopsy.

Tracheobronchial Papillomatosis

In juvenile laryngeal papillomatosis, multiple squamous papillomas involve the respiratory tree and are usually confined to the larynx. Tracheobronchial papillomatosis results from a multicentric viral infection with the human papilloma virus. The presence of solitary papillomas in some patients and diffuse papillomatosis in others suggests a variable host response to the human papilloma virus. Rarely, papillomas may spread distally to the trachea, bronchi, and lung (Fig. 12-17 on page 361). Distal disease in the absence of laryngeal disease is more common in adults than in children.

Clinically, laryngeal disease presents with hoarseness. Disseminated airway disease presents with wheezing, atelectasis, or recurrent pneumonia. Histologically, papil-

lomas in the airway are polypoid or sessile masses with central fibrovascular cores and layers of well-differentiated squamous epithelium. In the lung, sheets of squamous cells proliferate within alveoli. Central necrosis leads to cavitation. Transformation of the lesions into invasive squamous-cell carcinoma is well known.

Radiographically, diffuse papillomatosis manifests as diffuse nodularity of the involved airway (Fig. 12-18 on page 362). Characteristically, when the lung is involved pulmonary nodules, which may cavitate, are present.

Rhinosclerosis

Rhinosclerosis is a chronic granulomatous disorder of the upper respiratory tract associated with *Klebsiella rhinoscleromatis,* a gram-negative bacterium. This disease primarily affects the nose, paranasal sinuses, and pharynx. It involves the proximal trachea in less than 10% of patients, but it may involve the entire trachea and bronchi in some patients.

Either nodular masses or diffuse symmetric narrowing may develop and slowly progress over a period of 20 years. An initial catarrhal stage is followed by a nodular stage and a healing stage in which dense fibrous tissue and subsequent stenosis develop.

Tuberculous Tracheobronchial Stenosis

Tuberculous tracheobronchial stenosis may be caused by granulomatous changes in the airway wall or by extrinsic compression by peribronchial and paratracheal lymph nodes. The histopathologic changes include a hyperplastic stage in which tubercles form in the submucosal layer and there is ulceration and necrosis of the wall. A fibrostenotic stage follows in which a stenosis is formed. Bronchial involvement may result from contact of the mucosa with infected secretions, especially when parenchymal cavitation is present or may result from the submucosal spread of infection through the lymphatics from infected lymph nodes or lung. There is a high prevalence of lymphadenopathy with tuberculous bronchial lesions; this supports the concept of lymphatic spread of infection.

Radiographically, in the hyperplastic stage, the tracheobronchial walls will be irregularly thickened with variable degrees of luminal narrowing. There will often be associated hilar or mediastinal lymphadenopathy, which may demonstrate some contrast enhancement. Thick irregular cavities may be seen in lobes drained by the affected bronchi (Fig. 12-19 on page 363). In the fibrostenotic stage, the stenotic bronchi may remain thickened but they generally have a smooth appearance with associated luminal stenosis (Fig. 12-20 on page 363). Scarring, calcification, bronchiectasis, and atelectasis are often observed in the lung parenchyma. If the stenosis obstructs, complete collapse of the associated lobe will be present.

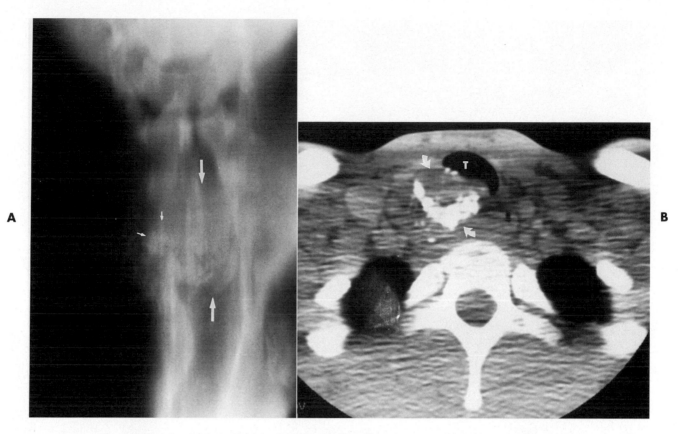

Fig. 12-13   Amyloidosis of the trachea, focal involvement. **A,** An anteroposterior tomogram of the trachea reveals a focal obstructing mass arising in the proximal trachea *(arrows).* The mass contains calcification *(small arrows)* and extends into the right paratracheal region. **B,** CT through the proximal trachea demonstrates pronounced tracheal narrowing *(T)* by a large calcified soft-tissue mass arising from the right posterolateral wall of the trachea *(arrows).* The mass enhanced with gadolinium on an MRI examination (not shown).

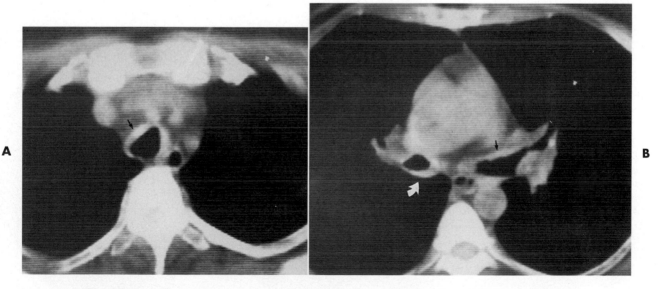

Fig. 12-14   Diffuse tracheobronchial amyloidosis. CT scans of the trachea, **A,** and bronchi, **B,** at the hilar level reveal diffuse thickening of the trachea and bronchi with slight nodularity of the walls *(black arrows).* Note involvement of the posterior wall of the bronchus intermedius *(white arrow).*

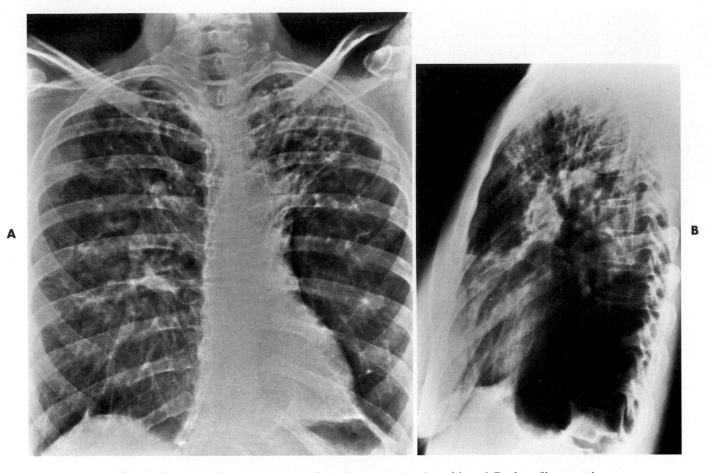

Fig. 12-15   Tracheal stenosis in sarcoidosis. Posteroanterior, **A,** and lateral, **B,** chest films reveal stenosis of the intrathoracic trachea. Note the coarse reticular opacities throughout the lungs, particularly in the upper lung zones. There is distortion of the lung parenchyma with upper lobe volume loss and traction bronchiectasis. The lower lobes are hyperinflated.

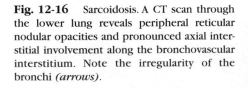

Fig. 12-16   Sarcoidosis. A CT scan through the lower lung reveals peripheral reticular nodular opacities and pronounced axial interstitial involvement along the bronchovascular interstitium. Note the irregularity of the bronchi *(arrows)*.

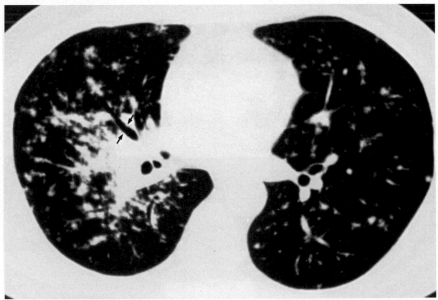

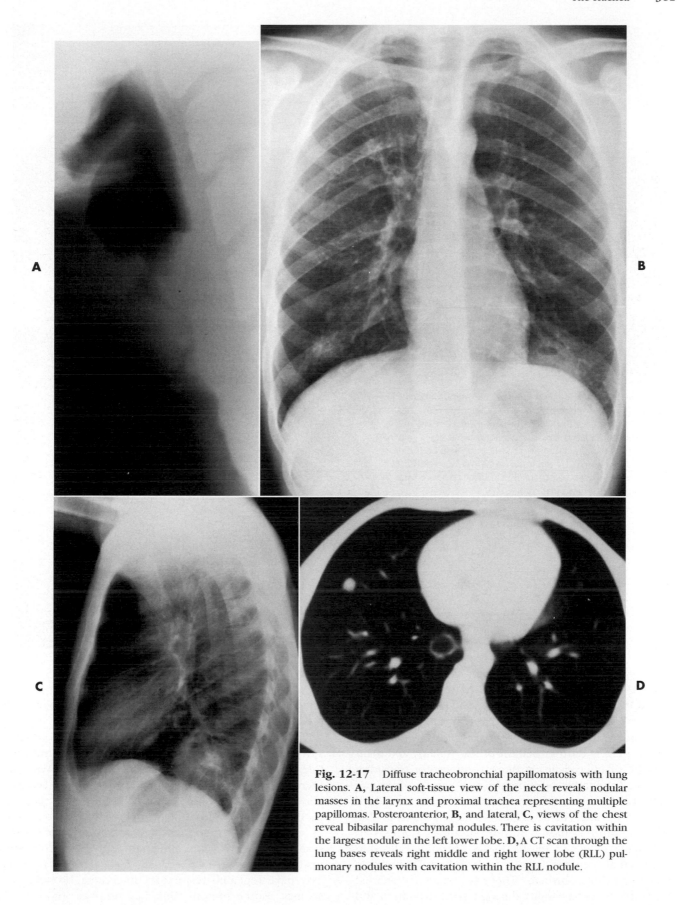

Fig. 12-17   Diffuse tracheobronchial papillomatosis with lung lesions. **A,** Lateral soft-tissue view of the neck reveals nodular masses in the larynx and proximal trachea representing multiple papillomas. Posteroanterior, **B,** and lateral, **C,** views of the chest reveal bibasilar parenchymal nodules. There is cavitation within the largest nodule in the left lower lobe. **D,** A CT scan through the lung bases reveals right middle and right lower lobe (RLL) pulmonary nodules with cavitation within the RLL nodule.

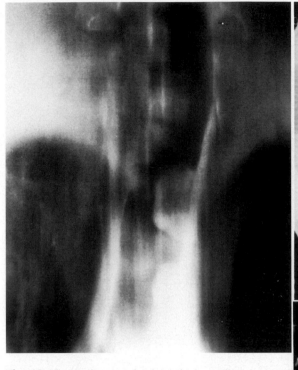

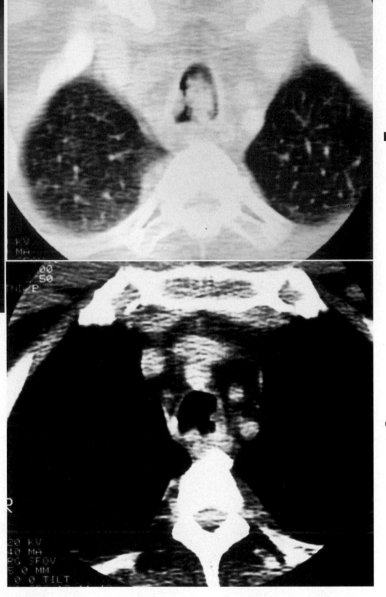

Fig. 12-18 Diffuse tracheobronchial papillomatosis. **A,** Anteroposterior tomogram of the trachea reveals multiple large polypoid and sessile masses within the trachea; the patient has obstructive symptoms. **B,** A scan through the proximal trachea reveals near obstruction of the tracheal lumen by irregular polypoid masses. **C,** A scan through the proximal trachea demonstrates nodular thickening of the tracheal wall.

TRACHEOBRONCHOMEGALY (MOUNIER-KUHN SYNDROME)

Mounier-Kuhn syndrome is a very rare condition in which there is diffuse dilation of the trachea and main bronchi. Characteristically there is an abrupt transition to normal-appearing peripheral airways at the segmental level. The disease occurs primarily in males in their third or fourth decade. The association with cutis laxis in children and Ehlos-Danlos syndrome in adults suggests an underlying defect in elastic tissue. Pathologically, thin atrophied muscular and elastic tissue is found in both the trachea and main bronchi. There is resultant increased flaccidity and collapsibility during forced expiration and cough. Most patients present in early childhood with recurrent respiratory infections.

The diagnosis of tracheobronchomegaly is usually apparent on chest radiographs, which demonstrate diffuse dilation of the trachea and main bronchi. Typically there is protrusion of the mucosa through the trachealis muscle between the cartilaginous rings (Fig. 12-21 on page 364). This finding, which can be detected on conventional tomograms, CT, or MRI, produces by a scalloped or corrugated appearance of the trachea and main bronchi (Fig. 12-22 on page 364). Because patients may have repeated respiratory infections, bronchiectasis may also be present (Box 12-2 on page 365).

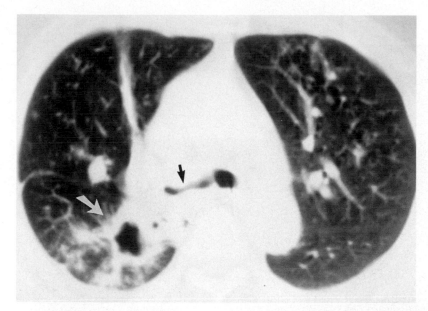

Fig. 12-19 Bronchial stenosis, hyperplastic stage. A CT scan demonstrates irregular stenosis of the right main and right upper lobe bronchus (*black arrow*). There is consolidation and cavitation in the superior segment of the right lower lobe (*white arrow*).

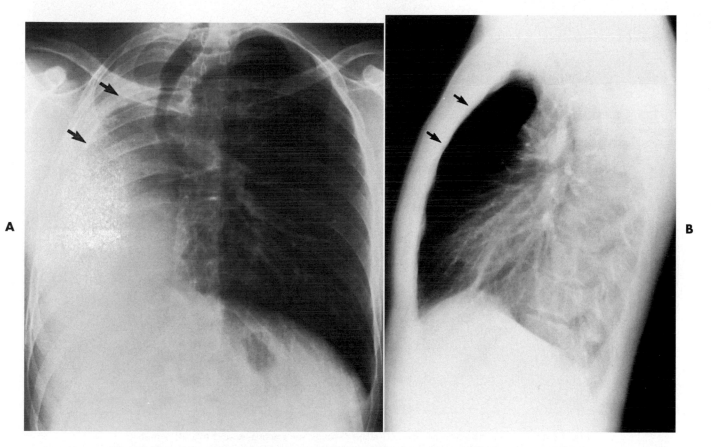

A

B

Fig. 12-20 Tuberculous tracheal stenosis, fibrotic stage. Posteroanterior, **A,** and lateral, **B,** chest radiograph demonstrates a diffuse smooth stenosis of the trachea with resultant collapse of the right lung. There is compensatory hyperinflation of the left lung and shift of the mediastinum to the right. Note the herniated left lung into the right hemithorax and anteriorly in the retrosternal space (*black arrows*).

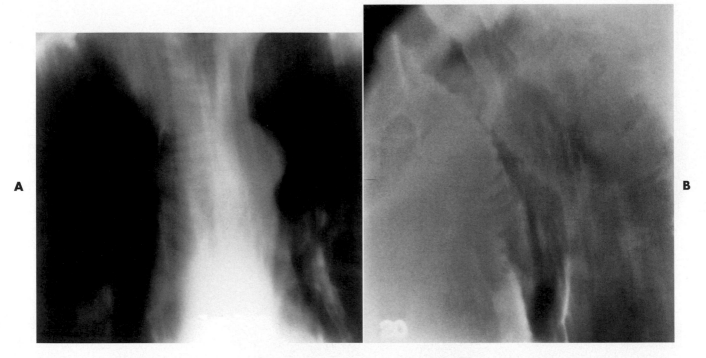

Fig. 12-21   Mounier-Kuhn syndrome. Anteroposterior, **A,** and lateral, **B,** tomograms demonstrate diffuse dilation of the trachea and bronchi. There is a corrugated appearance of the trachea caused by protrusion of mucosa through the trachealis muscle between the cartilaginous rings.

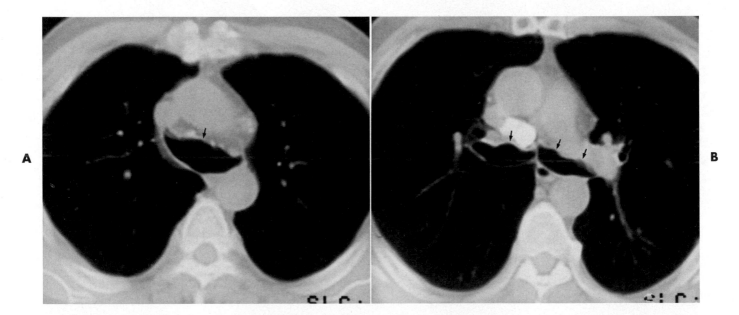

Fig. 12-22   Mounier-Kuhn syndrome. CT scans through the trachea, A, and hila, **B,** demonstrate pronounced dilation of the trachea and main bronchi. There is a scalloped appearance of the airway wall due to protrusion of the mucosa *(arrows)* between cartilaginous rings.

TRACHEAL TUMORS

Primary tracheal tumors are exceedingly rare, approximately one hundred times less common than bronchial tumors. Primary tracheal tumors present with equal fre-

quency in men and women, predominately between 30 and 50 years of age.

The clinical manifestations of tracheal tumors include shortness of breath and wheezing. These symptoms usually do not appear until the lumen has been reduced to one third of its width or less, because the luminal nar-

---

Box 12-2 Radiographic Findings in Mounier-Kuhn Syndrome

Increased flaccidity and collapsibility of trachea and bronchi
Diffuse dilation of trachea and main and lobar bronchi
Protrusion of mucosa between cartilaginous rings
Bronchiectasis

Box 12-3 Tracheal Tumors

MOST COMMON BENIGN TUMORS

Hemangioma
Papilloma
Hamartoma

MOST COMMON MALIGNANT TUMORS

Primary
    Squamous cell carcinoma
    Adenoid cystic carcinoma
Secondary
    Esophageal carcinoma
    Thyroid carcinoma

Box 12-4 Squamous-cell Carcinoma of Trachea

Male smokers over the age of 40
Slow-growing
Exophytic growth
Ulceration
Mediastinal invasion
Synchronous or metachronous tumors of the larynx, lungs, or esophagus

---

Box 12-5 Adenoid Cystic Carcinoma

Not smoking related
Males = females, fifth decade
Slow-growing
Endophytic growth with submucosal spread
Mediastinal extension

---

rowing is a gradual process. Approximately one third of patients with tracheal tumors are initially mistakenly treated for asthmatic bronchitis or bronchial asthma. Patients with a dyspnea that cannot be unequivocally attributed to cardiac or pulmonary disorders should be evaluated to exclude upper airway obstruction.

Tumors of the trachea can be classified as epithelial or mesenchymal lymphomatous. Although 90% of tracheal tumors in children are benign, malignant tumors predominate in adults. The most common benign tracheal tumors include hemangioma, papilloma (see previous section on Tracheobronchial Papillomatosis) and hamartoma (see Chapter 13). The most common primary malignant tracheal tumors are adenoid cystic carcinoma and squamous-cell carcinoma. The most common secondary malignant tumors include esophageal carcinoma and thyroid neoplasms both of which may cause direct tracheal invasion (Box 12-3).

Squamous-Cell Carcinoma

Squamous-cell carcinoma of the trachea accounts for approximately one half of all primary tracheal malignant tumors (Box 12-4). It predominates in male smokers over the age of 40, and it tends to grow slowly and

exophytically and commonly ulcerates. Squamous-cell carcinoma has a tendency to invade the mediastinum. Synchronous and metachronous squamous-cell carcinomas of the larynx, lungs, and esophagus are found in some patients.

Radiographically, the tracheal wall appears focally and circumferentially thickened and irregular. The lumen is secondarily narrowed by the tumor, which may be nodular in appearance. CT is valuable in demonstrating the primary tumor and extension into the adjacent mediastinal fat. Such direct extension will manifest as irregular soft-tissue opacity within the mediastinal fat or surrounding adjacent mediastinal vessels, bronchi, and esophagus. Lymph nodes that measures ≥1 cm in short axis identify mediastinal adenopathy.

Adenoid Cystic Carcinoma

Adenoid cystic carcinoma accounts for approximately one third of all primary tracheal malignant tumors (Box 12-5). Adenoid cystic carcinoma is unrelated to smoking, has no gender predilection, and is usually seen in the fifth decade. This tumor generally grows slowly with endophytic spread extending in the submucosal plane of the trachea and bronchi. Typically, on radiographs the trachea has a thickened and smooth or nodular appearance, with associated luminal narrowing (Fig. 12-23). Adenoid cystic carcinoma may spread into the surrounding tissues of the neck and mediastinum; it is seen on CT as soft-tissue

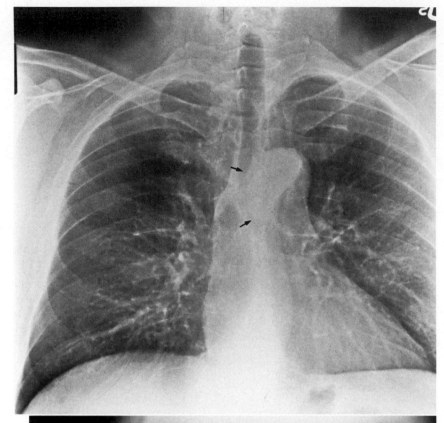

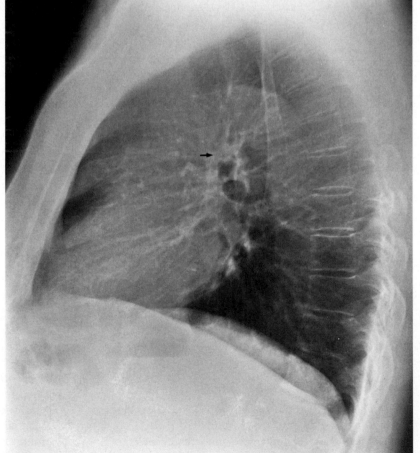

Fig. 12-23   Adenoid cystic carcinoma of the trachea and left main bronchus. Posteroanterior, **A,** and lateral, **B,** radiographs reveal a mass in the distal trachea and proximal left main bronchus *(arrows)*.

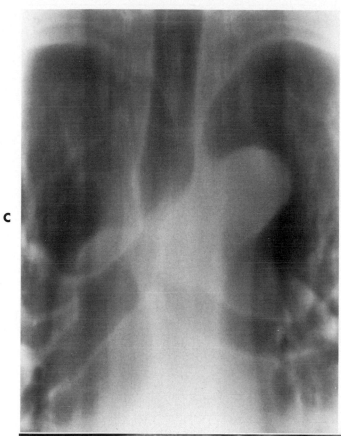

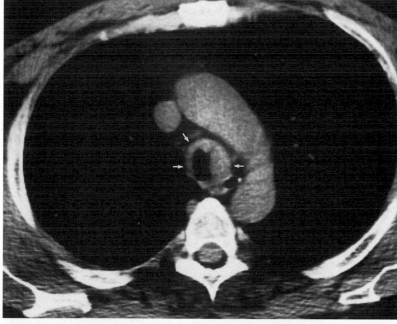

Fig. 12-23, cont'd.   C, An anteroposterior tomogram depicts more clearly the extent of the tumor, which is very smooth and well defined. **D,** A CT image reveals extensive submucosal extent of the tumor circumferentially within the trachea *(arrows)*.

extension into the adjacent mediastinal fat. Cervical and mediastinal lymph nodes are the first to be involved by metastases. Distant hematogenous metastases to lungs, liver, and bone do occur. When the tumor is localized, surgical resection and reconstruction is potentially curative. Adenoid cystic carcinoma is radiosensitive. Radiation therapy is indicated for nonresectable tumor. In such cases, the tumor will recur typically several years later.

Benign Tracheal Tumors

Radiographically, benign tracheal tumors generally present as a focal, well-defined, smooth or lobulated mass without evidence for contiguous tracheal or mediastinal invasion (Box 12-6) (Fig. 12-24). Benign lesions such as hamartomas and lipomas will contain fat density. Hamartomas and chondromas may demonstrate calcifi-

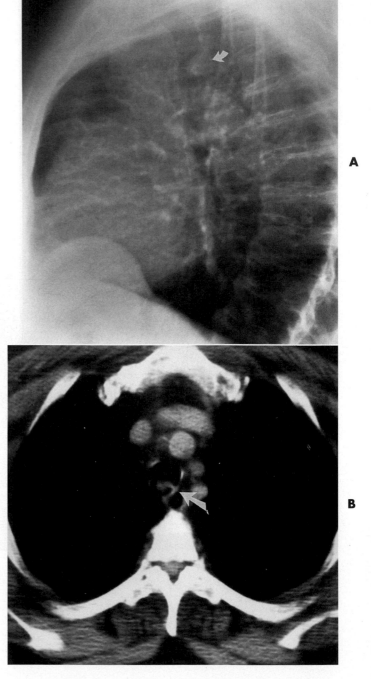

A

B

Fig. 12-24 Solitary benign papilloma of trachea. **A,** Lateral chest radiograph reveals a focal well-defined nodular mass *(arrow)* arising from the posterior wall of the trachea. The mass was not apparent on the PA view. **B,** CT scan through the upper trachea reveals a nodular mass arising from the tracheal wall on a pedicle *(arrow)*. There is no evidence for mediastinal invasion.

cation within the chondroid elements. In contrast, invasive malignant tracheal tumors may demonstrate contiguous circumferential tracheal-wall thickening with direct invasion of adjacent mediastinal fat planes and lymphadenopathy. While more advanced tumors may be readily apparent on chest radiographs as an intraluminal mass or a stenosis, early tracheal tumors are often initially missed on chest films. Chest CT is ideal for identifying both the endoluminal and mediastinal extent of tracheal neoplasms.

TRACHEOBRONCHOMALACIA

Tracheobronchomalacia refers to a weakness in the tracheal or bronchial walls and supporting cartilages with resultant collapsibility. The flaccidity of the trachea

or bronchi is usually most apparent during coughing or forced expiration. Primary malacia is associated with a congenital deficiency of the cartilage. Acquired malacia is found secondary to intubation, COPD, trauma, infection, and relapsing polychondritis. Focal areas of malacia can develop as a result of large goiters or mediastinal masses, aneurysms, or aberrant pulmonary vessels that compress the trachea or bronchus (Box 12-7).

The increased flaccidity of the airways results in an inefficient cough mechanism, retained mucus, infection, and bronchiectasis. Fluoroscopy (Fig. 12-25), cine CT, or

---

Box 12-6   Benign Tracheal Tumors

Focal mass
Smooth and well-defined margins
No mediastinal invasion

Box 12-7   Causes of Tracheobronchomalacia

PRIMARY

Congenital deficiency of cartilage

ACQUIRED

Intubation
Chronic obstructive pulmonary disease
Trauma
Infection
Relapsing polychondritis
Adjacent compression by mediastinal mass or vessel

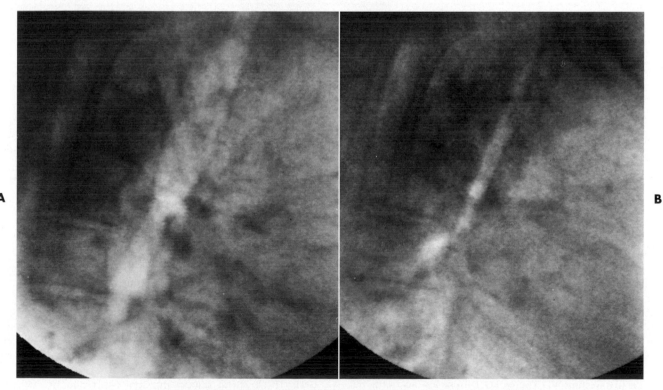

Fig. 12-25   Tracheobronchomalacia, fluoroscopy. Lateral views of the trachea during fluoroscopy on inspiration, **A,** and expiration, **B,** reveal collapse of the trachea on forced expiration.

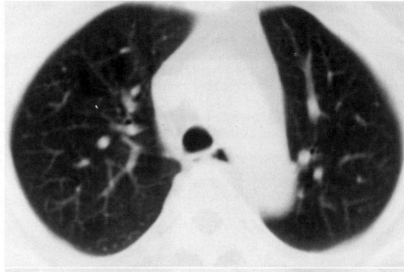

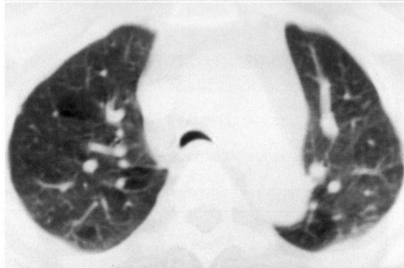

Fig. 12-26 Tracheobronchomalacia, inspiratory–expiratory chest CT. **A,** CT scans through the tracheal lumen on inspiration. On expiration, **B,** at the same table level, there is abnormal collapse of the tracheal wall with pronounced decrease in the tracheal lumen. Note the increased attenuation of the lung parenchyma on expiration compared with inspiration.

inspiration/expiration CT (Fig. 12-26) are the preferred imaging modalities for evaluation. The normal tracheobronchial lumen will decrease approximately 10% to 30% with expiration or coughing. A decrease of more than 50% of the lumen should be considered abnormal.

SUGGESTED READINGS

Case Records of the Massachusetts General Hospital: Case 1-1995, *N Engl J Med* 332(2):110-115, 1995.

Case Records of the Massachusetts General Hospital: Case 3-1992, *N Engl J Med* 326(3):184-191, 1992.

Case Records of the Massachusetts General Hospital: Case 46-1992, *N Engl J Med* 327(21):1512-1518, 1992.

Choe KO, Jeong HJ, Sohn HY: Tuberculous bronchial stenosis: CT findings in 28 cases, *AJR* 155:971-976, 1990.

Choplin RH, Wehunt WD, Theros EG: Diffuse lesions of the trachea, *Semin Roentgenol* 18(1):38-50, 1983.

Cordier JF, Loire R, Breene J: Amyloidosis of the lower respiratory tract, *Chest* 90(6):827-831, 1986.

Davis SD, Berkmen YM, King T: Peripheral bronchial involvement in relapsing polychondritis: demonstration by thin-section CT, *AJR* 153:953-954, 1989.

Di Benedetto RJ, Ribaudo C: Bronchopulmonary sarcoidosis, *Am Rev Respir Dis* 94:952-958, 1966.

Dolan DL, Lemmon GD, Teitelbaum SL: Relapsing polychondritis, *Am J Med* 41:285-299, 1966.

Dunne MG, Reiner B: CT features of tracheobronchomegaly, *J Comput Assist Tomogr* 12(3):388-391, 1988.

Feldman F, Seaman WB, Baker DC: The roentgen manifestations of scleroma, *AJR* 101:807-813, 1967.

Ferretti GR, Vining DJ, Knoplioch J et al: Tracheobronchial tree: three-dimensional spiral CT with bronchoscopic perspective, *J Comput Assist Tomogr* 20:777, 1996.

Fraser RG, Paré JAP, Paré PD, Fraser RS, Genereux GP editors: *Diagnosis of diseases of the chest*, vol 3, Philadelphia, 1990, WB Saunders.

Grillo HC: Tracheal tumors. In Choi NC, Grillo HC, editors: *Thoracic oncology*, New York, 1983, Lippincott-Raven.

Handousa P, Elivi AM: Some clinicopathological observations on scleroma. *J Laryngol Otol* 72:32-47, 1958.

Im J-G, Chung JW, Han SK, Han MC, Kim C-W: CT manifestations of tracheobronchial involvement in relapsing polychondritis, *J Comput Assist Tomogr* 12(5):792-793, 1988.

Jokinen K, Palva T, Nuutinen J: Bronchial findings in pulmonary tuberculosis, *Clin Otolaryngol* 2:139-148, 1977.

Katz M, Konen E, Rosenman J et al: Spiral CT and 3D image reconstruction of vascular rings and associated tracheobronchial anomalies, *J Comput Assist Tomogr* 19:564, 1995.

Katz I, LeVine M, Herman P: Tracheobroncheomegaly: the Mounier-Kuhn syndrome, *Am J Roentgenol Radium Ther Nucl Med* 88:1084-1094, 1962.

Kauczor H-U, Wolcke B, Fischer B et al: Three-dimensional helical CT of the tracheobronchial tree: evaluation of imaging protocols and assessment of suspected stenoses with bronchoscopic correlation, *AJR* 167:419, 1996.

Kwong JS, Müller NL, Miller RR: Diseases of the trachea and mainstem bronchi: correlation of CT with pathologic findings, *Radiographics* 12:645-657, 1992.

Lenique F, Brauner MW, Grenier P, Battesti JP, Loiseau A, Valeyre D: CT assessment of bronchi in sarcoidosis: endoscopic and pathologic correlations, *Radiology* 194:419-423, 1995.

McAdam LP, O'Hanlan MA, Bluestone R, Pearson CM: Relapsing polychondritis: prospective study of 23 patients and a review of the literature, *Medicine* 55:193-215, 1976.

Mendelson DS, Norton K, Cohen BA, Brown LK, Rabinowitz JG: Bronchial compression: an unusual manifestation of sarcoidosis, *J Comput Assist Tomogr* 7(5):892-894, 1983.

Mendelson DS, Som PM, Crane R, Cohen BA, Spiera H: Relapsing polychondritis studied by computed tomography, *Radiology* 157:489-490, 1985.

Miller RH, Shulman JB, Canalis RF et al: *Klebsiella rhinoscleromatis:* a clinical and pathogenic enigma, *Otolaryngol Head Neck Surg* 87:212-221, 1979.

Mounier-Khun P: Dilatation de la trachee: constellations radiographiques et bronchosopiques, *Lyon Med* 150:106-109, 1932.

Newmark GM, Conces DJ Jr, Kopecky KK: Spiral CT evaluation of the trachea and bronchi, *J Comput Assist Tomogr* 18:552, 1994.

Onitsuka H, Hirose N, Watanake K: Computed tomography of tracheopathia osteoplastica, *AJR* 140:268, 1983.

Poe RH, Utell MJ, Israel RH, Hall WJ, Eshleman JD: Sensitivity and specificity of the nonspecific transbronchial lung biopsy, *Am Rev Respir Dis* 119:25-31. 1979.

Quint LE, Whyte RI, Kazerooni EA Martinex FJ, Cascade PN, Lynch JP, Orringer-MB, Brunsting LA, Deeb GM: Stenosis of the central airways: evaluation by using helical CT with multiplanar reconstructions, *Radiology* 194:871-877, 1995.

Salkin D, Cadden AV, Edson RC: The natural history of tuberculous tracheobronchitis, *Am Rev Respir Dis* 47:351-369, 1943.

Sharma OP: Airway obstruction in sarcoidosis, *Chest* 73:6-7, 1978.

Shepard JO, Grillo HC, Bhalla M, Kuzo RS, McLoud TC: Inspiratory-expiratory chest CT in evaluation of large airway disease. Presented at the Radiological Society of North America Meeting, Chicago, Ill, *Radiology* 193(P):181, 1994.

Shin MS, Jackson RM, Ho K-J: Tracheobronchomegaly (Mounier-Kuhn Syndrome): CT diagnosis, *AJR* 150:777-779, 1988.

Spizarny DL, Shepard JO, McLoud TC, Grillo HC, Dedrick CG: CT of adenoid cystic carcinoma of the trachea, *AJR* 146:1129-1132, 1986.

Stern MG, Gamsu G, Webb WR, Stulbarg MS: Computed tomography of diffuse tracheal stenosis in Wegener granulomatosis, *J Comput Assist Tomogr* 10(5):868-870, 1986.

Unger JM, Schuchman GG, Grossman JE, Pellett JR: Tears of the trachea and main bronchi caused by blunt trauma: radiologic findings, *AJR* 153:1175-1180, 1989.

Urban BA, Fishman EK, Goldman SM, Scott WW, Jones B, Humphrey RL, Hruban RH: CT evaluation of amyloidosis: spectrum of disease, *Radiographics* 13:1295-1308, 1993.

Whyte RI, Quint LE, Kazerooni EA et al: Helical computed tomography for the evaluation of tracheal stenosis (abstract), *Radiology* 197:883, 1995.

Zeiberg AS, Silverman PM, Sessions RB et al: Helical (spiral) CT of the upper aiwway with three-dimensional imaging: technique and clinical assessment, *AJR* 166:293, 1996.

CHAPTER 13

The Bronchi

JO-ANNE O. SHEPARD

ANATOMY AND TERMINOLOGY

Air passes from the nasal and oral cavities to the gas exchange zone of the lung through the *conducting* or tracheobronchial airways, in which no gas exchange takes place. In humans, there is a *transitional zone* between the terminal bronchiole, the last purely conducting airway, and the gas-exchange region in which cells characteristic of conducting airways and gas-exchange area intermix. The *pulmonary acinus* represents the entire gas-exchange area distal to the terminal bronchiole.

The *trachea* divides into two primary or *main bronchi,* which give rise to the *lobar bronchi,* which branch further to become the *intrapulmonary bronchi.* The small branches of these bronchi are called *bronchioles.* They do not contain cartilage. The most distal bronchioles are the *terminal bronchioles,* which occur at the beginning of the alveolar gas-exchange area of the lung, and the *respiratory bronchioles,* which compose the transitional zone between the terminal bronchiole and the alveolar ducts. The *alveolar ducts* end in the *alveolar sacs.* An *alveolus* is a terminal air space whose wall is called an *interalveolar septa* and is comprised of gas-exchange tissue.

The *secondary pulmonary lobule* is the smallest portion of the lung that is surrounded by connective tissue septa. It contains 3 to 5 acini, is polyhedral in shape, and measures 10 to 25 mm in diameter. It is most visible in the subpleural portion of the lung on CT. A lobular bronchiole and a pulmonary artery branch are found in the center of the lobule. Pulmonary veins and lymphatics are found in the interlobular septa. The limit of CT visibility for a small bronchus or artery is 2 mm. Lobular bronchioles are beyond the limit of CT visibility because they measure less than 1 mm in diameter and their walls are less than 0.1 mm thick. Lobular bronchioles branch into 3 or more terminal bronchioles. Each terminal bronchiole supplies one acinus. An acinus consists of lung distal to one terminal bronchiole, 2 to 5 generations of respiratory bronchioles, alveolar ducts, alveolar sacs, and alveoli.

CT TECHNIQUE

The CT technique for evaluation of the central bronchi should include contiguous 5-mm scans through the hilar regions. All of the normal lobar and segmental bronchi should be identified routinely by this technique. Occasionally, evaluation of small and obliquely oriented bronchi such as the lingular bronchus may necessitate scanning with thinner sections or angling the gantry in the plane of the bronchus. High-resolution CT (HRCT) is the preferred technique for the evaluation of bronchiectasis and proliferative bronchiolitis. Paired inspiratory and expiratory scans performed at identical table levels are used to evaluate bronchomalacia and the presence of air trapping in patients with small-airways disease such as obliterative bronchiolitis. Measurement of attenuation values in endobronchial lesions is useful in identifying fat in hamartomas and calcification in hamartomas, chondromas, carcinoid tumors, and broncholiths.

ENDOBRONCHIAL LESIONS

Broncholithiasis

Broncholithiasis is a condition in which calcified material is present within a bronchus or adjacent cavity. Broncholiths arise from calcified peribronchial lymph nodes, the majority of which are due to *Histoplasma capsulatum*. However, other fungal infections, tuberculosis, sarcoidosis, or silicosis may predispose to broncholithiasis.

Radiographically, the key finding of a broncholith is a calcified endobronchial lesion or peribronchial lymph node, which may be associated with findings of bronchial obstruction (Box 13-1; Fig. 13-1).

Foreign Body

The majority of aspirated foreign bodies occur in children under the age of 10. Aspirated foreign bodies in adults are often seen in patients with altered mental status or poor dentition. Foreign bodies are most often aspirated into the lower-lobe bronchi. Aspirations into the right side are more common because of the more direct continuation of the right main bronchus with the trachea.

Air trapping is the most common finding following an acute aspiration of a foreign body with subsequent bronchial obstruction. The presence of air trapping may not be apparent, on inspiration films, but will be apparent on expiration chest films or expiratory CT scans and decubitus chest films. On expiration, the normal lung will become more opaque. Similarly, on decubitus films, the dependent lung will be hypoinflated and therefore more opaque. If air trapping is present, the obstructed lobe or lung will remain lucent and not decrease in volume on expiration or when in a dependent position, and the mediastinum will shift away from the side of air trapping (Figure 13-2). Hypoxic vasoconstriction may develop within an obstructed lobe or lung; this is manifested radiographically as hyperlucency of the lung and attenuation of the pulmonary vessels (Fig. 13-3 on page 377). In chronic obstruction, findings of atelectasis, pneumonia, or bronchiectasis may develop (Box 13-2). CT is very useful in identifying the endobronchial site of an aspirated foreign body. The presence of calcification in the foreign body may be a sign of an aspirated bone (Fig. 13-4 on page 378). MRI may be helpful in identifying aspirated peanuts, which characteristically have a high signal on T1-weighted images.

Bronchial Neoplasms

Hamartoma

Hamartomas are one of the most common benign tumors of the lung, representing 77% in a series by Arrigoni. Approximately 3% of these tumors arise within the bronchi. Bronchial hamartomas are generally slow-growing tumors within large bronchi. They contain elements of cartilage, fat, fibrous tissue, and epithelial components. The appearance of fat on CT will suggest the diagnosis. Calcification is present in approximately 25% of hamartomas (Box 13-3).

Text continued on p. 380

Box 13-2 Findings of Bronchial Obstruction

Air trapping
Hypoxic vasoconstriction with oligemia
Atelectasis
Pneumonia
Bronchiectasis

Box 13-1 Findings of Broncholithiasis

A calcified lymph node in a peribronchial location or that has eroded into a bronchus
Secondary findings of obstruction
No associated soft-tissue mass

Box 13-3 Bronchial Hamartomas

Slow-growing
Majority in lung periphery; minority found within large bronchi
CT identification of fat aids diagnosis
Calcification seen in 25%

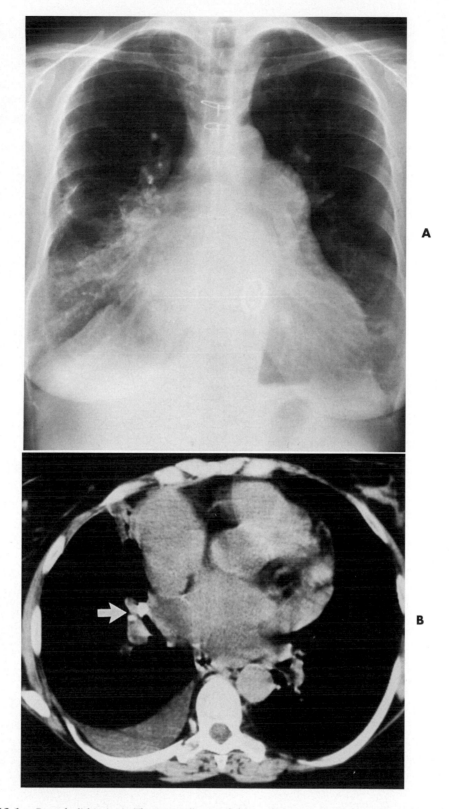

Fig. 13-1   Broncholithiasis. **A,** There is collapse of the medial segment of the right middle lobe and associated elevation of the right hemidiaphragm. **B,** A calcified broncholith *(arrow)* obstructs the right middle lobe bronchus.

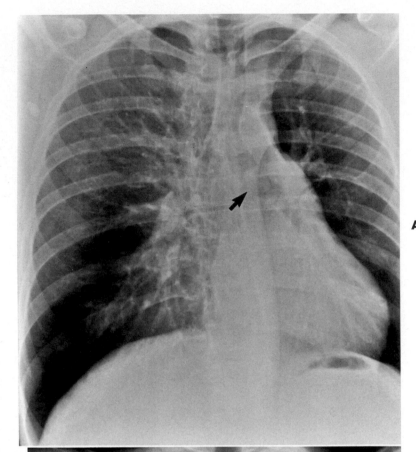

A

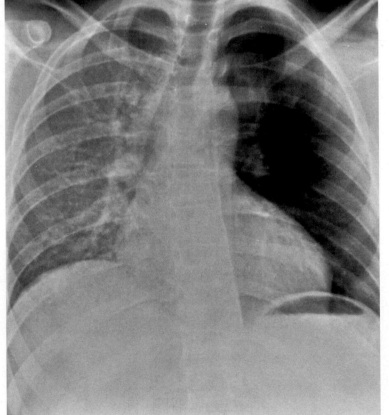

B

Fig. 13-2 Air trapping. Left main bronchus carcinoid. **A,** *Inspiratory* chest radiograph reveals an oval filling defect obstructing the left main bronchus *(arrow).* There is hyperlucency of the left lung and attenuation of the left pulmonary vasculature due to hypoxic vasoconstriction. There is slight volume loss in the left lung with shift of the mediastinum to the left. **B,** *Expiratory* chest radiograph demonstrates a normal decrease in right lung volume with elevation of the right diaphragm and shift of the mediastinum to the right, and crowding of right pulmonary vessels. There is hyperlucency and diffuse air trapping in the left lung without change in lung volume.

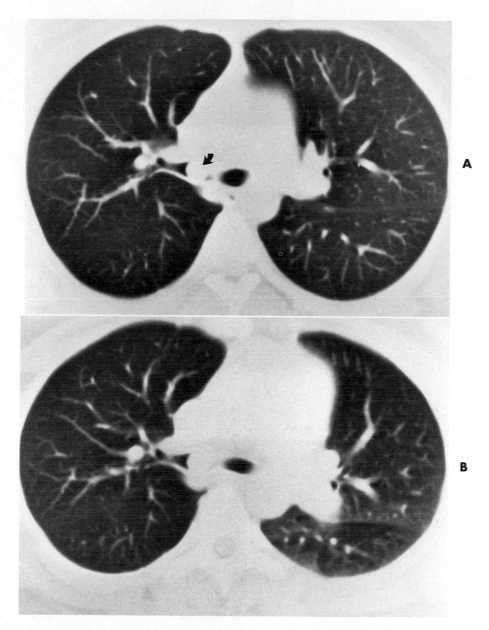

Fig. 13-3   Air trapping. Carcinoid tumor. **A,** *Inspiratory* CT demonstrates an obstructing carcinoid tumor in the right upper lobe bronchus *(arrow).* The right lung is more lucent than the left lung due to vascular attenuation from hypoxic vasoconstriction. **B,** *Expiratory* CT demonstrates normal decrease in the left lung volume and increased attenuation of the left lung. The right lung remains inflated and lucent.

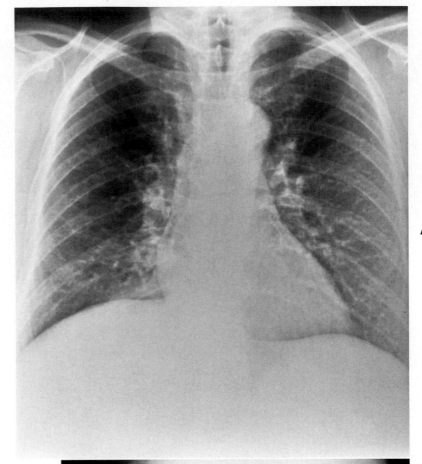

A

Fig. 13-4 Segmental obstruction due to aspirated turkey bone. **A & B,** A segmental pneumonia is present in the posterobasal segment of the right lower lobe.

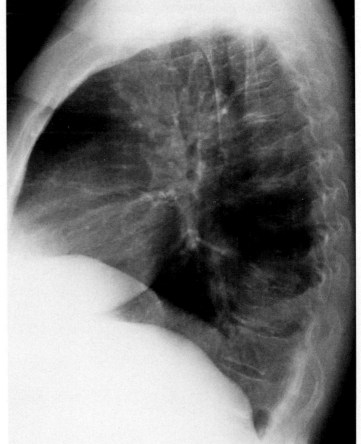

B

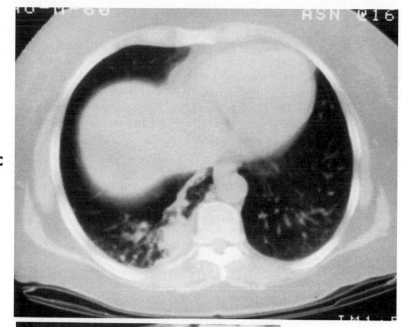

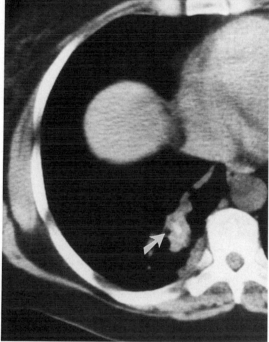

Fig. 13-4   Segmental obstruction due to aspirated turkey bone. **C,** CT demonstrates a focal consolidation in the posterobasal segment of the right lower lobe. **D,** A calcified foreign body is noted within the posterobasal segmental bronchus consistent with an aspirated turkey bone *(arrow).*

Carcinoid tumors

Carcinoid tumors are classified as neuroendocrine tumors of the lung. Typical carcinoid tumors represent the lowest grade subtype of a spectrum of neoplasms that include the more aggressive atypical carcinoid tumor and the extremely malignant small-cell carcinoma. The Kulchitsky cell is the cell of origin of these neuroendocrine tumors. It contains neurosecretory granules and is capable of producing seratonin, adrenocorticotropic hormone, and bradykinin.

The clinical differences between typical carcinoid, atypical carcinoid, and small-cell carcinoma lie in the prevalence of metastases and in the prognosis for each (Box 13-4). *Typical carcinoids* present in patients at an earlier age, usually 40 to 50 years. They are usually, smooth, round, well-defined masses that arise in the central bronchi (Fig. 13-5). Ten percent of carcinoids will present in the periphery of the lung (Fig. 13-6). *Atypical carcinoids* present in patients between 50 to 60 years of age. They tend to be larger than typical carcinoids at diagnosis, may be central or peripheral in location, and have a tendency to metastasize to hilar or mediastinal lymph nodes (Fig. 13-7). *Small-cell carcinoma* presents in older patients between 60 and 70 years of age. They are extremely malignant tumors that are most often associated with bulky hilar and mediastinal adenopathy. Small peripheral nodules representing the primary tumor are often found on CT. They metastasize commonly and have a strong association with smoking.

There are several distinguishing features of carcinoid tumors on imaging studies (Box 13-5). In addition to slow growth, carcinoids may demonstrate calcification (Fig. 13-5). Because they are highly vascular tumors, they will demonstrate marked contrast enhancement with iodinated contrast at CT (Fig. 13-6) and with gadolinium at MRI. Somatostatin receptors have been identified in a wide variety of human tumors with neuroendocrine characteristics including carcinoid tumors. ^{123}I-Tyr$_3$-octreotide and ^{111}In-octreotide are radionuclide-coupled somatostatin analogs that can be used to visualize somatostatin-receptor–bearing tumors (Fig. 13-8). Known tumor sites have been visualized in 86% of patients in whom histologically proven carcinoids were present. Endobronchial carcinoids often present as a nodule within a central bronchus and may be associated with distal pneumonia, atelectasis, and/or bronchiectasis.

Mucoepidermoid tumors

Mucoepidermoid tumors are uncommon, representing 0.2% of all lung tumors and 1% to 5% of bronchial tumors. The mean patient age at presentation is 36 years. There is no sex predilection, and smoking is not a risk factor. Mucoepidermoid tumors of the central airways may be of high- or low-grade malignancy, which is predictive of ultimate prognosis. The radiographic findings are usually of a focal endobronchial mass within a large central airway (Fig. 13-9 see page 384).

FIBROSING MEDIASTINITIS

Fibrosing mediastinitis, a rare disorder of the mediastinum, is a complication of a granulomatous mediastinitis resulting from infection due to *Histoplasma capsulatum* or *Mycobacterium tuberculosis*. It has also been associated with the use of methysergide. The inflammatory process is characterized by an exuberant proliferation of fibrous tissue in the mediastinum in which mediastinal structures are surrounded, invaded, or obliterated. Complications of the fibrosis may include tracheobronchial stenosis in addition to superior vena caval obstruction, esophageal obstruction, pulmonary artery occlusion, and obstruction of the pulmonary veins and thoracic duct.

Box 13-4   Spectrum of Neuroendocrine Tumors of Lung

TYPICAL CARCINOID

40–50 years of age
Round, smooth, well-defined nodule
90% in central bronchi, 10% in lung periphery
No tendency to metastasize

ATYPICAL CARCINOID

50–60 years of age
Larger nodule than typical carcinoid
Central or peripheral
Tendency to metastasize to hilar and mediastinal nodes

SMALL-CELL CARCINOMA

60–70 years of age
Small peripheral lung nodule often seen on CT
Bulky hilar and mediastinal adenopathy
Extrathoracic metastases common

Box 13-5   Imaging Features of Typical Carcinoid Tumors

Slow-growing
Calcification
Marked contrast enhancement
Octreotide uptake
Nodule or mass within a central bronchus associated with atelectasis, pneumonia, or bronchiectasis
10% present as a peripheral solitary pulmonary nodule

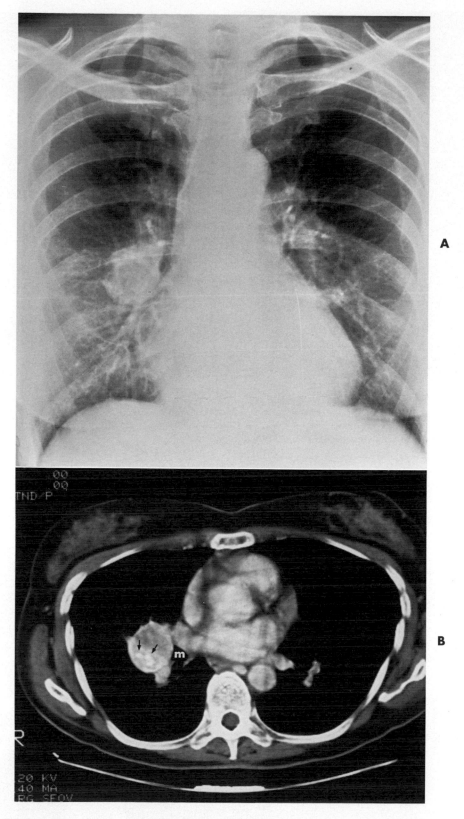

Fig. 13-5   Right middle lobe typical carcinoid tumor. **A,** A round well-defined right hilar mass is noted. **B,** On a contrast-enhanced CT, a well-defined mass is noted in the right hilum obstructing the right middle lobe bronchus (*m*). The tumor demonstrates heterogeneous enhancement and calcification *(arrows)*.

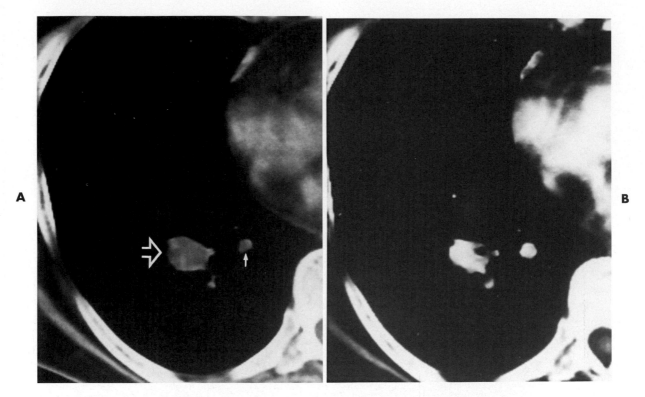

Fig. 13-6 Peripheral carcinoid tumor with contrast enhancement. **A,** A nonenhanced CT scan at the right lung base demonstrates a well-defined soft-tissue nodule *(open arrow)* lateral to a small lower lobe pulmonary artery *(small arrow).* **B,** Following contrast enhancement, there is dense uniform enhancement of the carcinoid tumor.

Fig. 13-7 Atypical carcinoid tumor. A contrast-enhanced CT scan demonstrates an irregular peripheral mass *(M)* in the right upper lobe abutting the pleura. There is a partially enhancing metastatic right hilar lymph node mass *(N).*

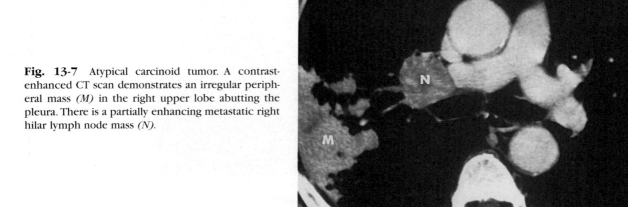

Patients with fibrosing mediastinitis most often have cough, dyspnea, and/or hemoptysis. The most common radiographic finding is widening of the mediastinum (Box 13-6). Calcification or calcified nodes may be identified within the mediastinal fibrosis, particularly on CT (Fig. 13-10). The mediastinal fibrosis will typically encase and narrow affected mediastinal and hilar structures including the bronchi. Contrast-enhanced CT or MRI is necessary to assess vascular patency of the superior vena cava or pulmonary artery.

If tracheobronchial obstruction is localized, surgical resection and reconstruction may be curative. However, in most cases, the obstruction is diffuse, and there is no effective treatment.

ESOPHAGOTRACHEOBRONCHIAL FISTULAS

Esophagotracheobronchial fistulas may be congenital or acquired (Box 13-7). Congenital esophagotracheobronchial fistulas are discussed elsewhere in Chapter 2. The majority of acquired fistulas result from tumors of the esophagus, tracheobronchial tree, thyroid, and mediastinal nodes. Of the nonmalignant esophagotracheobronchial fistulas, infection and trauma are the chief causes. Those caused by infection are the result of erosion of calcareous particles from peribronchial lymph nodes in which the infectious process is no longer active. Histoplasmosis may be responsible for many of these cases. Other infectious causes of esophagotracheobronchial fistula include tuberculosis, actinomycosis, and syphilis.

Box 13-6   Radiographic Features of Fibrosing Mediastinitis

Widened mediastinum
Calcification within mediastinal fibrosis and nodes
Encasement and narrowing of hilar and mediastinal
  structures

Box 13-7   Esophagotracheobronchial Fistula

CONGENITAL

ACQUIRED
Malignant Tumors

Esophageal
Tracheobronchial
Thyroid
Lymph node

Infectious Causes

Histoplasmosis (most common)
Tuberculosis
Actinomycosis
Syphilis

Traumatic Injury

Penetrating
Long-standing endotracheal and nasogastric tubes

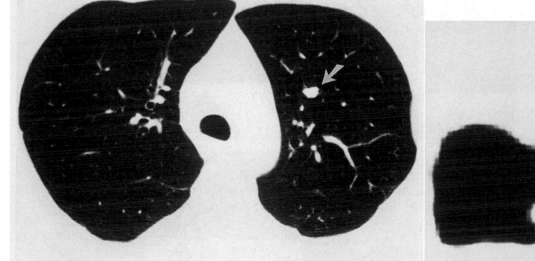
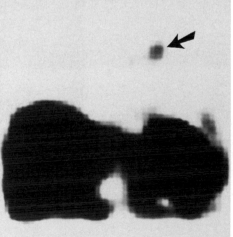

Fig. 13-8   Octreotide uptake within a carcinoid tumor. **A,** CT demonstrates a 6-mm left upper lobe nodule (*arrow*) **B,** Octreotide uptake is noted within the carcinoid tumor in the left upper lobe (*arrow*).

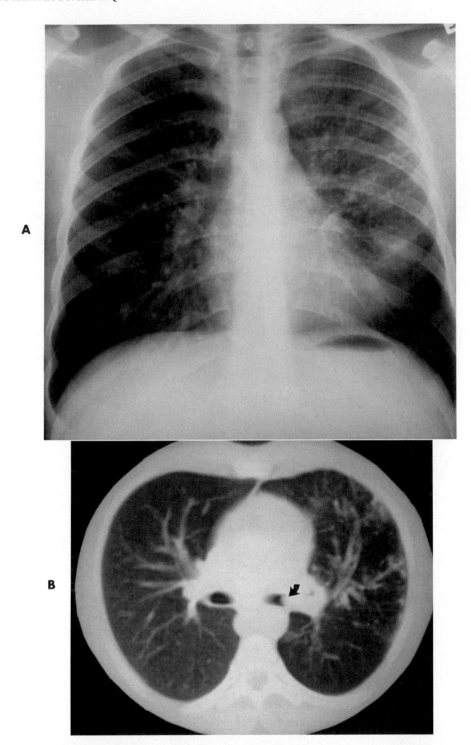

Fig. 13-9   Mucoepidermoid tumor. **A,** A chest radiograph demonstrates left upper lobe pneumonia partially obliterating the left heart border. **B,** A CT scan scan demonstrates a nodular lesion obstructing the left upper lobe bronchus *(arrow).* Some peripheral obstructive pneumonitis is present in the left upper lobe.

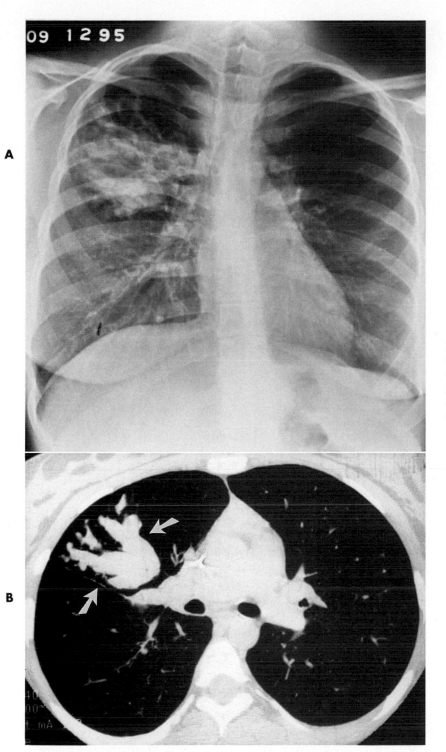

Fig. 13-19 Mucoid impaction. **A,** Large mass in the right upper lobe with nodular margins. **B,** CT demonstrates a branching tubular opacity in the posterior segment of right upper lobe with a "finger-in-glove" appearance representing a large mucoid impaction *(arrows).*

Whereas the lungs of infants with CF will appear normal on pathologic examination, older patients will demonstrate a multitude of findings including mucus plugging, pneumonia, abscess formation, obliterative bronchiolitis, bronchiectasis, focal atelectasis, and air trapping distal to obstructed segmental bronchi and pneumothorax (Fig. 13-20). Upper-lobe involvement predominates. Hilar and mediastinal adenopathy is often present.

Radiographically, the classic signs of bronchiectasis will be manifest as previously discussed (Box 13-11). Bronchiectasis involves all lobes in cystic fibrosis but is usually most severe in the upper lobes. The lungs are generally hyperinflated. Radiographic findings relating to obstruc-

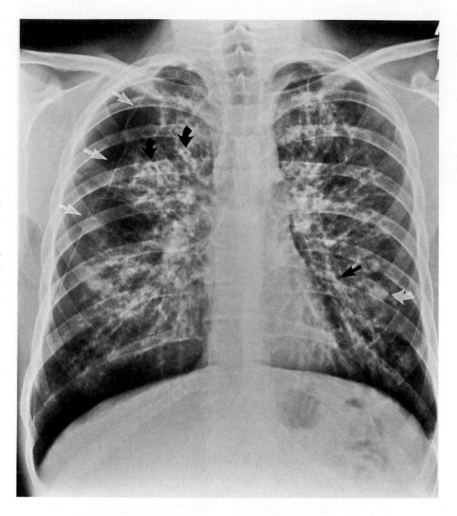

Fig. 13-20 Cystic fibrosis. The lungs are hyperinflated. Diffuse bronchiectasis is present, relatively sparing the lung bases. "Ring shadows" (*curved black arrows*) and "tram tracks" (*straight black arrow*) are present. Nodular opacities representing focal areas of mucoid impaction are noted (*curved white arrow*). A moderately large right-sided pneumothorax is present (*white arrows*).

tion of small- to medium-sized airways will be found including air trapping, atelectasis, and mucous plugging.

Clincially, patients will present with signs and symptoms of recurrent pulmonary infections. Hemoptysis and pneumothorax may occur. In the later stages of the disease, respiratory insufficiency and cor pulmonale develop. For many patients with CF, lung transplantation has been a life-saving procedure.

Dyskinetic Cilia Syndrome

Bronchiectasis is also a finding in dyskinetic cilia syndrome (DCS), a disorder characterized by abnormal ciliary structure and function. A subset of DCS is Kartagener's syndrome, which features situs inversus, sinusitis, and bronchiectasis (Fig. 13-21). In DCS there is an autosomal recessive pattern of inheritance, but there is considerable genetic heterogeneity and a discordance in phenotypic presentation. Diagnostic criteria include rhinitis and bronchial infections starting in early childhood, and one or more of the following findings: (1) situs inversus or dextrocardia in the patient or a sibling; (2) liv-

ing but immotile spermatazoa of abnormal appearance; (3) absent or nearly absent tracheobronchial clearance; and (4) nasal or bronchial biopsy demonstrating cilial ultrastructural defects.

Radiographic findings include bronchial wall-thickening, bronchiectasis, hyperinflation, and focal areas of consolidation and atelectasis. The findings are less severe than those seen in CF.

Allergic Bronchopulmonary Aspergillosis

Patients with allergic bronchopulmonary aspergillosis (ABPA) may demonstrate bronchiectasis. In ABPA, the aspergillus fungus is present in the airways and is responsible for (1) the presence of precipitating antibodies, (2) immediate and often delayed skin sensitivity, (3) the production of IgE, and (4) bronchial-wall and blood eosinophilia. The segmental and proximal subsegmental bronchi become dilated and filled with mucus that contains abundant eosinophils and fragmental fungal hyphae. Typically, radiographs and CT scans will show branching tubular opacities that emanate

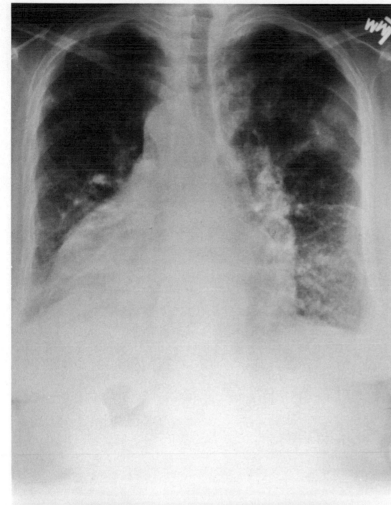

A

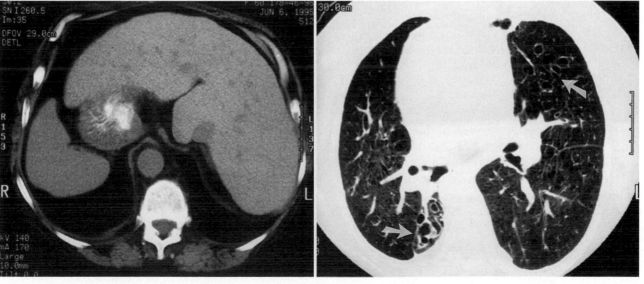

B   C

Fig. 13-21 Kartagener's syndrome. **A,** PA chest radiograph reveals complete situs inversus. The aortic arch and cardiac apex are on the right and the stomach bubble is in the right upper quadrant. Irregular parenchymal opacities noted bilaterally represent bronchiectasis. An incidental left upper lobe carcinoma is present. **B,** The spleen and stomach are in the right upper quadrant; the liver is left-sided. **C,** Cystic bronchiectasis is present bilaterally (*arrows*).

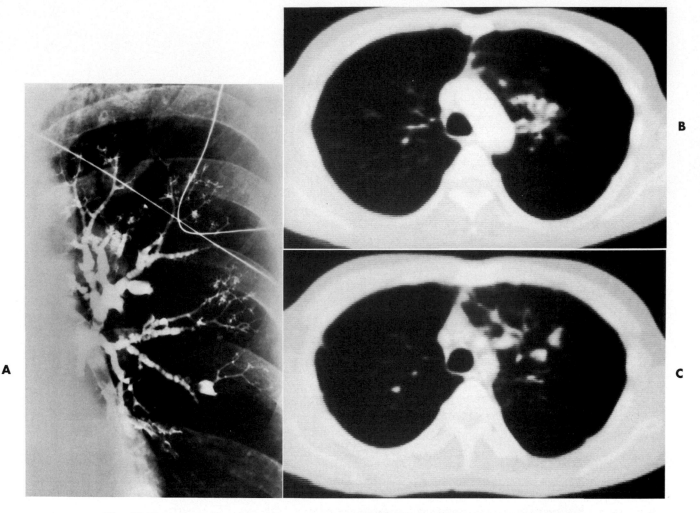

Fig. 13-22   Allergic bronchopulmonary aspergillosis (ABPA) in an asthmatic patient. **A,** AP view of the left lung on a bronchogram reveals central varicose bronchiectasis. **B & C,** CT scans demonstrate branching tubular opacities emanating from the left hilum in the distribution of left upper-lobe segmental and subsegmental bronchi representing mucoid impaction within central bronchiectasis.

from the hilum in the distribution of the segmental and central subsegmental bronchi, in the typical "finger-in-glove" appearance (Fig. 13-22). The mucous plugs may stay unchanged for weeks, or they may clear by expectoration, leaving central air-filled bronchiectasis (Fig. 13-16). Patients with asthma and CF are susceptible to ABPA.

Other Causes

There are other rare causes of bronchiectasis including *Young's syndrome* or obstructive azoospermia manifested by infertility and sinopulmonary infection. *Yellow nail syndrome* consists of a characteristic triad of yellow nails, lymphedema, and pleural effusion. In *familial dysautonomia,* an autosomal recessive trait seen exclu-

sively in those of Jewish descent, there is malfunction of the autonomic nervous system with consequent hypersecretion of the mucous glands and obstruction of the bronchi. Clinically, patients have recurrent pneumonias. Radiographic findings resemble those of CF.

DISEASES OF THE BRONCHIOLES

Plain-Film Findings

The bronchioles are not visible on standard chest radiographs. As a result, the plain radiographic findings of bronchiolar disease usually depend on indirect signs of airway obstruction, including hyperinflation and air trapping. The radiograph, however, is usually normal. When small airway disease extends into the interstitium,

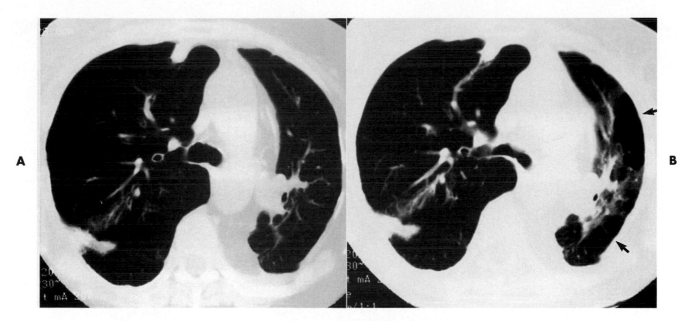

Fig. 13-23   Air trapping in obliterative bronchiolitis representing chronic rejection in a lung transplant recipient. **A,** *Inspiratory* CT scan in a patient with emphysema and a reduction pneumoplasty of the right lung, status post left lung transplantation. The left lung is of uniform lucency on inspiration. The right lung is hyperinflated due to emphysema. **B,** *Expiratory* CT scan reveals air trapping throughout the emphysematous right lung. Focal areas of lucency (*arrows*) representing air trapping in the transplanted left lung correspond to regions of bronchiolitis obliterans. The areas of increased attenuation in the left lung represent normal hypoinflated lung. Note the normal degree of collapse of the central bronchi on the expiratory scan.

such as in respiratory bronchiolitis or into the air space such as in bronchiolitis obliterans organizing pneumonia (BOOP), opacities may become radiographically apparent.

In bronchiolitis, dynamic signs of air trapping can be demonstrated at fluoroscopy, on standard chest radiographs, or on CT scans obtained at full inspiration and maximum expiration. Generalized air trapping can be manifest by a decrease in diaphragmatic excursion. Normally the diaphragmatic excursion is 3 to 4 cm, but when air trapping is present, it may be decreased to 1 to 2 cm. On expiratory films or CT scans, normal lung will deflate with an expected decrease in lung volume and an increase in the attenuation of the deflated lung. In an area of air trapping, the abnormal lung will remain lucent on expiration, and the volume of that portion of the lung will remain constant. The caliber of vessels within the region of air trapping may be attenuated as a result of hypoxic vasoconstriction.

When unilateral air trapping is present, contiguous structures such as the mediastinum will shift toward the contralateral side on expiration, and the diaphragm will remain depressed on the side of air trapping. When a patient cannot cooperate fully for inspiration and expiration films, bilateral decubitus films may demonstrate similar findings. Normal lung will deflate in the decubitus

position. If air trapping is present, the abnormal lung will remain hyperinflated and lucent in the decubitus position. Findings of hyperinflation and air trapping are often subtle on plain chest radiographs.

CT Findings

CT and particularly HRCT are much more sensitive examinations for bronchiolitis. Proper CT technique is important in imaging bronchiolitis. For HRCT, use 1- to 1.5-mm collimation, 10-mm intervals, and reconstruction with an edge-enhancing algorithm (i.e., bone). Use a window level of −700 HU and window width of 1000 to 1500 HU. Expiratory scanning facilitates assessment of air trapping. You should obtain at least six paired inspiratory and expiratory HRCT images performed at identical levels. During expiratory scanning, normal lung will demonstrate homogeneous increase in attenuation, whereas air trapping will have relatively decreased attenuation (Fig. 13-23).

The major disease entities in which bronchiolitis is found include acute infectious bronchiolitis; chronic inflammatory conditions of the bronchioles such as asthma, chronic bronchitis, and bronchiectasis; diffuse panbronchiolitis; respiratory bronchiolitis; bronchiolitis obliterans organizing pneumonia (BOOP); and obliterative or

Box 13-14 Disease Entities in Which Bronchiolitis is Found

PROLIFERATIVE BRONCHIOLITIS
Acute Infectious Bronchiolitis

Chronic Inflammatory Conditions of Bronchi

Asthma
Chronic bronchitis
Bronchiectasis

Diffuse Panbronchiolitis

Respiratory Bronchiolitis

Bronchiolitis Obliterans Organizing Pneumonia

OBLITERATIVE (CONSTRICTIVE) BRONCHIOLITIS

Toxic fumes
Postviral infections
Collagen vascular disease (rheumatoid arthritis)
Drugs (penacillamine)
Bone-marrow and lung transplants

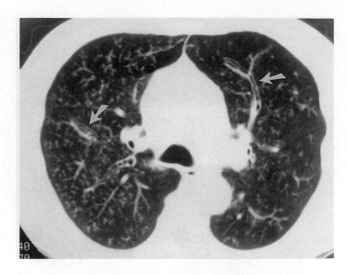

Fig. 13-24 Viral pneumonia. Small branching linear opacities and nodular opacities throughout the right lung in a "tree-in-bud" appearance. Cylindrical bronchiectasis is present in both upper lobes (*arrows*).

Box 13-15 Major CT Patterns of Bronchiolitis

NODULES AND BRANCHING LINEAR OPACITIES

Infectious bronchiolitis
Chronic bronchial diseases
Diffuse panbronchiolitis

GROUND-GLASS ATTENUATION AND CONSOLIDATION

Respiratory bronchiolitis
Bronchiolitis obliterans organizing pneumonia

MOSAIC PATTERN

Obliterative (constrictive) bronchiolitis

constrictive bronchiolitis (Box 13-14). The three major CT patterns of bronchiolitis include (1) nodules and branching linear opacities, (2) ground-glass attenuation and consolidation, and (3) mosaic pattern. (Box 13-15).

Proliferative bronchiolitis

Nodules and branching linear opacities

Nodules and branching linear opacities, also referred to as "tree-in-bud" appearance, are due to inflammatory cells in the walls of the small airways and inflammatory exudate and mucus in the lumina (Fig. 13-24). These findings are most often seen with *acute infectious bronchiolitis* from respiratory syncytial virus, adenovirus, or *mycoplasma* pneumonia. This form of acute proliferative bronchiolitis may lead to obliterative or constrictive

bronchiolitis (see below). Centrilobular nodular and linear opacities may also be seen in chronic inflammatory conditions of the bronchioles secondary to *primary bronchial diseases* such as asthma, chronic bronchitis, and bronchiectasis.

Nodular and linear opacities occur in *diffuse panbronchiolitis,* a disease of unknown origin. It is prevalent in Asians, particularly in Japanese men, and it is very rare in North America. Patients generally present with a chronic productive cough and progressive dyspnea. Histologically there is inflammation of the respiratory bronchioles with mononuclear cells and foamy macrophages found in bronchiolar lumina and alveoli. CT features include centrilobular nodules, branching linear opacities, bronchiolectasis, bronchiectasis, and air trapping. Although there may be a favorable initial response to treatment with erythromycin, the long-term prognosis is poor with progression of bronchiectasis.

Ground-glass attenuation and consolidation

Bronchiolar diseases presenting with CT findings of ground-glass attenuation and consolidation include respiratory bronchiolitis and BOOP. *Respiratory bronchiolitis,* otherwise known as smokers' bronchiolitis or smoker's lung, is a common incidental histologic finding in smokers, typically those 30 to 40 years of age. Patients are usually asymptomatic, but they may complain of cough or shortness of breath. The respiratory bronchioles are mainly involved. Histologically, mild chronic inflammation of the bronchioles is associated with pigmented macrophages in respiratory bronchioles and adjacent alveoli. CT demonstrates either ground-glass attenuation, or centrilobular micronod-

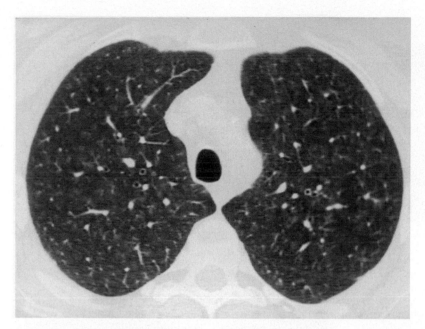

Fig. 13-25   Respiratory bronchiolitis. CT scan through the upper lobes reveals diffuse bilateral small ground-glass nodular opacities in a peribronchiolar distribution.

Table 13-1   Causes of Mosaic Pattern

	Vessel Size	Inspiration/ Expiration CT
Small airway disease	↓ Size and number in lucent lung	Air trapping
Vascular disease	↓ Size and number in lucent lung	No air trapping
Diffuse infiltrative disease producing patchy ground-glass attenuation	Similar size and number through-out lung	No air trapping

---

ules in the upper lung zones or in a diffuse distribution (Fig. 13-25).

Mosaic pattern

Low attenuation and mosaic pattern on CT are seen with obliterative bronchiolitis otherwise known as constrictive bronchiolitis. *Obliterative bronchiolitis* is characterized histologically by concentric narrowing of the bronchioles by submucosal and peribronchiolar fibrosis causing air-flow obstruction. Diseases associated with obliterative bronchiolitis include childhood viral infections; toxic-fume inhalation; rheumatoid arthritis; bone marrow transplantation secondary to a chronic graft versus host reaction; chronic rejection following lung transplantation and inflammatory bowel disease (Box 13-16). The radiographic features of obliterative bronchiolitis include variable degrees of hyperinflation, peripheral attenuation of vessels, and nodular or reticular nodular

pattern. However, the radiograph is usually normal. The most common CT finding is air trapping, which is accentuated on expiratory scans. A mosaic pattern of perfusion occurs as a result of hypoxic vasoconstriction in areas of bronchiolar obstruction resulting in redistribution of blood flow to normal areas of the lung. You can differentiate the mosaic pattern of air-trapping from that due to vascular disease or diffuse infiltrative lung disease by expiratory CT scanning. When air trapping is present, the affected lung will remain lucent. The pulmonary vessels are decreased in size in the low attenuation areas when air trapping and vascular disease are present, but they are normal in caliber with diffuse infiltrative lung disease. Diffuse infiltrative lung disease may produce patchy areas of ground-glass attenuation and therefore a mosaic pattern. These areas are abnormal, whereas the ground-glass areas in vascular disease and bronchiolitis represent normally perfused lung (Table 13-1). Bronchiectasis is

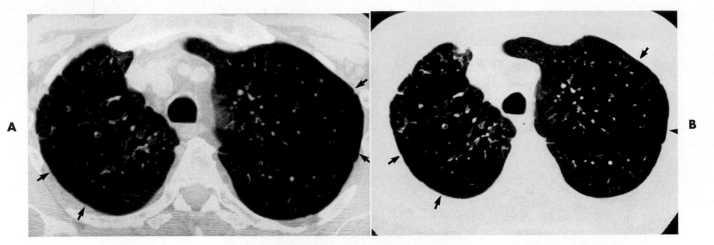

Fig. 13-26   Postinfectious obliterative bronchiolitis, Swyer-James syndrome. **A,** *Inspiratory* CT of upper lung zones reveals a right lung that is small in volume. There is bilateral bronchiectasis and areas of hyperlucency in the periphery of the upper lobes in which there is attenuation of vessels, most pronounced in the right lung (*arrows*). **B,** An *expiratory* CT scan demonstrates persistent lucency in areas of vascular attenuation, consistent with air trapping (*arrows*). The normal lung has increased in attenuation.

often associated with obliterative bronchiolitis. Rarely, bronchiolar wall-thickening and centrilobular branching are seen.

The *Swyer-James syndrome* is a variant of postinfectious obliterative bronchiolitis. It is related to an acute viral bronchiolitis in infancy or early childhood that prevents the normal development of the affected lung. It is manifested by a unilateral hyperlucent lung or lobe on standard films with normal or reduced volume during inspiration and air trapping on expiration. Typically the ipsilateral hilum is small because of decreased blood flow on the affected side. On CT the areas of bronchiolitis are usually not limited to a single lobe or lung, and patchy areas of air trapping can be observed bilaterally (Fig. 13-26).

SUGGESTED READINGS

Ahn JM, Im J-G, Seo JW, Han JW, Han HS, Yoon HK, Kim WS, Yoon KM: Endobronchial hamartoma: CT findings in three patients, *AJR* 163:49-50, 1994.

Akira M, Higashihara T, Sakatani M, Hara H: Diffuse panbronchiolitis: followup CT examination, *Radiology* 189:559-562, 1993.

Akira M, Kitatani F, Yong-Sikl, Kita N, Yamamoto S, Higashihara T, Morimoto S, Ikezoe J, Koguka T: Diffuse panbronchiolitis: evaluation with high-resolution CT, *Radiology* 168:433-438, 1988.

Arrigoni MG, Bernatz PE, Donoghue FE: Broncholithiasis, *J Thorac Cardiovasc Surg* 62:231-237, 1971.

Arrigoni MG, Woolner LB, Bernatz PE, Miller WE, Fontana RS, Minn R: Benign tumors of the lung: a ten-year surgical experience, *J Thorac Cardiovasc Surg* 60:589-599, 1970.

Burke CM, Theodore J, Dawking KD et al: Post-transplant obliterative bronchiolitis and other later sequelae in human heart-lung transplantation, *Chest* 86:824-825, 1989.

Choplin RH, Kowamoto EH, Dyer RB, Geisinger KR, Mills SE, Pope TL: Atypical carcinoid of the lung: radiographic features, *AJR* 146:665-668, 1986.

Conces DJ, Tarver RD, Vix VA: Broncholithiasis: CT features in 15 patients, *AJR* 157:249-253, 1991.

Dixon GF, Donnerberg RL, Schonfeld, Whitcomb ME: Advances in the diagnosis and treatment of broncholithiasis, *Am Rev Respir Dis* 129:1028-1030, 1984.

Douek PC, Simoni L, Revel D, Cordier JF, Amiel M: Diagnosis of bronchial carcinoid tumor by ultrafast contrast-enhanced MR imaging, *AJR* 163:563-564, 1994.

Eber CD, Stark P, Bertozzi P: Bronchiolitis obliterans on high-resolution CT, *J Comput Assist Tomogr* 17(6):853-856, 1993.

Epler GR, Colby TV: The spectrum of bronchiolitis obliterans, *Chest* 83:161-162, 1983.

Epler GR, Colby TV, McLoud TC, Carrington CB, Gaensler EA: Bronchiolitis obliterans organizing pneumonia, *N Engl J Med* 312:152-158, 1985.

Ferretti GR, Vining DJ, Knoplioch J, et al: Tracheobronchial tree: three-dimensional spiral CT with bronchoscopic perspective, *J Comput Assist Tomogr* 20:777, 1996.

Garg K, Lynch DA, Newell JD, King TE: Proliferative and constrictive bronchiolitis: classification and radiologic features, *AJR* 162:803-808, 1994.

Glazer HS, Anderson DJ, Sagel SS: Bronchial impaction in lobar collapse: CT demonstration and pathologic correlation, *AJR* 153:485, 1989.

Grenier P, Maurice F, Musset D, Menu Y, Nahum H: Bronchiectasis: assessment by thin section CT, *Radiology* 161:95-99, 1986.

Grote TH, Macon WR, Davis B, Greco FA, Johnson DH: Atypical carcinoid of the lung: a distinct clinicopathologic entity, *Chest* 93(2):370-375, 1988.

Gruden JF, Webb WR: CT findings in a proved case of respiratory bronchiolitis, *AJR* 161:44-46, 1993.

Hansell DM, Wells AU, Rubens MB, Cole PJ: Bronchiectasis: functional significance of areas of decreased attenuation at expiratory CT, *Radiology* 193:369-374, 1994.

Heitmiller RF, Mathisen DJ, Ferry JA, Mark EJ, Grillo HC: Mucoepidermoid lung tumors, *Ann Thorac Surg* 47:394-399, 1989.

Katz M, Konen E, Rosenman J, et al: Spiral CT and 3D image reconstruction of vascular rings and associated tracheobronchial anomalies, *J Comput Assist Tomogr* 19:564, 1995.

Kauczor H-U, Wolcke B, Fischer B, et al: Three-dimensional helical CT of the tracheobronchial tree: evaluation of imaging protocols and assessment of suspected stenoses with bronchoscopic correlation, *AJR* 167:419, 1996.

Lentz D, Bergin CJ, Berry GJ, Stoehr C, Theodore J: Diagnosis of bronchiolitis obliterans in heart-lung transplantation patients: importance of bronchial dilatation on CT, *AJR* 159:463-467, 1992.

Loubeyre P, Revel D, Delignette A, Wiesendanger Philit F, Bertocchi M, Loire R, Mornex J-F: Bronchiectasis detected with thin-section CT as a predictor of chronic lung allograft rejection, *Radiology* 194:213-216, 1995;.

Lynch DA, Newell JD, Tschomper BA, Ank TM, Newman LS, Bethel R: Uncomplicated asthma in adults: comparison of CT appearance of the lungs in asthmatic and healthy subjects, *Radiology* 188:829-833, 1993.

MacLeod EM: Abnormal transradiancy of one lung, *Thorax* 9:147-153, 1954.

Marti-Bonati L, Perales RF, Catala F, Mata J, Calonge E: CT findings in Swyer-James syndrome, *Radiology* 172:477-480, 1989.

Marti-Bonmati L, Catala FJ, Ruiz PF: Computed tomography differentiation between cystic bronchiectasis and bullae, *J Thorac Imaging* 7:83-85, 1991.

Martin KW, Sagel SS, Siegel BA: Mosaic oligemia simulating pulmonary infiltrates on CT, *AJR* 147:670-673, 1986.

McGuinness G, Naidich DP, Garay S, Leitman BS, McCauley DI: AIDS associated bronchiectasis: CT features, *J Comput Assist Tomogr* 17(2):260-266, 1993.

McLoud TC, Epler GR, Colby TV, Gaensler EA, Carrington CB: Bronchiolitis obliterans, *Radiology* 159:1-8, 1986.

Mendelsohn SL, Fagelman D, Zwanger-Mendelsohn S: Endobronchial lipoma demonstrated by CT, *Radiology* 148:790, 1983.

Moore ADA, Godwin JD, Dietrich PA, Verschakelen JA, Henderson WR: Swyer-James syndrome: CT findings in eight patients, *AJR* 158:1211-1215, 1992.

Morrish WF, Herman SJ, Weisbrod GL, Chamberlain DW: Bronchiolitis obliterans after lung transplantation: findings at chest radiography and high resolution CT, *Radiology* 179:487-490, 1991.

Müller NL, Miller RR: Neuroendocrine carcinomas of the lung, *Semin Roentgenol* 25(1):96-104, 1990.

Müller NL, Bergin CJ, Ostrow DN, Nichols DM: Role of computed tomography in the recognition of bronchiectasis, *AJR* 143:971-976, 1984.

Müller NL, Miller RR: Diseases of the bronchioles: CT and histopathologic findings, *Radiology* 196:3, 1995.

Müller NL, Staples CA, Miller RR: Bronchiolitis obliterans organizing pneumonia: CT features in 14 patients, *AJR* 154:983-987, 1990.

Müller NL, Thurlbeck WM: Thin-section CT, emphysema, air trapping, and airway obstruction, *Radiology* 199:621, 1996.

Naidich DP, McCauley DI, Khouri NF, Stitik FP, Siegelman SS: Computed tomography of bronchiectasis, *J Comput Assist Tomogr* 6(3):437-444, 1982.

Newmark GM, Conces DJ Jr, Kopecky KK: Spiral CT evaluation of the trachea and bronchi, *J Comput Assist Tomogr* 18:552, 1994.

O'Uchi T, Tokumaru A, Mikami I, Yamasoba T, Kikuchi S: Value of MR imaging in detecting a peanut causing bronchial obstruction, *AJR* 159:481-482, 1992.

Phillips MS, Williams MP, Flower CDR: How useful is computed tomography in the diagnosis and assessment of bronchiectasis, *Clin Radiol* 321-325, 1986.

Pugatch RD, Gale ME: Obscure pulmonary masses: bronchial impaction revealed by CT, *AJR* 141:909, 1983.

Reid LM: Reduction in bronchial subdivision in bronchiectasis, *Thorax* 5:233-247, 1950.

Remy-Jardin M, Remy J, Boulenguez C, Sobaszek A, Edme J-L, Furon D: Morphologic effects of cigarette smoking on airways and pulmonary parenchyma in healthy adult volunteers: CT evaluation and correlation with pulmonary function tests, *Radiology* 186:107-115, 1993.

Remy-Jardin M, Remy J: Comparison of vertical and oblique CT in evaluation of bronchial tree, *J Comput Assist Tomogr* 12(6):956-962, 1988.

Sakai F, Sone S, Kujono K et al: MR of pulmonary hamartoma: pathologic correlation, *J Thorac Imaging* 9:51-55, 1994.

Schmidt HW, Clagett OT, McDonald JR: Broncholithiasis, *J Thorac Cardiovasc Surg* 62:226-245, 1950.

Shin MS, Berland LL, Myers JL, Clary G, Zorn GL: CT demonstration of an ossifying bronchial carcinoid simulating broncholithiasis, *AJR* 153:51-52, 1989.

Silverman PM, Godwin JD: CT/bronchographic correlations in bronchiectasis, *J Comput Assist Tomgr* 11(1):52-56, 1987.

Skeens JL, Fuhrman CR, Yousem SA: Bronchiolitis obliterans in heart-lung transplantation patients: radiologic findings in 11 patients, *AJR* 153:253-256, 1989.

Stern EJ, Frank MS: Small-airway diseases of the lungs: findings at expiratory CT, *AJR* 163:37-41, 1994.

Sugiyama Y, Tukeuchi K, Yotsumoto H, Takaku F, Maeda H: A case of panbronchiolitis in a second generation Korean male, *Jpn J Thorac Dis* 24:183-187, 1986.

Swyer PR, James GCW: A case of unilateral pulmonary emphysema, *Thorax* 8:133-136, 1953.

Tarver RD, Conces DJ, Godwin JD: Motion artifacts on CT simulate bronchiectasis, *AJR* 151:1117-1119, 1988.

Watanabe Y, Nishiyama Y, Kanayama H, Enomoto K, Kato K, Takeichi M: Congenital bronchiectasis due to cartilage deficiency: CT demonstration, *J Comput Assist Tomogr* 11(4):701-703, 1987.

Weissberg D, Swartz I: Foreign bodies in the tracheobronchial tree, *Chest* 91(5):730-733, 1987.

Westcott JL, Cole SR: Traction bronchiectasis in end-stage pulmonary fibrosis, *Radiology* 161:665-669, 1986.

Yousem SA, Burke CM, Billingham ME: Pathological pulmonary alterations in long-term human heart-lung transplantation, *Human Pathol* 16:911-925, 1985.

Yousem SA, Hochholzer L: Mucoepidermoid tumors of the lung, *Cancer* 60:1346, 1987.

Zwiebel BR, Austin JH, Grimes MM: Bronchial carcinoid tumors: assessment with CT of location and intratumoral calcification in 31 patients, *Radiology* 179:483-486, 1991.

The radiologic appearance of the pulmonary vessels is dependent on both anatomic and physiologic parameters. In previous chapters, we have reviewed the normal pulmonary vascular anatomy on radiographs and on computed tomography (CT) scans. In addition to a knowledge of normal vascular anatomy, you should be aware of the physiologic effects of gravity on the radiologic appearance of the pulmonary vascularity. Gravitational differences in the lung are posturally dependent and are most striking in the erect position. Gravity has an important effect on the distribution of pulmonary blood flow, resulting in an increase in blood flow from the lung apices to the lung bases in an upright position. When interpreting erect chest radiographs, you will notice a gradual increase in the diameter of pulmonary vessels from the lung apices to the lung bases; this increase corresponds to the increasing distribution of pulmonary blood flow.

Gravitational effects are also evident in other positions. In the supine position, there is a gradient between the anterior and posterior portions of the lung, which results in increased blood flow to the dependent, posterior portions. However, in contrast to the upright position, blood flow is fairly equivalent in the upper and lower lung zones. Therefore, on supine chest radiographs, you will notice that the caliber of vessels in the upper and lower lung zones are nearly equal. In the decubitus position, gravitational effects result in increased blood flow to the lung in the dependent position. A consequence of this phenomenon is the occurrence of unilateral pulmonary edema in the dependent lung of a patient who has been lying in a decubitus position.

In this chapter, we will review the characteristic radiologic findings in a number of pulmonary vascular entities, including pulmonary artery hypertension, pulmonary venous hypertension, congestive heart failure, and pulmonary thromboembolism. As you examine the pulmonary vasculature on a chest radiograph, always consider the posturally dependent effect of gravity. Keep in mind that subtle alterations in the pulmonary vasculature may only be detectable as a change in appearance from prior radiographs. Whenever possible, you should compare current radiographs with prior studies that were performed in the same position.

PULMONARY ARTERY HYPERTENSION

Definition

Pulmonary artery hypertension (PAH) is defined as a condition of sustained elevation of pulmonary artery pressure. The diagnostic criteria for pulmonary artery hypertension are a systemic pulmonary artery pressure greater than 30 mm Hg or a mean pulmonary artery pressure greater than 20 mm Hg.

Box 14-1 Etiologies of Pulmonary Artery Hypertension

INCREASED PULMONARY BLOOD FLOW

Left-to-right shunts (ASD, VSD, PDA)
Increased total blood volume (thyrotoxicosis, anemia, pregnancy)

DECREASED CROSS-SECTIONAL AREA OF THE PULMONARY VASCULATURE
Secondary to Primary Disease in the Arterial Wall or Lumen

Chronic pulmonary embolism
Primary pulmonary hypertension
Peripheral pulmonary stenosis
Eisenmenger's syndrome
Pulmonary vasculitis

Secondary to Pulmonary or Pleural Disease

Emphysema
Diffuse lung disease
    Fibrosis
        Idiopathic pulmonary fibrosis
        Collagen-vascular disease
        Sarcoidosis
        Pneumoconiosis
    Granulomatous infections
    Bronchiectasis (cystic fibrosis)
    Neoplasm
Postpneumonectomy
Fibrothorax
Chest wall deformity (thoracoplasty, kyposcoliosis)

Secondary to Vasoconstriction from Hypoventilation

Obesity/hypoventilation syndrome
Upper airway obstruction
High altitude
Neuromuscular disorders

INCREASED RESISTANCE TO PULMONARY VENOUS DRAINAGE

Pulmonary vein abnormalities
    Pulmonary venoocclusive disease
    Congenital narrowing or anomalous drainage
Left atrial abnormalities
    Cor triatriatum
    Left atrial myxoma or thrombus
Mitral valve disease (stenosis or regurgitation)
Left ventricular failure
Constrictive pericarditis
Fibrosing mediastinitis

ASD, atrial septal defect; *PDA,* patent ductus arteriosus; *VSD,* ventricular septal defect.

Causes

In general, PAH may occur secondary to one of three basic mechanisms: (1) increased flow of blood through the pulmonary vessels, (2) decreased cross-sectional area of the pulmonary vasculature, and (3) increased resistance to pulmonary venous drainage. These mechanisms provide a convenient framework for categorizing and understanding the large number of causes of PAH (Box 14-1). Another common way to categorize causes of PAH is to broadly divide them into precapillary causes (entities that result in increased blood flow or decreased cross-sectional area of the pulmonary vasculature) and postcapillary causes (entities that result in increased resistance to pulmonary venous drainage).

Most cases of PAH occur secondary to a known cause; these are collectively referred to as secondary PAH. In a minority of cases, the cause remains unknown, and this is referred to as primary PAH. Primary PAH usually affects women younger than 40 years of age. A small percentage of patients with primary PAH have a familial form, which is inherited as an autosomal dominant trait. Affected patients usually present with symptoms of progressive dyspnea and easy fatigability. Approximately 10% of patients present with symptoms of Raynaud's phenomenon. Because of the nonspecific presenting symptoms and the subtlety of clinical findings early in the course of the disease, the diagnosis is often delayed. Treatment of primary PAH consists of supportive medical therapy and transplantation (lung or combined heart-lung). Interestingly, pulmonary vascular disease with clinical and radiologic manifestations similar to primary PAH has been described in association with portal hypertension, HIV infection, cocaine abuse, and appetite-suppressant drugs.

Radiographic Findings

Despite the wide variety of causes of PAH, the salient radiologic features are similar, regardless of the specific cause. There is usually marked enlargement of the main and hilar pulmonary arteries, which rapidly taper as they course distally (Fig. 14-1). Indeed, the most striking feature of PAH is the disparity in size between the central and peripheral pulmonary arteries. Right-ventricular cardiac enlargement, best demonstrated on the lateral chest radiograph may be present.

On chest radiographs, enlargement of the main pulmonary artery results in a prominent convex contour. Be aware, however, that the degree of pulmonary artery enlargement varies considerably among different patients and conditions. In fact, significant PAH may be present in the setting of a normal chest radiograph. Compared with chest radiographs, CT scans allow a more accurate determination of the size of the main pulmonary artery, and a diameter greater than 3 cm on CT is generally considered abnormal (Fig. 14-2).

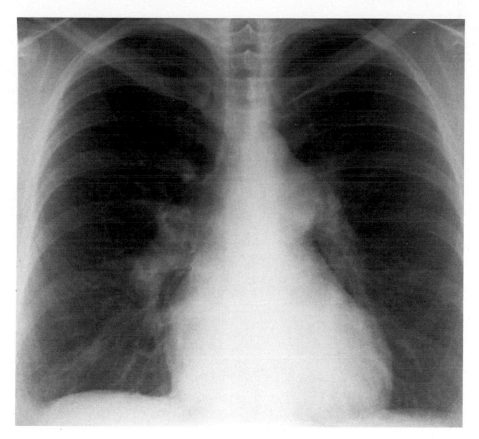

Figure 14-1   Primary pulmonary artery hypertension. A frontal chest radiograph demonstrates significant enlargement of the main and hilar pulmonary arteries, which rapidly taper as they course distally.

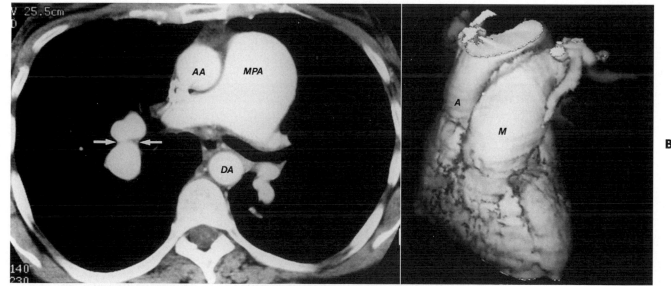

Figure 14-2   Pulmonary artery hypertension secondary to multiple peripheral pulmonic stenoses. **A,** A contrast-enhanced helical CT image of the chest reveals significant enlargement of the main pulmonary artery (MPA), which measures approximately 4.5 cm in diameter. There is also a weblike stenosis of the right interlobar pulmonary artery *(arrows)*, with associated poststenotic dilatation. Numerous additional sites of stenosis were evident on other images. *(AA,* ascending aorta; *DA,* descending aorta). **B,** A three-dimensional shaded-surface display image that was reconstructed from a helical CT acquisition shows the marked disparity in size between the enlarged main pulmonary artery *(M)* and the normal caliber ascending aorta *(A)*.

The evaluation of the hilar vessels on chest radiographs is usually a subjective assessment. An objective assessment of hilar vessel enlargement is the measurement of the diameter of the right interlobar artery.

On PA erect chest radiographs, the normal transverse diameter of the right interlobar artery as it descends adjacent to the bronchus intermedius is less than or equal to 16 mm.

In the setting of longstanding, severe PAH, the enlarged central pulmonary arteries may develop peripheral, atherosclerotic calcification. This is an unusual finding and is most frequently seen in patients with PAH secondary to Eisenmenger's syndrome (Fig. 14-3), a condition characterized by a reversal in the direction of a longstanding severe left-to-right shunt.

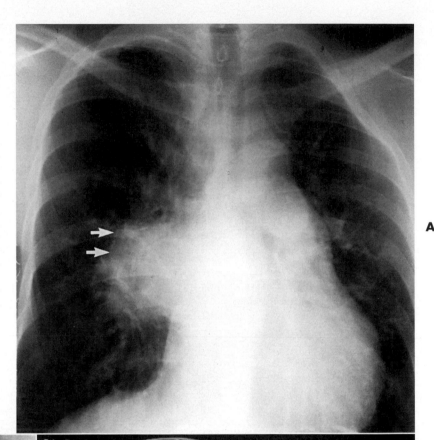

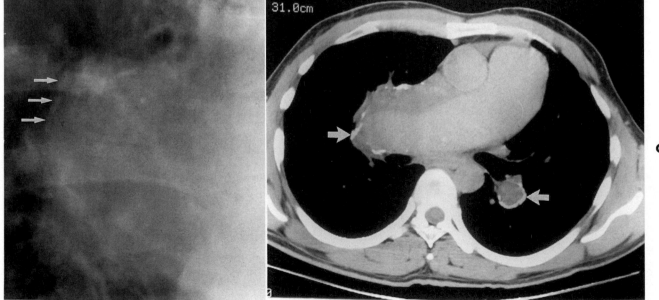

Figure 14-3 Pulmonary artery hypertension secondary to Eisenmenger's syndrome. **A,** A frontal chest radiograph reveals massive enlargement of the main and hilar pulmonary arteries. Note the presence of peripheral calcification *(arrows)* within the right interlobar pulmonary artery. The peripheral calcification is seen in greater detail on the coned-down image of the right hilum, **B. C,** An axial image from an unenhanced CT of the chest in the same patient demonstrates peripheral calcifications of both pulmonary arteries *(arrows)*. Atheromatous calcification is an unusual finding in PAH, and it is most frequently seen in patients with Eisenmenger's syndrome.

In cases of PAH that occur secondary to the mechanism of increased resistance to pulmonary venous return (postcapillary causes), you will also see radiographic findings of pulmonary venous hypertension. The most notable finding is cephalization of the pulmonary vasculature, also referred to as recruitment of upper lobe vessels. These terms refer to an increased caliber of the upper lobe vessels, which occurs secondary to a diversion of blood flow. As you will recall, this is a reversal of the gravity-dependent increased caliber of lower lobe vessels seen in upright radiographs of normal individuals. Therefore, cephalization is best evaluated on upright radiographs.

An objective method for assessing cephalization is to examine the relative sizes of the anterior segment artery of either upper lobe and its adjacent bronchus, both of which are usually seen "end-on" on a PA erect chest radiograph. In normal individuals, the diameter of the artery is about the same as the adjacent bronchus. Cephalization is present when the diameter of the artery is larger than the adjacent bronchus.

However, cephalization of blood flow is not seen exclusively in postcapillary causes of PAH. You may also encounter cephalization in cases of PAH that occur secondary to precapillary causes. In precapillary PAH, recruitment of upper lobe vessels occurs secondary to increased resistance in lower lobe pulmonary arteries.

In addition to cephalization, there are several other radiographic findings that may be associated with pulmonary venous hypertension, including interstitial edema (described in the next section), hemosiderosis, and pulmonary fibrosis. Hemosiderosis is related to recurrent episodes of alveolar hemorrhage. When these episodes are severe, you may detect hemosiderosis on chest radiographs as tiny punctate opacities in the middle- and lower-lung zones. Pulmonary fibrosis is related to recurrent episodes of pulmonary edema and hemorrhage. Radiographically, it is characterized by reticular opacities in the middle- and lower-lung zones.

It is important to identify the underlying cause of PAH, because each case has a different treatment regimen. For example, the treatment of patients with primary PAH is a transplant procedure, and the treatment for patients with secondary PAH from chronic thromboembolism is thromboendarterectomy. In some cases, a careful examination of the chest radiograph for ancillary cardiac, pulmonary, and pleural findings may provide clues to the underlying cause of PAH. In many cases, however, additional imaging studies such as echocardiography, ventilation-perfusion imaging, and pulmonary angiography are necessary to diagnose the precise cause of PAH. In cases of suspected chronic thromboembolic disease, CT and MR imaging can also be helpful. This is discussed in detail later in this chapter.

CONGESTIVE HEART FAILURE

Pulmonary edema refers to the presence of excess extravascular fluid within the interstitial and alveolar compartments of the lung. Under normal conditions, these compartments are kept relatively dry by two main factors: (1) a balance between capillary pressure and plasma oncotic pressure, and (2) maintenance of normal capillary wall permeability. Therefore, pulmonary edema generally occurs secondary to one of two mechanisms: (1) elevated pulmonary microvascular pressure, or (2) increased capillary membrane permeability. The former is referred to as cardiogenic or hydrostatic pulmonary edema, and the latter is referred to as noncardiogenic pulmonary edema.

We will focus on cardiogenic pulmonary edema in this chapter. The most common cause of elevated pulmonary microvascular pressure is an elevation in pulmonary venous pressure secondary to diseases of the left side of the heart. Examples include left ventricular failure, diseases of the mitral valve, and left atrial abnormalities (see Box 14-1).

Interstitial Edema

Pulmonary edema usually follows a typical course. It begins in the interstitial compartment of the lung and extends into the alveolar compartment as it increases in severity. The first phase of pulmonary edema involves the interstitial compartment. It contains two major components: the peribronchovascular sheath and the interlobular septa. Fluid within the peribronchovascular sheath results in indistinctness of the pulmonary vessels and peribronchial cuffing (Fig. 14-4). Fluid within the interlobular septa results in the presence of Kerley lines (Table 14-1, Fig. 14-5).

As interstitial edema progresses in severity, fluid may also accumulate within the subpleural space of the interlobar fissures. This is referred to as subpleural edema, and it results in thickening of the interlobar fissures on chest radiographs.

Table 14-1 Kerley A and B Lines		
	Location	**Length**
Kerley A Lines	Central Radiate from hila	2–6 cm
Kerley B Lines	Peripheral Adjacent to costophrenic sulcus	< 2 cm

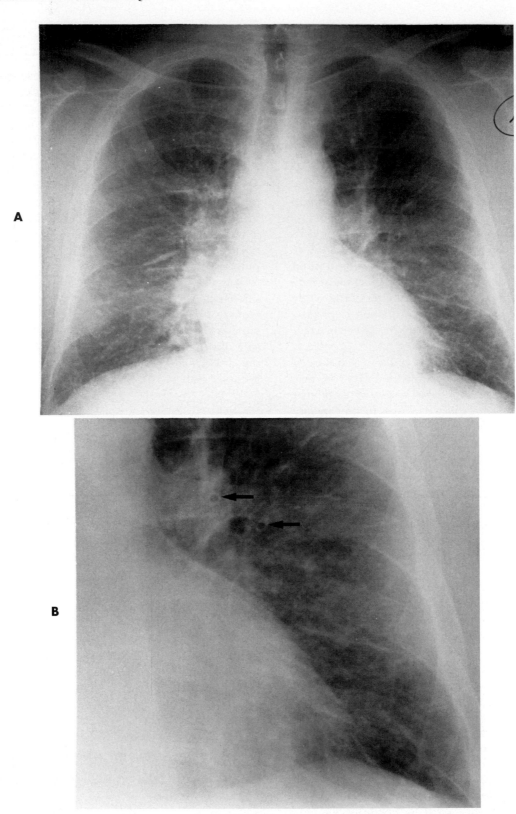

Figure 14-4 Interstitial pulmonary edema. **A,** A frontal chest radiograph reveals the presence of interstitial pulmonary edema, manifested by peribronchial cuffing, indistinctness of the pulmonary vessels, Kerley lines, and subpleural edema. **B,** The peribronchial cuffing *(arrows)* and Kerley lines are seen in greater detail on the coned-down image of the left lung.

A

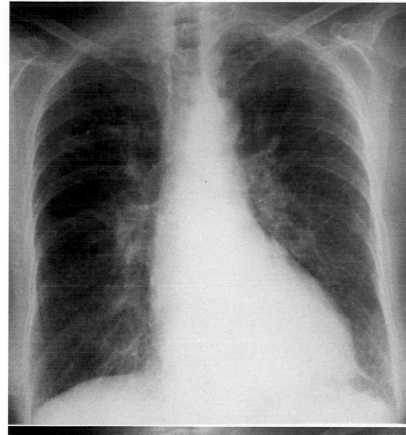

B

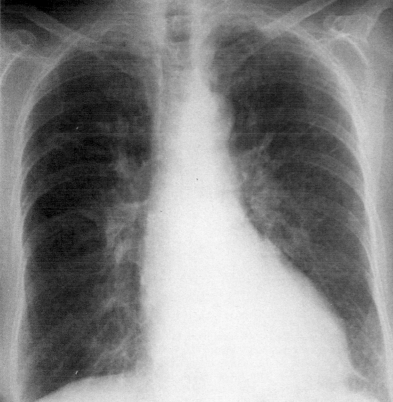

Figure 14-5 Interstitial pulmonary edema. **A,** A frontal chest radiograph reveals several linear opacities throughout both lungs. The linear opacities are referred to as Kerley lines, and they represent fluid-filled interlobular septae. The Kerley lines are more apparent when compared with the patient's baseline radiograph, **B**.

Continued

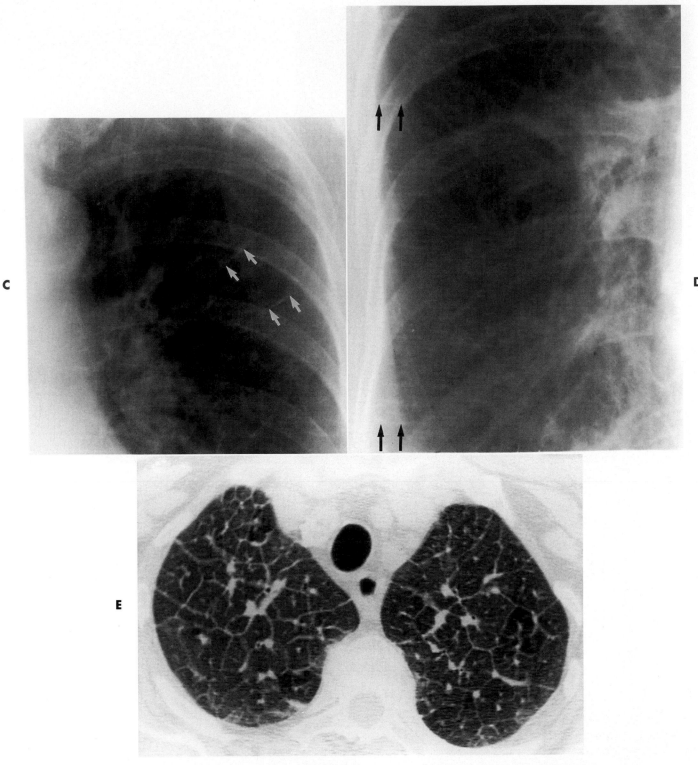

Figure 14-5, cont'd **C,** A coned-down image of the left upper lobe demonstrates linear opacities radiating from the hilar, consistent with Kerley A lines *(white arrows).* Note that Kerley A lines do not extend to the pleural surface. **D,** A coned-down image of the right mid- and lower-lung zones reveals linear opacities in the lung periphery, consistent with Kerley B lines *(black arrows).* Note that Kerley B lines extend to the pleural surface. **E,** A high-resolution CT scan image of the chest demonstrates smooth interlobular septal thickening, which outlines the secondary pulmonary lobules of the lungs. Interlobular septal thickening corresponds to the plain radiographic finding of Kerley lines. Also note the presence of ground-glass parenchymal opacities, peribronchovascular interstitial thickening, and increased vascular diameter. These are characteristic high-resolution CT findings of hydrostatic pulmonary edema.

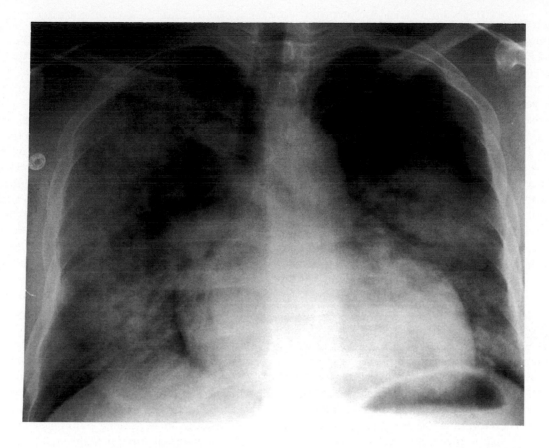

Figure 14-6 Alveolar edema. A frontal chest radiograph demonstrates the presence of bilateral air-space consolidation, which is more prominent in the right lung than in the left. When asymmetric, pulmonary edema is usually more severe in the right lung. Radiographs obtained during prior episodes of pulmonary edema (not shown) demonstrated a similar pattern of asymmetric airspace consolidation.

Alveolar Edema

The second phase of pulmonary edema involves the extension of fluid into the alveolar spaces of the lung. You can detect airspace involvement by identifying the presence of poorly defined nodular opacities, which represent the presence of fluid within the alveoli. As increasing amounts of fluid fill the alveoli, these opacities will coalesce to produce airspace consolidation, which is usually most prominent in the central, perihilar regions of the lungs.

Although the distribution of pulmonary edema is often bilateral and symmetric, you should know that there is considerable variability in its distribution. When asymmetric, pulmonary edema is usually more severe in the right lung (Fig. 14-6). An atypical pattern of pulmonary edema is often observed in patients with underlying lung disease. For example, patients with severe upper lobe emphysema will often demonstrate a basilar predominance of pulmonary edema. Although the appearance of pulmonary edema may vary among patients, there is often a strikingly similar pattern in an individual patient from episode to episode. You may find it helpful

to compare the current radiograph to one obtained during a prior episode of pulmonary edema, particularly for patients who present with an asymmetric or atypical distribution. Additional characteristic features of alveolar pulmonary edema include: (1) a fairly rapid onset, (2) an often dramatic shift in distribution with varying patient positions, and (3) a relatively quick resolution in response to adequate therapy. These features can be helpful in distinguishing asymmetric pulmonary edema from diffuse pneumonia.

Although we have presented the findings of interstitial and alveolar edema as separate entities, you should know that radiographic findings of both often coexist. Because the interstitial compartment is affected first, interstitial edema may be present without alveolar edema. On the other hand, if alveolar edema is present, then the interstitial compartment must also be edematous (even if it is not radiographically apparent).

Physiologic Correlation

The characteristic radiographic findings of pulmonary venous hypertension and congestive heart failure have been shown to correlate with physiologic parameters such as pulmonary venous wedge pressures (PVWP). The normal PVWP is less than 12 mm Hg. As the PVWP rises between 12 mm Hg and 17 mm Hg, you will see cephalization of the pulmonary vessels. At levels above 17 mm Hg, you should expect to see Kerley lines. Once the PVWP rises above 20 mm Hg, you may see a pleural effusion, which is usually right-sided. At pressures greater than 25 mm Hg, you should expect to see airspace consolidation. Keep in mind, however, that these values are relative. For example, you may occasionally see acinar opacities at PVWP levels of 20 to 25 mm Hg. Moreover, as pulmonary edema resolves, the radiographic findings may lag behind the clinical improvement of the patient. In this setting, you may see persistent radiographic evidence of pulmonary edema despite the fact that hemodynamic measurements have returned to normal.

PULMONARY THROMBOEMBOLISM

Acute pulmonary thromboembolism (PE) is an important cause of mortality, particularly among hospitalized patients. Although PE is a highly treatable condition, there are risks associated with its treatment—anticoagulation therapy. Therefore, it is essential that the diagnosis of acute PE is made promptly and accurately. Unfortunately, however, the diagnosis of acute PE is often delayed or goes unrecognized, in large part secondary to the nonspecific nature of its presenting symptoms, clinical signs, and laboratory test findings.

Because of the difficulty of diagnosing acute PE on the basis of clinical and laboratory data, imaging studies have come to play a primary diagnostic role in the evaluation of patients with suspected PE. Ideally, an imaging test for acute PE would be highly accurate, safe, noninvasive, readily available, and cost-effective. The traditional imaging techniques used for diagnosing acute PE—ventilation-perfusion (VQ) imaging and angiography—do not fully meet these criteria.

In recent years, there have been advances in the development of new, noninvasive imaging techniques for diagnosing acute PE. These techniques include spiral and electron-beam CT, MR angiography, and nuclear medicine imaging with thrombus-avid radiopharmaceutical drugs. Preliminary investigations with CT and MRI have generated considerable excitement regarding their potential as diagnostic tests for acute PE. Their precise roles in the diagnostic algorithm for acute PE are just now evolving.

In the next section, the basic pathophysiology of pulmonary emboli is reviewed. Also, the imaging findings related to acute pulmonary thromboembolism on chest radiographs, VQ scans, pulmonary angiograms, MR angiography, and spiral CT scans are described.

Pathophysiology of Pulmonary Thromboemboli and Infarction

Pulmonary thromboembolism refers to the transport of venous thrombus to the pulmonary circulation with subsequent dislodgement of thrombus within a pulmonary artery. Thrombi may dislodge in the main, lobar, segmental, or subsegmental pulmonary arteries.

The majority of thrombi arise from clots within the deep venous system of the lower extremities. Other sites of origin include the inferior vena cava, pelvic veins, right atrium, right ventricle, and veins of the head, neck, and upper extremities. Risk factors for venous thrombosis (and therefore PE) include: stasis (e.g., bed rest), endothelial damage (e.g., trauma), and coagulation abnormalities (e.g., coagulopathy).

Pulmonary thromboemboli are often multiple, and they have a predilection for the lower lobes of the lungs. Their distribution is likely related to increased pulmonary blood flow in the lower lobes. Only a minority of pulmonary thromboemboli (approximately 15%) result in pulmonary infarction. In general, infarction occurs when the combined pulmonary and bronchial circulation is inadequate. This happens most often when emboli dislodge in peripheral pulmonary artery branches, and when emboli affect patients with underlying cardiovascular disease.

In the majority of cases, the emboli resolve secondary to lysis, and the affected pulmonary vessels subsequently return to normal. In some patients, however, the emboli do not fully resolve. Following repeated bouts of thromboemboli, the patient may develop PAH.

Imaging Features of Pulmonary Thromboembolism and Infarction

Chest radiograph

Before describing the CXR features of pulmonary emboli and infarction, it is important to state that most episodes of pulmonary emboli do not result in radiographic abnormalities. In fact, you should consider the diagnosis of acute PE whenever a patient in acute respiratory distress presents with a normal chest radiograph!

The CXR has two primary roles in the evaluation of a patient with suspected acute PE. The first role is to evaluate for the presence of other thoracic abnormalities that may mimic PE clinically. For example, pleuritic chest pain and shortness of breath are common symptoms of acute PE, but they may also occur in a patient with a pneumothorax. The second role is to assist in the interpretation of ventilation-perfusion scans.

The CXR manifestations of pulmonary thromboembolic disease can be divided into those related to pul-

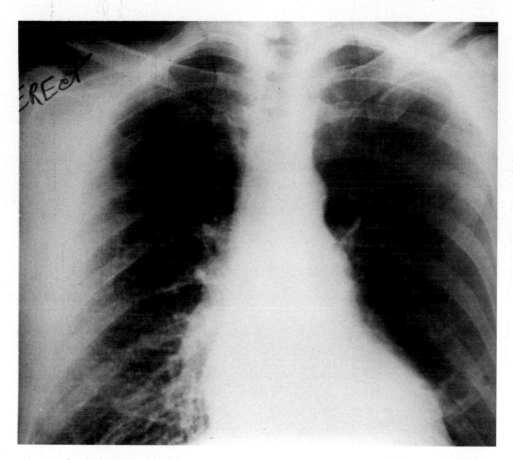

Figure 14-7 Westermark's sign. A frontal radiograph of the chest reveals asymmetry of the pulmonary vascularity of the two lungs, with diminished vascularity throughout the left lung. In this patient the asymmetry is most apparent in the middle- and lower-lung zones because of the presence of bilateral upper lobe vascular attenuation secondary to emphysema. A pulmonary angiogram (not shown) demonstrated occlusive thrombus in the left main pulmonary artery.

monary embolus and those related to pulmonary infarction (Box 14-2).

CXR findings in pulmonary embolus without infarction are uncommon. When present, they are usually associated with a large, central pulmonary embolus. *Westermark's sign* refers to the presence of oligemia distal to an obstructing embolus (Fig. 14-7). It is most evident when a large embolus occludes the main pulmonary artery of one lung. Enlargement of a central hilar artery with abrupt tapering, also referred to as the *knuckle sign,* represents vascular distention secondary to intraluminal thrombus. Vascular abnormalities from acute PE are best appreciated in the context of a change in appearance from prior radiographs.

Volume loss may accompany PE with or without infarction, but it is more commonly seen in the setting of infarction. Volume loss occurs secondary to surfactant depletion related to decreased pulmonary artery perfusion and bronchoconstriction. It is usually manifested on radiographs by an elevated hemidiaphragm and/or a displaced fissure.

Box 14-2 Radiographic Findings in Pulmonary Embolism

CHEST RADIOGRAPHIC SIGNS OF PE WITHOUT INFARCTION

Oligemia (Westermark's sign)
Increase in hilar vessel size with abrupt tapering (knuckle sign)
Volume loss

CHEST RADIOGRAPHIC SIGNS OF PE WITH INFARCTION

Consolidation (Hampton's lump)
Discoid atelectasis
Volume loss
Pleural effusion

PE, pulmonary embolism.

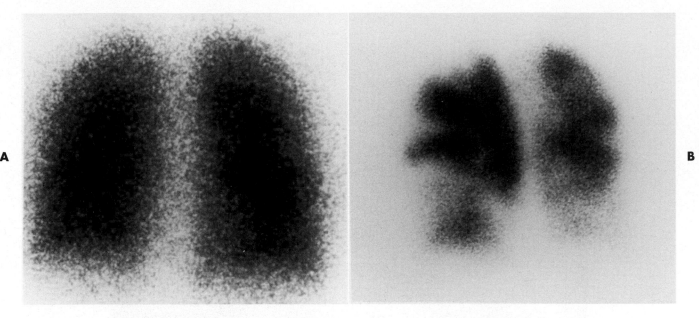

Figure 14-8 Multiple pulmonary emboli. **A,** A posterior image from the ventilation portion of a VQ scan demonstrates homogenous ventilation to both lungs, without evidence of ventilation defects. **B,** A right anterior oblique image from the perfusion portion of a VQ scan in the same patient reveals multiple subsegmental and segmental perfusion defects in both lungs consistent with multiple pulmonary emboli.

Additional chest radiograph signs of PE with infarction include consolidation, discoid atelectasis, and pleural effusion. Consolidation represents the presence of hemorrhage and/or necrosis. Areas of consolidation are usually segmental, homogeneous, and peripheral. They are often multiple, and there is a lower lobe predominance. The term Hampton's hump refers to the presence of a wedge-shaped, peripheral area of consolidation. Its base abuts the pleural surface of the lung and its apex is directed toward the hilum. This finding is highly suggestive of a pulmonary infarct.

The resolution of pulmonary infarction has a variable time course, but averages approximately 3 weeks. In some cases, however, resolution occurs over several months. The pattern of resolution can be helpful in distinguishing infarction from pneumonia. In general, pulmonary infarcts tend to decrease in size while maintaining their original shape and homogeneous appearance. This pattern of resolution, which has been compared to a melting ice cube, contrasts sharply with the heterogeneous appearance of a resolving pneumonia.

Discoid atelectasis refers to the presence of linear parenchymal opacities. They are often horizontal in position and are usually basilar in distribution.

Pleural effusions are a relatively common radiographic manifestation of pulmonary infarction. When present, they are usually small and unilateral. Although often accompanied by consolidation or atelectasis, a pleural effusion may be the sole radiologic abnormality of pulmonary infarction.

We have reviewed a variety of radiographic signs that are associated with PE and pulmonary infarction. You should know, however, that an analysis of the chest radiographic findings in patients with acute PE from the PIOPED (Prospective Investigation of Pulmonary Embolism Diagnosis) study revealed that these radiographic signs are all poor predictors of PE. Based on their results, the investigators of this study concluded that the chest radiographic findings in patients with suspected PE do not provide sufficient information to accurately establish or exclude the diagnosis of acute PE.

Ventilation-Perfusion Scan

The VQ scan is a nuclear medicine study that examines pulmonary ventilation and perfusion. It is performed by administering an inhaled ventilation agent (usually Xenon-133) and an intravenously injected perfusion agent (technetium 99m-macroaggregated human albumin). A VQ scan does not permit direct visualization of a PE. Rather, it relies on indirect evidence of PE: a ventilation-perfusion mismatch (Fig. 14-8). You should know that a V–Q mismatch is not specific for acute PE, because it may occur secondary to other causes including neoplasm, vasculitis, and pulmonary artery stenosis or atresia. When interpreting VQ scans, it is important to always compare the study with a current chest radiograph.

Although there are several interpretive schemes for diagnosing acute PE with VQ imaging, the most common criteria are those determined from the PIOPED study. This study, a landmark prospective multiinstitutional investigation, assessed the value of the VQ scan in diag-

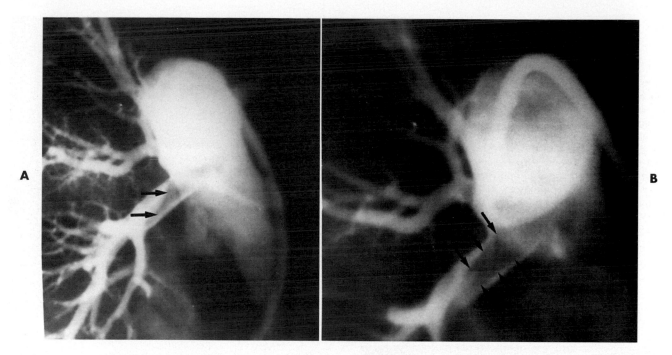

Figure 14-9   Acute PE. **A,** An oblique projection from a left pulmonary artery angiogram demonstrates the presence of an intravascular filling defect within the superior segment artery *(arrows),* consistent with an acute PE. The filling defect *(arrows)* is seen in better detail on the coned-down image of this vessel, **B**. *(Case courtesy of Dr. David Ball, Temple University.)*

nosing acute PE using pulmonary angiography as the gold standard. Using the PIOPED interpretive scheme, a VQ scan is categorized as (1) normal, (2) low probability for PE, (3) intermediate probability for PE, or (4) high probability for PE.

In general, a normal VQ scan reliably excludes the diagnosis of acute PE, and a high-probability VQ scan is considered sufficient evidence to treat a patient for acute PE. Unfortunately, however, the majority of VQ scan interpretations do not fall into these two categories. Based on their results, the PIOPED investigators recommended that patients with a high clinical suspicion for PE and either "low" or "intermediate" probability scans should be evaluated with additional diagnostic studies such as pulmonary angiography to exclude PE. Subsequent studies have shown, however, that clinicians infrequently adhere to these recommendations.

An in-depth discussion of VQ imaging is provided in *Nuclear Medicine: The Requisites,* and you are encouraged to consult this textbook or another nuclear medicine reference for more detailed information on this subject.

Angiography

Pulmonary angiography is currently considered to be the most accurate imaging test for diagnosing acute PE. It involves the percutaneous advancement of a catheter into the pulmonary arteries under fluoroscopic guidance with subsequent injection of contrast media. The complication rate of the procedure is relatively low, estimated at 1% to 5%. Complications include arrhythmias, cardiac arrest, cardiac perforation, and contrast reactions. The estimated mortality of the procedure is approximately 0.2%, increasing to approximately 2% in patients with severe pulmonary artery hypertension.

There are two major angiographic signs of acute PE: an intravascular filling defect and an abrupt vascular cutoff (Fig. 14-9). In general, a negative high-quality pulmonary angiogram is considered sufficient evidence to exclude acute PE.

Spiral and Electron-Beam CT

The advent of spiral (helical) and electron-beam CT has resulted in improved visualization of the pulmonary arteries on the basis of faster scan times and volumetric data acquisition. Several preliminary investigations have demonstrated a relatively high sensitivity and specificity of these techniques for diagnosing acute PE in the main, lobar, and segmental arteries. However, the reported accuracies have been considerably lower for the detection of PE in the subsegmental pulmonary arteries. Although it is estimated that isolated subsegmental PE occurs in approximately 5% of patients, the clinical significance of this estimate is unknown.

On CT, the diagnosis of acute PE is made by the direct visualization of thrombus, which appears as soft-tissue

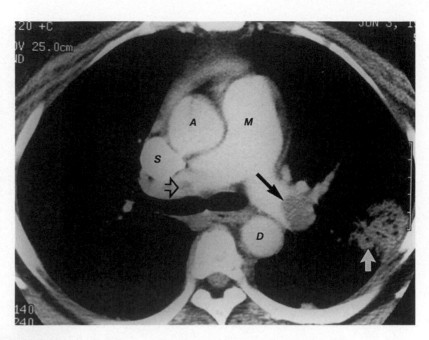

Figure 14-10 Acute PE. A contrast-enhanced helical CT image of the chest reveals the presence of soft-tissue attenuation thrombus within both the distal left main pulmonary artery *(solid black arrow)* and the right pulmonary artery *(open black arrow)*. Acute pulmonary emboli in these vessels were confirmed at angiography. Note the presence of peripheral consolidation in the left upper lobe *(white arrow)*, suggestive of pulmonary infarction. (*A*, ascending aorta; *D*, descending aorta; *M*, main pulmonary artery; *S*, superior vena cava). *(Case courtesy of Dr. Elizabeth Drucker, Massachusetts General Hospital.)*

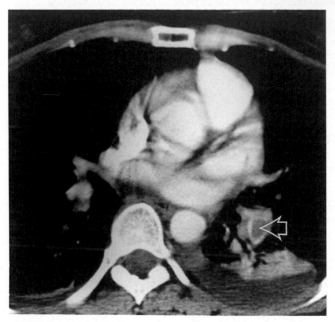

Figure 14-11 Acute PE. A contrast-enhanced helical CT image of the chest demonstrates the presence of soft-tissue attenuation thrombus *(arrow)* outlined by contrast within the left descending pulmonary artery. Angiography confirmed the presence of acute thrombus in this vessel. Note the presence of atelectasis and a small left pleural effusion.

attenuation material within the contrast-opacified vessel (Figs. 14-10 and 14-11). Thrombus may be identified as a partial or complete filling defect, or as free-floating soft-tissue attenuation material within the vascular lumen.

You should know that performing spiral CT in patients with suspected PE requires careful attention to technical parameters in order to obtain maximal contrast opacification and optimal visualization of the pulmonary arteries. Moreover, interpreting spiral CT scans for acute PE requires a thorough knowledge of normal pulmonary bronchovascular anatomy and normal hilar and intersegmental lymph node anatomy.

A potential advantage of CT in the evaluation of patients with suspected PE is its ability to detect other thoracic abnormalities that may mimic PE clinically. Therefore, CT may occasionally provide an alternative diagnosis to explain a patient's symptoms.

In addition to the characteristic vascular findings described in acute PE, you may also see abnormalities in the lung parenchyma, particularly in cases of pulmonary infarction. Pulmonary infarcts typically appear as peripheral, wedge-shaped areas of consolidation, with their bases abutting the visceral pleura. They are often multiple, and they have a lower-lobe predominance. Be aware that a wedge-shaped peripheral lesion is not specific for pulmonary infarct; it may also be seen in cases of pneumonia, neoplasm, and hemorrhage. When present, a feeding vessel directed toward the apex of the wedge-shaped consolidation is a feature more typical of infarction than these other entities. Another characteristic CT feature of pulmonary infarcts is the presence of foci of low attenuation within the area of consolidation; this corresponds to the presence of "spared," uninfarcted, secondary pulmonary lobules (Fig. 14-12).

MR Angiography

Currently, MRI techniques using fast scanning times and dynamic enhancement with gadolinium provide the ability to perform high-resolution pulmonary angiography during a single suspended inspiration. A recent preliminary investigation reported a high sensitivity and specificity of MR angiography for diagnosing acute PE.

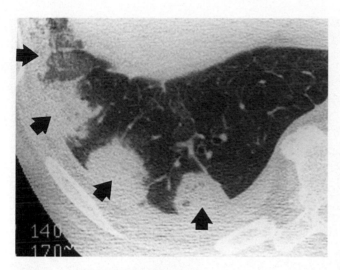

Figure 14-12 Pulmonary infarcts. A coned-down image of the right lung base from a high-resolution CT of the chest reveals multiple peripheral areas of consolidation *(arrows)* representing pulmonary infarcts. Note the presence of several foci of low attenuation within the consolidation, which correspond to focal areas of "spared" uninfarcted lung parenchyma. There is also a small pleural effusion present.

The diagnosis of acute PE on MR angiography is based on direct visualization of thrombus, which appears as an intravascular filling defect (Fig. 14-13). In comparison with CT, there are several potential advantages of MR angiography. First, MR angiography does not use iodinated contrast media. Therefore, it can be performed in patients with a history of contrast reaction and in those with depressed renal function. Second, MR does not involve ionizing radiation. This is an important consideration when imaging pregnant patients and children with suspected PE. Third, MR has the ability to image the pelvic and lower extremity veins for the presence of venous thrombosis. Therefore, in one setting, a patient may undergo both MR angiography to assess for PE, and MR venography to evaluate for residual deep venous thrombosis. A disadvantage of MR angiography is that a small number of patients will be excluded on the basis of contraindications to MR imaging.

The eventual roles of CT and MR imaging in the diagnostic algorithm for acute PE will likely be dependent on several factors, including improved technical parameters for optimal pulmonary artery visualization; increased experience at interpreting these studies; and further assessment of their accuracy in large prospective outcome trials.

Chronic Pulmonary Thromboembolism

As mentioned earlier in this chapter, recurrent episodes of PE may result in PAH. Interestingly, affected patients usually do not provide a history suggestive of

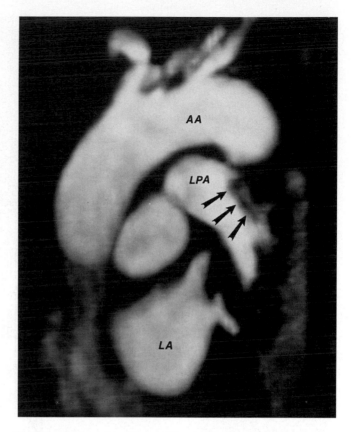

Figure 14-13 Acute PE. An oblique mean-planar reconstruction image from a magnetic resonance angiography study demonstrates a filling defect *(arrows)* within the left descending pulmonary artery consistent with an acute PE. (*AA,* aortic arch; *LPA,* left pulmonary artery; *LA,* left atrium). *(Case courtesy of Dr. James Meaney, Leeds General Infirmary, Leeds, U.K.)*

acute PE. Rather, they frequently present with symptoms of PAH, including progressive dyspnea and easy fatigability. In contrast to acute PE, which is treated with anticoagulation therapy, the treatment of chronic PE is thromboendarterectomy.

Characteristic imaging findings of chronic PE have been described for pulmonary angiograms and, more recently, for MR angiography and CT. In contrast, the VQ scan findings in chronic PE are similar to those in acute PE: multiple segmental VQ mismatches.

On pulmonary angiograms, the characteristic features of chronic PE are the presence of mural thrombi (eccentric thrombi contiguous with the vessel wall), multiple webs and stenoses, irregular vascular occlusions, and varying calibers of the pulmonary vessels.

On MR angiography, the characteristic vascular features of chronic PE are similar to those described for conventional angiography. A recent study suggests that MR angiography can reliably distinguish between patients with PAH secondary to chronic PE and those with primary PAH by comparing the caliber of the segmental pulmonary arteries. In cases of chronic PE, the segmental pulmonary arteries usually demonstrate vary-

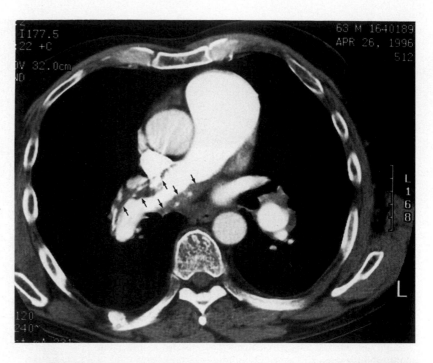

Figure 14-14 Chronic PE. A contrast-enhanced helical CT image of the chest at the level of the main pulmonary artery (MPA) demonstrates the presence of soft-tissue attenuation mural thrombus within the right pulmonary artery *(arrows)*. Note the presence of calcifications within the thrombus, a finding that is often associated with chronic PE. The main pulmonary artery is markedly enlarged in this patient with PAH secondary to chronic PE. *(Case courtesy of Dr. Colleen Bergin, University of California at San Diego.)*

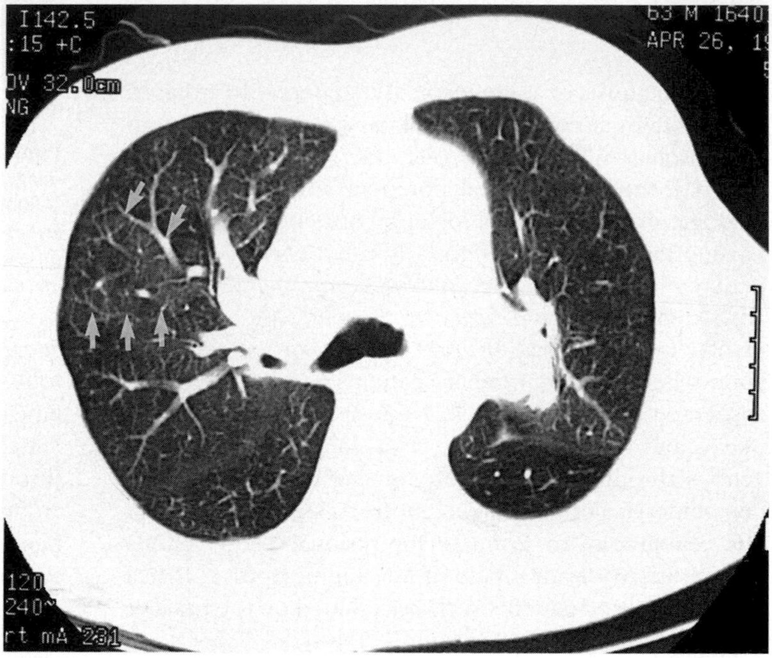

Figure 14-15 Mosaic perfusion secondary to chronic PE. An axial CT image of the lungs (from the same patient as shown in Figure 14-13) demonstrates areas of variable lung attenuation within the right upper lobe. One of the high-attenuation areas is marked *(arrows)*. Notice the subtle decrease in the caliber and number of vessels within the low-attenuation areas in comparison with the high-attenuation areas. *(Case courtesy of Dr. Colleen Bergin, University of California at San Diego.)*

ing calibers; in contrast, in primary PAH, the segmental pulmonary arteries appear more uniform in size.

On CT scans of patients with chronic PE, you may see characteristic vascular and parenchymal abnormalities. The most valuable vascular finding is the identification of mural thrombus (Fig. 14-14). An assessment of the morphologic features of intravascular thrombus may help you to distinguish acute PE from chronic PE. Acute thrombus is usually smoothly marginated, and it is at least partially surrounded by contrast material. Conversely, chronic thrombus is usually adherent to the vas-

cular wall; it has irregular margins, and it may contain calcification.

On conventional and high-resolution CT images of the lungs in patients with chronic PE, you may detect a mosaic pattern of lung attenuation, that is, the presence of areas of variable lung attenuation in a lobular or multilobular distribution. This pattern may be caused by a number of entities, including primary vascular diseases, small-airways diseases, and primary parenchymal diseases.

Although a mosaic pattern may be observed on conventional CT images, it is best evaluated with high-resolution CT. In cases that occur secondary to vascular disease and small-airways disease, the lower-attenuation areas of the lung show a decrease in number and caliber of vessels when compared with the higher-attenuation areas of lung. In contrast, a mosaic pattern from primary parenchymal disease reveals a uniform distribution and caliber of vessels in both the lower- and higher-attenuation areas. Expiratory CT imaging will allow you to distinguish between small-airways disease and primary vascular disease. On expiratory scans, you will see air-trapping only in cases of small-airways disease. A mosaic pattern of lung attenuation that occurs secondary to primary vascular lung disease such as chronic PE is referred to as mosaic perfusion or mosaic oligemia (Fig. 14-15).

SUGGESTED READINGS

Bergin CJ, Hauschildt J, Rios G, et al: Accuracy of MR angiography compared with radionuclide scanning in identifying the cause of pulmonary artery hypertension, *AJR* 168:1549-1555, 1997.

Bergin CJ, Rios G, King MA, et al: Accuracy of high-resolution CT in identifying chronic pulmonary thromboembolic disease, *AJR* 166:1371-1377, 1996.

Fraser RG, Pare JA, Pare PD, Fraser RS, Genereaux GP: Embolic and thrombotic diseases of the lungs. In Fraser et al, editors: *Diagnosis of diseases of the chest,* Philadelphia, 1990, WB Saunders: 1701-1782.

Fraser RG, Pare JA, Pare PD, Fraser RS, Genereaux: Pulmonary hypertension and edema. In Fraser et al, editors: *Diagnosis of diseases of the chest,* Philadelphia, 1990, WB Saunders; pp 1823-1968.

Greaves SM, Hart EM, Brown K, Young DA, Batra P, Aberle DR: Pulmonary thromboembolism: Spectrum of findings on CT, *AJR* 165:1359-1363, 1995.

Gurney J: Physiology. In Freundlich IM, Bragg DG, editors: *A radiologic approach to diseases of the chest,* Baltimore, 1992, Williams & Wilkins; pp 8-25.

Hansell DM, Peters AM: Pulmonary vascular diseases and pulmonary edema. In Armstrong P, Wilson AG, Dee P et al, editors: *Imaging of diseases of the chest,* ed 2, St. Louis, 1995, Mosby Inc.; pp 369-425.

Henschke CI, Mateescu I, Yankelevitz DF: Changing practice patterns in the diagnosis of pulmonary embolism, *Chest* 107:940-945, 1995.

Knight LC, Maurer AH, Romano JE: Comparison of Iodine-123-disintegrins for imaging thrombi and emboli in a canine model, *J Nucl Med* 37:476-482, 1996.

Meaney JFM, Weg JG, Chenevert TL et al: Diagnosis of pulmonary embolism with magnetic resonance angiography, *N Engl J Med* 336:1422-1427, 1997.

Miller SW: The elements of cardiac imaging. In *Cardiac radiology: The requisites,* St. Louis, 1997, Mosby, Inc.; pp 23-36.

PIOPED Investigators: Value of the ventilation/perfusion scan in acute pulmonary embolism. Results of the prospective investigation of pulmonary embolism diagnosis (PIOPED), *JAMA* 263:2753-2759, 1990.

Ralph DD: Pulmonary embolism: The implications of the prospective investigation of pulmonary embolism diagnosis, *Adv Chest Radiol,* 32:679-687, 1994.

Randall PA, Heitzman ER, Groskin SA, Scalzetti EM: Pulmonary arterial hypertension. In Freundlich IM, Bragg DG, editors: *A radiologic approach to diseases of the chest,* Baltimore, 1992, Williams & Wilkins. pp 151-162.

Remy-Jardin M, Remy J, Deschildre F, et al: Diagnosis of pulmonary embolism with spiral CT: Comparison with pulmonary angiography, *Radiology* 200:699-706, 1996.

Remy-Jardin M, Remy J, Artaud D, et al: Spiral CT of pulmonary embolism: Technical considerations and diagnostic pitfalls, *J Thorac Imaging* 12:103-117, 1997.

Roberts HC, Kauczor H-U, Schweden F, Thelen M: Spiral CT of pulmonary hypertension and chronic thromboembolism, *J Thorac Imaging* 12:118-127, 1997.

Rubin LJ: Primary pulmonary hypertension, *N Engl J Med* 336(2):111-117, 1997.

Sostman HD, Pope CJ: *Venous thromboembolic disease.* In Putman CE, Ravin CE, editors: *Textbook of diagnostic imaging,* ed 2, Philadelphia, 1994, WB Saunders, pp 546-562.

Stern EJ, Swensen SJ, Hartman TE, Frank MS: CT mosaic pattern of lung attenuation: Distinguishing different causes, *AJR* 165:813-816, 1995.

Teigen CL, Maus TP, Sheedy PF, et al: Pulmonary embolism: Diagnosis with contrast-enhanced electron beam CT and comparison with pulmonary angiography, *Radiology* 194:313-319, 1995.

Thrall JH, Ziessman HA: Pulmonary system. In *Nuclear medicine: The requisites,* St. Louis, 1995, Mosby, Inc.; pp 129-147.

Woodward PK: Pulmonary arteries must be seen before they can be assessed, *Radiology* 204:11-12, 1997.

Worsley LF, Alavi A, Aronchick JM, et al: Chest radiographic findings in patients with acute pulmonary embolism: Observations from the PIOPED study, *Radiology* 189:133-136, 1993.

CHAPTER 15

The Mediastinum: Normal Anatomy and Approach to Evaluating Focal Mediastinal Abnormalities

PHILLIP M. BOISELLE

The mediastinum is an anatomic region bounded laterally by the two lungs, anteriorly by the sternum, posteriorly by the vertebrae, superiorly by the thoracic inlet, and inferiorly by the diaphragm. A wide variety of focal and diffuse abnormalities occurs in the mediastinum. Computed tomography (CT) and magnetic resonance imaging (MRI) have improved our ability to detect, define, and characterize these abnormalities. In certain cases, the imaging features of a mediastinal mass allow a specific diagnosis to be made radiographically.

THE 4 D'S OF MEDIASTINAL MASSES

The classic differential diagnosis of an anterior mediastinal mass, the "4 T's," is one of the best known radiologic differential diagnoses among medical students and first-year radiology residents. However, before arriving at this seemingly simple differential diagnosis, you must first make several important observations and deductions. These include the following *4 D's of mediastinal masses:* (1) *detection* of an abnormality, (2) *description* of the abnormality, (3) placement of the abnormality into the appropriate anatomic *division* of the mediastinum, and finally, (4) generation of a limited *differential diag-nosis* based on the descriptive features and anatomic location.

For discussion of focal mediastinal masses and diffuse mediastinal abnormalities, please see the following two chapters.

Detection: Mediastinal Landmarks

To detect a mediastinal abnormality, one must be thoroughly familiar with both the normal radiographic anatomy and with the characteristic changes produced by abnormalities within various portions of the mediastinum. The radiographic landmarks of normal mediastinal anatomy are the lines, stripes, and interfaces produced when the x-ray beam passes tangential to an edge formed between tissues of differing attenuation (Box 15-1).

Lines

A line is a longitudinal opacity no greater than 2 mm in width. Examples include the anterior and posterior junction lines, which are formed by the close apposition of the visceral and parietal layers of pleura of both lungs as they approximate anteriorly and posteriorly to the mediastinum (Fig. 15-1). The anterior portion of the thorax begins at the thoracic inlet. Therefore, the anterior junction line begins at the undersurface of the clavicles; it courses inferiorly toward the left in an oblique orientation to the level of the heart. Because the posterior portion of the thorax extends more superiorly than the anterior portion, the posterior junction line can be seen as it extends above the level of the clavicles. It frequently appears as a straight line and often projects through the tracheal air column. You will not always see the anterior and posterior junction lines on all radiographic examinations. However, detection of a displaced junction line allows both identification of a mediastinal abnormality and localization as either anterior or posterior.

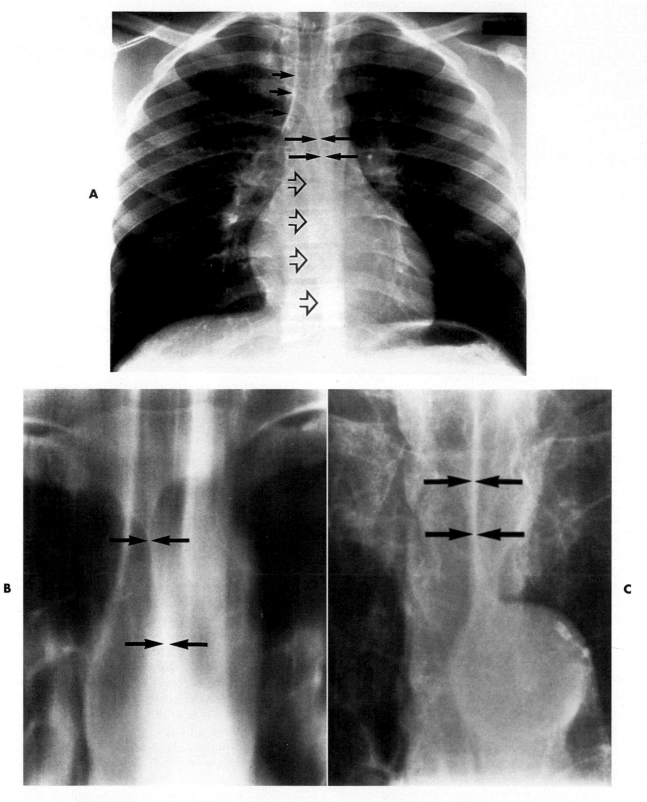

Figure 15-1   Mediastinal lines, stripes and interfaces. **A,** Frontal CXR demonstrates anterior junction line (*long black arrows*), right paratracheal stripe *(short black arrows),* and azygoesophageal interface *(open arrows).* **B,** AP tomogram demonstrates anterior junction line *(arrows).* Note that the anterior junction line begins below the level of the clavicles. **C,** Frontal CXR demonstrates posterior junction line *(arrows).* Note that the posterior junction line extends superiorly above the level of the clavicles.

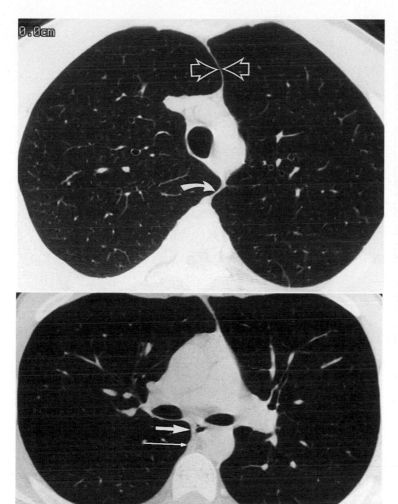

Figure 15-1, cont'd.   D, Axial high-resolution CT image demonstrates the anterior *(open arrows)* and posterior *(curved arrow)* junction lines. **E,** Axial CT image demonstrates the azygoeophageal interface, formed by the juxtaposition of aerated lung and the lateral walls of the azygous vein *(long, thin arrow)* and esophagus *(short arrow).*

Box 15-1   Detection: Mediastinal Landmarks

LINES

Anterior junction line
Posterior junction line
Right and left paraspinal lines

STRIPES

Right paratracheal stripe

INTERFACES

Azygoesophageal interface
Descending aortic interface

Two additional mediastinal lines are the right and left paraspinal lines, which are each about 1 mm wide. You can see these best on AP thoracic spine films. The left paraspinal line extends superiorly from the level of the aortic arch and inferiorly to the level of the diaphragm

and parallels the lateral margin of the vertebral bodies. An important relationship to keep in mind is the one between the left paraspinal line and the descending aortic interface (see section on interfaces). The left paraspinal line normally lies medial to the descending aortic interface. Displacement of the left paraspinal line lateral to the descending aortic interface signals the presence of a posterior mediastinal abnormality (Fig. 15-2). The right paraspinal line is less frequently visualized; when seen, it is often only identified over a portion of its course, generally between the eighth and twelfth thoracic vertebral levels. Both paraspinal lines are normally straight and maintain a constant relationship with the adjacent vertebral bodies, except when displaced laterally by osteophytes. An ectatic aorta may displace the left paraspinal line laterally.

Stripe

A stripe is a longitudinal composite opacity 2 to 5 mm in width. The right paratracheal stripe is formed by the apposition of the right upper lobe pleura and the right lateral tracheal wall. You can identify it on the majority of

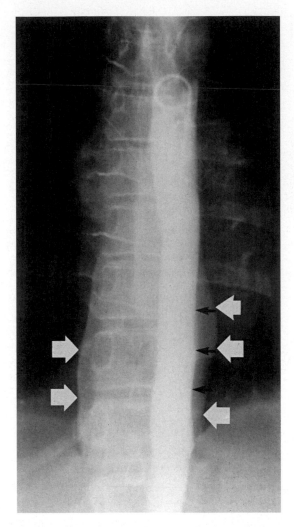

Figure 15-2 AP radiograph from an aortagram demonstrates contrast-opacification of the aorta and bilateral lateral displacement of the paraspinal lines *(white arrows)* in a patient with posterior mediastinal lymphadenopathy from lymphoma. Note that the left paraspinal line *(white arrows)* is displaced lateral to the descending aortic interface *(short black arrows)*.

chest radiographs. The normal right paratracheal stripe is identified as a smooth stripe adjacent to the right lateral border of the tracheal air column, extending inferiorly to the level of the azygous vein (Fig. 15-1). In normal individuals, it is seen as a smooth stripe of uniform width, measuring less than or equal to 3 mm in diameter. Widening of the right paratracheal stripe is a sign of middle mediastinal pathology, such as right paratracheal lymphadenopathy (Fig. 15-3).

Interfaces

An interface is the common boundary between the shadows of two juxtaposed tissues of differing opacity; for example, between the lungs and heart. Two interfaces that are important landmarks of normal mediastinal anatomy are the azygoesophageal interface and the descending aortic interface. The azygoesophageal interface

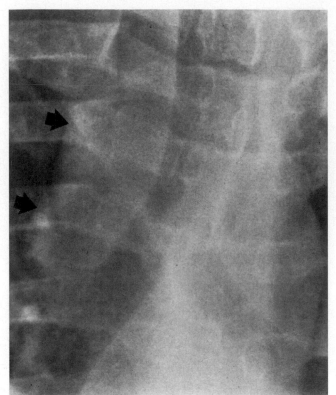

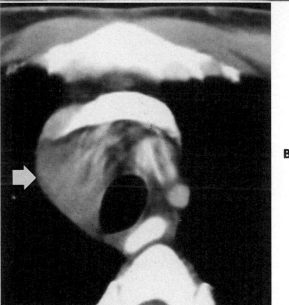

Figure 15-3 Right paratracheal lymphadenopathy. **A,** PA CXR demonstrates widening of the right paratracheal stripe *(arrows)*. **B,** Axial contrast-enhanced CT demonstrates right paratracheal lymphadenopathy *(white arrow)*.

is formed by the juxtaposition of aerated lung within the right lower lobe and the soft-tissue opacity of the right lateral margin of the azygous vein and/or esophagus (Fig. 15-1). You can frequently identify the azygoesophageal recess on well-penetrated PA chest radiographs as an interface beginning superiorly at the level of the azygous

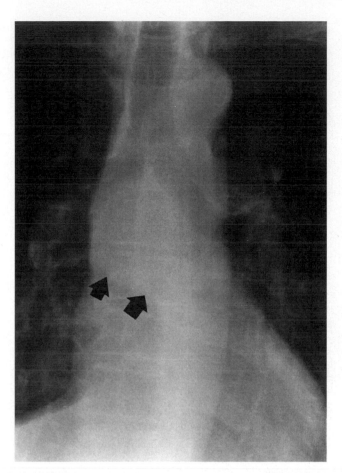

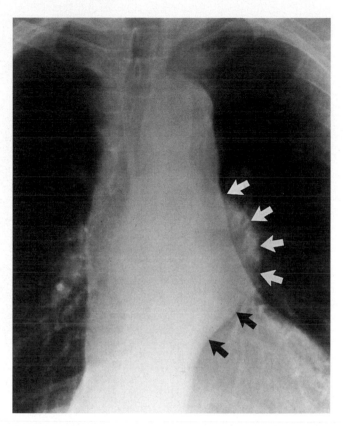

Figure 15-4   Bronchogenic cyst. PA CXR demonstrates an abnormal convex contour of the azygoesophageal interface *(arrows)* secondary to a subcarinal mass. Compare to the normal azygoesophageal interface in Fig. 15-1A.

Figure 15-5   Descending thoracic aortic aneurysm. PA CXR reveals convexity of the descending thoracic aortic interface *(white and black arrows),* corresponding to the presence of an aneurysm.

arch and extending inferiorly to the level of the diaphragm. The azygoesophageal interface normally produces a gentle concave slope as it curves slightly toward the left; a focal convexity of the azygoesophageal interface signals the presence of a mediastinal abnormality. Subcarinal masses such as bronchogenic cysts and esophageal abnormalities such as achalasia frequently produce abnormalities in the contour of the azygoesophageal interface (Fig. 15-4). The descending aortic interface is formed by the juxtaposition of aerated lung and the soft-tissue opacity of the left lateral margin of the descending thoracic aorta; it is usually visible from the top of the aortic arch to the level of the diaphragm inferiorly. Because the descending thoracic aorta is a posterior structure, abnormalities in the descending aortic interface imply pathology within the posterior mediastinum. A descending thoracic aortic aneurysm is a common cause for an abnormal contour of the descending aortic interface (Fig. 15-5).

In addition to a familiarity with the normal lines, stripes, and interfaces of the mediastinum, you should

also have a knowledge of the normal mediastinal contours on the frontal radiograph of the chest (Fig. 15-6). You should also carefully assess the lateral chest radiograph. Keep in mind that there are normally two "clear" spaces: retrosternal, between the sternum and ascending aorta; and retrocardiac, between the heart and spine. Midline anterior mediastinal masses are often best visualized on lateral chest radiographs as opacification within the normally clear retrosternal space (Fig. 15-7).

A thorough knowledge of normal mediastinal anatomy and of the changes produced by abnormalities within various portions of the mediastinum is important for both detection and localization of mediastinal abnormalities. A displaced mediastinal line, a widened stripe, and an abnormal contour of an interface are all important signs of mediastinal pathology.

It is extremely important to compare with previous radiographs. You can most easily see subtle changes in the lines, stripes, and interfaces of the mediastinum as a change in appearance on serial examinations.

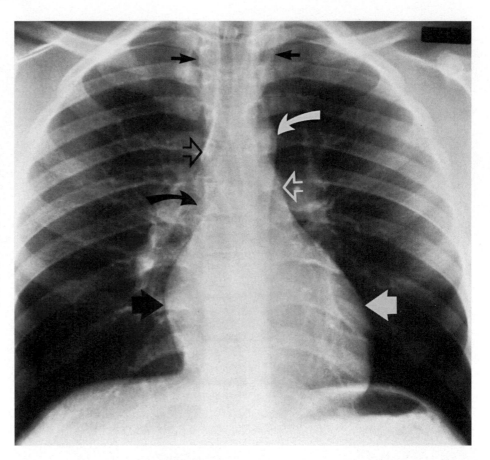

Figure 15-6 Normal mediastinal contours. The normal structures that comprise the mediastinal contours on the frontal chest radiograph have been labeled as follows (from superior to inferior): (1) brachiocephalic vessels, *small black arrows* (left and right); (2) aortic arch, *curved white arrow;* (3) azygous arch, *open black arrow;* (4) main pulmonary artery, *open white arrow;* (5) ascending aorta, *curved black arrow;* (6) right atrium, *large, short black arrow;* and (7) left ventricle, *large, short white arrow.*

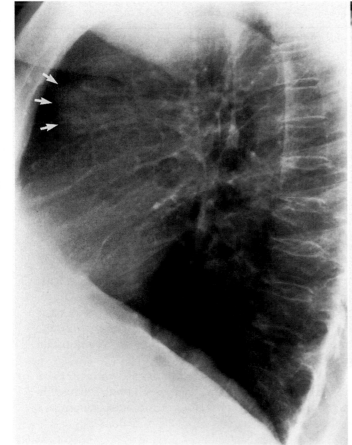

A

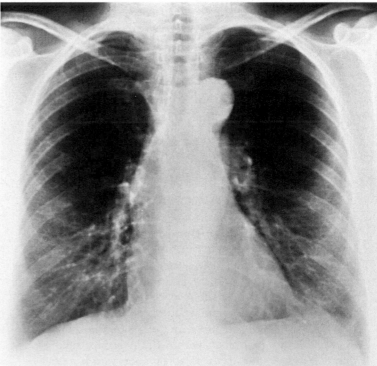

B

Figure 15-7 Thymoma.**A,** An anterior mediastinal mass is easily visualized on the lateral CXR as a sharply defined, round opacity *(arrows)* in the retrosternal space, but is difficult to identify on the frontal CXR, **B.** Because the mass is not in direct contact with structures that form the normal mediastinal contours on the frontal radiograph, it does not obliterate the margins of these structures.

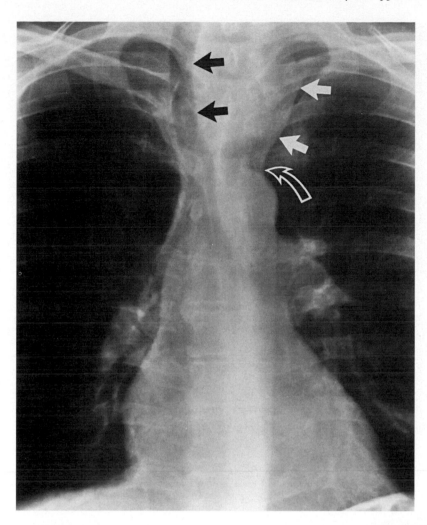

Figure 15-8 Thyroid adenoma. Frontal CXR demonstrates a large mass at the thoracic inlet that demonstrates four features suggestive of a mediastinal origin: smooth, sharp margins *(short white arrows);* obtuse angles with adjacent lung *(curved open arrow);* epicenter in the mediastinum; and an intimate effect on mediastinal structures (displacement of the trachea, *black arrows*).

Descriptive Features of Mediastinal Masses

Once detected, it is often difficult to determine whether a centrally located mass is mediastinal, pleural, or parenchymal in origin. Heitzman lists three primary descriptive features that are commonly seen in masses of mediastinal origin.

Intimate effect on mediastinal structures

The first feature, an intimate effect on mediastinal structures, is considered the most important feature in determining whether a centrally located mass is mediastinal in origin (Fig. 15-8). Displacement or compression of mediastinal structures, particularly a localized effect, strongly suggests that a mass is mediastinal in origin. Therefore, carefully inspect the tracheal air column and barium-filled esophagus for signs of displacement or compression when evaluating a centrally located mass.

Smooth, sharp margins

The second descriptive feature of mediastinal masses is smooth, sharp margins (Fig. 15-9). Smooth margins are created by displacement of the adjacent visceral and parietal layers of pleura, which surround the lateral mar-

Table 15-1 Mediastinal Mass versus Lung Mass	
Mediastinal mass	**Lung mass**
Smooth sharp margins	Usually irregular margins
Obtuse angles	Acute angles
Intimate effect on mediastinal structures	Does not usually produce an intimate effect on mediastinal structures

gin of a mediastinal mass. If a mass demonstrates irregular margins, it is more likely to originate in the lung than in the mediastinum.

Obtuse angles with adjacent lung

The third descriptive feature is formation of obtuse angles between the margins of the mass and adjacent lung (Fig. 15-9). Masses originating within the lung more often demonstrate acute angles. However, because there is considerable overlap between mediastinal and lung masses, it is better to combine criteria to determine whether a mass originates within the mediastinum or lung (Table 15-1).

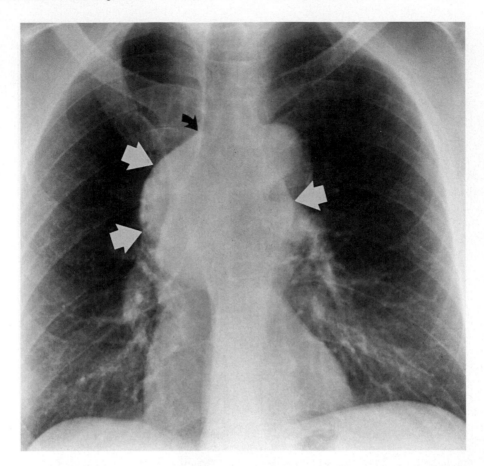

Figure 15-9 Posterior mediastinal mass. Frontal CXR shows a large, centrally located, posterior mass. This demonstrates three features suggestive of a mediastinal mass: smooth, sharp margins *(white arrows);* obtuse angles with adjacent lung *(small curved black arrow);* and epicenter within the mediastinum.

Table 15-2 Divisions of the mediastinum

Division	Boundaries	Normal structures
Anterior	Bounded anteriorly by the sternum posteriorly by the anterior margins of the pericardium, aorta, and brachiocephalic vessels	Thymus gland Lymph nodes Fat Internal mammary vessels
Middle	Bounded by posterior margin of anterior division and anterior margin of posterior division	Heart and pericardium Ascending and transverse aorta Brachiocephalic vessels SVC and IVC Main pulmonary vessels Trachea and main bronchi Lymph nodes Fat
Posterior	Bounded anteriorly by the posterior margins of the pericardium and great vessels and posteriorly by the thoracic vertebral bodies	Descending thoracic aorta Esophagus Thoracic duct Azygous/hemiazygous Autonomic nerves Lymph nodes Fat

Modified from Fraser RG, Pare JAP, Pare PD, Fraser FS, Genereux GP: *Diagnosis of diseases of the chest,* ed 3, Philadelphia, 1998, WB Saunders.

Additional features that can be helpful in determining that a mass is mediastinal include: epicenter in the mediastinum, bilaterality; and movement with swallowing rather than movement with respiration.

Divisions of the Mediastinum

Once you have detected an abnormality and decided it is mediastinal in origin, localizing the abnormality within a specific anatomic division of the mediastinum is the next most important step in generating a limited differential diagnosis. There are several different classification systems of the mediastinum, and these classifications are based on landmarks on the lateral chest radiograph rather than true anatomic fascial planes. The classification described here, a modified classification as proposed by Fraser and Paré, has been chosen for its simplicity and wide recognition (Table 15-2).

In this classification system, the mediastinum is divided into three compartments: anterior, middle, and posterior (Fig. 15-10).

Some classification systems include a fourth compartment, the superior mediastinum, which is bounded inferiorly by a line drawn from the sternal angle to the fourth intervertebral disc. Rather than containing structures unique to one compartment, this compartment contains structures that are continuous with compartments below it.

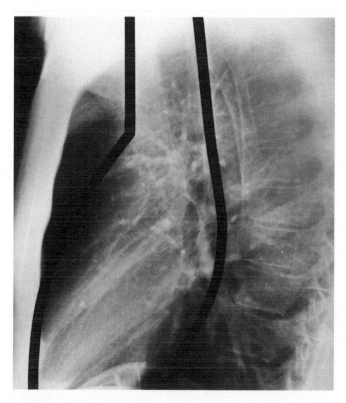

Figure 15-10 Mediastinal compartments. Lateral chest radiograph demonstrates boundaries of anterior, middle, and posterior compartments of the mediastinum.

Differential Diagnosis

Using a compartmental division of the mediastinum allows you to easily generate a limited differential diagnosis for a focal mediastinal abnormality. Based on location, you can consider lesions that are likely to occur in a specific division and exclude abnormalities that are unlikely to occur within that division.

First, consider abnormalities of the normal structures that reside in a given compartment (Table 15-2). For example, for a mass localized within the anterior mediastinum, consider abnormalities of the thymus gland, lymph nodes, and anterior mediastinal fat, as well as in the internal mammary vessels. Abnormalities of the thymus gland, specifically thymoma, account for the majority of anterior mediastinal masses in adults in most series. Abnormalities of the lymph nodes, especially Hodgkin's lymphoma, are also a common cause of anterior mediastinal masses. A knowledge of other common masses that occur within the anterior mediastinum, such as germ-cell neoplasms and thyroid abnormalities, will help you complete the list of diagnostic considerations in most cases.

Table 15-3 summarizes the common differential diagnoses for each of the three mediastinal compartments. As you review these lists, notice that the majority of diagnoses relate to abnormalities of structures normally located within each compartment. These differential diagnoses are based on the statistical likelihood of a mass occurring within a given compartment. Be aware that many of these entities can occur in any of the three compartments but are much more likely to occur in the one

Table 15-3	Differential diagnosis of mediastinal masses
Anterior mediastinum	**Thymoma**
	Lymphoma
	Germ cell neoplasms
	Thyroid abnormalities*
Middle mediastinum	**Lymphadenopathy**
	Bronchogenic cyst
	Vascular abnormalities
	Pericardial cyst
	Tracheal tumor
Posterior mediastinum	**Neurogenic tumors**
	Paravertebral abnormalities
	Vascular abnormalities
	Esophageal abnormalities
	Lymphadenopathy
	Neurenteric cyst
	Bochdalek hernia
	Extramedullary hematopoeisis

Bold print signifies most common entity in each compartment.
*Thyroid abnormalities frequently extend into middle and posterior compartments as well.

noted. For example, although bronchogenic cysts have been described in all three mediastinal compartments, the vast majority occur in the middle mediastinum.

Careful analysis of imaging features and correlation with clinical data such as patient age and symptoms can effectively narrow the differential diagnosis and in some cases can lead to a specific diagnosis. For imaging features and demographic characteristics of the common mediastinal masses in each compartment, see the following chapter.

SUGGESTED READINGS

Davis RD, Oldham HN, Sabiston DC: Primary cysts and neoplasms of the mediastinum: recent changes in clinical presentation, methods of diagnosis, management and results, *Ann Thorac Surg* 44:229-237, 1987.

Felson B: *Chest roentgenology,* Philadelphia, 1973, WB Saunders.

Fraser RG, Pare JAP, Pare PD et al: *Diagnosis of diseases of the chest,* ed 3, Philadelphia, 1988, WB Saunders.

Heitzman ER: The mediastinum: radiologic correlations with anatomy and pathology, ed 2, Berlin, Germany, 1988, Springer-Verlag.

McLoud TC, Ragozzino MW: MR imaging of the thorax. In Edelman RR, Hesselink JR, editors: *Clinical magnetic resonance imaging,* Philadelphia, 1990, WB Saunders, pp 731-744.

Naidich DP, Zerhouni EA, Siegelman SS: Computed tomography and magnetic resonance of the thorax, ed 2, New York, 1991, Raven Press.

Pierson DJ: Disorders of the pleura, mediastinum and diaphragm. In Wilson JD, Braunwald E, Isselbacher KJ et al, editors: *Harrison's principles and practices of internal medicine,* ed 12, vol 2, New York, 1991, McGraw-Hill, pp 1111-1116.

Reed JC: Chest radiology: plain film patterns and differential diagnoses, ed 3, St. Louis, Mo, 1991, Mosby-Year Book.

Shaffer K, Pugatch RD: Diseases of the mediastinum. In Freundlich IM, Bragg DG, editors: *Radiologic approach to diseases of the chest,* Baltimore, 1992, Williams & Wilkins, pp 171-185.

Vail CM, Ravin CE: Mediastinal masses. In Freundlich IM, Bragg DG, editors: *Radiologic approach to diseases of the chest,* Baltimore, 1992, William & Wilkins, pp 360-373.

Webb WR: Diseases of the mediastinum. In Putman CE, Ravin CE, editors: *Textbook of diagnostic imaging,* ed 2, Philadelphia, 1994, WB Saunders, pp 428-447.

CHAPTER *16*

Mediastinal Masses

PHILLIP M. BOISELLE

DIAGNOSTIC IMAGING WORKUP OF MEDIASTINAL MASSES

Radiologic examination of a mediastinal mass can generally narrow the differential diagnosis to two or three likely entities. In some cases, imaging features allow you to make a specific diagnosis. The radiologic work up varies depending on the location of the mass (Fig. 16-1) (Box 16-1).

For masses localized within the anterior compartment of the mediastinum, computed tomography (CT) is a good diagnostic choice. It provides information concerning the precise location of a mass and its relationship to adjacent mediastinal structures. CT can also determine whether a mass is cystic or solid, and whether it contains calcium or fat. In many cases, noncontrast CT will be sufficient. In certain cases, however, contrast-enhanced CT will provide important information concerning enhancement of the mass and the relationship of the mass to adjacent vascular structures. You may find correlative nuclear medicine studies helpful in suspected cases of Hodgkin's lymphoma (gallium scan) and substernal goiter (radioiodine scan).

CT is also the preferred imaging modality for further evaluation of a middle mediastinal mass. Contrast-enhanced CT is preferred for the evaluation of middle mediastinal masses, especially when you suspect a vascular abnormality. Magnetic resonance imaging (MRI) is superior to contrast-enhanced CT in assessing the relationship of a mass to vascular structures and in deter-

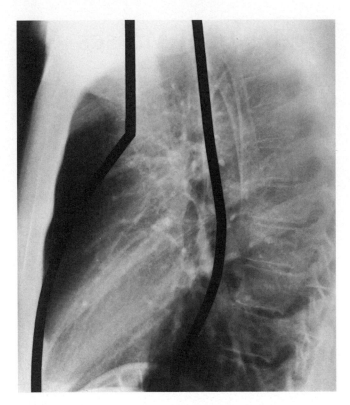

Figure 16-1 Mediastinal compartments. A lateral chest radiograph demonstrates the boundaries of the anterior, middle, and posterior mediastinal compartments.

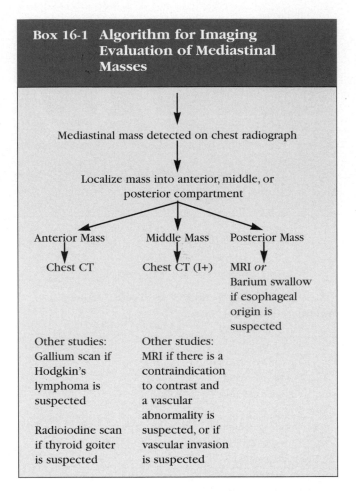

Box 16-1 Algorithm for Imaging Evaluation of Mediastinal Masses

Mediastinal mass detected on chest radiograph

Localize mass into anterior, middle, or posterior compartment

Anterior Mass	Middle Mass	Posterior Mass
Chest CT	Chest CT (I+)	MRI *or* Barium swallow if esophageal origin is suspected

Other studies: Gallium scan if Hodgkin's lymphoma is suspected

Radioiodine scan if thyroid goiter is suspected

Other studies: MRI if there is a contraindication to contrast and a vascular abnormality is suspected, or if vascular invasion is suspected

mining vascular invasion. MRI should be the first cross-sectional imaging study for patients with a suspected vascular abnormality who have a contraindication to intravenous contrast.

For masses localized within the posterior mediastinum, MRI is usually preferred because of its superior ability to assess the relationship of the mass to the adjacent spine. An exception occurs when a posterior mediastinal mass is suspected to be of esophageal origin. In this situation, a barium swallow should be obtained.

You should be aware that the algorithm presented in this chapter is a general guideline. The decision to obtain a CT or an MRI may vary, depending on several factors. These include the availability of MRI, patient factors (contraindication to intravenous contrast or contraindications to MRI), and institutional practices. In some cases, CT and MRI will provide complementary information, and both may be indicated.

ANTERIOR MEDIASTINAL MASSES

Thymic Abnormalities

The thymus is a bilobed structure that is normally located within the anterior mediastinum. The thymus reaches its maximum weight at puberty and subsequent-ly undergoes fatty involution over a 5- to 15-year period. There are a wide variety of thymic abnormalities that may present as an anterior mediastinal mass.

Thymoma

The most common thymic abnormality to present as an anterior mediastinal mass is *thymoma*, a neoplasm arising from thymic epithelium (Box 16-2).

Thymomas account for the majority of anterior mediastinal masses in adults and typically occur as incidental findings in otherwise healthy individuals. However, thymomas may also occur in association with other abnormalities, including myasthenia gravis, red cell aplasia, and hypogammaglobulinema. The association with myasthenia gravis is the most common of the three; roughly 15% of patients with myasthenia gravis have a thymoma, while roughly 50% of patients with thymomas have myasthenia gravis.

As with other midline anterior mediastinal masses, plain radiographic findings are often limited to the lateral chest radiograph, which may demonstrate a well-defined mass in the normally clear retrosternal space. Small masses may not be detectable on plain radiographs, but CT will often help assess the presence of a thymoma in patients with myasthenia gravis. Characteris-

Box 16-2   Thymoma

DEMOGRAPHICS

Age

Usually 40–60; unusual in patients less than 30

Gender

Male and females, equally

Associations

Myasthenia gravis, hypogammaglobulinemia, red cell aplasia

DESCRIPTIVE FEATURES

Thymoma (Noninvasive)

Well-defined, round, soft-tissue density mass, usually located anterior to the junction of the heart and great vessels
Curvilinear calcification in 20%

Invasive Thymoma

Additional findings of invasion of adjacent mediastinal structures, chest wall invasion, or contiguous spread along pleural surfaces (usually unilaterally)

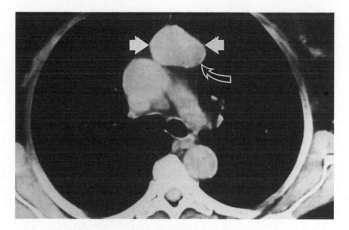

Figure 16-2   Thymoma. Axial CT image demonstrates an oval, homogeneous soft-tissue mass *(short closed arrows)* in the anterior mediastinum, with a thin rim of peripheral calcification posteriorly *(open curved arrow)*. Calcification occurs in approximately 20% of thymomas.

Box 16-3   Thymic Hyperplasia—Associated Systemic Abnormalities

Hyperthyroidism
Acromegaly
Addison's disease
Myasthenia gravis
Systemic lupus erythematosis
Scleroderma
Rheumatoid arthritis

tic CT imaging features include a well-defined, round, or oval mass, usually of homogeneous soft-tissue density, located within the anterior mediastinum (Fig. 16-2). Although they are most commonly located anterior to the junction of the heart and great vessels, thymomas may occur at any level from the thoracic inlet to the diaphragm. In roughly 20% of cases, there is evidence of calcification, which is typically curvilinear.

The majority of thymomas are benign lesions confined within a fibrous capsule, but roughly 30% of thymomas are more aggressive and demonstrate invasion through the fibrous capsule. Interestingly, both forms appear similar histologically. Malignancy is therefore based on demonstration of invasion through the fibrous capsule, often first detected at surgery, rather than on the histologic features of the neoplasm. The term "invasive" thymoma is preferred to "malignant" thymoma. Invasive thymomas typically spread locally (Fig. 16-3), and metastases outside of the thorax are rare.

Thymic Hyperplasia

Thymic hyperplasia (Box 16-3) is associated with a wide variety of systemic abnormalities, including hyperthyroidism. You will often see "rebound" thymic hyperplasia in patients who have been treated with chemotherapy.

Thymic hyperplasia is usually identified on CT as enlargement of the thymus gland, which maintains its normal bilobed, "arrowhead" configuration (Fig. 16-4). In contrast, most other thymic abnormalities appear as a discrete mass rather than as uniform glandular enlargement.

Thymic Carcinoid

Thymic carcinoid tumor is rare and is thought to arise from thymic cells of neural crest origin. Patients with thymic carcinoid tumors often present with endocrine abnormalities, including Cushing's syndrome; the syndrome of inappropriate antidiuretic hormone secretion (SIADH); hyperparathyroidism; and multiple endocrine neoplasia (MEN I) syndrome.

There are no distinguishing radiologic features of thymic carcinoid, and the diagnosis is often suspected on the basis of the presence of endocrine abnormalities in a patient with an anterior mediastinal mass.

Thymic Carcinoma

Thymic carcinoma is a recently described rare neoplasm that occurs in adult patients. Because the thymus gland may also be a site of metastatic disease, particularly from breast and lung cancer, a diagnosis of primary thymic carcinoma is made by excluding a primary carci-

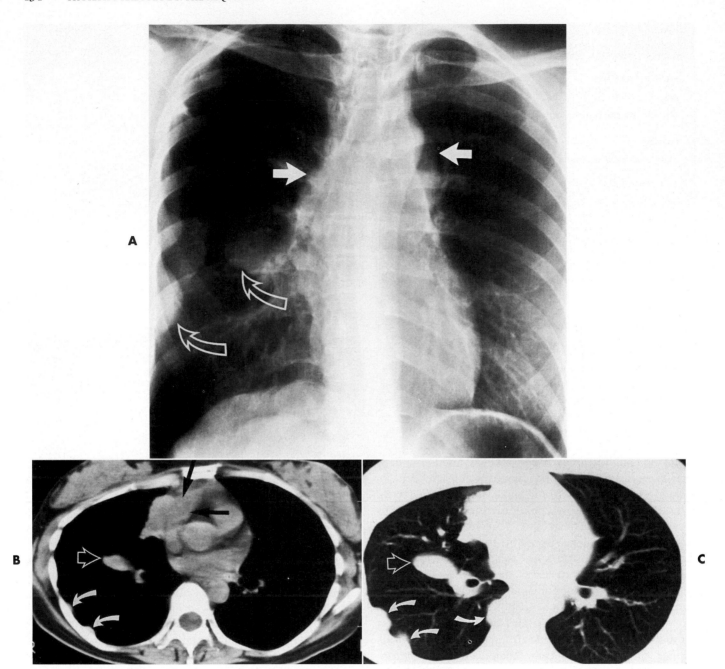

Figure 16-3   Invasive thymoma. **A,** PA chest radiograph demonstrates a lobulated anterior medi-astinal mass *(closed white arrows)* as well as multiple pleural masses in the right hemithorax *(curved open arrows)*. **B,** Axial CT image of the chest (filmed in soft-tissue windows) demonstrates an anterior mediastinal mass *(closed black arrows)* and multiple unilateral pleural masses *(curved white arrows)*. Note that one of the pleural masses is located within the minor fissure *(open white arrow)*. **C,** Axial CT image of the chest (filmed in lung windows) again demonstrates multiple pleu-ral masses *(curved closed arrows)*, including a pleural mass within the minor fissure *(open white arrow)*. The presence of an anterior mediastinal mass and unilateral pleural masses is highly sug-gestive of invasive thymoma.

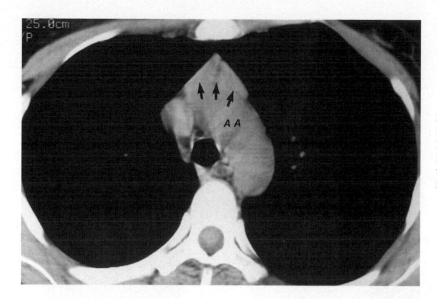

Figure 16-4 Thymic hyperplasia secondary to hyperthyroidism. Axial CT image of the chest at the level of the aortic arch *(AA)* demonstrates enlargement of the thymus gland *(short black arrows),* which maintains its normal bilobed "arrowhead" configuration.

thymic carcinoma is made by excluding a primary carcinoma elsewhere.

Radiographically, thymic carcinoma usually presents as a solid mass with poorly defined margins. It is a very aggressive lesion and is often locally invasive. In contrast to invasive thymomas, which rarely metastasize outside the thorax, thymic carcinomas may metastasize hematogenously to distant organs.

Thymic Cyst

Thymic cysts may be congenital or acquired. Acquired thymic cysts are most often associated with Hodgkin's disease following radiation therapy.

Radiographically, a thymic cyst usually appears as a well-defined, cystic mass with an imperceptible wall. The CT attenuation values are typically consistent with fluid; however, the appearance may vary if hemorrhage or infection complicate the cyst. Curvilinear calcification of the cyst wall occurs in a minority of cases.

Thymic Lymphoma

Thymic involvement may occur in up to a third of patients with Hodgkin's lymphoma and is usually accompanied by involvement of mediastinal lymph nodes.

Thymic lymphoma usually presents as a homogeneous, round, soft-tissue density mass without calcification. The presence of associated enlarged mediastinal lymph nodes may suggest the diagnosis.

Thymolipoma

Thymolipoma is rare. It is a benign thymic neoplasm composed primarily of fat, but it also contains strands of thymic tissue. Thymolipomas most often occur in younger patients and are usually identified on chest radiographs as incidental findings.

Because of their soft, pliable nature, thymolipomas commonly drape around the heart and other mediastinal

---

Box 16-4 Hodgkin's Lymphoma

DEMOGRAPHICS

Age

Bimodal distribution, with initial peak in young adults and second peak after age 50

Gender

Male predominance, especially among younger patients

DESCRIPTIVE FEATURES

Variable appearance, ranging from a single spherical soft-tissue mass to a large lobulated mass
Margins may be well-defined or irregular
The mass may be homogeneous or heterogeneous soft-tissue attenuation
Calcification is rare in untreated cases

---

structures. They are often quite large at the time of presentation, and they may mimic cardiac enlargement on chest radiographs. Identification of fat within the mass on either CT or MRI suggests the diagnosis (Fig. 16-5).

Hodgkin's Lymphoma

The majority of patients with Hodgkin's lymphoma (Box 16-4) present with mediastinal lymphadenopathy. Although most of these patients present with multiple sites of lymph node involvement, isolated anterior mediastinal lymphadenopathy is the most common site of a localized nodal mass, particularly in the subset of patients with nodular sclerosing type. Within the anterior mediastinum, Hodgkin's lymphoma often involves both anterior mediastinal lymph nodes and the thymus; how-

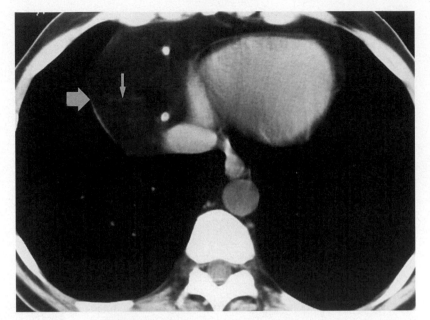

Figure 16-5 Thymolipoma. Axial CT image of the chest demonstrates a right cardiophrenic angle mass, which is predominately fat attenuation. Note thin strands of soft-tissue attenuation *(white arrow)* within the mass, representing strands of thymic tissue, as well as foci of calcification.

ever, isolated thymic involvement without associated lymph node involvement is unusual.

Imaging features vary, ranging from a single, spherical soft-tissue mass in the anterior mediastinum to a large lobulated mass representing a conglomeration of lymph nodes. On CT, the mass may be of homogeneous soft-tissue density or may appear heterogeneous: the low-attenuation areas represent necrosis. Whereas anterior mediastinal masses from lymphoma typically demonstrate well-defined margins, invasion of adjacent lung parenchyma may result in irregular margins. Invasion into the chest wall may also occur (Fig. 16-6). When presenting as a solitary, spherical mass, lymphoma may be indistinguishable from thymoma. Correlative nuclear medicine gallium imaging may be helpful because the majority of Hodgkin's lymphomas are gallium-avid.

Associated lymphadenopathy in other compartments of the mediastinum and associated extrathoracic lymphadenopathy each suggest the diagnosis of lymphoma. An important discriminating feature is the absence of calcification in untreated lymphoma. Although the presence of calcification strongly suggests a diagnosis other than lymphoma, calcification frequently occurs in cases of treated lymphoma, but only rarely in untreated cases.

Germ-Cell Neoplasms

Primary germ-cell neoplasms (GCN) arise from rests of primitive germ cells that were left within the mediastinum during their migration from the yolk sac to the urogenital ridge. The anterior mediastinum is the most common extragonadal site of GCN.

There are a variety of benign and malignant GCN (Box 16-5). The majority of GCN (70%) are benign, comprising mostly teratomas and dermoid cysts. Dermoid cysts contain only ectodermal layer elements, but teratomas contain elements of all three germinal layers. A variety of malignant GCN occur within the anterior mediastinum, including seminoma; choriocarcinoma; embryonal cell carcinoma, and yolk sac tumors, the most aggressive GCN. Teratomas are almost always benign, but carcinoma may rarely develop within one of the germinal layer elements.

Patients with GCN may be asymptomatic or may have symptoms from compression or invasion of adjacent mediastinal structures. Because GCNs grow rapidly and have a propensity to invade mediastinal structures, patients with malignant GCN are more likely to be symptomatic.

Box 16-5 Germ-Cell Neoplasms

DEMOGRAPHICS

Age

Young patients, usually third decade

Gender

Malignant germ cell neoplasms—male predominance

DESCRIPTIVE FEATURES

Benign GCN (Teratoma, Dermoid Cyst)

Heterogeneous, predominately cystic mass with solid components
Well-defined margins
Calcification common
Presence of fat is suggestive; identification of a tooth, while rare, is diagnostic

Malignant GCN (Seminoma, Choriocarcinoma, Embryonal Cell Carcinoma, Yolk Sac Tumor)

Heterogeneous, solid mass
Irregular margins
Calcification uncommon

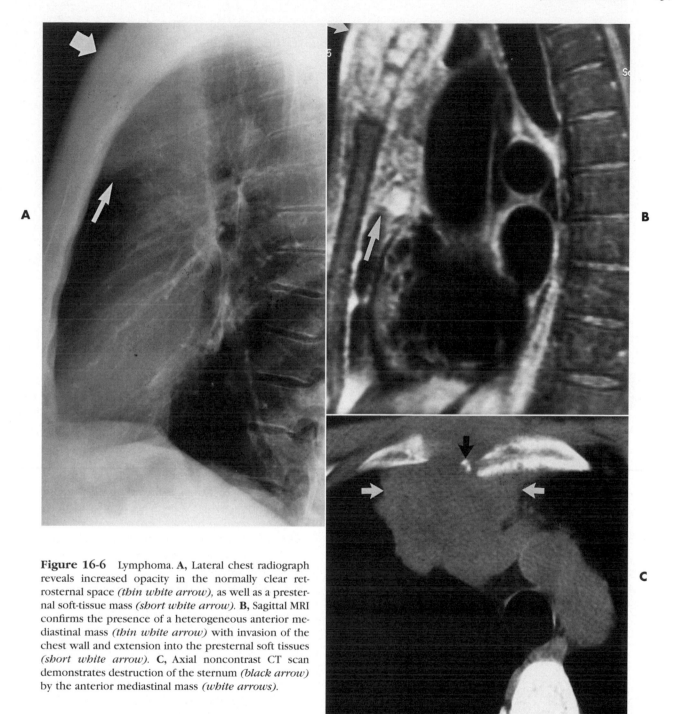

Figure 16-6 Lymphoma. **A,** Lateral chest radiograph reveals increased opacity in the normally clear retrosternal space *(thin white arrow)*, as well as a presternal soft-tissue mass *(short white arrow).* **B,** Sagittal MRI confirms the presence of a heterogeneous anterior mediastinal mass *(thin white arrow)* with invasion of the chest wall and extension into the presternal soft tissues *(short white arrow).* **C,** Axial noncontrast CT scan demonstrates destruction of the sternum *(black arrow)* by the anterior mediastinal mass *(white arrows).*

Dermoid cysts and teratomas have similar imaging features. Both typically appear as heterogeneous, predominately cystic masses with well-defined margins, and both frequently contain calcification. The presence of foci of fat or a fat-fluid level is highly suggestive of a dermoid cyst or teratoma (Fig. 16-7). Although rare, the identification of a tooth within the mass is diagnostic.

Surgical excision of teratomas and dermoid cysts is usually curative. In contrast, patients with malignant

GCN usually have a very poor prognosis, with the exception of those with seminoma. Mediastinal seminomas are usually radiosensitive and patients have an overall survival of roughly 75%.

Thyroid Abnormalities

Thyroid abnormalities (Box 16-6) account for the majority of thoracic inlet masses in adults. They may ex-

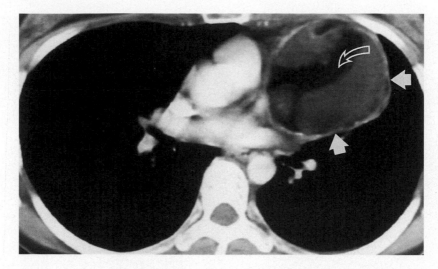

Figure 16-7 Teratoma. Axial contrast-enhanced CT image reveals a large heterogeneous anterior mediastinal mass with a calcified rim *(short white arrows)*. Note the presence of fat attenuation within the mass *(curved open arrow)*, highly suggestive of a teratoma.

Box 16-6 Thyroid Masses

DEMOGRAPHICS

Age

Usually >30 years of age

Gender

Female predominance

DESCRIPTIVE FEATURES

CXR Features Include

Well-defined mass that extends from above the thoracic inlet

Displacement and/or compression of the trachea

Foci of calcification may occasionally be visible

CT Features Include

Continuity with the cervical thyroid gland

Foci of high attenuation on noncontrast images

Intense enhancement following intravenous contrast administration

Cystic areas and foci of calcification are common

---

tend inferiorly into the anterior, middle, and posterior compartments of the mediastinum. When located in the anterior mediastinum, thyroid masses are almost always located posterior to the great vessels, usually in a paratracheal location. However, most other anterior mediastinal masses are commonly located anterior to the great vessels. Therefore, a mediastinal mass located anterior to the great vessels in a retrosternal location is unlikely to be of thyroid origin.

The majority of mediastinal masses of thyroid origin represent thyroid goiters, and they almost always extend inferiorly from the thyroid gland. A truly ectopic thyroid goiter is rare. Other thyroid abnormalities, such as thyroid adenomas and malignant thyroid neoplasms, infrequently extend into the mediastinum.

Because thyroid goiters account for the majority of mediastinal masses of thyroid origin, the demographics of thyroid mediastinal masses are similar to those of thyroid goiter with tendency to occur predominately in middle-aged female patients. Most patients are asymptomatic, but symptoms may arise from compression of the trachea or esophagus.

The following are the CT imaging features of mediastinal thyroid goiters: (1) continuity of the mass with the cervical thyroid gland; (2) foci of high attenuation on noncontrast examination (reflecting high iodine content of thyroid tissue); (3) foci of heterogeneous attenuation (low attenuation cystic areas and high-attenuation foci of calcification); and (4) intense and prolonged enhancement following administration of intravenous contrast. As on plain radiographs, deviation or compression of the trachea is frequently identified on CT. Large thyroid masses, especially posterior-descending goiters, may also compress the esophagus.

The most important of these features is demonstration of continuity of the mass with the cervical thyroid gland. A combined CT examination of the lower neck and chest is best (Fig. 16-8), although you can also use MRI (Fig. 16-9). Nuclear medicine radioiodine scan may be confirmatory, with demonstration of radioiodine uptake from foci of functioning thyroid tissue within the mass.

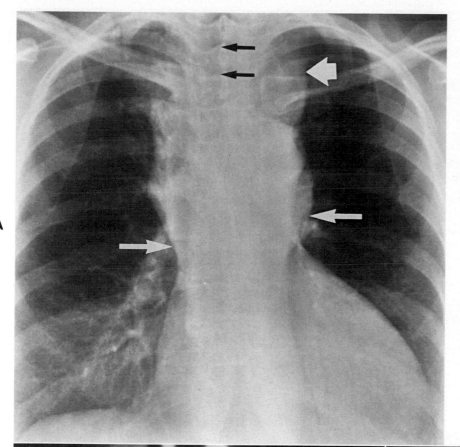

A

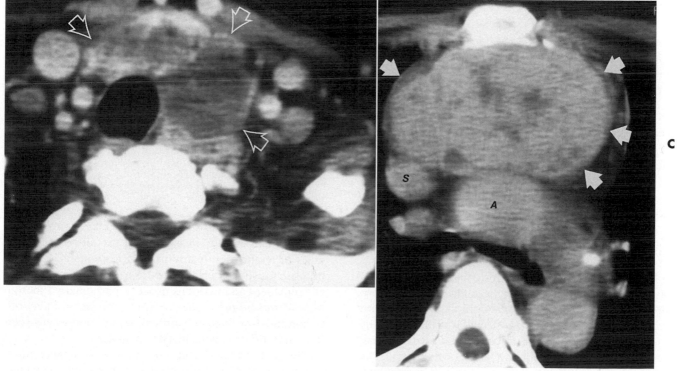

B   C

Figure 16-8 Thyroid goiter. **A,** PA chest radiograph demonstrates a large anterior mediastinal mass. The superior extent of the mass *(short white arrow)* extends above the thoracic inlet and is associated with rightward deviation of the trachea *(black arrows)*. The mass extends inferiorly to the level of the base of the heart *(thin white arrows)*. **B,** Axial contrast-enhanced CT image of the lower neck demonstrates a heterogeneous mass *(open white arrows)* that is continuous with the isthmus and left lobe of the thyroid gland. The mass contains foci of thyroid tissue that demonstrate intense enhancement, as well as foci of low attenuation consistent with cysts. **C,** Axial contrast-enhanced CT image at the level of the aortic arch demonstrates the large substernal component of the mass *(short white arrows)*, which displaces the ascending aorta *(A)* and superior vena cava *(S)* posteriorly.

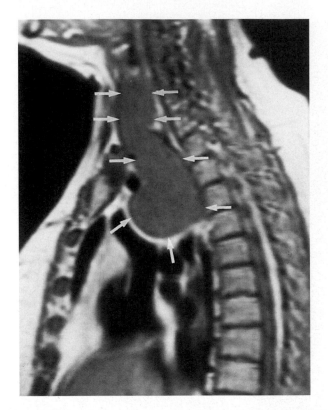

Figure 16-9 Thyroid goiter. Right parasagittal T1-weighted MRI image demonstrates a homogeneous mass *(arrows)* that extends inferiorly from the right lobe of the thyroid gland to involve the middle and posterior mediastinal compartments.

MIDDLE MEDIASTINAL MASSES

Lymphadenopathy

Lymphadenopathy (Box 16-7) is the most common cause of a middle mediastinal mass and may be neoplastic, inflammatory, or infectious in etiology (Box 16-8). Therefore, it is no surprise that there are no distinguishing demographic features for this cause.

You should consider lymphadenopathy in assessing a middle mediastinal mass when the mass is localized to a known anatomic lymph node site such as the azygous, subcarinal, or aortic-pulmonary window regions. Lymphadenopathy often presents as multiple discrete masses (Fig. 16-10), in contrast to most other causes of mediastinal masses, which usually present as a single mass. Therefore, the presence of multiple masses within known anatomic lymph node sites is highly suggestive of lymphadenopathy.

CT plays a role both in detecting and characterizing lymph nodes. Although lymph nodes often appear as homogeneous soft-tissue density on CT, they may also demonstrate calcification, low-density centers, or vascular enhancement. When present, these lymph-node characteristics allow you to shorten the lengthy differential diagnosis of mediastinal lymphadenopathy (Box 16-9).

Box 16-7 Lymphadenopathy

DEMOGRAPHICS

No general distinguishing demographic features

DESCRIPTIVE FEATURES

Single or multiple round or elliptical masses located within known anatomic sites of lymph nodes
Often homogeneous soft-tissue density on CT, but may demonstrate calcification, low-density centers, or vascular enhancement (see Box 16-9).

Box 16-8 Mediastinal Lymphadenopathy Differential Diagnosis

NEOPLASTIC

Metastatic disease (bronchogenic carcinoma or extrathoracic primary*)
Lymphoma
Leukemia

INFECTIOUS

Tuberculosis
Fungal infection (especially histoplasmosis)
Viral infection (measles, infectious mononucleosis)**
Bacterial infection**

DRUG REACTION

Diphenylhydantoin (dilantin)

INFLAMMATORY

Sarcoidosis
Castleman's disease
Angioimmunoblastic lymphadenopathy

*Extrathoracic primaries that commonly metastasize to mediastinal lymph nodes include genitourinary tumors, head and neck carcinomas, thyroid carcinomas, melanoma, and breast carcinoma.
**Lymphadenopathy infrequently detected on CXR but often seen on CT.

Identification of low-density mediastinal lymph nodes is particularly helpful in narrowing the differential diagnosis of lymphadenopathy in AIDS patients (Fig. 16-11) because low-density lymph nodes in an AIDS patient usually represent an infectious process, particularly tuberculosis, *M. avium-intracellulare* (MAI), or fungal infection. In contrast, low-density lymph nodes are not usually seen in neoplastic processes in AIDS patients.

Although calcified lymph nodes may occur secondary to many etiologies, the presence of peripheral calcification within a lymph node, referred to as "eggshell calcification," is suggestive of silicosis or coal worker's pneumoconiosis. However, eggshell calcification is not pathognomonic of these entities because it may also be an

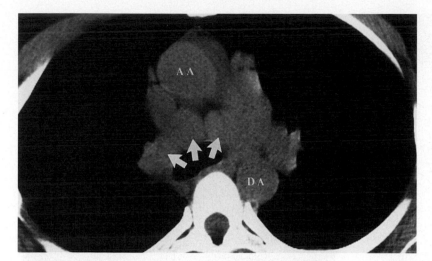

Figure 16-10 Sarcoidosis. Axial noncontrast CT image demonstrates discrete, round, soft-tissue masses *(arrows)* in the anterior subcarinal region, consistent with enlarged lymph nodes. Other images (not shown) demonstrated lymphadenopathy in the right paratracheal region and both hila, a characteristic distribution of lymphadenopathy in sarcoidosis. *AA=* ascending aorta; *DA=*descending aorta.

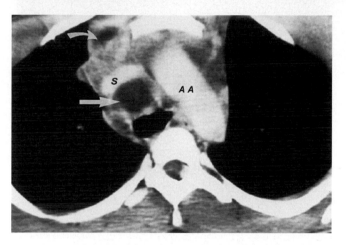

Figure 16-11 Mediastinal lymphadenopathy secondary to tuberculosis infection in an AIDS patient. Axial contrast-enhanced CT image demonstrates pretracheal *(straight white arrow)* and prevascular *(curved white arrow)* enlarged lymph nodes. Note the low attenuation of the lymph nodes and the peripheral enhancement, a characteristic appearance of tuberculosis lymphadenopathy in HIV-positive patients.

unusual manifestation of sarcoidosis, granulomatous infection, treated lymphoma, scleroderma, and amyloidosis.

The presence of associated hilar lymphadenopathy and its distribution (unilateral or bilateral) is also helpful in narrowing the differential diagnosis of lymphadenopathy (Box 16-10).

Bronchogenic Cyst

Bronchogenic cysts (Box 16-11) are the result of an abnormality in primitive foregut development. Although they occur in all three mediastinal compartments, the middle mediastinum is the most common site. The cysts are lined by respiratory epithelium and their walls contain cartilage, smooth muscle, or mucous glands.

You will usually detect bronchogenic cysts as an incidental finding in asymptomatic patients, but they occa-

---

Box 16-9 Mediastinal Lymphadenopathy: Characteristic Features

ISODENSITY LYMPH NODES

Infectious

Tuberculosis
M. avium-intracellulare (MAI) } May have low-density center

Fungal

Neoplastic

Metastases (seminoma, lung cancer)
Lymphoma (not commonly seen in AIDS-related lymphoma)

CALCIFIED LYMPH NODES

Infectious

Fungal (especially histoplasmosis)
Tuberculosis

Neoplastic

Hodgkin's lymphoma following radiation therapy
Metastases (especially mucinous adenocarcinoma)

Inflammatory

Sarcoidosis (5% of cases)

Inhalational

Silicosis (often eggshell appearance of calcification)

ENHANCING LYMPH NODES

Neoplastic

Metastases (especially renal-cell carcinoma, thyroid carcinoma, and small-cell lung cancer)

Inflammatory

Castleman's disease (benign lymph-node hyperplasia)
Sarcoidosis (rare)

Box 16-10 Hilar Lymphadenopathy Differential Diagnosis

UNILATERAL

Neoplastic

Metastatic (bronchogenic carcinoma, extrathoracic primary*)

Lymphoma

Infectious

Tuberculosis

Fungal

Viral

BILATERAL, ASYMMETRIC

Neoplastic

Lymphoma

Leukemia (chronic lymphocytic leukemia)

Metastases (bronchogenic carcinoma, extrathoracic primary*)

Infectious

Fungal

BILATERAL, SYMMETRIC

Inflammatory

Sarcoidosis

*Extrathoracic primary carcinomas that commonly metastasize to hilar lymph nodes include genitourinary tumors, head and neck carcinomas, thyroid carcinomas, melanoma, and breast carcinoma.

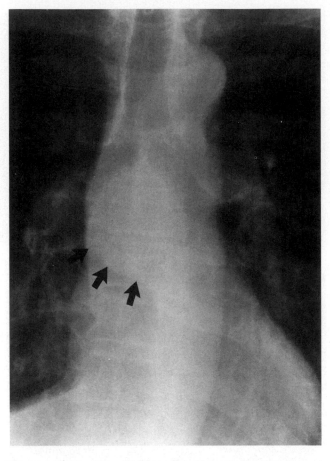

Figure 16-12 Bronchogenic cyst. Frontal chest radiograph demonstrates a well-defined, round, subcarinal mass. Note the focal convexity of the azygoesophageal interface *(arrows)*. The subcarinal region is the most common location of a bronchogenic cyst.

Box 16-11 Bronchogenic Cyst

DEMOGRAPHICS

Age

Often seen in younger patients, but may be detected at any age

Gender

Males and females equally

DESCRIPTIVE FEATURES

Subcarinal or right paratracheal location

Well-defined, homogeneous mass with imperceptible wall

Fluid or soft-tissue attenuation on CT

Variable appearance on MRI, depending on cyst contents: low signal on T1 and bright on T2, or bright signal or T1 and bright on T2 (if cyst contains mucin, protein, or hemorrhage)

sionally cause symptoms secondary to compression of adjacent structures. Infrequently, they may cause symptoms secondary to infection.

The most common location is subcarinal, and the presence of a well-defined subcarinal mass in an asymptomatic patient should suggest a bronchogenic cyst (Fig. 16-12). The right paratracheal region is the second most common location.

Imaging features include a well-defined, round, or oval homogeneous mass with a thin, often imperceptible wall. Air within the cyst is uncommon and suggests secondary infection and communication with the tracheobronchial tree. The CT and MRI characteristics vary, depending on the contents. In a significant number of cases, bronchogenic cysts appear as soft-tissue attenuation on CT and demonstrate bright signal on T1-weighted images (Fig. 16-13). These seemingly paradoxic imaging features of a cystic structure can be explained by the presence of proteinacious, mucinous, or hemorrhagic contents within the cyst. Calcification is uncommon but it may occur in the wall or within the cyst contents.

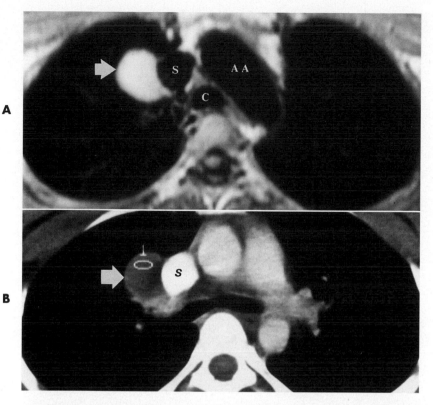

A

B

Figure 16-13 Bronchogenic cyst. **A,** Axial T$_1$-weighted MR image at the level of the carina *(C)* and aortic arch *(AA)* reveals an oval, well-defined mass *(short white arrow)* adjacent to the superior vena cava *(S)*. The mass demonstrates homogenous bright signal intensity. **B,** Axial contrast-enhanced CT image at the level of the main bronchi demonstrates a homogeneous mass *(short white arrow)* adjacent to the superior vena cava *(S)*. The mass measured 30 Hounsfield units, consistent with soft-tissue attenuation. When bronchogenic cysts contain mucin, protein, or hemorrhage, they will appear as soft-tissue attenuation on CT and as bright signal intensity on T1-weighted MRI images.

Box 16-12   Vascular Variants

DEMOGRAPHICS

No distinguishing demographic features

DESCRIPTIVE FEATURES

Aberrant Right Subclavian Artery

CXR: Oblique opacity coursing superiorly from left to right beginning at the superior margin of the aortic arch.

Barium swallow: Oblique indentation on the posterior wall of the esophagus

CT/MR: Vascular structure arising from the distal aortic arch and coursing obliquely behind the trachea and esophagus

Left-Sided Superior Vena Cava

CT/MR: Vascular structure located lateral to the left common carotid artery, which lies anterior to the left hilum as it courses caudally to drain into the right atrium via a dilated coronary sinus

Right-Sided Aortic Arch

CXR: Right-sided convex mediastinal contour with associated leftward deviation of the trachea; absent left-sided aortic arch

Barium swallow: Right-sided lateral impression on the esophagus; in the case of a right-sided aortic arch with an aberrant left subclavian artery, an oblique impression on the posterior wall of the esophagus will also be present

CT/MR: Vascular arch located to the right of the trachea

Double Aortic Arch

CXR: Convex mediastinal contours bilaterally, corresponding to two aortic arches—the right arch is usually larger and more cephalad than the left

Barium swallow: Bilateral impressions on the esophagus on the AP projection; posterior compression of the esophagus on the lateral projection

CT/MR: Bilateral vascular arches join posterior to the trachea and esophagus to form a single descending aorta

---

Vascular Structures

Vascular structures, including anatomic variants and acquired abnormalities, are a common cause of middle mediastinal masses. It is extremely important to consider that a mediastinal mass may be vascular in origin, particularly when a biopsy is being considered.

Vascular Anatomic Variants

The demographics and descriptive features of vascular variants are summarized in Box 16-12.

Aberrant right subclavian artery An aberrant right subclavian artery is a relatively common normal variant, occurring in approximately 1% of the population. The anomalous right subclavian artery arises as the last branch

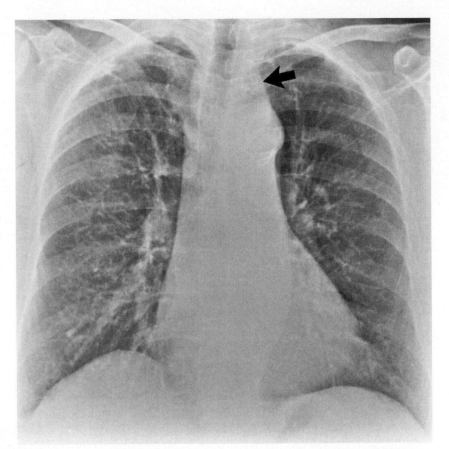

Figure 16-14 Aberrant right subclavian artery. Frontal radiograph of the chest reveals an oblique opacity *(arrow)* arising from the aortic arch and coursing superiorly from left to right.

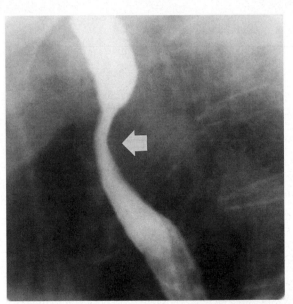

Figure 16-15 Aberrant right subclavian artery. Barium swallow demonstrates a posterior impression on the barium column, corresponding to an aberrant right subclavian artery.

of the aortic arch and courses obliquely from left to right behind the trachea and esophagus as it heads cephalad.

On chest radiographs, an aberrant right subclavian artery may appear as an oblique opacity coursing superiorly from left to right, beginning at the superior margin of the aortic arch (Fig. 16-14). On lateral chest radiographs, you may infrequently detect a posterior impression on the tracheal air column. Barium swallow examination will demonstrate an oblique indentation on the posterior wall of the esophagus (Fig. 16-15). An aberrant right subclavian artery is readily identified on MRI and CT (Fig. 16-16). It is often dilated at its origin, and the adjacent esophagus may be slightly displaced or compressed by the dilated vessel.

Left-sided superior vena cava A persistent left superior vena cava, which occurs in less than 0.5% of the population, is secondary to failure of embryologic regression of a portion of the left common and anterior cardinal veins. A persistent left superior vena cava usually drains the left jugular and left subclavian veins, the latter of which may be small or absent in these patients. Most often, the right superior vena cava is present.

The persistent left superior vena cava, located lateral to the left common carotid artery, courses inferiorly in a position analogous to the right-sided superior vena cava (Fig. 16-17). As it courses caudally, the left superior vena cava lies anterior to the left hilum and almost always drains into the right atrium by way of a dilated coronary sinus. On chest radiographs, you may see widening of the left superior mediastinal contour and a well-defined vertical opacity lateral to the aortic arch contour. The diagnosis is easily confirmed on CT or MRI. The key to diag-

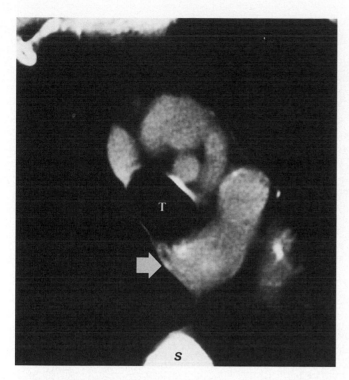

Figure 16-16 Aberrant right subclavian artery. Axial CT image of the chest reveals a vessel arising from the distal aortic arch and coursing posteriorly behind the trachea *(T)*, corresponding to an aberrant right subclavian artery. *S* = spine.

nosing this and other vascular anomalies on cross-sectional imaging is to carefully follow the course of the vessel on serial images.

Right-sided aortic arch Depending on the point of interruption of the aortic arch, at least five potential types of right-sided aortic arches are possible, but you will usually encounter only two. The most common type is a right-sided aortic arch with an aberrant left subclavian artery; this type of aortic arch is infrequently (10% incidence) associated with congenital heart disease. The second most common type is a right-sided aortic arch with mirror-image branching, an anomaly that has a very high (98%) incidence of associated congenital heart disease, especially tetralogy of Fallot.

On chest radiographs, you can identify a right-sided aortic arch in the majority of affected patients as an abnormal convex mediastinal contour located to the right of the trachea, analogous to that produced by the left-sided aortic arch (Fig. 16-18). The trachea is frequently deviated to the left at the level of the right-sided arch, and the normal left-sided aortic arch contour is absent. In the case of a right-sided aortic arch with an anomalous left-subclavian artery, you may also see on the lateral radiograph an impression on the posterior wall of the tracheal air column. Barium-swallow examination will demonstrate an impression on the right lateral wall of the esophagus from the right-sided aortic arch; in the case of a right-sided aortic arch with an aberrant left

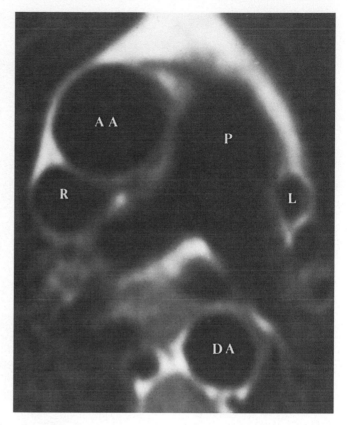

Figure 16-17 Left-sided superior vena cava. Axial T1-weighted MRI image demonstrates a left-sided superior vena cava *(L)* located lateral to the main pulmonary artery *(P)* in a position analogous to the right-sided vena cava *(R)*. On more caudal images, the left-sided superior vena cavae drained into a dilated coronary sinus (not shown). *AA* = ascending aorta; *DA* = descending aorta.

subclavian artery, it will also demonstrate an oblique impression along the posterior wall of the esophagus. CT or MRI easily confirms the presence of a right-sided aortic arch and the presence of an associated aberrant left-subclavian artery.

Double aortic arch A double aortic arch is an anomaly characterized by the presence of both a left- and a right-sided aortic arch, each of which gives rise to its own subclavian and common carotid arteries. The two arches join posteriorly to form a single descending aorta, thus forming a vascular ring around the trachea and esophagus. The right-sided arch is usually larger and is located more cephalad than the left-sided arch. Most often, both arches are patent and functioning; rarely, there is atresia of a portion of the left arch.

Because the two arches form a vascular ring, affected patients are often symptomatic secondary to tracheal and/or esophageal compression. The diagnosis of a double aortic arch may be suggested by chest radiography, which demonstrates both right- and left-sided mediastinal convex contours corresponding to the two arches. Barium swallow will demonstrate bilateral impressions on the AP view,

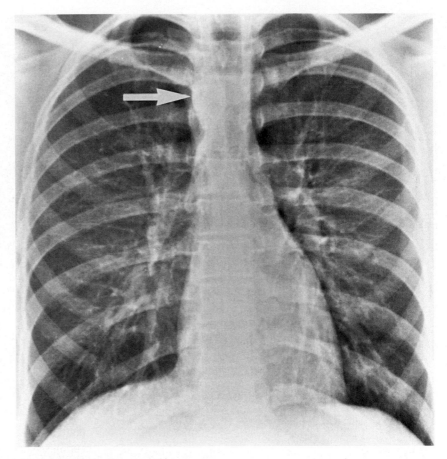

Figure 16-18 Right-sided aortic arch. Frontal chest radiograph reveals a convex contour to the right of the trachea *(arrow)*, corresponding to a right-sided aortic arch. Note the leftward deviation of the trachea and the absence of the normal left-sided aortic arch contour.

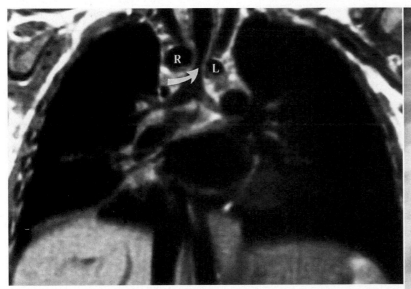

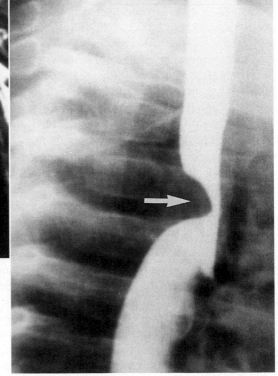

Figure 16-19 Double aortic arch in a male infant. **A,** A coronal T1-weighted MRI image of the chest demonstrates bilateral aortic arches. The right-sided arch *(R)* is larger and is located more cephalad than the left-sided arch *(L),* a common appearance in patients with double aortic arches. The two arches form a vascular ring around the trachea and esophagus. Note the narrowed coronal diameter of the trachea *(curved arrow).* **B,** Lateral radiograph from a barium swallow in the same patient reveals a posterior impression on the barium column, with pronounced narrowing of the AP diameter of the esophagus. On the AP view (not shown), there were bilateral impressions on the barium column from the two aortic arches.

Box 16-13   Aortic Aneurysms

DEMOGRAPHICS

Atherosclerosis the most common cause of aortic
aneurysms, usually affecting patients over the age
of 40

DESCRIPTIVE FEATURES

CXR

Mass—indistinguishable from the aortic contour
Curvilinear calcification (especially atherosclerotic
aneurysms)

CT/MR/Angiography

Mass contiguous with the aorta
Mass demonstrates characteristics of a vascular structure (enhancement, flow void, contrast opacification), unless thrombosed

CLASSIFICATION

Integrity of the Aortic Wall

True aneurysm has intact but dilated aortic wall
False aneurysm has disrupted aortic wall, contained by
surrounding tissues

Shape

fusiform aneurysm, characterized by cylindrical dilation
of entire aortic circumference
saccular aneurysm, characterized by a focal area of outpouching of the aorta

Location

Ascending
Transverse
Descending

---

and posterior compression on the lateral projection. MRI
(Fig. 16-19) or CT can confirm the diagnosis.

Acquired Aortic Abnormalities

Aortic aneurysm   A thoracic aortic aneurysm (Box
16-13) is an abnormal dilation of the aorta, generally
defined as an aortic lumen greater than 4 cm in diameter.

Aneurysms may be classified based on several features, including integrity of the aortic wall, aneurysm
shape, and aneurysm location.

Based on the integrity of the aortic wall, aneurysms
may be classified as *true* aneurysms, characterized by an
intact aortic wall, and *false* aneurysms, characterized by
a disrupted aortic wall, in which case the aneurysm is
contained by surrounding tissues.

Aneurysms may be further classified by their shape as
either *fusiform* or *saccular.* Fusiform aneurysms are
characterized by cylindrical dilation of the entire aortic

circumference, while saccular aneurysms are characterized by a focal area of outpouching of the aorta.

By location, aneurysms may be classified as occurring
within the ascending, transverse, and descending aorta.

Aneurysms that classically involve the ascending aorta
include those related to cystic medial necrosis and
syphilis. The latter, previously a common cause of ascending aortic aneurysms, is infrequently seen today. Aneurysms that commonly involve the descending thoracic
aorta include atherosclerotic, posttraumatic, and mycotic.
The transverse aorta, usually involved by processes similar to those in the descending thoracic aorta, is uncommonly affected by cystic medial necrosis.

The majority of thoracic aortic aneurysms are atherosclerotic and are true aneurysms. Because atherosclerosis generally affects long segments of the aorta, atherosclerotic aneurysms are usually fusiform in shape. They
most commonly affect the aortic arch and descending
thoracic aorta. Atherosclerotic aneurysms typically contain mural thrombus and calcification.

Aneurysms that occur secondary to connective tissue
disorders such as Marfan's syndrome and Ehlers-Danlos
syndrome most often affect the ascending aorta and are
secondary to cystic medial necrosis (Fig. 16-20). Complications of ascending aortic aneurysms include rupture, dissection, aortic insufficiency, and pericardial tamponade.

Posttraumatic aneurysms are usually the result of a
rapid deceleration injury, often secondary to a motor
vehicle accident. Of those patients that survive the initial
injury, the majority of aortic transections (80%) occur at
the level of the ligamentous arteriosum, which is located
just distal to the origin of the left subclavian artery. Posttraumatic aneurysms are classified as false aneurysms
and are an acute surgical emergency, because the associated mortality is very high. In fact, the majority of patients who sustain a traumatic transection of the aorta do
not survive the initial injury; of those who do survive,
prompt diagnosis and treatment are critical. Uncommonly, a patient may present with a chronic false
aneurysm from previous trauma; as in acute posttraumatic aneurysms, the most common location is at the
level of the ligamentum arteriosum.

Infectious aneurysms are also known as mycotic
aneurysms. They are classified as false aneurysms and are
usually saccular. Mycotic aneurysms may be associated
with periaortic inflammation and abscess formation.

On chest radiographs, you should suspect an aortic
aneurysm whenever a mediastinal mass is immediately
adjacent to the aorta, particularly if a border of the mass
is indistinguishable from the aortic contour. The presence of peripheral calcification within such a mass is
supportive evidence of a vascular etiology, particularly in
atherosclerotic aneurysms. You can confirm the diagnosis by either contrast-enhanced CT, MRI, or angiography.
Important information provided by these studies include

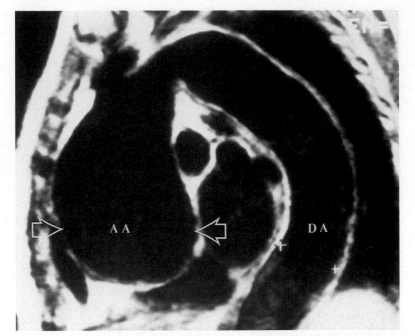

Figure 16-20 Ascending aortic aneurysm secondary to cystic medial necrosis. A sagittal-oblique T1-weighted MRI image of the chest demonstrates aneurysmal dilation *(open arrows)* of the ascending aorta *(AA)*, which does not extend into the descending aorta *(DA)*.

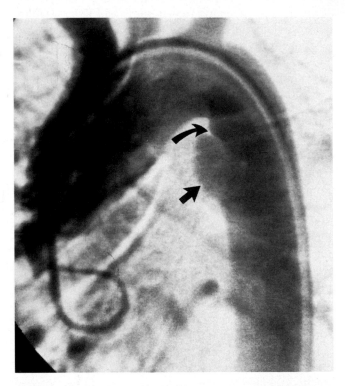

Figure 16-21 Acute aortic transection. Digital subtraction angiogram demonstrates a posttraumatic pseudoaneurysm *(straight arrow)* of the proximal descending thoracic aorta at the level of the ligamentum arteriosum. Note the presence of intimal disruption *(curved black arrow)*.

the precise location and size of the aneurysm; the relationship of the aneurysm to the great vessels; and the presence of complications, including aortic rupture and dissection. It is important to accurately measure the maximal diameter of an aortic aneurysm, because the incidence of rupture correlates with the size of the aneu-

rysm and increases significantly for aneurysms greater than 5 cm in diameter.

Contrast-enhanced CT, MRI, and angiography play an important role in imaging aortic aneurysms. You should consider both the location of the abnormality and the expected etiology when deciding which imaging modality to obtain for further evaluation. For abnormalities of the ascending aorta, MRI is usually preferred over CT. The multiplanar capability of MRI, including the ability to image in sagittal-oblique (LAO) and coronal projections, allows for precise measurement of an ascending aortic aneurysm; MRI is also able to accurately identify associated effacement of the sinotubular junction by an aortic root aneurysm. Contrast-enhanced CT is generally sufficient for the evaluation of aneurysms of the aortic arch and descending thoracic aorta. CT can accurately demonstrate aortic dilation, intramural thrombus, and the presence of perianeurysmal hemorrhage or infection. Be aware, however, that occasionally a tortuous aorta courses obliquely on a transaxial CT image and may be difficult to measure accurately. Angiography remains the preferred modality for evaluation of acute posttraumatic aortic transection (Fig. 16-21). However, CT may play an important role in screening for the presence of mediastinal hemorrhage in patients with a history of trauma and equivocal chest radiographic findings.

Aortic dissection   Aortic dissection (Box 16-14) is a life-threatening condition characterized by a tear in the intima of the aortic wall, followed by separation of the tunica media that creates two channels for the passage of blood, a true and false lumen. Aortic dissection is most commonly associated with systemic hypertension. It is also associated with a variety of other entities including cystic medial necrosis, syphilitic aortitis, coarctation of the aorta, and pregnancy. Affected patients most often

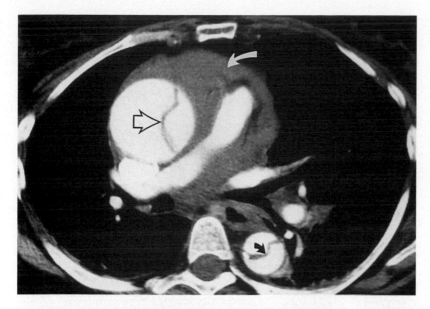

Figure 16-22 Stanford Type A aortic dissection with aortic rupture. Contrast-enhanced axial CT image demonstrates intimal flaps within the ascending aorta *(open arrow)* and descending aorta *(closed arrow)*. Note the presence of hemopericardium *(curved white arrow)* secondary to aortic rupture.

Box 16-14   Aortic Dissection

DEMOGRAPHICS

Systemic hypertension is the most common association with aortic dissection; usually occurs in patients over the age of 40

DESCRIPTIVE FEATURES

CXR

Widened mediastinum
Inward displacement of intimal calcifications
Diffuse aortic dilation

CT/MR/Transesophageal Echo/Angiography

Intimal flap
Differential flow between the true and false lumens
Pericardial effusion (suggests rupture)

Box 16-15   Aortic Dissection: Features to Identify on Imaging Studies

1. Identification of an intimal flap
2. Determination of the site of involvement, particularly whether or not there is involvement of the ascending aorta
3. Visualization of differential flow between the true and false lumens
4. Determination of whether the dissection extends into the origin of the great vessels
5. Assessment for the presence of associated pericardial or pleural effusion in cases complicated by rupture
6. Assessment for the presence of aortic regurgitation

---

present with acute onset of chest and back pain, and they are usually hypertensive.

Chest radiograph findings suggestive of aortic dissection include widening of the mediastinum, inward displacement of intimal calcifications, and diffuse aortic enlargement. The best way to appreciate these findings is by an interval change in appearance compared with previous chest radiographs (Box 16-15). The definitive diagnosis of dissection is dependent on identification of an intimal flap, for which contrast-enhanced CT, MRI, transesophageal echo, or angiography (Fig. 16-22) is useful. The decision of which imaging modality to choose is often based on several factors, including the stability of the patient and individual institutional practices.

Because management depends on the site of involvement, it is important to accurately localize the site of dissection. There are two main classification systems for aortic dissections, the DeBakey and Stanford classification systems, both of which are based on the site of aortic dissection (Box 16-16). Because of their propensity to rupture across the coronary ostia and into the aortic valve and pericardium, dissections that involve the ascending aorta (Debakey I and II, Stanford A) are treated surgically. Dissections that begin distal to the origin of the left subclavian artery (DeBakey III and Stanford B) are treated medically, by controlling the patient's hypertension.

Pericardial Cyst

Pericardial cysts are attached to the parietal pericardium and are lined by mesothelial cells. They usually contain clear fluid and do not communicate with the pericardial space.

Pericardial cysts are generally detected as incidental findings in asymptomatic patients, usually after age 30. There is no sexual prediliction.

The majority of pericardial cysts are in the anterior right cardiophrenic angle; but, they may occur in other locations, including the left cardiophrenic angle, in up to

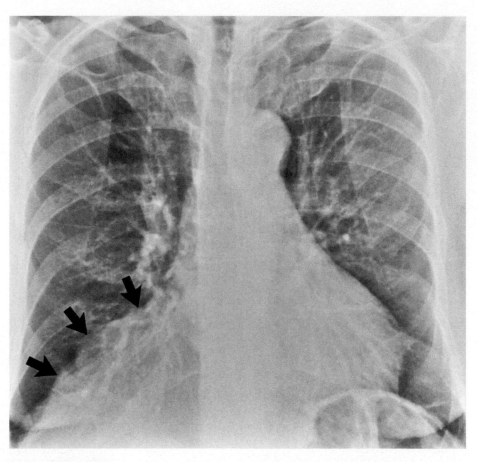

Figure 16-23   Pericardial cyst. Frontal chest radiograph demonstrates a large, well-defined mass in the right cardiophrenic angle. CT image (not shown) demonstrated fluid attenuation consistent with a pericardial cyst.

Box 16-16   Aortic Dissection: Classification Systems

DEBAKEY CLASSIFICATION

Type I: Dissection involves ascending and descending aorta

Type 2: Dissection involves ascending aorta only

Type 3: Dissection involves descending aorta only

STANFORD CLASSIFICATION

Type A: Dissection involves ascending aorta +/- descending aorta

Type B: Dissection involves descending aorta only

one third of cases. On plain radiographs, they appear as well-defined, round, or oval masses located in the normally clear cardiophrenic angle (Fig. 16-23). On CT, pericardial cysts typically demonstrate fluid attenuation; however, they may infrequently contain viscous fluid that measures soft-tissue attenuation. Similarly, the MR signal characteristics are typically that of water (low-signal T1, bright signal T2), but may vary depending on the cyst content.

Other Cardiophrenic Angle Masses

An important differential diagnosis is that of a cardiophrenic angle mass. Although the majority of etiologies of cardiophrenic angle masses are benign entities (lipoma, pericardial fat pad, foramen of Morgagni hernia, pericardial cyst), enlarged epicardial lymph nodes due to lymphoma or metastases may also present in this location. It may occasionally be difficult to distinguish a mediastinal cardiophrenic angle mass from a pleural mass such as a fibrous tumor of the pleura. Sometimes, a well-defined lung mass in the right middle lobe may also mimic a mediastinal cardiophrenic angle mass.

Pericardial fat pad and lipoma   A prominent pericardial fat pad may simulate a cardiophrenic angle mass. Large pericardial fat pads are often seen in obese patients, in patients receiving exogenous steroid therapy, and in patients with Cushing's syndrome. In many cases, excess fat deposition in the pericardial region is associated with generalized excess fat deposition throughout the mediastinum (mediastinal lipomatosis). A focal fatty mass, a benign lipoma, may also present as a cardiophrenic angle mass and may be indistinguishable from a prominent pericardial fat pad.

Previous radiographs are often helpful in the evaluation of patients with prominent pericardial fat pads, because they usually demonstrate a stable appearance over time. However, pericardial fat pads may occasionally increase in size in response to interval weight gain. CT plays an important role in such a case, because it can confirm that the mass is of fat-attenuation. It is helpful in differentiating a pericardial fat pad from epicardial lymph nodes, which

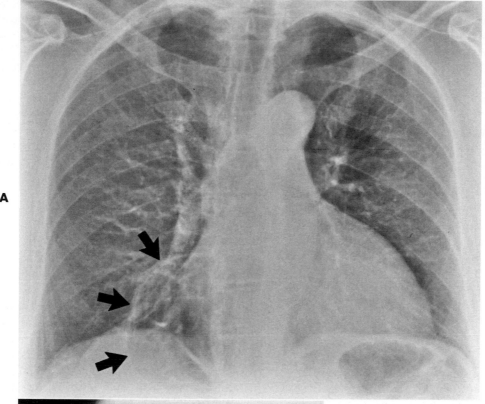

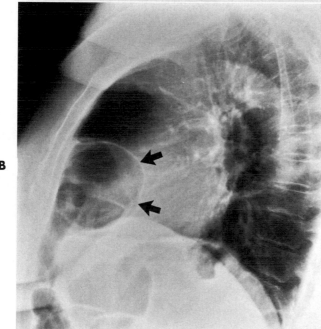

Figure 16-24 Foramen of Morgagni hernia. Frontal and lateral chest radiographs demonstrate a well-defined mass in the right cardiophrenic angle *(arrows)*, which contains gas-filled loops of bowel, an appearance diagnostic of a Morgagni hernia. When the hernia contains omental fat or liver without bowel, additional imaging studies such as CT are required for diagnosis.

demonstrate soft-tissue attenuation, and from pericardial cysts, which usually demonstrate fluid attenuation.

Foramen of Morgagni hernia Herniation of abdominal contents through the anteromedial diaphragmatic foramen of Morgagni may result in a cardiophrenic angle mass, most often on the right side.

The imaging features vary depending on the contents that herniate through the foramen. Most often, herniated contents include omentum, liver, or colon. When the her-

nia contains only omentum, the CT appearance is similar to that of a lipoma. However, the identification of fine linear densities representing omental vessels within the fat should suggest the diagnosis of herniated omental fat rather than a lipoma. Either CT or a nuclear medicine hepatobiliary scan can confirm the presence of herniated liver. Finally, when a Morgagni hernia contains bowel, you can often make the diagnosis by identifying gas-filled loops of bowel within the mass on chest radiographs (Fig. 16-24).

Epicardial lymph nodes Enlarged epicardial lymph nodes may also present as a cardiophrenic angle mass. Because epicardial lymph nodes are rarely enlarged from benign processes, you should suspect a neoplastic process, either lymphoma or metastatic disease. Epicardial lymph nodes are a common site of recurrence in patients with Hodgkin's lymphoma following radiation therapy.

On CT, epicardial lymph nodes will appear as single or multiple soft-tissue attenuation masses.

Tracheal Neoplasms

You should consider tracheal neoplasms in the differential diagnosis of a middle mediastinal mass, especially when a mass extends into or narrows the tracheal lumen. These are discussed in Chapter 12.

POSTERIOR MEDIASTINAL MASSES

Neurogenic Tumors

Neurogenic tumors (Box 16-17) are the most common cause of a posterior mediastinal mass. Roughly 70% of neurogenic tumors are benign. There are three main groups: (1) those arising from peripheral nerves (schwannoma, neurofibroma); (2) those arising from the sympathetic chain (ganglioneuroma, ganglioneuroblastoma, neuroblastoma); and (3) those arising from the paraganglia (pheochromocytoma, chemodectoma). The first group is the most common and the third group is the least common.

Neurogenic tumors typically occur in younger patients. Although most patients are asymptomatic, these tumors may cause neurologic symptoms such as radicular pain and neuresthesias. Intravertebral extension may result in symptoms of cord compression.

Tumors arising from the peripheral nerves tend to be round in shape, and those arising from the sympathetic chain are usually fusiform with a more vertical orientation. Neurogenic tumors generally occur in a paraspinal location. Benign neurogenic neoplasms typically appear homogeneous and have well-defined margins. Malignant neurogenic tumors are more likely to appear heterogeneous and have irregular margins. Associated bony abnormalities, including rib spreading and rib erosion, are commonly seen. These do not imply malignancy (Fig. 16-25). The presence of frank bone destruction, however, should raise the suspicion for malignancy.

MRI is the preferred cross-sectional imaging modality because of its superb ability to demonstrate the presence of intraspinal extension of tumor or the presence of an associated spinal-cord abnormality. On MRI, neurogenic tumors are typically well-defined masses of homogeneous appearance, demonstrating signal intensity slightly greater than that of skeletal muscle on T1-weighted images and markedly increased signal on T2-weighted images (Fig. 16-26). Neurogenic tumors typically enhance homogeneously following gadolinium administration.

Associated abnormalities of the vertebral bodies are well demonstrated on CT. Because nerve sheath tumors arise posterolaterally, they are often associated with widening of the neural foramen. In contrast, tumors arising from the sympathetic ganglia are located anterolateral to the vertebral bodies and more often result in vertebral body erosion.

Paravertebral Abnormalities

Infectious, malignant, and traumatic abnormalities of the thoracic spine may result in the presence of a posterior mediastinal mass.

Due to the wide variety of etiologies of paravertebral abnormalities (Box 16-18), they may occur in patients of any age and there is no sexual predilection. Patients with paravertebral posterior mediastinal masses often present with back pain. Patients with infectious processes may also have fever and leukocytosis. An important infectious etiology is Pott's disease, a paraspinal abscess from tuberculous infection. Malignant etiologies include metastatic disease and myeloma. Traumatic etiologies include vertebral fracture with associated paraspinal hematoma.

Box 16-17 Neurogenic Tumors

DEMOGRAPHICS

Age

Usually occur in younger patients, first 4 decades of life

Gender

Males and females equally affected

DESCRIPTIVE FEATURES

Nerve Sheath Tumors

Round, homogeneous, paraspinal mass
May be associated with widening of the neural foramen
MRI: slightly brighter than muscle on T1 and very
   bright on T2, homogeneous enhancement following
   gadolinium administration

Sympathetic Chain Tumors

Fusiform, homogeneous, paraspinal mass
May be associated with vertebral body erosion
MR characteristics similar to those of nerve sheath
   tumors

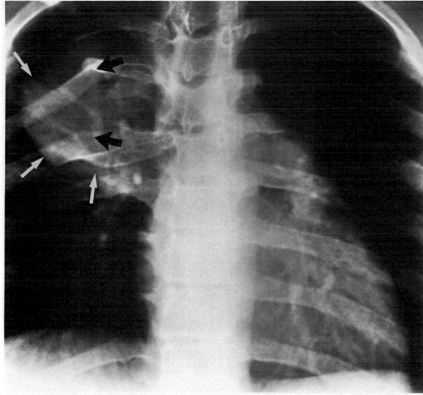

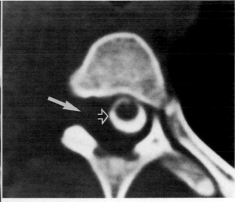

Figure 16-25   Ganglioneuroma. **A,** Frontal chest radiograph demonstrates a large posterior mediastinal mass *(white arrows)* with associated rib spreading and rib erosions *(black arrows)*. **B,** Axial image from a CT-myelogram demonstrates extension of the right paraspinal mass into the neural foramen *(closed white arrow),* with associated displacement of the thecal sac and spinal cord *(open white arrow).*

On imaging studies, paravertebral posterior mediastinal masses are often bilateral and fusiform. When present, bilaterality may help distinguish paravertebral masses from neurogenic tumors, which are usually unilateral paraspinal masses. An important exception is neurofibromatosis, which may present with multiple bilateral neurofibromas.

The presence of associated abnormalities of the vertebral bodies or intervertebral disc spaces suggests a paravertebral etiology. Disc space involvement can help distinguish between infectious and malignant etiologies. Narrowing of the intervertebral disc spaces and abnormalities of the adjacent vertebral body endplates suggest an infectious etiology. Malignant processes are associated with destruction of the vertebral body, but these usually spare the intervertebral disc spaces.

A posttraumatic paraspinal hematoma is generally associated with fracture of one or more thoracic vertebral bodies. MRI demonstrates signal characteristics of hemorrhage within the paraspinal mass, which vary depending on the stage of hemorrhage.

Vascular Abnormalities

The descending thoracic aorta and the azygous vein are both located within the posterior mediastinum, and

---

Box 16-18   **Paravertebral Abnormalities**

DEMOGRAPHICS

No general distinguishing demographic features

DESCRIPTIVE FEATURES

Paravertebral masses are often bilateral and fusiform
The presence of associated abnormalities of the vertebral bodies and/or intervertebral disc spaces is an important feature of paravertebral abnormalities
Involvement of the intervertebral disc is characteristic of an infectious etiology, while involvement of the vertebral body with sparing of the disc space is suggestive of a neoplastic process
Posttraumatic paravertebral abnormalities are characterized by the presence of a vertebral body fracture and paraspinal hematoma

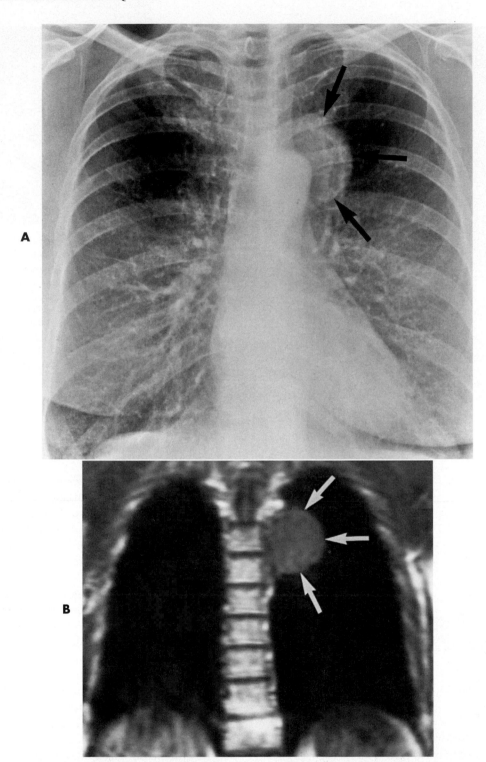

Figure 16-26 Schwannoma. **A,** Frontal chest radiograph reveals a well-defined, round, left paraspinal posterior mediastinal mass (*arrows*). **B,** Coronal T1-weighted MRI demonstrates homogeneous, intermediate signal intensity within the mass (*arrows*), which is slightly brighter than skeletal muscle. T2-weighted images (not shown) demonstrated homogeneous bright signal within the mass. These MRI signal characteristics are typical of neurogenic tumors.

Box 16-19 Vascular Abnormalities—Posterior Mediastinum

DEMOGRAPHICS

Aortic Aneurysms

Atherosclerosis is the most common cause of thoracic aortic aneurysms, usually affecting patients over the age of 40

Azygous Continuation of the Inferior Vena Cava

May be detected in patients of any age; associated with polysplenia and asplenia

Esophageal Varices

Usually seen in adult patients with a history of alcohol abuse and cirrhosis

DESCRIPTIVE FEATURES

Thoracic Aortic Aneurysm

CXR: Abnormal convex contour of the descending thoracic aortic interface; may contain peripheral calcification

CT/MR/Angio: Confirms vascular etiology; may detect complications, including rupture

Azygous Continuation of the Inferior Vena Cava

CXR: Enlargement of the azygous arch and lateral displacement of the azygoesophageal interface; decrease in size following Valsalva maneuver

CT/MR: Enlargement of the azygous arch and the paraspinal and retrocrural portions of the azygous vein; absence of the suprarenal portion of the inferior vena cava

Esophageal Varices

CXR: May present as a mass in the inferior aspect of the posterior mediastinum

Barium swallow: Demonstrates serpiginous defects in the barium column that change in configuration following Valsalva maneuver

CT/MR/Angiography: Confirms the vascular origin of the abnormality; CT/MR may also demonstrate a cirrhotic liver and splenomegaly

abnormalities of either of these structures may result in a posterior mediastinal mass (Box 16-19). Abnormalities of the descending thoracic aorta include atherosclerotic, mycotic, and posttraumatic aneurysms. Azygous vein enlargement may result from increased flow (obstruction of the superior or inferior vena cava) or from increased pressure (tricuspid insufficiency or right-sided heart failure); the azygous vein may also be enlarged in the congenital condition known as "azygous continuation of the inferior vena cava". Esophageal varices may also result in a posterior mediastinal mass.

The majority of thoracic aortic aneurysms are atherosclerotic in etiology, and therefore more common in older patients. Mycotic and posttraumatic aneurysms may be seen in any age group. Azygous continuation of the inferior vena cava is associated with polysplenia and asplenia, but it may also be an incidental finding. Esophageal and paraesophageal varices are associated with portal hypertension and cirrhosis and are often seen in patients with a history of alcohol abuse.

On chest radiographs, thoracic aortic aneurysms typically produce an abnormal contour of the descending thoracic aortic interface and often demonstrate curvilinear calcification (Fig. 16-27). The diagnosis may be confirmed with contrast-enhanced CT, MRI, or angiography.

Azygous continuation of the inferior vena cava may present with enlargement of the azygous arch and lateral displacement of the azygocsophageal interface (Fig. 16-28). You can readily confirm the diagnosis by contrast-enhanced CT, which demonstrates enlargement of the azygous arch and the paraspinal and retrocrural portions of the azygous vein, as well as absence of the suprarenal portion of the inferior vena cava.

Esophageal and paraesophageal varices may present as a mass in the inferior aspect of the posterior mediastinum. Barium swallow typically demonstrates serpiginous filling defects in the barium column; these change in configuration with the Valsalva maneuver. Contrast-enhanced CT, MRI, or angiography can confirm the vascular etiology of this abnormality. Associated findings on cross-sectional imaging include a cirrhotic liver and splenomegaly.

Esophageal Abnormalities

A wide variety of esophageal abnormalities (Box 16-20) may result in a posterior mediastinal mass. These include benign and malignant neoplasms, achalasia, hiatal hernia, and duplication cyst.

Because of the wide variety of etiologies, there are no general distinguishing demographic features. However, there are some helpful guidelines.

Even though many esophageal abnormalities may occur in patients of any age group, malignant esophageal neoplasms are more common in older males and are associated with smoking and alcohol abuse. Leiomyoma, the most common benign tumor of the esophagus, occurs in patients with a broad range in age from 20 to 60, with a male predominance. Achalasia usually occurs in patients 30 to 50 years of age, with equal frequency among men and women.

Malignant esophageal neoplasms tend to present with symptoms of dysphagia before they become large enough to result in the presence of a mediastinal mass. Obstructing esophageal malignancies may result in the

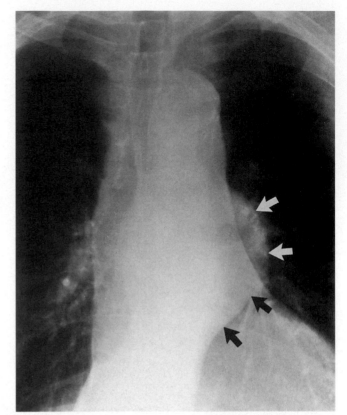

Figure 16-27   Descending thoracic aortic aneurysm. Frontal chest radiograph demonstrates a posterior mediastinal mass that is contiguous with the descending thoracic aortic interface *(white and black arrows)*. Angiography (not shown) revealed a large descending thoracic aortic aneurysm.

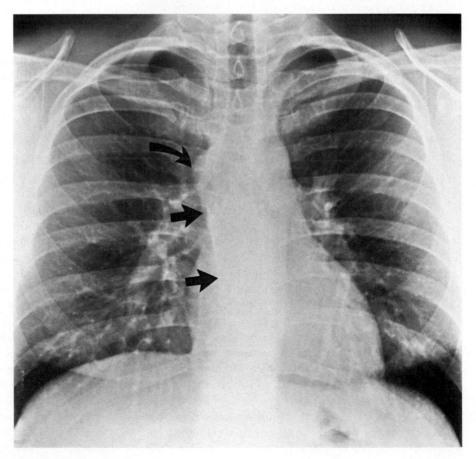

Figure 16-28   Azygous continuation of the inferior vena cava. Frontal chest radiograph reveals enlargement of the azygous arch contour *(curved arrow)* and lateral displacement of the azygoesophageal interface *(straight arrows)*, corresponding to the presence of an enlarged azygous vein.

Box 16-20 Esophageal Abnormalities

DEMOGRAPHICS

No general distinguishing demographic features

DESCRIPTIVE FEATURES

Malignant Esophageal Neoplasm

Obstructing lesions may present as thickening of the tracheoesophageal stripe on the lateral CXR; an air/fluid level may be identified within the esophagus

CT may demonstrate esophageal wall thickening, as well as the presence of nodal spread or distant metastases

Benign Esophageal Neoplasm

May present as a smooth mass that distorts the azygoesophageal interface

Achalasia

Typically presents as a longitudinal mass extending the length of the mediastinum with diffuse rightward lateral displacement of the azygoesophageal interface; an air/fluid level may be visible

Hiatal Hernia

Typically presents as a round, retrocardiac mass that causes a focal rightward lateral displacement of the inferior aspect of the azygoesophageal interface; an air/fluid level is often visible

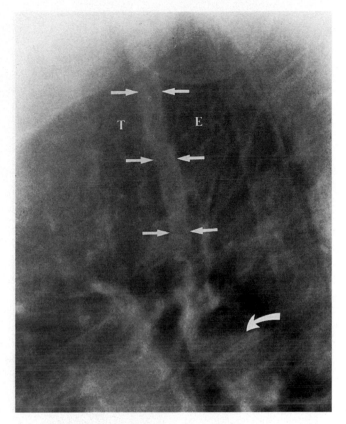

Figure 16-29 Esophageal carcinoma. Magnified image of a lateral chest radiograph demonstrates thickening of the tracheoesophageal stripe *(short white arrows)* and an air-fluid level within the midthoracic esophagus *(curved white arrow)* in a patient with esophageal obstruction secondary to squamous cell carcinoma. *T* = trachea; *E* = esophagus.

presence of an air/fluid level within the esophagus and thickening of the tracheoesophageal stripe (Fig. 16-29). In contrast, benign esophageal neoplasms are usually asymptomatic and larger than malignant neoplasms at diagnosis. Despite this fact, the majority of benign esophageal neoplasms are not detectable on chest radiographs.

Barium swallow is helpful for confirming the esophageal origin and in further characterizing the abnormality as mucosal or submucosal (Fig. 16-30).

Nonneoplastic esophageal abnormalities that may result in a posterior mediastinal mass include achalasia and hiatal hernia. Achalasia, a primary dysmotility disorder of the esophagus, results in aperistalsis of the esophagus below the level of the aortic arch, and subsequent diffuse esophageal dilation with retention of food and secretions. On chest radiographs, achalasia often appears as a longitudinal posterior mediastinal mass, extending the entire length of the mediastinum (Fig. 16-31). The azygoesophageal interface is typically laterally displaced and often demonstrates a rightward convexity. The presence of an air/fluid level within the mass is highly suggestive of achalasia. Barium swallow demon-

strates aperistalsis below the level of the aortic arch and a characteristic "bird's beak" appearance of the distal esophagus.

A hiatal hernia results from the extension of the stomach into the chest through the esophageal hiatus. On chest radiographs, hiatal hernias typically appear as rounded retrocardiac masses that often cause a focal rightward convexity in the inferior aspect of the azygoesophageal interface (Fig. 16-32 on p. 460). You will often identify an air/fluid level. Barium swallow is diagnostic.

Other Posterior Mediastinal Masses

Posterior Mediastinal Lymphadenopathy

Posterior mediastinal lymphadenopathy may be secondary to neoplastic etiologies, especially lymphoma and bronchogenic carcinoma, and inflammatory etiologies, including sarcoidosis. However, involvement of this lymph node group is an uncommon manifestation of these disorders. Posterior mediastinal lymphadenopathy typically results in bilateral paraspinal masses and may be seen as widening of the paraspinal lines on chest radiographs.

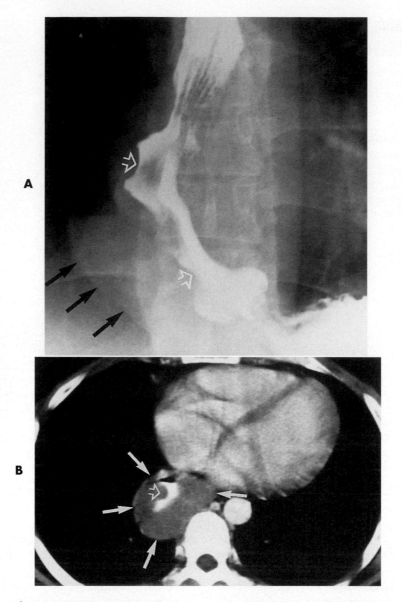

Figure 16-30 Leiomyoma. **A,** Coned-down image of the lower mediastinum from a barium esophagram reveals a posterior mediastinal mass *(black arrows)* with an associated submucosal impression on the barium-filled esophagus *(open white arrows).* **B,** Axial CT image obtained following administration of oral and intravenous contrast medium demonstrates a circumferential mass *(closed arrows)* arising from the esophageal wall. Note the submucosal impression on the esophageal lumen *(open arrow).*

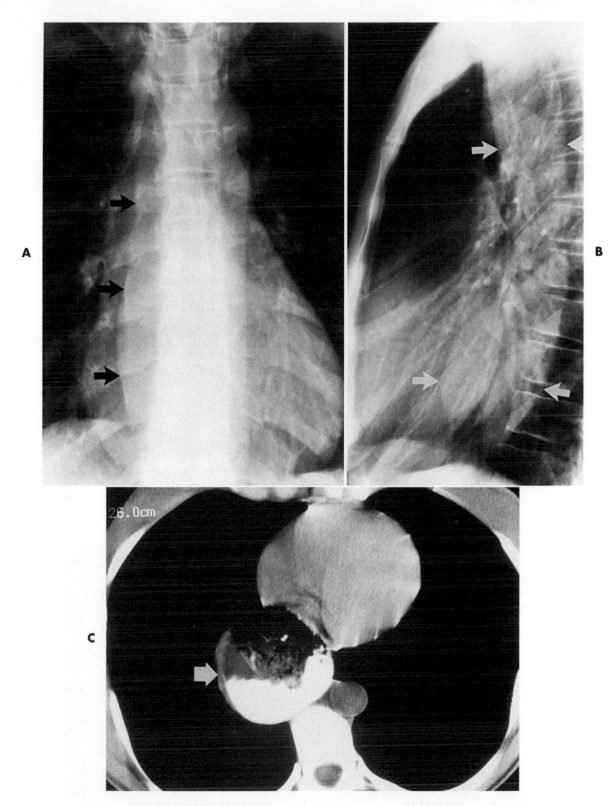

Figure 16-31   Achalasia. **A,** Frontal chest radiograph demonstrates lateral displacement of the azygoesophageal interface *(arrows)*. **B,** Lateral chest radiograph reveals a longitudinal posterior mediastinal mass that extends the entire length of the thorax *(paired arrows)*. **C,** Axial CT image of the chest obtained following administration of oral contrast medium demonstrates pronounced dilation of the esophagus *(arrow)*, characteristic of achalasia.

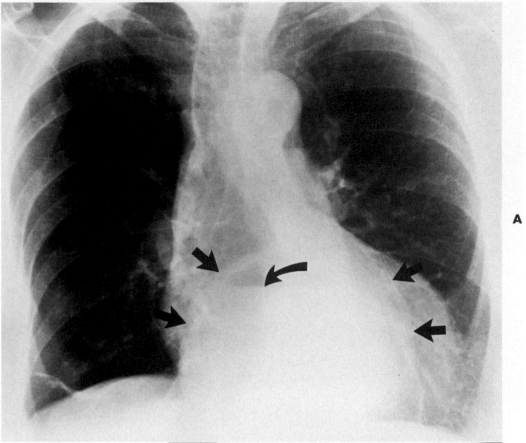

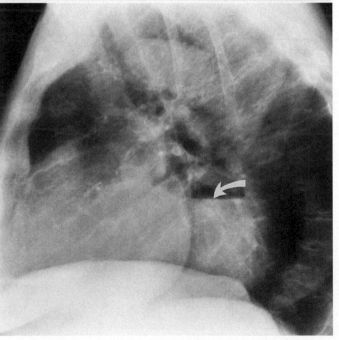

Figure 16-32 Hiatal hernia. Frontal and lateral chest radiographs reveal a large, round retrocardiac mediastinal mass *(straight arrows)* that contains an air/fluid level *(curved arrow)*. Note the lateral displacement of the azygoesophageal interface on the frontal radiograph.

Neurenteric cyst Neurenteric cysts are rare developmental anomalies that contain both neural and gastrointestinal elements. They are often painful, and they generally develop at a young age.

Often associated with vertebral anomalies and scoliosis, they typically present as a well-defined, homogeneous cystic mass. They rarely fill with contrast medium following myelography.

Meningocele Anterior and lateral meningoceles represent herniations of meninges through the neural foramina or through defects in the vertebral bodies. Meningoceles are usually asymptomatic and most often

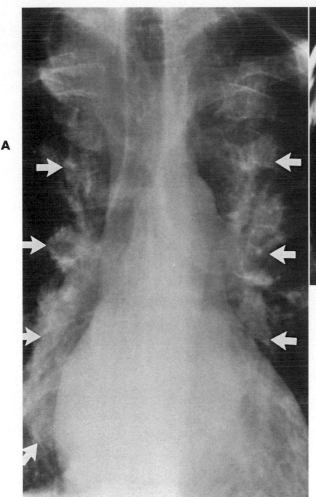

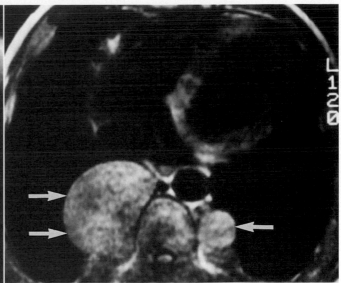

Figure 16-33 Extramedullary hematopoeisis in a patient with thalessemia. **A,** Frontal chest radiograph demonstrates bilateral, lobulated paraspinal masses *(arrows)* that extend the entire length of the mediastinum. Note widening of the ribs, consistent with marrow expansion. **B,** Axial T1-weighted MRI reveals bilateral, round, paraspinal masses of bright signal intensity *(arrow).*

present in adulthood. They are often associated with neurofibromatosis.

Meningoceles typically appear as well-defined, homogeneous, paraspinal masses. Like neurenteric cysts, they are often associated with vertebral anomalies and scoliosis. In contrast to neurenteric cysts, they frequently fill with contrast medium following myelography.

Bochdalek hernia Herniation of omental fat, kidney, or spleen through the foramen of Bochdalek may result in a posterior mediastinal mass. On chest radiographs, Bochdalek hernias usually present as a smooth bulge in the posterior aspect of the left hemidiaphragm. You can confirm the diagnosis by demonstration of a diaphragmatic defect on CT with herniated fat, kidney, or spleen.

Extramedullary hematopoeisis Extramedullary hematopoeisis is a rare compensatory response of marrow expansion. It is associated with severe anemias, particularly thalassemia intermedia.

Extramedullary hematopoeisis typically presents as longitudinal, bilateral, lobulated paraspinal masses (Fig. 16-33). Associated osseous findings of marrow expansion, including expanded ribs with narrowed rib interspaces, suggest the diagnosis.

SUGGESTED READINGS

Davis RD, Oldham HN, Sabiston DC: Primary cysts and neoplasms of the mediastinum: recent changes in clinical presentation, methods of diagnosis, management and results, *Ann Thorac Surg* 44:229-237, 1987.

Felson B: *Chest roentgenology,* Philadelphia, 1973, WB Saunders.

Fraser RG, Pare JAP, Pare PD, Fraser FS, Genereux GP: *Diagnosis of diseases of the chest,* ed 3, Philadelphia, 1988, WB Saunders.

Grillo HC, Mathieson DJ: Primary tracheal tumors: treatment and results, *Ann Thorac Surg* 49:69-77, 1990.

Halpert RD, Goodman P: *Gastrointestinal radiology: the requisites,* St. Louis, Mo., 1993, Mosby–Year Book.

Heitzman ER: The mediastinum: radiologic correlations with anatomy and pathology, ed 2, Berlin, 1988, Springer-Verlag.

McCarthy MJ, Rosado-de-Christenson ML: Tumors of the trachea, *J Thorac Imaging* 10:180-198, 1995.

McLoud TC, Ragozzino MW: MR imaging of the thorax. In Edelman RR, Hesselink JR, editors: *Clinical magnetic resonance imaging,* Philadelphia, 1990, WB Saunders; pp 731-744.

Nadler LM: The malignant lymphomas. In Wilson JD, Braunwald E, Issclbacher KJ, Petersdorf RF, Martin JB, Fauci AS, Root RK, editors: *Harrison's principles and practices of internal medicine,* ed 12, vol 2, New York, 1991, McGraw-Hill; pp. 1599-1612.

Naidich DP, Zerhouni EA, Siegelman SS: Computed tomography and magnetic resonance of the thorax, ed 2, New York, 1991, Raven Press.

Palmer EL, Scott JA, Strauss HW: *Practical nuclear medicine,* Philadelphia, 1992, WB Saunders.

Pierson DJ: Disorders of the pleura, mediastinum and diaphragm. In Wilson JD, Braunwald E, Isselbacher KJ, Petersdorf RG, Martin JB, Fauci AS, editors: *Harrison's principles and practices of internal medicine,* ed 12, vol 2, New York, 1991, McGraw-Hill; pp 1111-1116.

Reed JC: *Chest radiology: plain film patterns and differential diagnoses,* ed 3, St. Louis, Mo., 1991, Mosby–Year Book.

Shaffer K, Pugatch RD: Diseases of the mediastinum. In Freundlich IM, Bragg DG, editors: *Radiologic approach to diseases of the chest,* Baltimore, 1992, Williams & Wilkins; pp 171-185.

Vail CM, Ravin CE: Mediastinal masses. In Freundlich IM, Bragg DG editors: *Radiologic approach to diseases of the chest,* Baltimore, 1992, William & Wilkins; pp 360-373.

Webb WR: Diseases of the mediastinum. In Putman CE, Ravin CE editors: Textbook of diagnostic imaging, ed 2, Philadelphia, 1994, WB Saunders; pp 428-447.

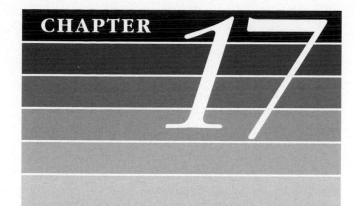

CHAPTER 17

Diffuse Mediastinal Abnormalities

PHILLIP M. BOISELLE

Unlike focal mediastinal masses, which usually can be localized within a single mediastinal compartment, diffuse mediastinal abnormalities almost always involve more than one compartment of the mediastinum and therefore preclude classification by the traditional compartmentalization method. The common feature among these entities is that they all may present with *diffuse mediastinal widening* on chest radiographs.

RADIOLOGIC APPROACH TO DIFFUSE MEDIASTINAL WIDENING

Recognition and evaluation of diffuse mediastinal widening on plain radiographs can be challenging, even for experienced radiologists. The first challenge is recognizing the abnormality. Accurate recognition is particularly difficult on anteroposterior (AP) portable supine radiographs because they result in magnification of normal mediastinal structures. You will often need to assess the mediastinum on portable radiographs, especially in trauma patients, even though posteroanterior (PA) and lateral chest radiographs are superior. Assessment of the mediastinum is also difficult in older patients with atherosclerotic vascular disease, because the mediastinum may appear wide secondary to tortuosity of the aorta

and great vessels. Comparison with prior radiographs is particularly helpful in this population.

Once you have recognized diffuse mediastinal widening, you need to attempt to determine its etiology, which can be a difficult task based on chest radiographic findings alone. Of particular importance is an assessment of the mediastinal contours and normal mediastinal landmarks. Subtle alterations are often best appreciated as a change in appearance from previous radiographs. The identification of diffuse mediastinal widening on plain radiographs, particularly when accompanied by abnormalities of the normal mediastinal landmarks, generally requires further evaluation with computed tomography (CT) or magnetic resonance imaging (MRI). Suspicion for aortic injury requires emergent angiography.

DIFFUSE MEDIASTINAL ABNORMALITIES

Mediastinal Lipomatosis

Mediastinal lipomatosis is the diffuse accumulation of excess unencapsulated fat within the mediastinum. This benign condition is usually seen in adult patients and may be associated with Cushing's syndrome, exogenous steroid use, and obesity.

Fat accumulation is usually most prominent in the anterior and superior portions of the mediastinum, where it surrounds the great vessels and results in lateral displacement of the pleural reflections. You may also detect it in other parts of the mediastinum, including the cardiophrenic angles, paravertebral regions, retrocrural, and subcostal regions.

The appearance on chest radiographs and CT depends on the distribution of excess fat deposition. Accumulation of fat in the anterior and superior portions of the mediastinum results in smooth widening of the anterior and superior mediastinal contours as seen on chest radiographs (Fig. 17-1). An important feature is the lack of mass effect on the trachea and esophagus, structures that are often displaced or compressed by other mediastinal abnormalities. Excess fat deposits within the cardiophrenic angles result in the presence of cardiophrenic angle "masses," and excess fat within the paravertebral regions may result in bilateral lateral displacement of the paraspinal lines.

A definitive diagnosis of mediastinal lipomatosis may be made at CT (Fig. 17-2). Fat is recognized on CT by its low CT numbers, which typically vary from negative 70 to negative 130 Hounsfield units (HU). Although CT is generally considered the imaging modality of choice, you can also make the diagnosis by MRI. On MRI, fat demonstrates bright signal intensity on T1-weighted images. Using a fat-suppression sequence will result in suppression of the normally bright T1 signal from fat tissue and help you differentiate it from other tissues with bright T1 signal. An important feature of mediastinal lipomatosis on either CT or MRI is a homogeneous appearance of the mediastinal fat. An inhomogeneous appearance, such as the presence of high-attenuation foci within the fat,

should raise the suspicion of a superimposed process such as mediastinal hemorrhage or neoplastic infiltration.

Mediastinitis

Diffuse mediastinitis may be either acute or chronic. Both are most often infectious in etiology: acute mediastinitis is often the result of a bacterial infection; chronic mediastinitis is more often related to a granulomatous infection such as histoplasmosis. Patients with acute mediastinitis usually present with an acute onset of symptoms, including fever and leukocytosis, while patients with chronic mediastinitis are often asymptomatic. If symptoms occur, they usually arise secondary to compression of mediastinal structures.

Acute mediastinitis

Acute mediastinitis may occur following esophageal perforation, secondary to extension of an infectious process from thoracic and extrathoracic structures (especially from the neck), and as an infrequent compli-

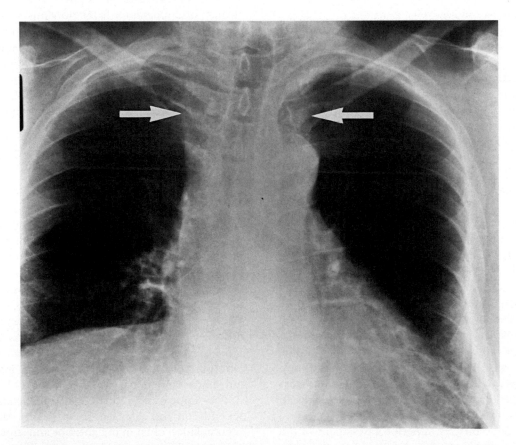

Fig. 17-1 Mediastinal lipomatosis. Frontal chest radiograph reveals smooth widening of the superior mediastinum *(arrows)*. Note the absence of mass effect on the trachea, which is midline in position.

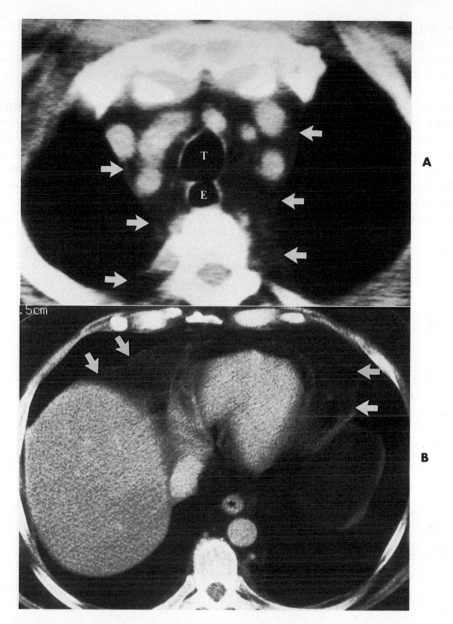

Fig. 17-2   Mediastinal lipomatosis. **A,** Axial noncontrast CT image of the chest at the level of the brachiocephalic vessels demonstrates a large amount of fat within the mediastinum that surrounds the vessels and results in lateral displacement of the pleural reflections *(arrows).* Note the normal midline position of the trachea *(T)* and esophagus *(E).* **B,** Axial CT image of the chest at the level of the diaphragm reveals excess fat within the cardiophrenic angles *(paired arrows).*

cation of cardiac surgery (Box 17-1). The vast majority occur secondary to esophageal perforation.

Esophageal perforation Clinically, patients with esophageal perforation frequently present with fever, leukocytosis, dysphagia, and retrosternal chest pain, which often radiates into the neck. On physical examination, these patients may demonstrate subcutaneous emphysema and Hamman's sign, a finding on auscultation heard over the cardiac apex that is associated with pneumomediastinum.

Chest radiographic findings include diffuse widening of the mediastinum and pneumomediastinum (Fig. 17-3). Associated pleural abnormalities are usually left-sided and include pneumothorax and empyema. In cases in which the diagnosis is delayed, complications may include mediastinal abscess formation as well as rupture of the abscess into the adjacent bronchus (esophagobronchial fistula) and pleura (esophagopleural fistula). You can confirm the diagnosis of esophageal perforation by fluoroscopic examination following administration of water-soluble contrast medium, which will demonstrate extravasation of contrast at the site of perforation (Fig. 17-4). In complicated cases that have progressed to mediastinal abscess formation, CT may be helpful in identifying the precise location and extent of fluid collections (Fig. 17-5).

Prompt diagnosis and treatment of esophageal perforation are critical. There is a very high morbidity and mortality rate associated with delay in diagnosis beyond 24 hours.

Other causes of acute mediastinitis Other causes of acute mediastinitis are much less common. They include: 1) extension of infection from adjacent thoracic structures, including the lungs, pleura, pericardium and mediastinal lymph nodes; 2) extension of infection from adjacent anatomic regions, especially from the neck; 3) following traumatic tracheobronchial rupture, and 4) following cardiac surgery (an infrequent postoperative complication).

Chest radiographs may demonstrate diffuse mediastinal widening and findings associated with a mediastinal abscess, including gas bubbles or an air/fluid level. Pneumomediastinum and pneumothorax, findings frequently associated with esophageal perforation, are not usually seen with other causes of acute mediastinitis. An important exception is traumatic tracheobronchial rupture, which frequently presents with pneumomediastinum and pneumothorax.

You will find CT helpful in diagnosing acute mediastinitis, because it is more sensitive than chest radiographs for detecting the presence and extent of mediastinal fluid collections and the presence of extraluminal gas. Because mediastinitis may result from extension of infection from adjacent thoracic and extrathoracic structures, CT can determine the relationship of mediastinal fluid collections to these structures. Finally, CT may play a role in guiding drainage procedures of mediastinal fluid collections.

Chronic mediastinitis

Chronic mediastinitis is the result of chronic inflammation of the mediastinum, which may progress to diffuse mediastinal fibrosis. In patients with chronically enlarged inflammatory lymph nodes, rupture of lymph nodes may incite an inflammatory response that results in diffuse fibrosis. Over time, enlarged mediastinal lymph nodes and adjacent fibrous tissue may compress adjacent mediastinal and hilar structures, including arteries, veins, the trachea and bronchi, and the esophagus.

There are a variety of causes of chronic mediastinitis (Box 17-2). The majority of cases are secondary to granulomatous processes, including infections such as histoplasmosis, coccidiomycosis, and tuberculosis, and, less commonly, noninfectious granulomatous processes such as sarcoidosis. Sclerosing mediastinitis refers to a noninfectious, nongranulomatous cause of chronic mediastinitis, which is frequently associated with other sites of fibrosis, including the retroperitoneum (retroperitoneal fibrosis), thyroid gland (Riedel's struma), the orbit (orbital pseudotumor), and the cecum (ligneous perityphlitis). Chronic mediastinitis has also been associated with immunologic abnormalities (systemic lupus, erythematosus rheumatoid arthritis, Raynaud's phenomenon), and drugs (methysergide).

Histoplasmosis is the most common cause of chronic mediastinitis and mediastinal fibrosis. Endemic areas in North American for the organism *H. capsulatum* include

---

Box 17-1   Etiologies of Acute Mediastinitis

ESOPHAGEAL PERFORATION

Iatrogenic (following esophagoscopy or following esophageal dilation)
Impacted foreign body (chicken bone, sharp objects)
Obstructing esophageal neoplasm
Trauma (penetrating trauma more than blunt trauma)
Repeated episodes of vomiting (Boerhaave's syndrome)

EXTENSION OF INFECTION FROM ADJACENT SPACES

Pharynx (retropharyngeal or nasopharyngeal abscess)
Retroperitoneum (pancreatic pseudocyst)
Abdomen (subphrenic abscess)

EXTENSION OF INFECTION FROM ADJACENT THORACIC STRUCTURES

Lung
Lymph nodes
Pleura (empyema)
Pericardium

POSTOPERATIVE COMPLICATION FOLLOWING CARDIAC SURGERY
TRAUMATIC RUPTURE OF THE AIRWAY

the Ohio, Mississippi, and St. Lawrence river valleys, Histoplasmosis can be acquired during even a brief stay in an endemic area. Individuals of all ages and both genders may be affected.

Patients with chronic mediastinitis are often asymptomatic. The diagnosis of chronic mediastinitis is frequently suggested following the incidental detection of characteristic abnormalities on chest radiographs. When present, symptoms usually arise as a result of compression of mediastinal structures, including vascular structures (superior vena cava, pulmonary arteries, pulmonary veins), the airway, and the esophagus. Mediastinal fibrosis, particularly from histoplasmosis, should be considered in the differential diagnosis of superior vena cava obstruction. The most common etiology of superior vena caval obstruction is neoplastic (especially bronchogenic carcinoma), and mediastinal fibrosis is the most common benign cause of superior vena caval obstruction.

On chest radiographs, mediastinal fibrosis may present as diffuse widening of the mediastinal contours or as a localized mass. When it occurs as a localized mass, it is most common in the right paratracheal region (Fig. 17-6). In cases that occur secondary to granulomatous infections such as histoplasmosis or tuberculosis, calcifications are frequently identified within enlarged mediastinal and hilar lymph nodes (Fig. 17-7) CT is more sensitive than chest radiographs for detecting enlarged mediastinal lymph nodes, fibrosis, and the presence of calcification. In addition to detecting the presence of mediastinal fibrosis, CT plays an important role in evaluating the effect of fibrosis on adjacent mediastinal structures. Contrast-enhanced CT is helpful in evaluating the presence of vascular compression, including obstruction of the superior vena cava, pulmonary arteries, and pulmonary veins (Fig. 17-8). CT will also detect the presence of airway narrowing and obstruction.

Lung abnormalities may also be identified in patients with chronic mediastinitis and may occur secondary to the underlying granulomatous process (fungal or tuberculous infection, sarcoidosis) or secondary to complications of mediastinal fibrosis. For example, pulmonary artery or vein compression may result in the presence of pulmonary infarcts, and bronchial obstruction may result in the presence of postobstructive pneumonitis and atelectasis.

Mediastinal fibrosis is often suggested on CT by the findings of abnormal fibrous tissue and multiple calcified mediastinal lymph nodes. The diagnosis may be more difficult to make in cases that present as diffuse fibrosis without calcification. In such cases, the appearance of mediastinal fibrosis may be difficult to distinguish from diffuse mediastinal involvement by malignancy, including lymphoma and metastatic carcinoma. MRI plays an important diagnostic role in such cases, because benign mediastinal fibrosis will demonstrate low signal intensity on both T1- and T2-weighted images (Fig. 17-9 on p. 471) and malignant processes will typically demonstrate bright signal intensity on T2-weighted images. MRI is also helpful for assessing vascular patency in cases of suspected vascular obstruction, particularly in patients who have contraindications to intravenous contrast.

Diffuse Mediastinal Lymphadenopathy

When lymphadenopathy involves multiple lymph node sites, it may result in the presence of diffuse mediastinal widening. This is especially true of diffuse neoplastic mediastinal lymphadenopathy, particularly secondary to lymphoma (Fig. 17-10 on p. 472) and small-cell lung cancer. Metastases from extrathoracic neoplasms that may present with diffuse mediastinal lymphadenopathy include poorly differentiated neoplasms; tumors arising in the head and neck, genitourinary tract, and breast; and melanoma (especially seminoma) (Box 17-3).

Box 17-2 Etiologies of Chronic Mediastinitis

INFECTION

Fungal (histoplasmosis, coccidiomycosis)
Tuberculosis

INFLAMMATORY

Sarcoidosis

IMMUNOLOGIC

Systemic lupus erythematosus
Rheumatoid arthritis
Raynaud's phenomenen

DRUGS

Methysergide

TRAUMATIC

Mediastinal hemorrhage (rare)

IDIOPATHIC

Sclerosing mediastinitis

Box 17-3 Diffuse Neoplastic Mediastinal Lymphadenopathy

Lymphoma (especially Hodgkin's lymphoma)
Bronchogenic carcinoma (especially small-cell carcinoma)
Extrathoracic primary neoplasm (especially poorly differentiated neoplasms; neoplasms of the head and neck, genitourinary tract, and breast; and melanoma)

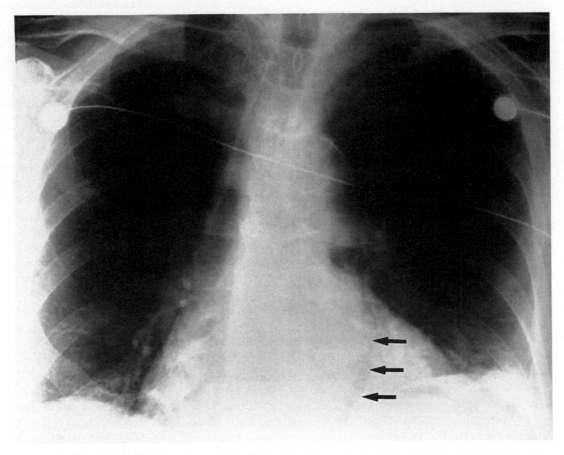

Fig. 17-3 Acute mediastinitis secondary to esophageal perforation (Boerhaave's syndrome). Frontal radiograph of the chest reveals an abnormal linear lucency *(arrows)* adjacent to the descending aortic interface, consistent with pneumomediastinum.

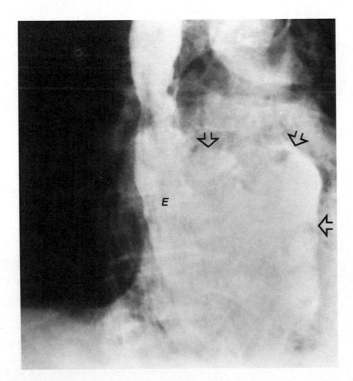

Fig. 17-4 Acute mediastinitis secondary to esophageal perforation (Boerhaave's syndrome) Coned-down image of the distal esophagus following administration of water-soluble contrast media demonstrates extravasation of contrast *(open arrows)* from the distal esophagus, consistent with an esophageal perforation.

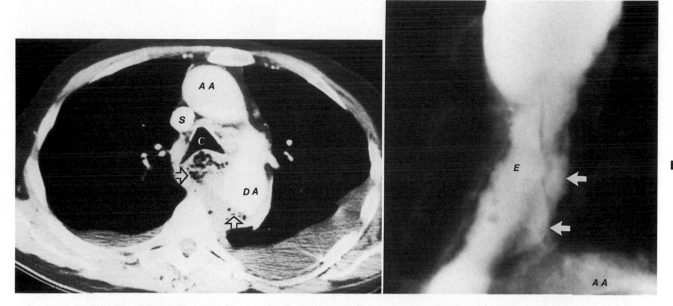

Fig. 17-5   Mediastinal abcess following esophageal perforation from penetrating trauma. **A,** Axial contrast-enhanced CT of the chest at the level of the carina *(C)* reveals a large subcarinal fluid collection *(arrows)* containing foci of gas, consistent with a mediastinal abcess. *AA* ascending aorta; *DA,* descending aorta; *S,* superior vena cava. **B,** Coned-down image of the upper thoracic esophagus following administration of water-soluble contrast media demonstrates extravasation of contrast *(arrows)* consistent with esophageal perforation. *AA,* aortic arch.

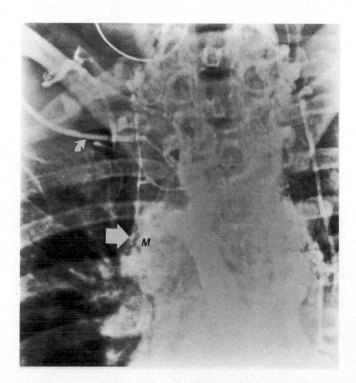

Fig. 17-6   Mediastinal fibrosis secondary to histoplasmosis. Coned-down image of the chest following contrast injection into a right subclavian vein catheter *(small curved arrow)* demonstrates obstruction of the superior vena cava secondary to a large calcified right paratracheal mass *(arrow, M)*. Note the opacification of extensive venous collaterals throughout the chest. Histoplasmosis is the most common benign cause of superior vena caval obstruction.

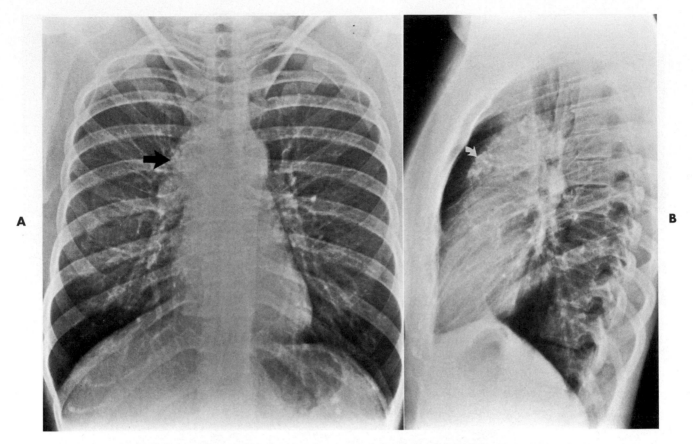

Fig. 17-7   Mediastinal fibrosis secondary to histoplasmosis. **A,** Frontal radiograph of the chest demonstrates a large calcified right paratracheal mass *(arrow)*. **B,** Lateral chest radiograph reveals calcified anterior mediastinal lymph nodes *(curved arrow)*.

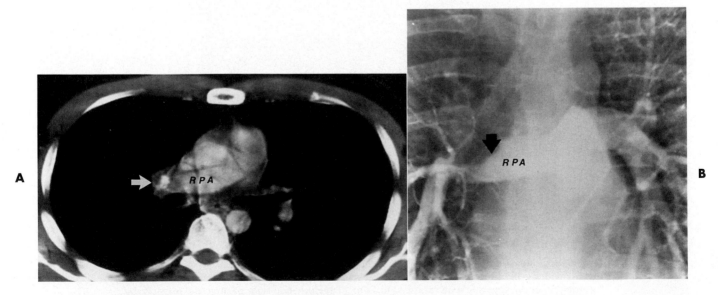

Fig. 17-8   Mediastinal fibrosis secondary to histoplasmosis. **A,** Axial contrast-enhanced CT image demonstrates a calcified nodal mass *(arrow)* compressing the distal right pulmonary artery (RPA). **B,** Pulmonary artery angiogram reveals obstruction of the truncus anterior branch of the right pulmonary artery (RPA). Note the contour deformity of the distal right pulmonary artery *(arrow)* secondary to extrinsic compression from the calcified nodal mass.

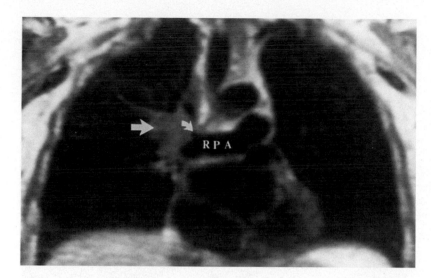

Fig. 17-9   Mediastinal fibrosis secondary to histoplasmosis. Coronal T1-weighted MRI (same patient as in Fig. 17-7). The nodal mass *(straight arrow)* is characterized by relatively low signal intensity. The truncus anterior *(curved arrow)* is obstructed just distal to its origin from the right pulmonary artery (RPA). The nodal mass also demonstrated low signal intensity on T2-weighted images (not shown), a characteristic feature of mediastinal fibrosis.

Table 17-1   Mediastinal lymphadenopathy, radiographic findings

Lymph Node Station	Radiographic Findings
ANTERIOR MEDIASTINAL	
Internal mammary	Lobulated upper retrosternal opacity on lateral CXR; parasternal mass on PA CXR (Fig. 17-11)
Prevascular	
Left prevascular	Partial or complete obscuration of the aortic knob (Fig. 17-12)
Right prevascular	Usually not demonstrated on CXR
Aorticopulmonary window	Convex bulge at junction of the descending aorta and left pulmonary artery (Fig. 17-13)
Anterior diaphragmatic	Cardiophrenic angle mass on PA CXR (Fig. 17-14)
MIDDLE MEDIASTINAL	
Paratracheal	
Right paratracheal	Thickened right paratracheal stripe (>3 mm) (Fig.17-15)
Left paratracheal	Usually not demonstrated on CXR
Azygous	Enlarged azygous diameter (>10 mm) (Fig. 17-12)
Subcranial	Lateral convex bulge in the azgoesophageal interface; widened subcranial angle (Fig. 17-15)
POSTERIOR MEDIASTINAL	
Paraesophageal	Usually not demonstrated on CXR
Paraaortic	Usually not demonstrated on CXR
Paravertebral	Lateral displacement of the paraspinal lines (see Fig.15-2, Chapter 15)

CXR, chest x ray.

Identification of enlarged lymph nodes on chest radiographs is dependent on recognition of characteristic alterations in the normal mediastinal landmarks. Table 17-1 reviews the typical radiographic findings associated with lymph node enlargement in various lymph node stations. Characteristic radiographic appearances of lymphadenopathy with CT correlation are illustrated in Figures 17-11 through 17-15 on pages 473-477.

Multiple mediastinal contour abnormalities corresponding to known anatomic lymph node sites suggest the diagnosis of diffuse lymphadenopathy. On CT, it usually presents as multiple discrete masses located in known lymph node sites, such as the azygous, subcarinal, and aorticopulmonary window regions. CT is helpful both for detecting enlarged lymph nodes and for further characterizing them (Fig. 17-16 on page 478).

Text continues on p. 479

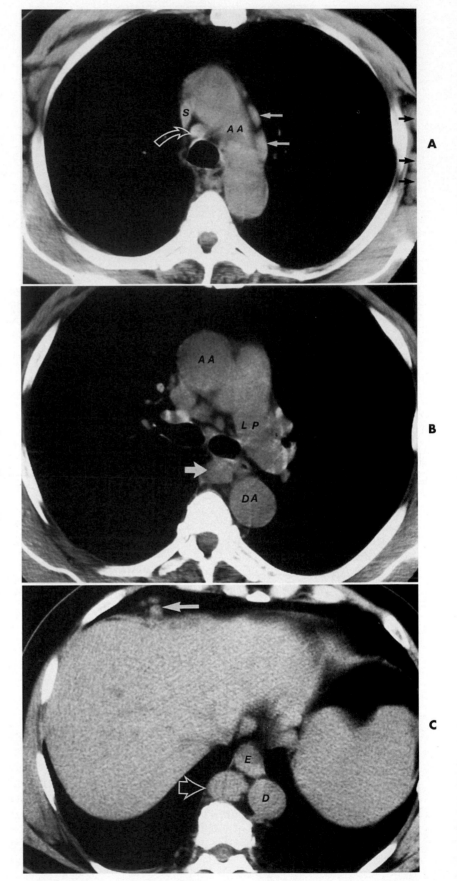

Fig. 17-10 Diffuse lymphadenopathy secondary to lymphoma. **A,** Axial noncontrast CT image of the chest at the level of the aortic arch *(AA)* demonstrates prevascular *(closed white arrows)*, pretracheal *(open curved white arrow)* and left axillary *(black arrows)* lymphadenopathy. *S,* superior vena cava. **B,** Axial CT image of the chest at the level of the left pulmonary artery (LP) reveals an enlarged posterior mediastinal lymph node *(arrow)*. *DA,* descending aorta. **C,** Axial CT image at the level of the diaphragm demonstrates additional lymph nodes anterior to the liver *(closed arrow)* and in the paraaortic region *(open arrow)*. *D,* descending aorta; *E,* esophagus.

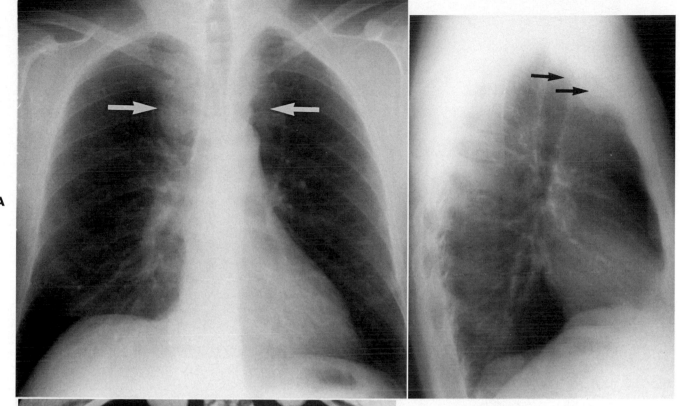

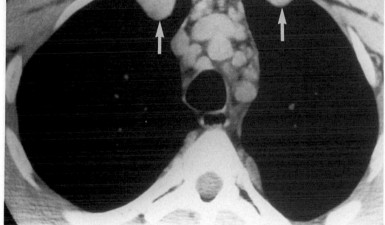

Fig. 17-11 Internal mammary lymph node enlargement secondary to lymphoma. **A,** Frontal radiograph of the chest reveals a large right parasternal mass and a subtle left parasternal mass *(white arrows)*. Internal mammary nodes must be considerably enlarged before they are detectable on frontal radiographs. **B,** Lateral chest radiograph demonstrates lobulated upper retrosternal opacities *(black arrows)*. Internal mammary node enlargement is usually easier to detect on the lateral projection. **C,** Axial noncontrast CT image at the level of the great vessels reveals bilateral lobulated soft-tissue masses *(white arrows)* representing enlarged internal mammary lymph nodes. They are most commonly enlarged in patients with lymphoma and metastatic breast cancer. Also note the presence of extensive lymphadenopathy in the prevascular, paratracheal, and paravertebral regions.

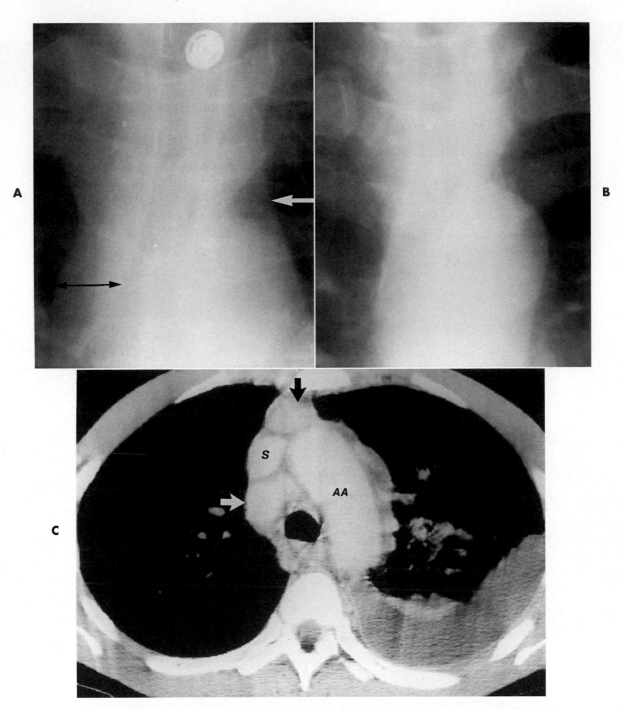

Fig. 17-12 Diffuse mediastinal lymphadenopathy secondary to metastatic carcinoma. **A & B,** Coned-down image of the mediastinum (A) demonstrates widening of the left supraaortic mediastinal contour *(white arrow)* and indistinctness of the superior aspect of the aortic arch, corresponding to the presence of enlarged left prevascular lymph nodes. These abnormalities are more apparent when you compare with a normal radiograph of the same patient (B) obtained several years earlier. Also note widening of the right paratracheal stripe and enlargement of the azygous contour *(black arrows).* **C,** Contrast-enhanced axial CT image at the level of the aortic arch *(AA)* demonstrates enlarged enhancing lymph nodes in the azygous *(white arrow)* and right prevascular *(black arrow)* regions. Enlarged right prevascular lymph nodes are not usually apparent on chest radiographs (*S,* superior vena cava).

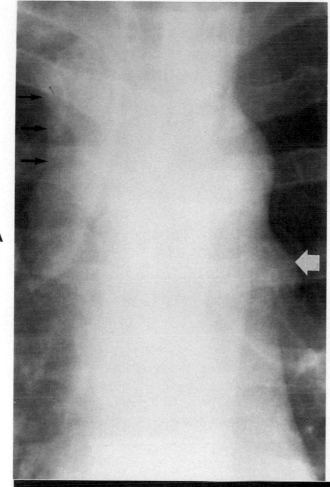

Fig. 17-13 Diffuse mediastinal lymphadenopathy secondary to metastatic carcinoma. **A,** Coned-down image of the mediastinum demonstrates a convex bulge *(short white arrow)* at the junction between the descending aorta and left pulmonary artery (the "aortic-pulmonary window"). Also note the presence of thickening of the right paratracheal stripe *(small black arrows)* and enlargement of the azygous contour. **B,** Axial noncontrast CT image at the level of the origin of the right and left mainstem bronchi reveals a large nodal mass *(short white arrow)* in the aorticopulmonary region. Also note the presence of an enlarged lymph node in the anterior subcarinal region *(curved white arrow),* located posterior to the superior vena cava *(S)* and ascending aorta *(A)* *(D, descending aorta).*

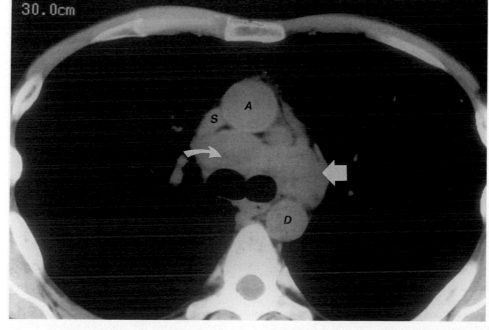

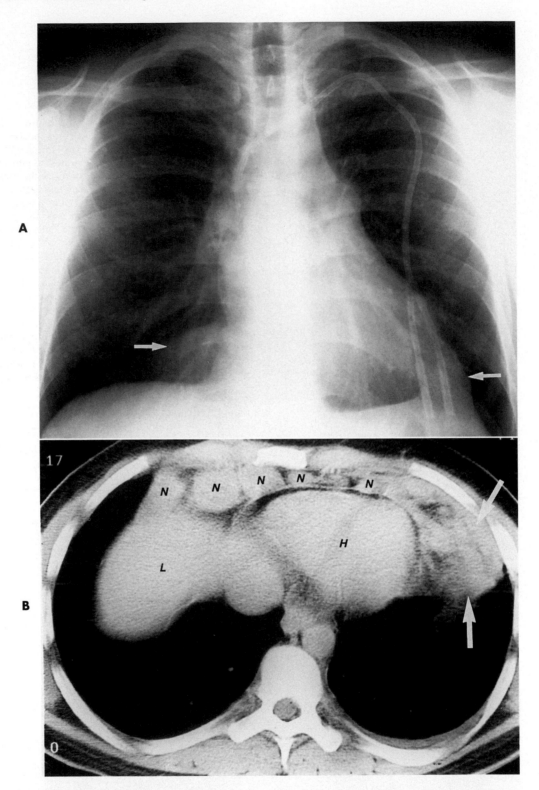

Fig. 17-14   Anterior diaphragmatic lymph node enlargement secondary to recurrent Hodgkin's lymphoma. **A,** Frontal chest radiograph reveals bilateral cardiophrenic angle masses *(arrows)*. **B,** Axial contrast-enhanced CT image at the level of the diaphragm demonstrates multiple discrete enlarged lymph nodes *(N)* and a large nodal mass *(arrows)* along the superior surface of the diaphragm anterior to the heart *(H)* and liver *(L)*. The most medial of these nodes are referred to as pericardiac lymph nodes. Anterior diaphragmatic lymph nodes are most frequently involved by lymphoma. This is a frequent site of recurrence in patients with Hodgkin's disease.

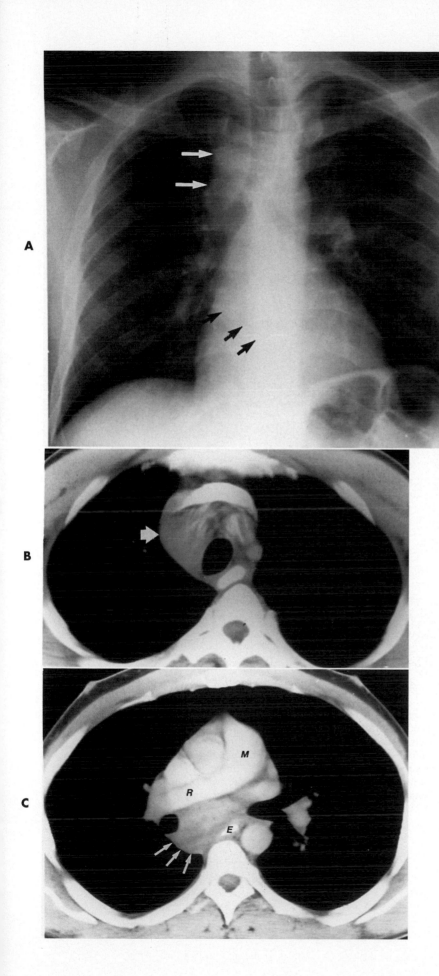

Fig. 17-15 Diffuse mediastinal lymphade-nopathy secondary to lymphoma. **A,** Frontal chest radiograph demonstrates widening of the right paratracheal stripe *(paired white arrows)* corresponding to the presence of enlarged right paratracheal lymph nodes. There is also an abnormal lateral convex bulge in the azygo-esophageal interface *(black arrows)* corre-sponding to enlarged subcarinal lymph nodes. **B,** Contrast-enhanced CT image at the level of the great vessels reveals an enlarged right para-tracheal lymph node *(arrow).* **C,** CT image at the level of the main pulmonary artery *(M)* demonstrates a large nodal mass in the subcari-nal region *(arrows),* accounting for the lateral-ly displaced azygoesophageal interface on CXR *(R,* right pulmonary artery, *E,* esophagus).

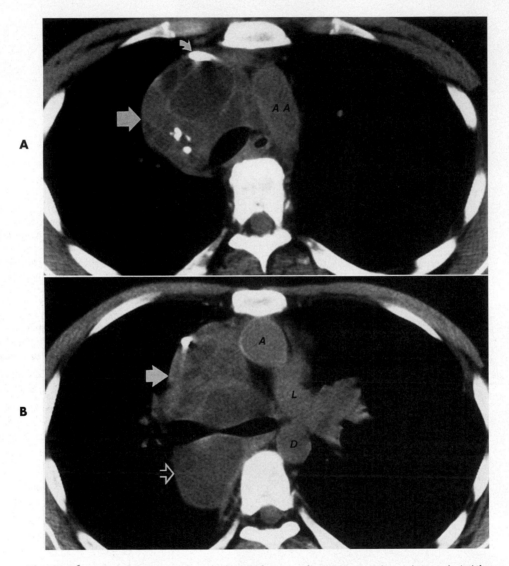

Fig. 17-16   Diffuse mediastinal lymphadenopathy secondary to metastatic seminoma. **A,** Axial non-contrast CT image of the chest at the level of the aortic arch *(AA).* There is a large heterogeneous right paratracheal mass *(arrow),* which demonstrates central foci of low attenuation consistent with necrosis as well as several dense foci of calcification. A central venous catheter *(small curved arrow)* is present within the anteriorly displaced superior vena cava. **B,** Axial noncontrast CT image of the chest at the level of the left pulmonary artery *(L)* demonstrates the inferior extent of the right paratracheal mass *(closed arrow)* as well as an additional low-attenuation lymph node mass *(open arrow)* posteriorly. Low-attenuation lymph nodes are a characteristic feature of metastatic seminoma.

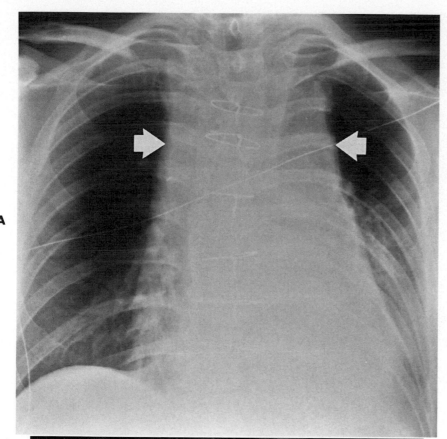

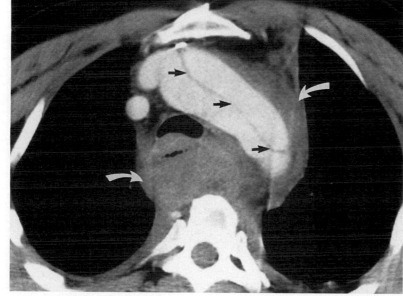

Fig. 17-17 Mediastinal hemorrhage secondary to aortic rupture. **A,** Frontal chest radiograph reveals diffuse widening of the mediastinum (*arrows*) and a left pleural effusion in a patient who is status post median sternotomy and aortic valve replacement. **B,** Axial contrast-enhanced CT image of the chest at the level of the aortic arch. An intimal flap is present within the aortic arch (*black arrows*) consistent with aortic dissection. There is extensive high-attenuation fluid throughout the mediastinum (*curved arrows*), consistent with diffuse mediastinal hemorrhage.

Mediastinal Hemorrhage

Mediastinal hemorrhage may occur secondary to a variety of etiologies, including traumatic, iatrogenic, and spontaneous (Box 17-4). It is often secondary to abnormalities of the thoracic aorta, including traumatic aortic transection and rupture of a thoracic aortic aneurysm. However, mediastinal hemorrhage may also result from abnormalities of other vascular structures in the thorax, including veins and arteries, or following trauma to the cervical and thoracic spine. Spontaneous mediastinal hemorrhage is an uncommon complication of coagulopathies. The most common chest radiographic finding of hemorrhage is diffuse mediastinal widening (Fig. 17-17).

Because trauma is the most common cause of mediastinal hemorrhage, we will focus the remainder of our discussion on traumatic transection of the aorta. Aortic transection is a life-threatening complication of trauma and is usually the result of a rapid deceleration injury,

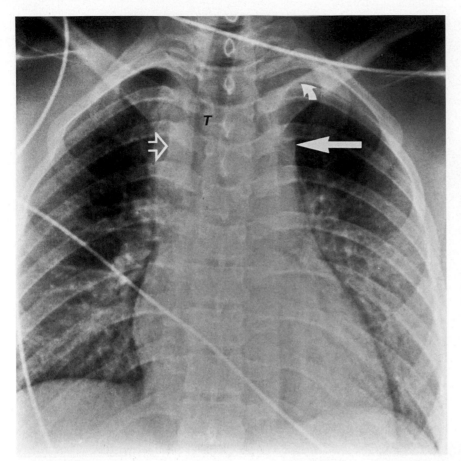

Fig. 17-18 Mediastinal hemorrhage secondary to traumatic aortic transection. Supine portable chest radiograph demonstrates several radiographic signs of mediastinal hemorrhage: mediastinal widening, rightward deviation of the trachea (*T*), widening of the right paratracheal stripe (*open arrow*), indistinctness of the aortic arch (*closed straight arrow*) and a left apical cap (*small closed curved arrow*). Angiography (not shown) revealed a transection of the aorta at the level of the ligamentum arteriosum.

Box 17-4 Etiologies of Mediastinal Hemorrhage

TRAUMATIC

Aortic transection

Laceration of branch vessels of aorta and thoracic venous structures

Fracture of cervical or thoracic vertebral bodies

IATROGENIC

Transection of subclavian artery or vein during central venous catheter placement

Transection of adjacent vascular structures during sternal marrow aspiration, pericardiocentesis, arteriography, and cervical and thoracic surgical procedures

AORTIC, ANEURYSM RUPTURE

SPONTANEOUS HEMORRHAGE

Coagulopathy (rare)

Box 17-5 Chest Radiographic Signs of Aortic Injury

Mediastinal widening

Abnormal aortic knob contour (indistinct or irregular) and loss of the aortic pulmonary window

Rightward deviation of the trachea

Depression of the left main bronchus

Rightward deviation of the nasogastric tube

Widening of the right paratracheal stripe

Displacement of the paraspinal lines

Left apical cap

Left pleural effusion

---

often secondary to a motor vehicle accident. There are three common sites of occurrence of aortic transections: (1) at the level of the ligamentum arteriosum, (2) at the level of the aortic root, and (3) at the level of the diaphragm. In patients who survive the initial injury, the majority of aortic transections (80%) occur at the level of the ligamentum arteriosum, which is located just distal to the origin of the left subclavian artery.

There are a variety of radiographic signs (Box 17-5; Fig. 17-18). You should know that no single radiographic sign is highly specific for aortic injury. The most reliable signs are mediastinal widening and an abnormal aortic contour. Thus, a careful evaluation of the mediastinal width and aortic contour is critical in the radiologic assessment of a trauma patient. Unfortunately, the mediastinum is often difficult to assess in these patients because radiographs are frequently obtained using a portable supine technique that magnifies the normal

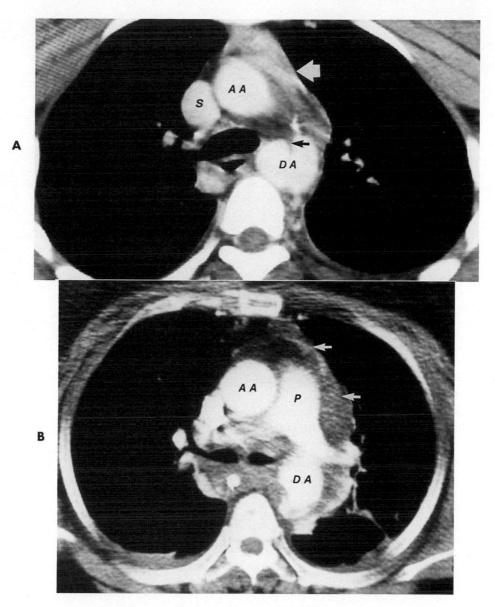

Fig. 17-19 Mediastinal hemorrhage secondary to traumatic aortic transection in two different patients. **A,** Axial contrast-enhanced CT image of the chest reveals a focal high-attenuation mass in the anterior mediastinum (*white arrow*) consistent with a mediastinal hematoma. Note the presence of an intimal flap (*black arrow*) within the proximal descending thoracic aorta (*DA*). Angiography confirmed the presence of an aortic transection. *AA,* ascending aorta; S, superior vena cava. **B,** Axial contrast-enhanced CT in another patient demonstrates a heterogenous appearance of the mediastinal fat, with diffuse high-attenuation stranding of the fat (*arrows*) secondary to mediastinal hemorrhage. Note the contour deformity of the descending thoracic aorta (*DA*). Transection of the proximal descending thoracic aorta was confirmed at angiography. *AA,* ascending aorta; *P,* main pulmonary artery.

mediastinal structures. In addition, trauma patients may be unable to achieve a full inspiration, resulting in further magnification of the mediastinal contours. Trauma patients may also have coexisting radiographic abnormalities, such as pulmonary contusion, atelectasis, aspiration, and paramediastinal pleural fluid collections, that obscure the mediastinal contours. Finally, there may be superimposed devices such as a trauma board, oxygen tubing, and monitoring devices, which can obscure visualization of the mediastinal structures.

Diagnostic evaluation is controversial. It is generally agreed that the presence of chest radiographic findings such as mediastinal widening and indistinctness of the aortic knob should lead to emergent angiography. In many cases, however, chest radiographic findings are equivocal. In such instances, CT plays an important role in screening for the presence of mediastinal hemorrhage. On CT, hemorrhage may be identified as abnormal foci of increased attenuation within the normally homogeneous low-attenuation mediastinal fat,

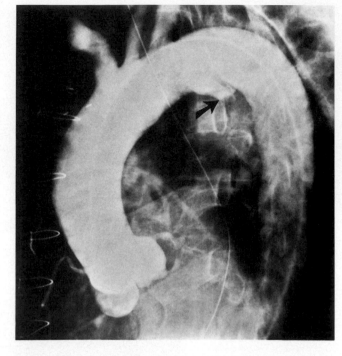

Fig. 17-20 Traumatic aortic transection. Thoracic aortagram reveals a posttraumatic pseudoaneurysm of the proximal descending thoracic aorta at the level of the ligamentum arteriosum. This is the most common site of aortic transection in patients who survive the initial injury.

either in the form of diffuse stranding of the fat (hemorrhage) or a focal mass (hematoma) (Fig. 17-19). Although aortic injuries can be detected by identification of a focal contour abnormality or an intimal flap on contrast-enhanced CT, angiography remains the study of choice for the evaluation of traumatic aortic transection (Fig. 17-20).

SUGGESTED READINGS

Fraser RG, Paré JAP, Paré PD, Fraser FS, Genereux GP: *Diagnosis of diseases of the chest,* ed 3, Philadelphia, 1988, WB Saunders.

Gavant ML, Menke PG, Fabian T, et al: Blunt traumatic aortic rupture: detection with helical CT of the chest, *Radiology* 197:125-133, 1995.

Halpert RD, Goodman P: *Gastrointestinal radiology: the requisites,* St. Louis, 1993, Mosby–Year Book.

Heitzman ER: *The mediastinum: radiologic correlations with anatomy and pathology,* ed 2, Berlin, Germany, 1988, Springer-Verlag.

Libshitz HI: Intrathoracic lymph nodes. In Freundlich IM, Bragg DG, editors: *A radiologic approach to diseases of the chest,* Baltimore, 1992, Williams & Wilkins; pp 100-114.

Naidich DP, Zerhouni EA, Siegelman SS: *Computed tomography and magnetic resonance of the thorax,* ed 2, New York, 1991, Raven Press.

Reed JC: *Chest radiology: plain film patterns and differential diagnoses,* ed 3, St. Louis, 1991, Mosby–Year Book.

Rholl KS, Levitt RG, Glazer HS: Magnetic resonance imaging of fibrosing mediastinitis, *AJR* 145:255-259, 1985.

Richardson P, Mirvis SE, Scorpio R et al: Value of CT in determining the need for angiography when findings of mediastinal hemorrhage on chest radiographs are equivocal, *AJR* 156:273-279, 1991.

Shaffer K, Pugatch RD: Diseases of the mediastinum. In Freundlich IM, Bragg DG (eds): *A radiologic approach to diseases of the chest,* Baltimore, 1992, Williams & Wilkins; pp 171-185.

Webb WR: Diseases of the mediastinum. In Putman CE, Ravin CE (eds). *Textbook of diagnostic imaging,* ed 2, Philadelphia, 1994, WB Saunders; pp 428-447.

Woodring JH, Loh FK, Kryscio RJ: Mediastinal hemorrhage: an evaluation of radiographic manifestations, *Radiology* 151:15-21, 1984.

A number of different imaging modalities are frequently used to image the pleural space. The most important is chest radiography, which remains the initial examination in the assessment of pleural disease. Other imaging techniques that may be used include computed tomography (CT) and ultrasound. Magnetic resonance (MR) imaging currently plays a limited role in the assessment of pleural abnormalities.

ANATOMY AND PHYSIOLOGY OF THE PLEURAL SPACE

The pleura consists of a visceral and parietal layer that is composed of a continuous surface epithelium of mesothelial cells and underlying connective tissue. The visceral pleura covers the lungs and interlobar fissures whereas the parietal pleura lines the ribs, diaphragm, and mediastinum. A double fold of pleura extends from the hilum to the diaphragm to form the inferior pulmonary ligament. There is no communication between the two pleural cavities. The pleural space is a potential space that contains 2 to 10 ml of pleural fluid in the normal individual. The pleura can produce up to 100 ml of fluid in an hour, and the absorption capacity of the pleural surface is approximately 300 ml per hour. The parietal pleura is supplied by systemic capillary vessels and drains into the right atrium by way of the azygos, hemiazygos, and internal mammary veins. The visceral pleura is supplied by pulmonary arterioles and capillaries and drains mainly into the pulmonary veins. Fluid is usually produced at the level of the parietal pleura and is drained by the visceral pleura. Lymphatics also play a role in the clearance of pleural fluid in health and disease. Lymphatic drainage occurs through the parietal pleural lymphatics and ultimately reaches the thoracic duct. The lymphatic drainage of the pleural space begins within lymphatic stomata located mainly in the mediastinal, intercostal, and diaphragmatic portions of the parietal pleura. These eventually drain into larger lymphatic channels. The visceral subpleural space is in continuity with the interlobular septa of the pulmonary interstitium. In contrast with the parietal pleura there is no communication between lymphatic channels of the visceral pleura and the pleural space. Lymph from the visceral pleura flows centripetally toward the hila.

The main manifestations of disease in the pleura include pleural effusion, pleural thickening (which may or may not be calcified), pleural air (i.e., pneumothorax), and pleural neoplasms. Primary disease of the pleura is rare. Most pleural abnormalities occur subsequent to disease processes in other organs.

PLEURAL EFFUSIONS

General Considerations and Clinical Features

Pleural effusions occur when the rates of entry and exit for pleural liquid and protein are no longer in equilibrium. Increased pleural fluid may result from one of six mechanisms (Box 18-1): (1) increase in hydrostatic pressure in the microvascular circulation, for example, in congestive heart failure (CHF); (2) decrease in osmotic pressure in the microvascular circulation as seen in patients with hypoalbuminemia and cirrhosis; (3) decrease in pressure in the pleural space as occurs in atelectasis; (4) increased permeability of the microvascular circulation such as seen in inflammatory and neoplastic processes in the pleura; (5) impaired lymphatic drainage from the pleural space due to blockage of the lymphatic

system by tumor or fibrosis; and (6) transport of fluid from the peritoneal space by way of diaphragmatic lymphatic vessels or through diaphragmatic defects as may occur in patients with ascites.

Pleural effusions may either be transudates or exudates (Box 18-2). Transudates are usually caused by increased capillary hydrostatic pressure or decreased osmotic pressure such as in CHF, hypoalbuminemia, hepatic cirrhosis, and nephrotic syndrome. Management of transudates usually consists of treatment of the underlying cause such as CHF. Exudates on the other hand are secondary to inflammatory and neoplastic processes involving the pleura. Other examples include pulmonary infarction and collagen vascular diseases. The presence of an exudate requires a clinical investigation to determine the cause of the pleural effusion. Exudates are characterized by the following criteria: (1) a pleural fluid protein concentration divided by the serum protein concentration greater than 0.5; (2) a pleural fluid lactate dehydrogenase (LDH) level divided by the serum LDH level greater than 0.6; or (3) a pleural fluid LDH level greater than two thirds of the upper limit of normal for the serum LDH level. An exudative effusion with frank pus is referred to as an empyema. Hemothoraces may arise from traumatic laceration of vessels adjacent to the pleura. A pleural fluid hematocrit greater than 50% of the peripheral blood hematocrit establishes the diagnosis. Hemorraghic effusions may also occur with neoplasms, tuberculosis, and infarction. Rupture or obstruction of major lymphatic channels such as the thoracic duct may result in a chylothorax, suggested by the presence of elevated triglyceride and cholesterol levels in the pleural fluid. Pleural effusions may also contain a high proportion of eosinophils. Causes include drug hypersensitivity, pneumonia, and pulmonary infarction. Intraabdominal abnormalities may lead to pleural effusions such as ascites, benign ovarian fibroma (Meig's syndrome), hydronephrosis, and pancreatitis.

Predominantly left-sided effusions may be caused by pancreatitis, distal thoracic duct obstruction, Dressler's syndrome, and postpericardiotomy syndrome. Predominantly right-sided effusions occur in proximal thoracic duct obstruction and ascites related to hepatic or ovarian disease and in endometriosis.

Box 18-1 Physiologic Mechanisms In the Development of Pleural Effusions

Increase in hydrostatic pressure in microvascular circulation (CHF)
Decrease in osmotic pressure in microvascular circulation
  Hypoalbuminemia
  Cirrhosis
Decrease in pleural pressure
  Atelectasis
Increase in permeability of microvascular circulation
  Inflammatory conditions
  Neoplasms
Impaired lymphatic drainage
  Tumor
  Fibrosis
Transport of fluid from abdomen
  Ascites

CHF, congestive heart failure.

Box 18-2 Types of Effusions

Transudates
Exudates
  Empyema
  Hemothorax
  Chylothorax

Radiologic Features

Standard radiographs

On an upright chest radiograph a free pleural effusion will demonstrate a "meniscus" sign, that is, a concave upward sloping that occurs at the costophrenic angle (Figs. 18-1 and 18-2). Usually approximately 200 ml of fluid is necessary to blunt the lateral costophrenic angle, although smaller amounts, that is, greater than 75 ml, will produce a meniscus that blunts the posterior costophrenic angle on the lateral view (Fig. 18-3). A lateral decubitus view of the chest is much more sensitive than the upright view in the detection of pleural effusion, and as little as 5 ml of fluid can be demonstrated on decubitus views (Fig. 18-4).

In the upright position in the normal individual, a small amount of pleural fluid will accumulate in a subpulmonic position. In certain individuals a large amount of free-flowing pleural fluid may accumulate in this position before spilling into the costophrenic angles. On the frontal view, this produces a characteristic appearance with elevation of the apparent ipsilateral hemidiaphragm, flattening of the medial aspect, and displacement of the peak of the diaphragm laterally. On the left side this is easy to recognize because of separation of the stomach bubble from the apparent left hemidiaphragm (Fig. 18-5). A massive effusion will produce a complete or nearly complete opacification of a hemithorax with displacement of the mediastinum to the opposite side (Fig. 18-6). This appearance contrasts with complete atelectasis of the lung where the shift of the mediastinum is toward the side of the opaque hemithorax. Moderate to large amounts of pleural effusion may be missed on supine radiographs. Such effusions will layer posteriorly and produce a generalized increase in opacity of the hemithorax, through which the pulmonary vessels can still be visualized (Fig. 18-7). There may be blunting of the costophrenic angle and on occasion the fluid will track over the apex of the lung producing an apical cap.

Fluid may occasionally accumulate within fissures. Such accumulations may produce the appearance of a mass or "pseudotumor" (Fig. 18-8). The differentiation from a mass can be easily made because the fluid is free and will shift on decubitus views.

Pleural effusions frequently loculate (Fig. 18-9), that is, they do not shift freely in the pleural space because of adhesions between the visceral and parietal pleura. Loculation of fluid occurs in exudative effusions but particularly in empyema and hemothorax.

Text continues on p. 491

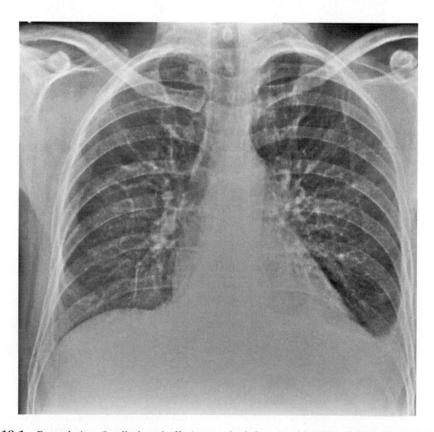

Fig. 18-1   Frontal view. Small pleural effusion on the left causes blunting of the left costophrenic sulcus producing a meniscus.

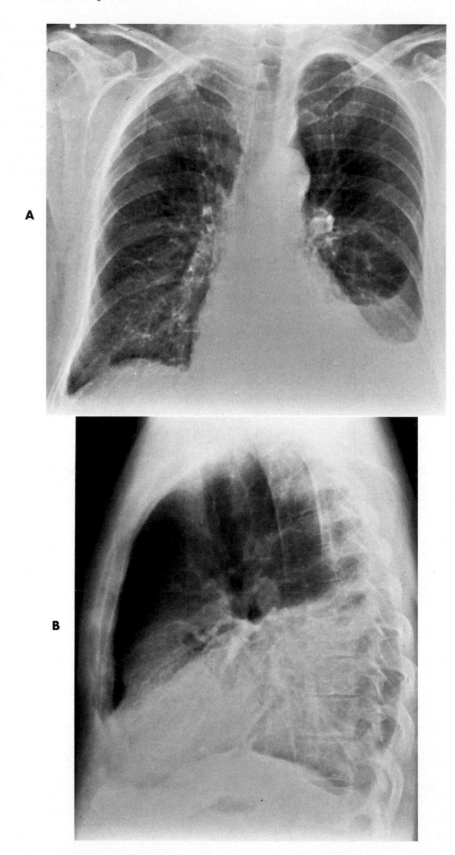

Fig. 18-2   A, Frontal view demonstrates a meniscus in the left costophrenic angle. The effusion extends upward along the left lateral chest wall. **B,** On the lateral view the fluid extends anteriorly but reaches a higher level posteriorly than anteriorly.

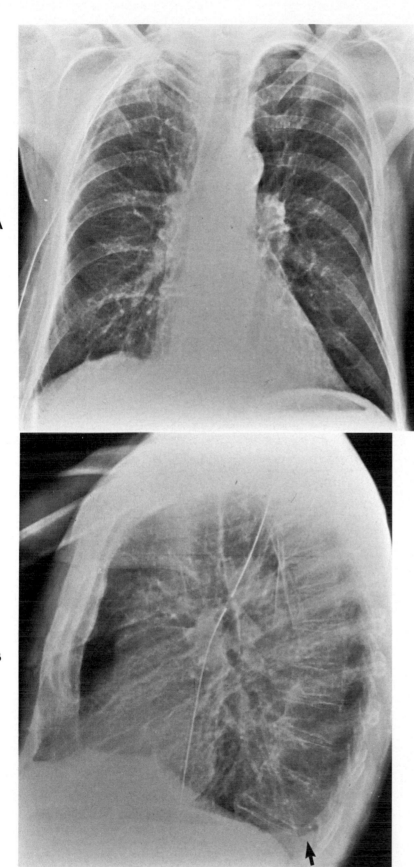

Fig. 18-3.   Small pleural effusion seen only on the lateral view. **A,** On the frontal PA radiograph the costophrenic angle on the right is sharp. **B,** The lateral view demonstrates minimal blunting of the right costophrenic angle *(arrow).*

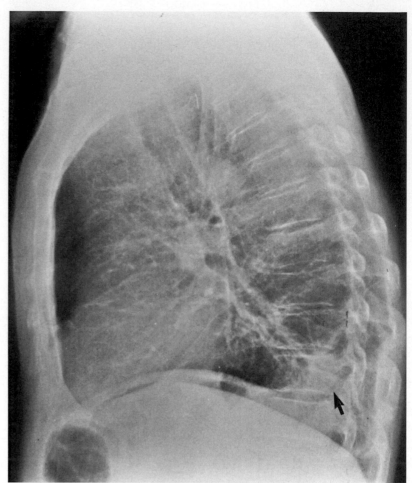

A

Fig. 18-4 **A,** Lateral view shows blunting of the costophrenic angle posteriorly *(arrow).* **B,** Left side down decubitus radiograph demonstrates fluid layering along the left lateral chest wall *(arrows).*

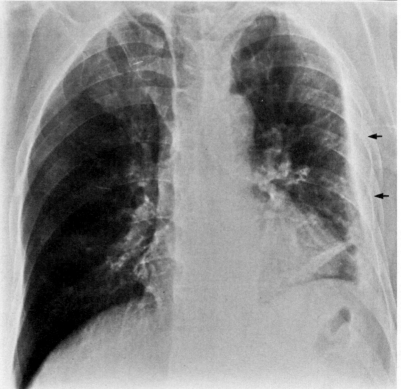

B

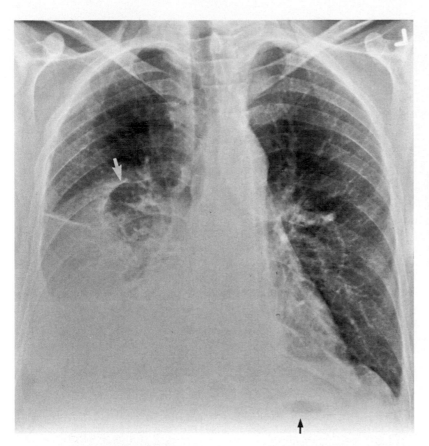

Fig. 18-5 Subpulmonic effusion. On the left there is separation of the apparent hemidiaphragm from the stomach bubble *(black arrow)*. There is also minimal blunting of the lateral costophrenic angle. On the right a large effusion extends to the major fissure subtending a lucent area that represents the superior segment of the right lower lobe *(white arrow)*.

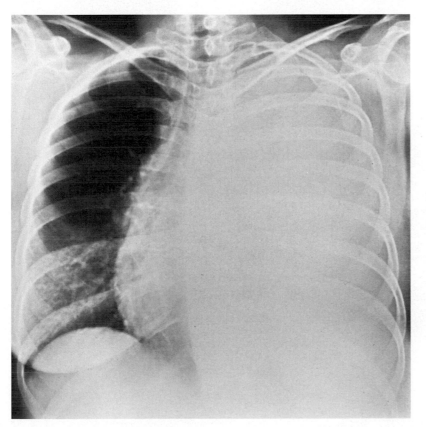

Fig. 18-6 Massive effusion. There is mediastinal shift to the opposite side and a completely opaque left hemithorax.

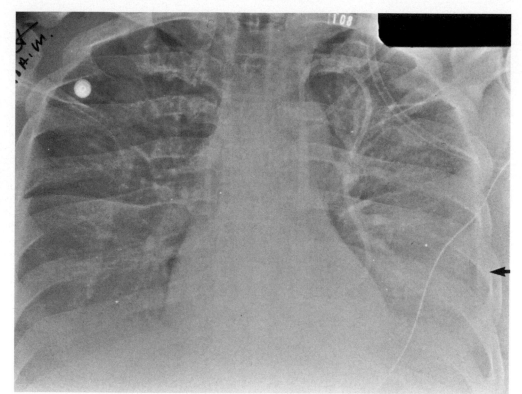

Fig. 18-7 Bilateral effusions. Supine position. Hazy opacification is noted in both hemithoraces caused by fluid layering posteriorly in the pleural spaces. The pulmonary vessels can still be visualized through the fluid. Fluid is present laterally on the left *(arrow)* and in the minor fissure.

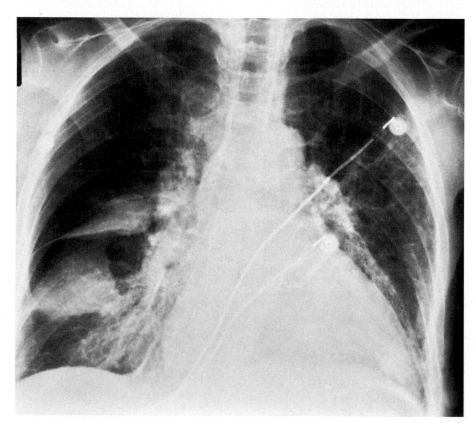

Fig. 18-8 Pseudotumor. Fluid is seen in both the upper and lower portions of the major fissure on the right and it extends into the minor fissure. Fluid in the fissure may have a tapered or spindle-shaped configuration as demonstrated in the more cephalad collection.

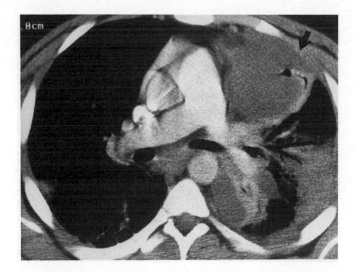

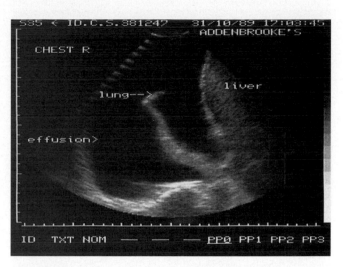

Fig. 18-9   Loculated effusion. CT demonstrates a large collection of pleural fluid in an anterior nondependent location *(arrow).* There is also a lenticular collection of fluid lateral to the spine that displaces the enhancing lung parenchyma of the left lower lobe.

Fig. 18-10   Anechoic pleural fluid collection. Sonogram shows collapsed right lower lobe surrounded by a large pleural effusion. *(From McLoud TC, Flower CD: Imaging of the pleura: Sonography, CT and MR imaging,* AJR *156:1145-1153, 1991.)*

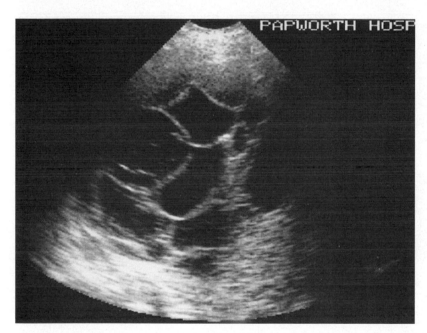

Fig. 18-11   Empyema with multiple loculations. There is a transonic space divided into multiple secondary loculations by curvilinear septa. *(From McLoud TC, Flower CD: Imaging of the pleura: Sonography, CT and MR imaging,* AJR *156:1145-1153, 1991.)*

Ultrasound

Ultrasound may be used to detect pleural abnormalities and to differentiate solid pleural masses from pleural effusions. However, ultrasound is most frequently used in severely ill patients and in the intensive care unit because of the ready availability for bedside imaging. Ultrasound is useful not only in detecting the presence of pleural fluid but as a guide to aspiration.

Pleural fluid collections may be either anechoic or echoic and may change shape during respiration. The majority of collections are anechoic (Fig. 18-10) and are delineated by an echogenic line of visceral pleura and lung. Anechoic effusions are usually transudates where-

as effusions that contain septations represent exudates in approximately 80% of cases (Fig. 18-11).

Computed tomography

Free-flowing pleural fluid produces a sickle-shaped opacity in the most dependent part of the thorax posteriorly on CT scanning (Fig. 18-12). CT allows very small amounts of pleural fluid to be detected. Loculated fluid collections are seen as lenticular opacities in fixed position (Fig. 18-9). CT is of limited value in differentiating transudates from exudates or in the diagnosis of chylous pleural effusions. Acute pleural hemorrhage however can be identified either by the presence of a fluid-fluid

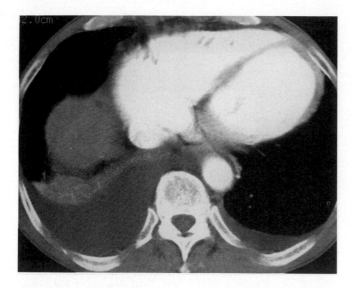

Fig. 18-12 Contrast-enhanced CT. There are bilateral pleural effusions, right greater than left. Both are of low attenuation and form sickle-shaped opacities posteriorly.

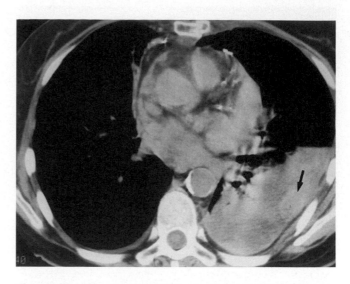

Fig. 18-13 Hemothorax following median sternotomy. There are multiple areas of increased attenuation in the fluid collection *(arrow)*.

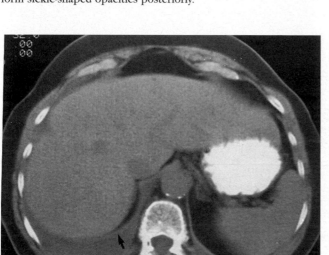

Fig. 18-14 Pleural fluid "displaced crus" sign. Pleural fluid lies inside the crus of the diaphragm *(arrow)* and displaces it away from the spine. *(From McLoud TC, Flower CD: Imaging of the pleura: Sonography, CT and MR imaging,* AJR *156:1145-1153, 1991.)*

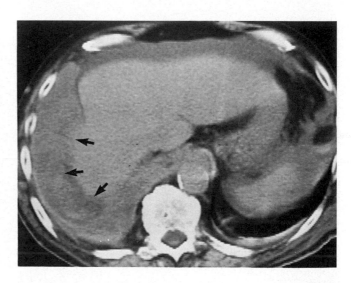

Fig. 18-15 "Interface" sign. Pleural fluid and ascites. A hazy indistinct interface is seen between the pleural effusion and liver laterally *(arrows)*. Ascites is present anteriorly. *(From McLoud TC, Flower CD: Imaging of the pleura: Sonography, CT and MR imaging,* AJR *156:1145-1153, 1991.)*

Box 18-3 Computed Tomography: Pleural Fluid versus Ascites

PLEURAL FLUID	ASCITES
Displaced crus	
Ill-defined interface with liver and spleen	Sharp interface with liver or spleen
Fluid outside diaphragm contour	Fluid inside diaphragm contour
	Fluid excluded from bare area of liver

---

level or because of increased attenuation of the pleural fluid collection (Fig. 18-13).

Pleural fluid can be distinguished from ascites by several CT features (Box 18-3). These include the "displaced crus" sign, the "interface" sign, the "diaphragm" sign, and the "bare area" sign. If the diaphragmatic crus is displaced away from the spine by an abnormal fluid collection, the fluid is located in the pleural space (Fig. 18-14). Ascites, on the other hand, lies lateral and anterior to the crus. The "interface" sign describes a sharp interface that can be identified between fluid and the liver or spleen when ascites is present. In ascites the interface is sharp, whereas in pleural effusion the interface is ill-defined (Fig. 18-

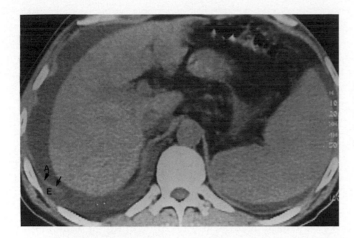

Fig. 18-16 Pleural fluid and ascites. "Diaphragm" sign. Ascites *(A)* lies inside the diaphragm (small arrows) and produces a sharp interface with the liver. The effusion *(E)* is visualized outside the diaphragm. *(From McLoud TC, Flower CD: Imaging of the pleura: Sonography, CT and MR imaging, AJR 156:1145-1153, 1991.)*

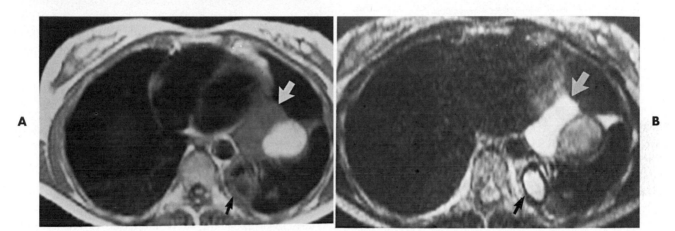

Fig. 18-17 **A,** (T1W) and **B,** (T2W) images. MRI of complex pleural effusion. There is typical pleural fluid abutting the heart of water content *(white arrows)* that is of low signal intensity on T1W images and bright signal intensity on T2W images. There is also a subacute hematoma *(black arrows)* that on the T2W image has bright internal signal characteristics and a dark concentric ring due to hemosiderin. The high signal intensity collection in the major fissure on the T1W image is due to fat (chylous effusion). There is T2 shortening similar to subcutaneous fat. *(From McLoud TC, Flower CD: Imaging of the pleura: Sonography, CT and MR imaging, AJR 156:1145-1153, 1991.)*

15). If the diaphragm is identifiable adjacent to an abnormal fluid collection in the right upper quadrant, then the "diaphragm" sign is probably the most reliable means of differentiating fluid from ascites (Fig. 18-16). The location of the diaphragm is readily visible in patients with ascites, but may not be identified in patients with pleural effusions. Pleural effusion is visualized outside the hemidiaphragm whereas ascites is seen within the hemidiaphragmatic contour. The bare area is the portion of the right lobe of the liver that lacks peritoneal covering. Restriction of peritoneal fluid by the coronary ligaments from that area is another useful distinguishing sign. To distinguish pleural effusions from intraabdominal fluid collections, all four signs should be assessed in each case. There can be certain pitfalls in the attempt to differentiate ascites from pleural effusion. A large pleural effusion, particularly on the left side, may cause inversion of the diaphragm resulting in the pleural fluid being located centrally rather than peripherally.

CT is helpful in the assessment and management of loculated pleural effusions (Fig. 18-9). Accurate localization of such loculated collections is useful prior to drainage. Loculated effusions have a lenticular configuration with smooth margins and displace the adjacent parenchyma. This is a typical appearance for any pleural process and this distinguishing feature can help differentiate a pleural from parenchymal process.

Magnetic resonance imaging

The role of MR imaging in the evaluation of the pleura is somewhat limited. MR does provide certain advantages because of its ability to image the thorax directly in the axial, sagittal, and coronal planes. MR may be slightly superior to CT in the characterization of pleural fluid (Fig. 18-17). Typically fluid collections in the pleural cavity show a low signal intensity on T1-weighted images and a high relative signal intensity on T2-weighted images because of their water content. It may be possible to differentiate transudates, simple exudates, and exudates with the use of a triple-echo pulse sequence. Complex exudates have greater signal intensity than simple exudates, which in turn are brighter than transudates. Preliminary results also suggest chylothorax may have distinctive findings on MR with signal intensity characteristics similar to those of subcutaneous fat. Subacute or chronic hematomas demonstrate typical signal intensity on MR with a "concentric ring" sign; this consists of an outer dark rim composed of hemosiderin and bright signal intensity in the center because of the T1 shortening effects of methemoglobin.

EMPYEMA

Clinical Features

An empyema may be defined as an exudative effusion with pus in the pleural cavity. There are a number of criteria that are used for the diagnosis of empyema and they include the following (Box 18-4): (1) grossly purulent fluid; (2) organisms identified on the basis of gram stain or culture; (3) a white blood cell count in the pleural fluid greater than 5×10^9 cells per liter; (4) a pH below 7 or glucose level less than 40 mg/ml. The natural progression of an empyema consists of several phases from an exudative to a fibropurulent phase and finally to an organizing phase that results in the development of a thickened pleura or "fibrin peel". Early diagnosis and treatment is therefore imperative.

Most empyemas are the result of acute bacterial pneumonias or abscesses, but they may occur following thoracic surgery, trauma, or very occasionally from hematogenous dissemination from extrapulmonary sites or direct spread through the diaphragm from a subphrenic abscess. Empyemas are frequently associated with a communication from the lung, that is, a bronchopleural fistula, which will produce air in the pleural space. Empyemas may drain into the chest wall producing an empyema necessitans.

Radiologic Features

See Box 18-5.

Standard radiographs

Most empyemas present as a classic pleural effusion. However, they tend to loculate early and as a result may not change with patient position, or they may not have a classic "meniscus" sign. Loculated collections will have a lenticular shape that forms obtuse angles with the chest wall. If a bronchopleural fistula is present, an air/fluid level will be identified in the empyema space prior to any thoracentesis (Fig. 18-18). On standard radiographs, the air/fluid level will vary in length on radiographs taken at 90 degrees to each other; that is, there may be a short air/fluid level on the frontal radiograph and a long air/fluid level on the lateral radiograph. This is in contradistinction to lung abscesses in which the length of the air/fluid level is usually equal on both views.

Computed tomography

CT is particularly helpful in establishing the diagnosis of empyema and helping to distinguish empyemas from lung abscesses. The most reliable sign is the so-called "split pleura" sign, which is usually identified during the organizing phase of an empyema (Fig. 18-19). After intravenous administration of a bolus of contrast medium, both the parietal and visceral pleura will enhance vigorously most likely due to the increased vascular supply in the inflamed pleura. In an empyema, both the parietal and visceral pleura will be thickened, and the extrapleural fat between the empyema space and the chest wall may be increased in size, particularly if the empyema is chronic, and the fat may also be increased in attenuation because of surrounding edema.

CT is the best method to differentiate empyemas from lung abscesses. Both may contain air/fluid levels. Characteristic features of empyema include a lenticular shape and compression of the surrounding lung by the empyema space such that the pulmonary vessels and bronchi are displaced and draped around the pleural

---

Box 18-4 Fluid Characteristics of Empyema

Grossly purulent
Organisms on stain or culture
WBC > 5×10^9 cells/liter
pH < 7.0
Glucose < 40 mg/ml

Box 18-5 Radiologic Features of Empyema

Standard radiographs
  Loculation
  Air/fluid level (BPF) varies in length on PA and lateral
Computed tomography
  Lenticular shape
  Compression of surrounding lung
  "Split pleura" sign

BPF, bronchopleural fistula.

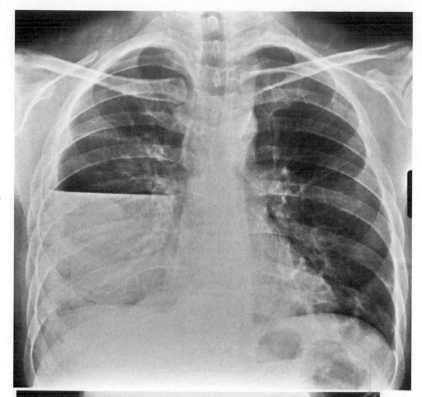

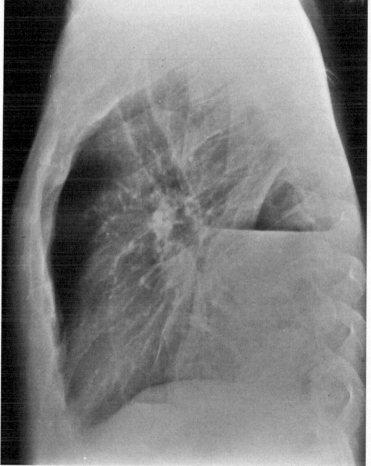

Fig. 18-18 Empyema with bronchopleural fistula. **A,** Frontal radiograph demonstrates an air/fluid level extending from the lateral chest wall to the mediastinum. **B,** Lateral view. The air/fluid level is considerably shorter in length and located posteriorly.

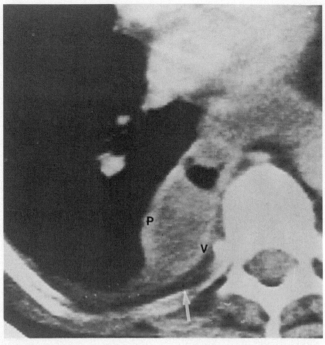

Fig. 18-19 "Split pleura" sign. Empyema. Enhancement and separation of the visceral (v) and parietal (p) pleura in a loculated posterior empyema. There is also an increase in extrapleural fat (arrow). (From McLoud TC, Flower CD: Imaging of the pleura: Sonography, CT and imaging, AJR 156:1145-1153, 1991.)

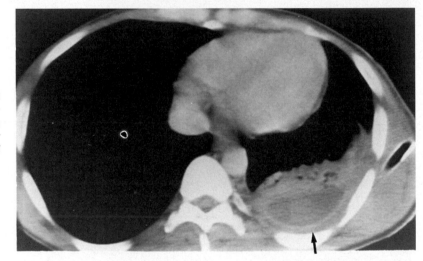

Fig. 18-20 Empyema. Lenticular fluid collection posteriorly. Adjacent lung is compressed and displaced by the empyema space. There is an increase in extrapleural fat (arrow). (From McLoud TC, Flower CD: Imaging of the pleura: Sonography, CT and imaging, AJR 156:1145-1153, 1991.)

fluid collection (Fig. 18-20). Abscesses on the hand often have a rounded shape and lack a distinct boundary with the adjacent lung parenchyma. The bronchi and vessels of the adjacent lung appear to end abruptly at the margins of the abscess. The "split pleura" sign can also be useful in differentiating empyemas from lung abscesses, although none of the above criteria are absolutely reliable.

CT is also a very useful guide to the treatment and drainage of empyemas, particularly when the empyema contains multiple areas of loculation. Imaging-guided interventional methods for the treatment of empyema are discussed in the next chapter.

PNEUMOTHORAX

Pneumothorax (Box 18-6) may be defined as the presence of air or gas within the pleural space. A pneumothorax is considered to be under tension if pleural pressure exceeds alveolar pressure. In such situations the pressure may reach atmospheric levels. Air may be combined with different types of fluid in the pleural space producing a hydropneumothorax, hemopneumothorax, or pyothorax respectively. Routes of entry of air into the pleural space include the lung and the mediastinum from pneumomediastinum. In the case of penetrating injury the route may be from outside the chest.

Epidemiology and Etiology

Spontaneous pneumothorax is the most common etiology, and it occurs predominantly in apparently healthy males during the third and fourth decades of life. It is associated with the presence of blebs that are gas pockets within the elastic fibers of the visceral pleura. This abnormality is localized and not necessarily associated with generalized pulmonary emphysema. Rupture of such a bleb produces spontaneous pneumothorax.

In addition to apical blebs there are many other causes of pneumothorax that are related to underlying lung disease or trauma. Chronic obstructive pulmonary disease, especially chronic bronchitis and emphysema, account for a second peak in the incidence of pneumothorax that occurs between 45 and 65 years of age. In these conditions the pneumothorax results from rupture of peripheral emphysematous areas. Recurrent pneumothorax may be associated with chronic infiltrative lung disease of any cause, but the prevalence is particularly high in two diseases, Langerhans' cell histiocytosis (histiocytosis X) and lymphangioleiomyomatosis. However, pneumothorax may be seen as a complication of late stages of other types of infiltrative lung disease that are associated with fibrosis and honeycombing.

Malignant neoplasms, particularly metastatic sarcoma, are occasional causes of spontaneous pneumothorax. The most common tumor type is metastatic osteogenic sarcoma. Pneumothorax may also be an occasional complication of septic infarcts and lung abscess. Catamenial pneumothorax is a rare but interesting manifestation of intrathoracic endometriosis.

A more common cause of pneumothorax is open or closed chest trauma. In blunt trauma, pneumothorax may occur without evidence of rib fracture, although rib fractures are commonly present. In such cases the lung may be lacerated by a rib fragment. Pneumothorax along with pneumomediastinum may occur in cases of tracheal, bronchial and esophageal rupture. This is discussed in more detail in Chapter 6. Penetrating thoracic injuries from knife or bullet wounds can also produce pneumothorax. Finally iatrogenic pneumothorax may be produced as a result of subclavian line placement, liver biopsy, percutaneous needle aspiration biopsy of the lung and renal biopsies. Pneumothorax is the most common form of barotrauma, occurring in about 25% of patients maintained on mechanical ventilation and positive-end expiratory pressure. Pneumothorax associated with mechanical ventilation may be antedated by the development of interstitial or mediastinal emphysema. It is frequently bilateral and under tension.

Clinical Features

The clinical features of pneumothorax, particularly the spontaneous variety, are characterized by the development of dyspnea and chest pain, which is aggravated by deep breathing and body movement. Occasionally asymptomatic pneumothorax is discovered incidentally. Bilateral pneumothorax is rare. In patients with chronic obstructive pulmonary disease, pneumothorax may potentially be lethal and lead to respiratory failure. Pneumothorax should always be suspected as a possible cause of sudden clinical deterioration in a patient with chronic obstructive pulmonary disease.

Radiologic Features

The radiologic findings of pneumothorax vary considerably depending on the degree of pulmonary collapse, the presence of tension, and other associated conditions (Box 18-7). The basic observation consists of recognizing that the outer margin of the visceral pleura and lung is separated from the parietal pleura and chest wall by a lucent gas space devoid of pulmonary vessels (Fig. 18-21). Typically in the upright patient the pneumothorax occurs at the lung apex. When a suspected pneumothorax is not definitely seen on an inspiration study, then an expiration radiograph may be diagnostic. The constant volume of the pneumothorax gas is accentuated by an overall reduction in the size of the hemithorax on expiration. Similar accentuation of a small pneumothorax can be obtained with lateral decubitus studies of the appropriate side. There are some pitfalls in the diagnosis of pneumothorax. These include skinfolds, clothing, tubing artifacts, and abnormalities of the chest wall as well as cavitary and bullous lung disease. A skinfold can be particularly troublesome (Fig. 18-22). The density characteristics of a skinfold are quite different from those of the visceral pleural tangent. The lung opacity of a skinfold progressively increases until it reaches a maximum at its tangent and then it abruptly becomes lucent.

Box 18-7 Radiologic Features Of Pneumothorax

STANDARD RADIOGRAPHS

Visceral pleural line separated from chest wall by gas space devoid of vessels

Apex when upright

Lung opaque only with complete collapse

Tension

    Mediastinal shift

    Depression of hemidiaphragm

Supine

    Medial recess—juxtacardiac

    Deep sulcus sign

    Subpulmonic

    Retrocardiac lucent triangle medially

ANCILLARY VIEWS

Expiratory

Decubitus

PITFALLS

Skinfolds

Clothing

Tubing artifacts

Bullae

CT

More sensitive in detection of small pneumothoraces

More accurate in determining size

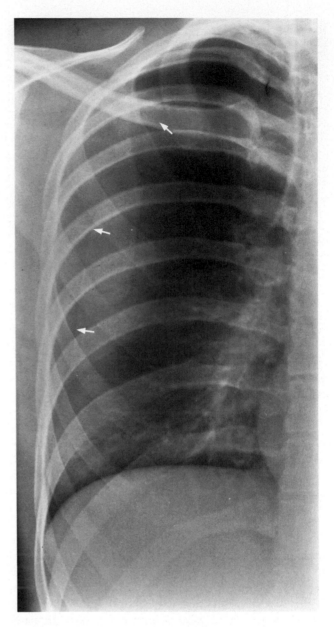

Fig. 18-21 Pneumothorax in an upright patient. The extremely thin visceral pleural line can be seen extending along the lateral aspect of the lung to the apex *(arrow)*. Exterior to the line is a gas space devoid of vessels.

This is quite different from the uniform lucency of the pneumothorax lung and pleural space interrupted by a thin visceral pleural tangent. Large avascular bullae or thin-walled cysts have concave rather than convex inner margins and do not exactly conform to the normal shape of the costophrenic sulcus when they occur at the lung base (Fig. 18-23).

When lung collapse is nearly complete from pneumothorax, the lung hangs limply from the hilum, and the margins of the separate lobes can often be seen (Fig. 18-24). The collapsed lung will be uniformly opaque. This is in contrast to a small pneumothorax where the lung, although partially collapsed, usually does not change in density. When a flap-like pleural defect results in a tension pneumothorax the pleural space becomes expanded. Manifestations of tension pneumothorax include mediastinal shift, diaphragmatic depression, and rib cage expansion at maximum inspiration (Fig. 18-24). The degree of lung collapse is not a dependable sign for or against tension. Underlying lung disease may prevent total collapse even if tension is present. Little if any mediastinal shift will be noted in patients maintained on positive airway pressure despite the presence of a tension pneumothorax.

In the supine patient identification of a pneumothorax is more difficult than in the erect patient because air will often accumulate along the long ventral surface of the lung rather than at the apex (Fig. 18-25). The medial pleural recess is a common site for pleural air to accumulate, and air can often be identified along the juxtacardiac area. Anteromedial air in the pleural space may produce a deep anterior costophrenic sulcus often referred to as the "deep sulcus" sign, which outlines the medial hemidiaphragm under the heart. Air in such a location often produces an appearance of a lucency projected in the right or left upper abdominal quadrants.

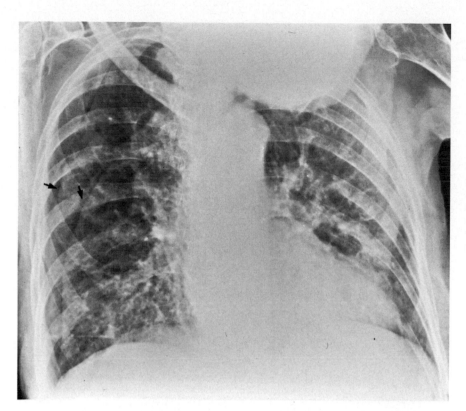

Fig. 18-22 Skinfolds. There are two skinfolds on the right *(arrows)*. Note the increasing opacification that they produce with an abrupt transition to lucency laterally. Skinfolds often produce an edge rather than the crisp visceral pleural line produced by a pneumothorax.

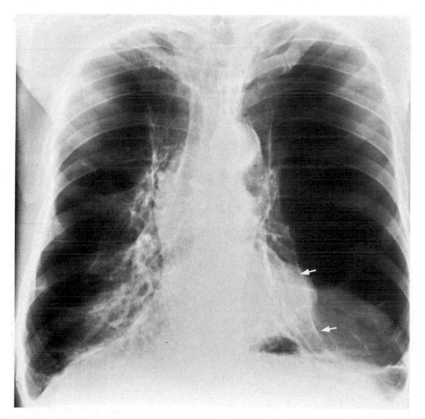

Fig. 18-23 Large bullae simulating pneumothorax. The left lung is lucent, devoid of vessels and almost completely replaced by bullae. The bullae have concave margins *(arrows)*, in contradistinction to pneumothorax where the lung margin is convex and parallels the chest wall.

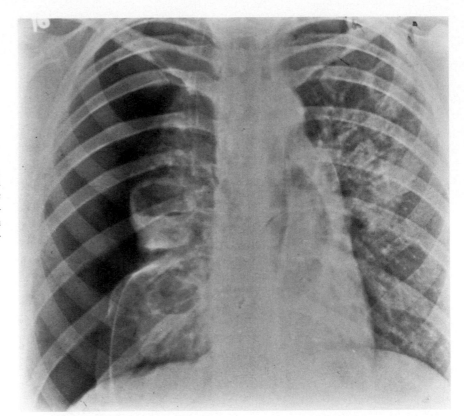

Fig. 18-24 Large tension pneumothorax. There is large pneumothorax on the right with almost complete collapse of the right lung. The margins of the lobes can be seen. There is evidence of tension with shift of the mediastinum to the left and depression of the right hemidiaphragm.

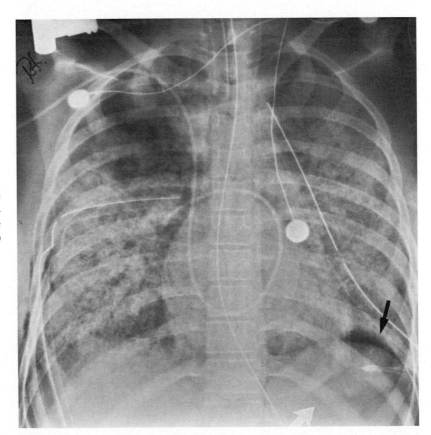

Fig. 18-25 Pneumothorax in a supine patient. Portable AP radiograph demonstrates a subpulmonic pneumothorax *(black arrow)* as well as lucency projecting in the area of the left upper quadrant in the anterior costophrenic sulcus ("deep sulcus" sign) *(white arrow)*.

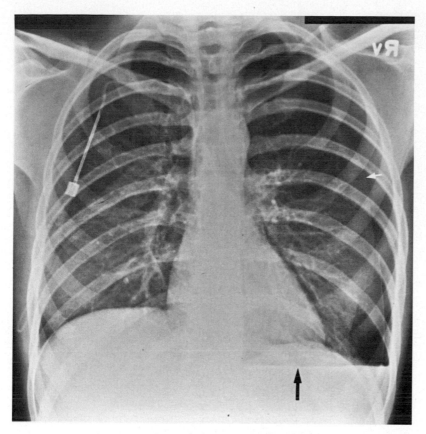

Fig. 18-26 Hydropneumothorax. Erect frontal view demonstrates an air/fluid level at the base of the left pleural space *(black arrow)*. The pneumothorax can also be seen extending along the lateral chest wall and at the apex *(white arrow)*.

Pneumothorax may also accumulate in a subpulmonic location. This will produce a sharply outlined hemidiaphragm that is well defined and a deep lateral costophrenic sulcus (Fig. 18-25). Occasionally pneumothorax will accumulate posteromedially in supine patients and will appear as a lucent triangle located medially at the lung base. This appearance was previously thought to be due to air in the pulmonary ligament. However, recent CT studies suggest that air at this location is usually posterior to the ligament and actually represents a pneumothorax. Occasionally pneumothorax air may be identified in either the major or minor fissures.

You should remember to carefully search for subtle signs of pneumothorax in intubated patients maintained on positive pressure ventilation. Rapid increase in size of a pneumothorax may occur with the development of tension and result in respiratory arrest. Heart-lung transplantation, bilateral lung transplantation, and emphysema volume lung reduction surgery may create a communication between the right and left pleural spaces so that air or fluid can move from one side to the other.

The presence of fluid of any type in the pleural space accompanying a pneumothorax will produce an air/fluid level if the film is taken with the patient in the erect position (Fig. 18-26). In the supine patient the diagnosis of hydropneumothorax is more difficult. A hydrothorax or hemothorax frequently coexists with a pneumothorax. When the pneumothorax is small and pleural con-

tact is maintained at the lung base the fluid will appear as a meniscus on the erect radiograph. When the pneumothorax is large a typical air/fluid interface will be identified.

Other imaging studies are rarely used for the evaluation of pneumothorax. A ventilation scan may be helpful in distinguishing bullae from pneumothoraces because bullae will have delayed wash-in and prolonged wash-out of xenon, and a pneumothorax will fail to show evidence of ventilation. CT is much more sensitive than plain films in detecting small pneumothoraces, particularly in the supine patient. Unsuspected small pneumothoraces are frequently detected at the bases of the lungs in patients who have sustained trauma and who undergo abdominal CT.

Accurately estimating the size of a pneumothorax is very difficult. It is not often realized that a pneumothorax that occupies the peripheral inch of the lung amounts to about 30% of total lung volume. Percentage estimations are generally speaking inaccurate and most often underestimate the true size of the pneumothorax.

FOCAL PLEURAL DISEASE

The most common focal pleural abnormalities include pleural plaques, localized pleural tumors, and local extension of bronchogenic carcinoma.

Box 18-8   Fibrous Tumors of Pleura

CLINICAL FEATURES

< 5% of pleural tumors
Equal sex incidence
50% asymptomatic
Hypertrophic pulmonary osteoarthropathy
Episodic hypoglycemia (4% to 5%)

PATHOLOGIC FEATURES

80% visceral pleura, 20% parietal pleura
Encapsulated, pedunculated
60% benign, 40% malignant
Malignant—invade chest wall and recur locally; pleural
    effusion

RADIOLOGIC FEATURES

Standard radiographs
    Round or lobulated
    Slow growth
    Variable size
    May be mobile

COMPUTED TOMOGRAPHY

Displace lung parenchyma
Enhancement after contrast
Acute angles with chest wall
Malignant
    Large
    Chest-wall invasion
    Pleural effusion

Pleural Plaques

Pleural plaques are discussed in the chapter dealing with pneumoconiosis (Chapter 8).

Localized Pleural Tumors

Localized pleural tumors are relatively uncommon. They usually fall into one of two types: fibrous tumors of the pleura or lipomas. Liposarcomas are extremely rare, but the pleura may commonly be invaded locally by adjacent bronchogenic carcinoma. CT is the imaging modality most commonly used for the assessment of localized pleural tumors because of its ability to determine the tissue composition (i.e., lipoma) and to determine extension into the lungs or chest wall.

Fibrous tumors of the pleura

Clinical features   Fibrous tumors of the pleura (Box 18-8) were previously referred to as "benign fibrous mesotheliomas". They account for less than 5% of all pleural tumors and have an equal sex incidence. The peak incidence occurs in the sixth to seventh decades. They are not related to asbestos exposure. Approximately 50% of individuals will be asymptomatic. These tumors can occasionally reach extremely large size and produce symptoms that consist of cough, dyspnea, and chest pain.

These tumors have a high incidence of associated hypertrophic osteoarthropathy and episodic hypoglycemia may be present in 4% to 5% of cases.

Pathologic features   Eighty percent of these tumors arise from the visceral pleura and 20% from the parietal pleura. They usually are encapsulated and frequently pedunculated with a broad-based pleural attachment. Vascular structures are present in the tumor pedicle. Microscopically approximately 60% of the localized fibrous tumors of the pleura are benign, and 40% are malignant. They all, however, have a good prognosis; all benign tumors and 45% of malignant tumors are cured by means of surgical resection. The malignant tumors may invade the chest wall and then after surgical excision recur locally, but they do not metastasize widely. Some of the malignant lesions are associated with pleural effusion. As mentioned previously these tumors may reach enormous sizes and tumors greater than 10 cm in diameter are more likely to be malignant. Calcification is present in 5% or less of cases.

Radiologic features   Fibrous tumors of the pleura usually appear as round or lobulated pleural masses that show evidence of slow growth and variable size (Fig. 18-27). Those that are attached to the visceral pleura by a pedicle may be mobile and will change location over time on serial chest radiography or when the position of the patient is altered.

CT findings are similar to those observed on plain radiography (Fig. 18-28). When these tumors are large it may be difficult to determine that they arise from the pleura although they typically displace the lung parenchyma. Enhancement of tumor following contrast administration is a frequent finding. On CT scans most of the tumors form acute angles with the chest wall. Lesions may be heterogeneous due to necrosis and hemorrhage. The malignant pleural fibrous tumors are usually greater than 10 cm, may invade the chest wall, and can be associated with pleural effusion. Central necrosis is common in the larger tumors. Calcification, however, is rare.

On MR imaging, these lesions often have relatively low signal intensity on both T1W and T2W images because of the high fibrous content (Fig. 18-29).

Lipomas and liposarcomas

Lipomas may occur either in the pleural space or mediastinum. These lesions are asymptomatic and are usually discovered incidentally on chest radiographs. Some are purely intrathoracic but others may be transmural and involve the chest wall. A definitive diagnosis is usually not possible on standard films. However, CT clearly delineates

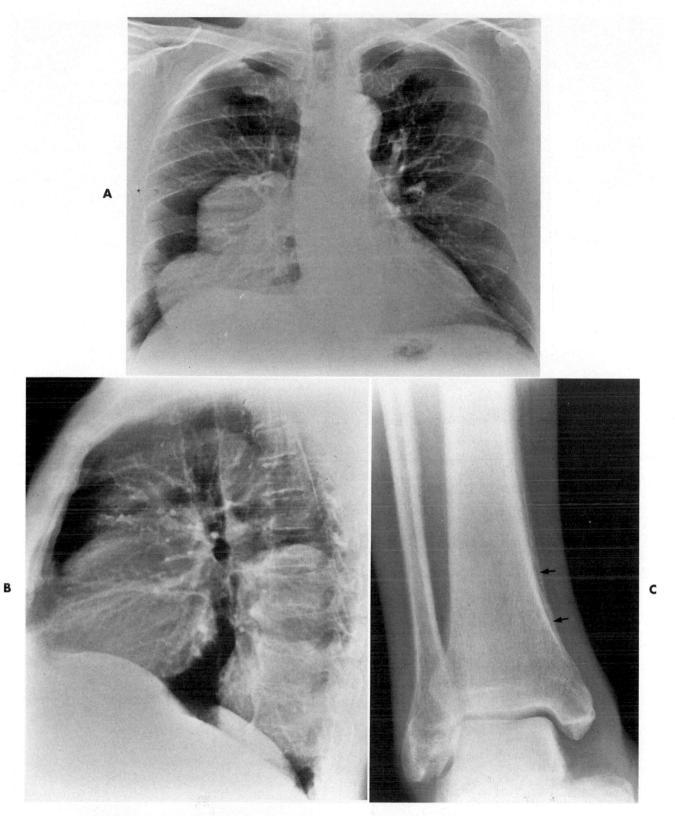

Fig. 18-27   Fibrous tumor of the pleura. **A** and **B**, PA and lateral views demonstrate a large bulky mass medially and posteriorly in the right hemithorax. The origin from the pleura can be suspected, because the mass is longer than it is wide and conforms to the shape of the pleural space. **C,** Right lower leg. There is periosteal reaction along the medial surface of the distal tibia indicating hypertrophic pulmonary osteoarthropathy *(arrows).*

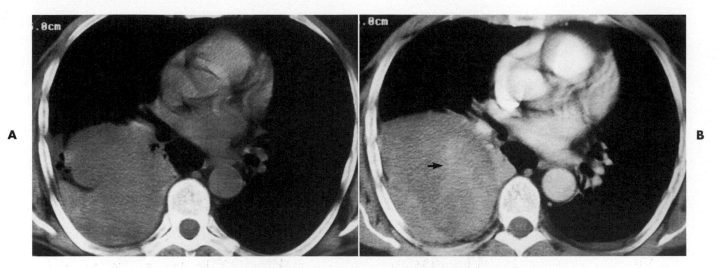

Fig. 18-28.   CT—fibrous tumor of the pleura. **A,** Precontrast scan shows a mass posteriorly of fairly uniform attenuation that makes an acute angle with the lateral chest wall. **B,** After the administration of contrast, focal areas of enhancement can be appreciated *(arrow)*.

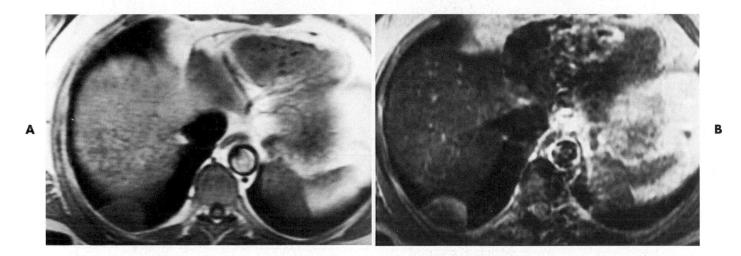

Fig. 18-29   MRI—fibrous tumor of the pleura. **A,** Spin-echo T1W image shows a mass posteriorly of signal intensity equal to muscle. **B,** On the T2W image most of the mass remains of low signal intensity with a slightly bright rim.

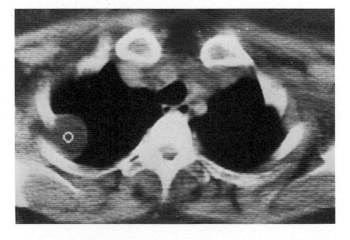

Fig. 18-30   Lipoma. CT demonstrates intrapleural tumor of fatty composition (-90 HU). *(From McLoud TC, Flower CD: Imaging of the pleura: Sonography, CT and MR imaging, AJR 156:1145-1153, 1991.)*

the pleural origin of these lesions in the majority of cases and their fatty composition (–50 to –150 Hounsfield Units [HU]) (Fig. 18-30). Benign lipomas have a completely uniform fatty density although linear soft-tissue strands due to fibrous stroma may be present. When the tumor is heterogeneous and has higher attenuation greater than –50 HU, a liposarcoma should be suspected. Liposarcomas usually contain a mixture of fat and soft-tissue attenuation. These are extremely rare tumors.

Pleural extension of bronchogenic carcinoma

The features of pleural extension of bronchogenic carcinoma are discussed in Chapter 11 on neoplasms.

DIFFUSE PLEURAL DISEASE

Both benign and malignant diseases may cause diffuse pleural abnormalities. Causes include fibrothorax as well as malignant tumors such as malignant mesothelioma and metastatic carcinoma.

The radiographic definition of diffuse pleural thickening is somewhat arbitrary, and there is no general consensus on such a definition. However, it has been suggested that diffuse pleural thickening consists of a smooth uninterrupted pleural opacity extending over at least a fourth of the chest wall with or without obliteration of the costophrenic angles. The CT definition that has been used in describing asbestos-related changes consists of thickening that extends more than 8 cm in the craniocaudal direction and 5 cm laterally, and a pleural thickness more than 3 mm.

Fibrothorax

Definition and clinical features

Common causes of fibrothorax or diffuse pleural fibrosis (Box 18-9) include organized hemorrhagic effusions,

tuberculous effusions, pyogenic empyema, and benign asbestos-related pleurisy. When it is bilateral it may produce a restrictive defect leading to respiratory compromise and occasionally respiratory failure.

One of the common causes of diffuse pleural thickening is asbestos exposure. This is discussed in Chapter 8 on pneumoconioses.

Radiologic features

A number of radiologic features, particularly CT features, may permit a diagnosis of the etiology of fibrothorax. Underlying parenchymal disease can be seen in patients who have had tuberculosis or empyema previously. Extensive calcification of the visceral pleura favors previous tuberculosis or empyema (Fig. 18-31). Calcification is seldom seen with asbestos-related pleurisy. When pleural thickening occurs as a sequela of a benign asbestos pleurisy there are usually bilateral pleural abnormalities detected, whereas other causes of diffuse pleural thickening usually lead to unilateral pleural abnormalities (Fig. 18-32).

CT may be helpful in the differentiating benign from malignant pleural thickening (Box 18-10) (Figs. 18-33 and 18-34). Benign fibrothorax seldom involves the mediastinal pleura. Involvement of the mediastinal pleura on the other hand is common with malignant mesothelioma and metastatic adenocarcinoma. Malignant thickening is more frequently nodular and masslike (Fig. 18-34). CT is also helpful in the assessment of the underlying lung when there is extensive pleural thickening present. The pleural thickening may interfere with the diagnosis of subtle parenchymal lung abnormalities such as interstitial disease due to asbestosis.

Malignant Mesothelioma

Clinical features

Diffuse malignant mesothelioma (Box 18-11) is a rare primary pleural neoplasm. Approximately 2000 to 3000 cases per year are reported in the United States. Ap-

---

Box 18-9 Fibrothorax

ETIOLOGY

Hemorrhagic effusions
Tuberculous effusion
Pyogenic empyema
Benign asbestos pleurisy

RADIOLOGIC FEATURES

Standard film
 > 1/4 chest wall in length
CT
 ≥ 8 cm in length
 > 5 cm laterally
 > 3 mm thick

Box 18-10 Benign versus Malignant Pleural Thickening

BENIGN	MALIGNANT
< 1 cm thick	> 1 cm thick
Does not involve entire pleura	Circumferential
Spares mediastinal surface	Involves mediastinal surface
Smooth	Nodular

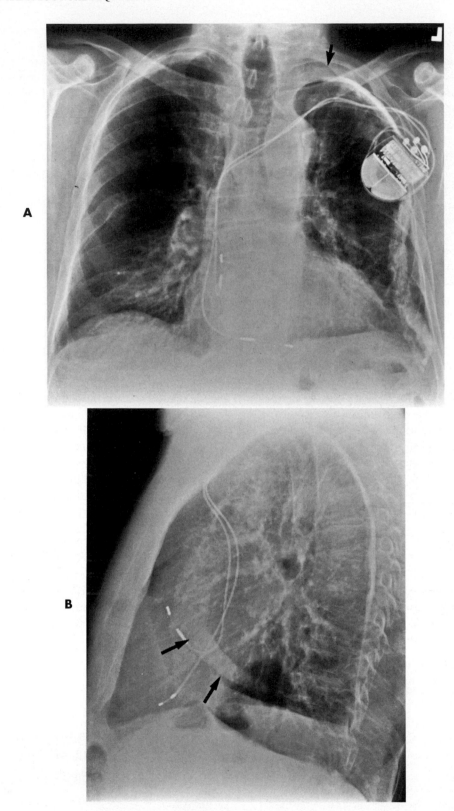

Fig. 18-31   **A** and **B,** Calcified fibrothorax in a patient treated many years ago with pneumothorax for tuberculosis. There is extensive calcification surrounding the entire lung. On the frontal view the calcification can be easily localized to the visceral pleura *(arrow).* On the lateral view the pleura is markedly thickened anteriorly *(arrows).*

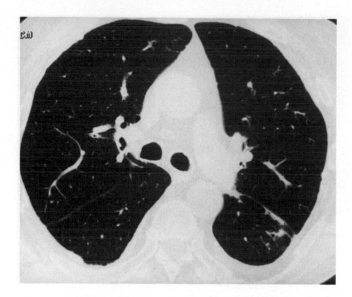

Fig. 18-32 Asbestos related pleural thickening. CT shows bilateral diffuse thickening. No calcification is noted.

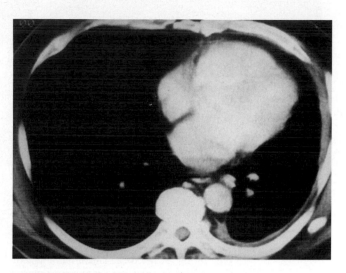

Fig. 18-33 Benign diffuse pleural thickening post empyema. CT demonstrates smooth thickening without nodularity involving the lateral and posterior but not the mediastinal pleural surfaces.

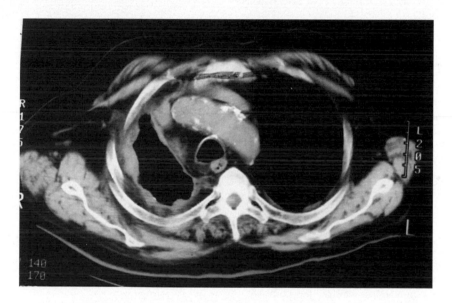

Fig. 18-34 Malignant mesothelioma. There is diffuse pleural thickening on the right which is nodular and extends along the mediastinal pleural surface. The volume of the right hemithorax is reduced. Plaques are present on the left.

proximately 80% of these lesions occur in individuals exposed to asbestos. The amphibolic asbestos fibers are the most carcinogenic or tumorogenic. There is usually a 30- to 40-year latency period between the time of initial exposure and the development of malignant mesothelioma. The incidence is highest in cities with shipyards and asbestos plants. It usually occurs in the sixth to eighth decades of life with a male to female predominance of approximately 4 to 1. Clinical symptoms are frequently present 6 to 8 months prior to diagnosis and consist mainly of chest pain, although dyspnea, cough, and weight loss may also be present. Prognosis is

extremely poor in this tumor with a median survival of 10 months or less.

Pathologic features

There are three major histologic types of malignant mesothelioma: epithelial, sarcomatous or mesenchymal, and mixed. The epithelial type is the most common and accounts for 50%. The major differential diagnosis for the pathologist is metastatic adenocarcinoma, and a generous biopsy specimen that allows for immunohistochemistry and ultrastructural analysis is usually required to make the differentiation. The classic gross features include sheets,

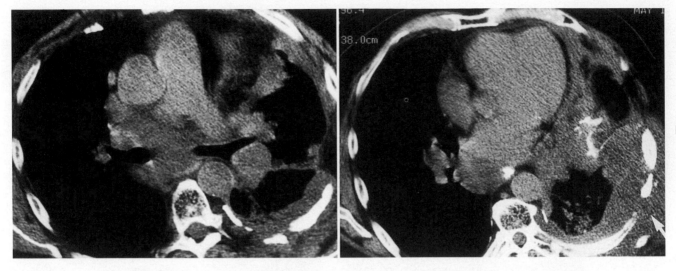

Fig. 18-35   **A** and **B,** Malignant mesothelioma. There is diffuse pleural thickening on the left, which is lobular. The tumor involves the major fissure and extends into the chest wall *(arrow).*

Box 18-11   Malignant Mesothelioma

CLINICAL FEATURES

Rare—2000 to 3000 cases/year
80%—history of asbestos exposure
30- to 40-year latency
6th to 8th decades of life
Men more than women, 4:1
Symptoms
  Chest pain
  Dyspnea; weight loss

PATHOLOGIC FEATURES

Types
  Epithelial (50%)
  Sarcomatous
  Mixed
Gross features
  Encasement of lung
  Growth of tumor into lung, chest wall, mediastinum,
  diaphragm

RADIOLOGIC FEATURES

Standard radiographs
  Diffuse pleural thickening
    Nodular
    Encases lung
  Pleural effusion
  Pleural mass
  Decrease in size of hemithorax, shift of mediastinum to
  affected side
  Plaques
CT
  Staging
  Extent
  Chest wall, mediastinal diaphragmatic invasion
MR
  Improved staging

---

plaques, and masses of tumor that coat the pleural surface. There is involvement of both the parietal and visceral pleura in most cases. The lung is encased and tumor grows into the fissures and the interlobular septa eventually producing parenchymal involvement. Crossover to the opposite pleural space and invasion of the mediastinum, chest wall, and diaphragm may occur.

Radiologic features

The most common radiologic feature is diffuse pleural thickening that is irregular and nodular with or without an associated pleural effusion (Fig. 18-34). In a minority of cases effusion alone or a pleural mass will be detected. Pro-

gressively the irregular pleural surface will enlarge producing multiple pleural masses. Frequently the diffuse pleural involvement results in decrease in the size of the hemithorax with restriction of the underlying lung and shift of the mediastinum toward the side of the disease (Fig. 18-34). Other findings of asbestos-related pleural disease (e.g., plaques), occur in only 20% to 25% of cases. Occasionally pleural effusions and mesothelioma may be associated with marked contralateral shift of the mediastinum.

CT is particularly helpful in assessing both the presence and the staging of malignant mesothelioma. CT findings include pleural thickening (92%), thickening of the interlobular fissures (86%), pleural effusion (74%), loss of vol-

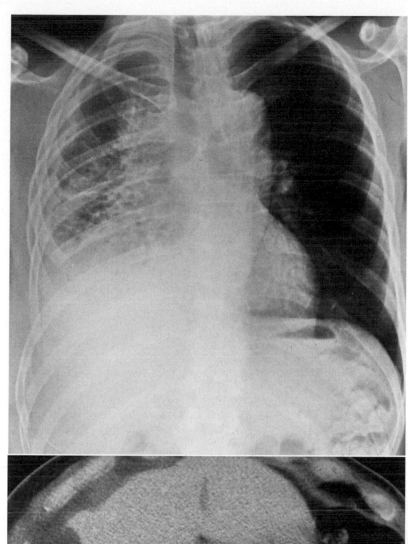

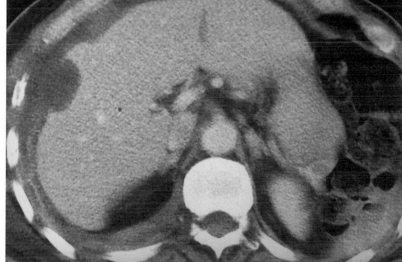

Fig. 18-36 Malignant mesothelioma. **A,** Standard radiograph demonstrates diffuse pleural thickening on the right with contracture of the right lung. **B,** CT shows involvement of the peritoneum and liver.

ume of the involved hemithorax (42%), pleural calcification (20%), and invasion of the chest wall 18% (Fig. 18-35). Metastases from malignant mesothelioma may occur to hilar and mediastinal nodes, but distant metastases are much less common. On CT the pleural thickening is typically circumferential and involves the mediastinal pleural surface. It is nodular and the thickness of the pleura almost always exceeds 1 cm. However, malignant mesothelioma cannot be reliably differentiated from pleural metastases.

Extrapleural pneumonectomy is occasionally used in an attempt to produce a cure. Although the results are somewhat disappointing, CT can be helpful in the preoperative staging of patients with this disease. CT may identify unresectable disease such as direct chest wall and mediastinal invasion; spread to the contralateral thorax or mediastinal lymph nodes; or spread through the diaphragm to the abdomen (Fig. 18-36). CT is also useful in the follow-up of patients who have undergone

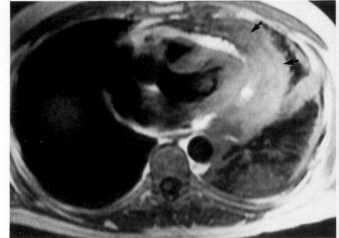

A

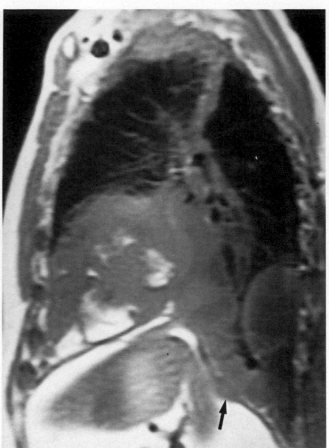

B

Fig. 18-37 MRI of malignant mesothelioma. Extensive left mesothelioma involving the pericardium, **A,** *(arrows)* and diaphragm, **B** *(arrow)*.

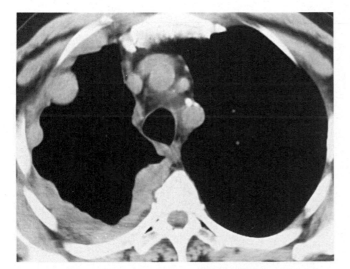

Fig. 18-38 Metastatic disease to the right pleural space from renal cell carcinoma. Note the nodular pleural thickening. *(From McLoud TC, Flower CD: Imaging of the pleura: Sonography, CT and MR imaging, AJR 156:1145-1153, 1991.)*

Box 18-12 Pleural Metastases

Origins
  Lung
  Breast
  Ovary
  Stomach
  Lymphoma
Manifestations
  Malignant effusion
  Diffuse thickening
  Focal seeding

tumor resection, often suggesting the presence of tumor recurrence before there is other radiologic or clinical evidence.

MR findings typically consist of tumor showing minimally increased signal on T1 and moderately increased signal on T2. MR may be superior to CT in determining the extent of disease because it allows better evaluation of apical tumor, diaphragmatic and infradiaphragmatic extension, and the relationship of tumors to mediastinal structures (Fig. 18-37).

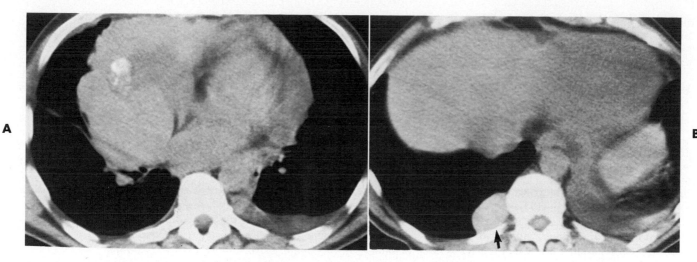

Fig. 18-39. Malignant thymoma. **A,** There is a large anterior mediastinal mass. **B,** A nodular pleural mass is noted posteriorly and inferiorly on the right *(arrow).* Proven pleural seeding. *(From McLoud TC, Flower CD: Imaging of the pleura: Sonography, CT and MR imaging,* AJR *156:1145-1153, 1991.)*

Pleural Metastases

Pleural metastases (Box 18-12) are the most common pleural neoplasm, accounting for 95% of cases. Metastases to the pleura are usually adenocarcinoma with sites of origin including the lung, breast, ovary, and stomach. Lymphoma may also involve the pleural space. There are three major manifestations of pleural metastases with pleural effusion being by far the most common. However, occasionally pleural metastases may produce diffuse pleural thickening with masses similar to malignant mesothelioma and involvement of the pleura may occasionally occur due to direct pleural seeding from tumors within the thorax such as malignant thymoma.

Malignant pleural effusion

Malignant pleural effusion is the most common manifestation of metastatic involvement. Metastatic disease to the pleura is probably only second to congestive heart failure as a cause of pleural effusion in patients over the age of 50, and it is the most common cause of an exudative effusion. The most common cause of a malignant pleural effusion is an underlying lung cancer. This occurs in 15% of patients at initial evaluation and 50% of patients with disseminated disease. Breast cancer is the second most common cause of malignant effusion (25%), followed by lymphoma (10%) and ovarian and gastric carcinoma (5% or less). In approximately 10% of patients with malignant pleural effusion, the primary site is unknown.

Diffuse pleural thickening

Diffuse pleural thickening due to solid pleural metastases may occur with peripheral lung adenocarcinoma but also secondary to adenocarcinomas arising elsewhere. Lymphoma can manifest as plaquelike or nodular thicken-

ing of the pleura or large pleural masses. Extensive pleural thickening similar to that of malignant mesothelioma may occur with metastatic disease to the pleura (Fig. 18-38). Diffuse encasement of the underlying lung occurs with shift of the mediastinum to the ipsilateral side.

Pleural seeding

Solid pleural metastases may occur by means of direct seeding (Fig. 18-39). This is usually from primary intrathoracic tumors, the most common being malignant thymoma. In those patients in whom malignant thymoma has been resected, careful follow-up with CT is recommended to determine the presence of recurrence involving the pleura. This will typically appear as small plaquelike areas of pleural thickening.

SUGGESTED READINGS

Aberle DR, Gamsu G, Ray CS: High-resolution CT of benign asbestos related diseases: Clinical and radiographic correlation, *AJR* 151:883-891, 1988.

Antman KH, Corson JM: Benign and malignant pleural mesothelioma, *Clin Chest Med* 6:127-140, 1985.

Bressler EL, Francis IR, Glazer GM, Gross BH: Bolus contrast medium enhancement for distinguishing pleural from parenchymal lung disease: CT features, *J Comput Assist Tomogr* 11:436-440, 1987.

Craighead JE: Current pathogenetic concepts of diffuse malignant mesothelioma, *Human Pathol* 18:544-557, 1987.

Dedrick CG, McLoud TC, Shepard JO, Shipley R: Computed tomography of localized pleural mesothelioma, *AJR* 144:275-280, 1985.

Dwyer A: The displaced crus: A sign for distinguishing between pleural fluid and ascites on computed tomography, *J Comput Assist Tomogr* 2:598-599, 1978.

England DM, Hochholzer L, McCarthy MJ: Localized benign and malignant fibrous tumors of the pleura: A clinicopathologic review of 223 cases, *Am J Surg Pathol* 13:640-658, 1989.

Epler GR, McLoud TC, Munn CS, Colby TV: Pleural lipoma: Diagnosis by computed tomography, *Chest* 90:265-268, 1986.

Evans AR, Wolstenholte RJ, Shettar SP, Yogish H: Primary pleural liposarcoma, *Thorax* 40:554-555, 1985.

Fleischner FG: Atypical arrangement of free pleural effusion, *Radiol Clin North Am* 1:347-362, 1963.

Fraser RG, Paré JAP, Paré PD, Fraser RS, Genereux GP: *Diagnosis of diseases of the chest*, ed 3, Philadelphia, 1991, WB Saunders; pp. 2712-2793.

Friedman AC, Fiel SB, Radecki PD, Lev-Toaff AS. Computed tomography of benign pleural and pulmonary parenchymal abnormalities related to asbestos exposure, *Semin Ultrasound, CT, MR* 11:393-408, 1990.

Friedman PJ, Hellekant CAG: Radiologic recognition of bronchopleural fistula, *Radiology* 124:289-295, 1977.

Friedman RL: Infrapulmonary pleural effusions, *Am J Roentgenol Radium Ther Nucl Med* 71:613-623, 1954.

Greene R, McLoud TC, Stark P: Pneumothorax, *Semin Roentgenol* 12:313-325, 1977.

Griffin DJ, Gross BH, McCracken S, Glazer GM: Observation on CT differentiation of pleural and peritoneal fluid, *J Comput Assist Tomogr* 8:24-28, 1984.

Halvorsen RA, Fedyshin PJ, Korobkin M, Foster WL Jr, Thompson WM: Ascites or pleural effusion? *RadioGraphics* 6:135-149, 1986.

Henschke CI, Davis SD, Romano PM, et al: Pleural effusions: Pathogenesis, radiologic evaluation and therapy, *J Thorac Imaging* 4:49-60, 1989.

Henschke CI, Yankelevitz DT, Davis SD, et al: Diseases of the pleura. In Freundlich IM, Bragg DG, editors: *A radiologic approach to diseases of the chest*, Baltimore, 1992, Williams & Wilkins; pp. 225-234.

Jones RN, McLoud T, Rockoff SD: The radiographic pleural abnormalities in asbestos exposure: Relationship to physiologic abnormalities, *J Thorac Imaging* 3:56-66, 1988.

Kawashima A, Libshitz HI: Malignant pleural mesothelioma: CT manifestations in 50 cases, *AJR* 155:965-969, 1990.

Lee KS, Im JG, Choe KO, Kim CJ, Lee BH: CT findings in benign fibrous mesothelioma of the pleura: Pathologic correlation in nine patients, *AJR* 158:983-986, 1992.

Leung AN, Müller NL, Miller RR: CT in differential diagnosis of diffuse pleural disease, *AJR* 154:487-492, 1990.

Light RW, MacGregor MI, Luchsinger PC, et al: Pleural effusions: The diagnostic separation of transudates and exudates, *Ann Intern Med* 77:507-513, 1972.

Lipscomb DJ, Flower CDR, Hadfield JW: Ultrasound of the pleura: An assessment of its clinical value, *Clin Radiol* 32:289-290, 1981.

Lorigan JG, Libshitz HI: MR imaging of malignant pleural mesothelioma, *J Comput Assist Tomogr* 13:617-620, 1989.

Malatskey A, Fields S, Libson E: CT apppearance of primary pleural lymphoma, *Comput Med Imaging Graphics* 13:165-167, 1989.

McLoud TC, Flower CD: Imaging the pleura: Sonography, CT and MR imaging, *AJR* 156:1145-1153, 1991.

McLoud TC, Woods BO, Carrington CB, Epler GR, Gaensler EA: Diffuse pleural thickening in an asbestos-exposed population: Prevalence and causes, *AJR* 144:9-18, 1985.

McLoud TC. The pleura and chest wall. In Haaga JR, Lanzieri CF, Sartoris DJ, Zerhouni EA, editors: *Computed tomography and magnetic resonance imaging of the whole body*, St. Louis, 1994, Mosby; pp 772-787.

Mendelson DS, Meary E, Buy JN, Pigeau I, Kirschner PA: Localized fibrous pleural mesothelioma: CT findings, *Clin Imaging* 15:105-108, 1991.

Mirvis S, Dutcher JP, Haney PJ, Whitley NO, Aisner J: CT of malignant pleural mesothelioma, *AJR* 140:665-670, 1983.

Montalvo BM, Morillo G, Sridhar K, Christoph C: MR imaging of malignant pleural mesotheliomas (abstract), *Radiology* 181(P):109, 1991.

Moskowitz H, Platt RT, Schachar R, Mellins H: Roentgen visualization of minute pleural effusion, *Radiology* 109:33-35, 1973.

Müller NL: Imaging the pleura, *Radiology* 186:297-309, 1993.

Munk PL, Müller NL: Pleural liposarcoma: CT diagnosis, *J Comput Assist Tomogr* 12:709-710, 1988.

Naidich DP, Megibow AJ, Hilton S, Hulnick DH, Siegelman SS: Computed tomography of the diaphragm: Peridiaphragmatic fluid localization, *J Comput Assist Tomogr* 7:641-649, 1983.

Naidich DP, Zerhouni EA, Siegelman SS: Pleura and chest wall. In Naidich DP, Zerhouni EA, Siegelman SS, editors: *Computed tomography and magnetic resonance of the thorax*, ed 2, New York, 1991, Raven-Lippincott; pp 407-471.

O'Moore PV, Mueller PR, Simeone JF, et al: Sonographic guidance in diagnostic and therapeutic interventions in the pleural space, *AJR* 149:1-5, 1987.

Rigler LG: Roentgenologic observations on the movement of pleural effusions, *Am J Roentgenol* 25:220-229, 1931.

Rusch VW, Godwin JD, Shuman WP: The role of computed tomography scanning in the initial assessment and the follow-up of malignant pleural mesothelioma, *J Thorac Cardiovasc Surg* 96:171-177, 1988.

Ruskin JA, Gurney JW, Thorsen MK, Goodman LR: Detection of pleural effusions on supine chest radiographs, *AJR* 148:681-683, 1987.

Saifuddin A, Da Costa P, Chalmers AG, Carey BM, Robertson RJH: Primary malignant localized fibrous tumours of the pleura: Clinical, radiological and pathological features, *Clin Radiol* 45:13-17, 1992.

Schwartz DA, Fuortes LJ, Galvin JR, et al: Asbestos-induced pleural fibrosis and impaired lung function, *Am Rev Respir Dis* 141:321-325, 1990.

Shuman LS, Libshitz HI: Solid pleural manifestations of lymphoma, *AJR* 142:269-273, 1984.

Silverman SG, Mueller PR, Saini S, et al: Thoracic empyema: Management with image-guided catheter darainage, *Radiology* 169:5-9, 1988.

Sohn SA. The pleura, *Am Rev Respir Dis* 138:184-234, 1988.

Stark DD, Federle MP, Goodman PC, Podrasky AE, Webb WR: Differentiating lung abscess and empyema: Radiography and computed tomography, *AJR* 141:163-167, 1983.

Staub NC, Wiener-Kronish JP, Albertine KH: Transport through the pleura: Physiology of normal liquid and solute exchange in the pleural space. In Chretien J, Bignon J, Hirsch A, editors: *The pleura in health and disease*, New York, 1985, Marcel-Dekker; pp. 169-193.

Teplick JG, Teplick SK, Goodman L, Haskin ME: The interface sign: A computed tomographic sign for distinguishing pleural and intra-abdominal fluid, *Radiology* 144:359-362, 1982.

Tocino I, Miller MH, Frederick PR, Bahr AL, Thomas F: CT detection of acute pneumothorax in head trauma, *AJR* 143:989-990, 1984.

van Sonnenberg E, Nakamoto SK, Mueller PR, et al: CT- and ultrasound-guided catheter drainage of empyemas after chesttube failure, *Radiology* 151:349-353, 1984.

Vix VA: Roentgenographic manifestations of pleural disease, *Semin Roentgenol* 12:277-286, 1977.

Yang PC, Luh KT, Chang DB, Wu HD, Yu CJ, Kuo SH: Value of sonography in determining the nature of pleural effusion: Analysis of 320 cases, *AJR* 159:29-33.

Zerhouni EA, Scott WW, Baker RR, Wareham MD, Siegelman SS: Invasive thymomas: Diagnosis and evaluation by computed tomography, *J Comput Assist Tomogr* 6:92-100, 1982.

CHAPTER 19

Interventional Techniques

THERESA C. McLOUD

A number of interventional techniques are performed in thoracic radiology. The most important is percutaneous transthoracic needle biopsy (TNB) of lung and mediastinal lesions. Other interventional procedures that are mostly related to the pleura include drainage of fluid collections, catheter drainage of pneumothoraces, and sclerotherapy.

TRANSTHORACIC NEEDLE BIOPSY

Indications

Transthoracic needle biopsies (Box 19-1) are performed most commonly for the diagnosis of an indeter-minate solitary pulmonary nodule. Not all solitary pulmonary nodules that are suspect for bronchogenic carcinoma require biopsy. If the pretest probability is very high for lung cancer or a biopsy is unlikely to have any impact on management, TNB should not be performed. For example, if a patient presents with a long smoking history and a new irregular spiculated nodule in the lung, the likelihood is extremely high that this represents a lung cancer, and it is perfectly reasonable to proceed directly to staging and resection. Other indications for TNB include undiagnosed mediastinal masses, a hilar mass when bronchoscopy is negative, single or multiple pulmonary nodules in a patient with a known extrathoracic malignancy or a suspicion of metastatic disease, and suspected infectious lesions presenting as solitary nodules, masses or very focal areas of consolidation, particularly in the immunocompromised host.

There are a number of diagnostic alternatives to TNB. The most important is bronchoscopy. However, bronchoscopy is preferred for central lesions, particularly if a prebronchoscopy CT scan shows evidence of endobronchial involvement. Transthoracic biopsy may be used to diagnose hilar masses when bronchoscopy is negative and extraluminal compression of the airway is noted. Transbronchial needle aspiration (Wang needle) is primarily used to establish metastatic malignancy in mediastinal nodes for the purposes of staging lung cancer. A needle is inserted via the bronchoscope through the tracheal wall or carina to facilitate the biopsy of such nodes. In the absence of a visible endobronchial lesion, the diagnostic yield for bronchoscopy in peripheral nodules is low in the range of 58% to 80% and is lowest for nodules less than 2 cm in diameter. Video-assisted thoracoscopy allows the diagnosis of peripheral subpleural pulmonary lesions. However, this is an operative procedure that requires an inpatient stay and general anesthesia, and that is more expensive than either bronchoscopy or transthoracic needle aspiration biopsy.

Box 19-1   Indications for TNB

Indeterminate solitary pulmonary nodule
Undiagnosed mediastinal mass
Hilar mass when bronchoscopy is negative
Single or multiple nodules when metastases are suspect
Probable infectious lesions presenting as nodules or
    masses

TNB, transthoracic needle biopsy.

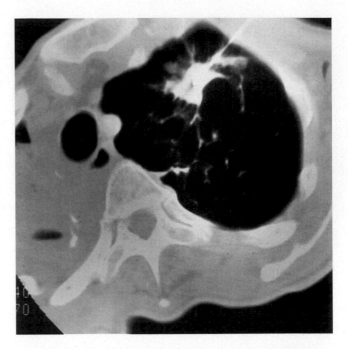

Fig. 19-1   Anterior approach to a lesion in the left upper lobe. The patient was placed in a slightly oblique position, and an oblique anterior approach was chosen to avoid bullae surrounding the mass.

Contraindications

Most contraindications to TNB are relative rather than absolute (Box 19-2). The most important is a bleeding diathesis. A prebiopsy prothrombin time, partial thromboplastin time, and platelet count are recommended. A careful history of coagulation abnormalities or the ingestion of drugs such as aspirin, which may lead to abnormal platelet function, should be obtained. Patients with low platelets who require an emergent biopsy, such as an immunocompromised patient with pulmonary infection, can receive platelet transfusions. Other relative contraindications include pulmonary hypertension. Needle biopsy can be safely attempted in patients with mild pulmonary hypertension if the nodule is peripheral. In the case of deep nodules or hilar masses it is not recommended. Patients should be cooperative and be able to maintain a certain position. Many patients will be biopsied in the prone position. Uncooperative patients may undergo biopsy under conscious sedation. Other relative contraindications include mechanical ventilation, bullae or severe emphysema in the path of the lesion to be biopsied, vascular lesions such as an arteriovenous malformation, severe chronic obstructive pulmonary disease (COPD) (a forced expiratory volume in one second [FEV_1] of less than 1 liter), and intractable cough.

Box 19-2   Relative Contradictions to TNB

Bleeding diathesis
Pulmonary hypertension
Uncooperative patient
Mechanical ventilation
Bullae
Severe COPD ($FEV_1 \leq 1.0$)
Intractable cough

COPD, chronic obstructive pulmonary disease; *FEV_1,* forced expiratory volume in one second.

Technique

Prebiopsy imaging

A CT is highly recommended prior to TNB. The exception may be extremely large and obviously malignant masses within the lung. CT is useful in providing a specific benign diagnosis in certain instances, for example, a calcified granuloma or hamartoma, and it can also provide information concerning the optimal approach to the lesion (Fig. 19-1). Areas of necrosis within large masses can be identified. Such areas should be avoided because they often produce nondiagnostic samples (Fig. 19-2). Vascular lesions such as aneurysms or arterial venous malformations can be easily recognized on contrast-enhanced CT.

Imaging guidance

Fluoroscopy or CT can be used for imaging guidance. Ultrasound is occasionally used for chest wall or peripheral lesions abutting the pleura. Fluoroscopically guided biopsies are usually reserved for large masses (Fig. 19-3). Fluoroscopy allows real-time moment to moment visualization and often permits the biopsy to be performed in less time than that required for a CT-guided biopsy. However, we prefer to use CT for imaging guidance in all of our transthoracic needle biopsies. It allows for a more complex approach, and safe and accurate sampling of hilar or mediastinal masses is possible. CT also provides better visualization of severe emphysematous areas or bullae, which may lie within the path of a needle. Real-

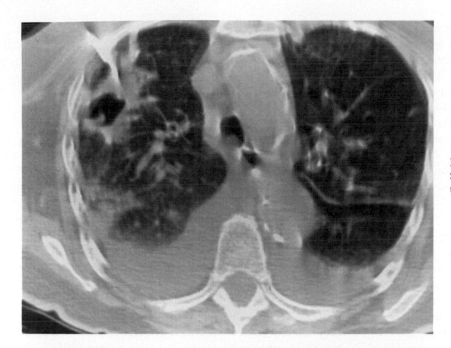

Fig. 19-2 Cavitary lesion right upper lobe. Specimens were taken from the wall of the lesion to avoid nondiagnostic areas of necrosis.

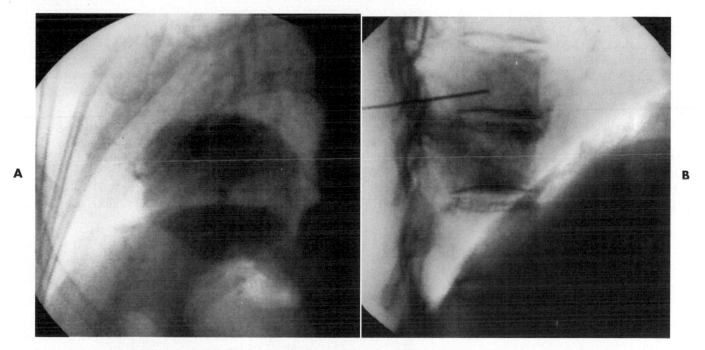

Fig. 19-3 **A** and **B,** Fluoroscopically guided biopsy of a large right lower lobe mass. A C-arm or biplane fluoroscopic unit should be used for such procedures.

time continuous CT fluoroscopy is currently available and combines the advantages of standard fluoroscopy with CT guidance.

Needle selection

There are a variety of needles that can be used for TNB. Small-bore 18- to 22-gauge needles are preferred because larger bore needles have been associated with high complication rates, particularly bleeding and pneu-

mothorax. Aspirating needles commonly used include Chiba and Greene varieties. Such needles only provide cytologic material from aspirates. Automatic biopsy devices, sometimes referred to as "biopsy guns," which provide small cores of tissue, are now available.

On-site pathology

The high diagnostic accuracy of TNB can be attributed to improved radiologic techniques such as CT guidance, but even more importantly to advances in cytologic techniques and interpretation. The transthoracic needle biopsy technique should be a cooperative effort between the cytologist and the radiologist. We prefer to have a cytologic technician available during the biopsy. Quick stains can be performed, and a cytologist can be called to provide a rapid interpretation of the specimen. This allows for rebiopsy if the specimen is nondiagnostic or inadequate and also permits the use of core-needle specimens as a supplement to the aspiration when the diagnosis cannot be obtained from the aspirated sample.

Technical factors

The shortest, most vertical biopsy path should be chosen based on the prebiopsy CT scan (Fig. 19-4). Interlobar fissures, pulmonary vessels, bullae, and areas of severe emphysema should be avoided (Fig. 19-1). The patient is placed in a position that provides such an approach—prone, supine, or, occasionally, decubitus—as indicated. After a scanogram is performed, thin-section 3 to 5 mm CT slices are obtained through the lesion with a localizing grid in place on the skin overlying the lesion. A desired skin puncture site is identified using the grid, and the patient is prepped and draped in the usual manner.

Although the biopsy needle may be introduced alone, we prefer a coaxial technique. A 19-gauge introducer spinal needle is placed by way of the skin and chest wall through the pleura just adjacent to or into the lesion to be biopsied. A smaller gauge, 21- or 22-gauge aspirating needle is then used for the actual biopsy and is placed by way of the introducer needle. Ultrathin 19-gauge introducer needles are now available that accommodate 20-gauge automatic biopsy devices for core specimens. The coaxial technique allows several specimens to be obtained with only one pleural puncture.

After the introduction of local anesthesia, a small puncture is made in the skin and subcutaneous tissues with a scalpel. The introducer 19-gauge needle is then advanced through the chest wall using intermittent CT scans to verify the position of the needle. It is important when performing TNB that the introducer needle is perfectly aligned with the lesion prior to the pleural puncture. It is very difficult to reposition or reorient the path of the needle once the lung is entered. Attempting to do so often produces a pleural tear.

Once the introducer needle has been correctly positioned immediately adjacent to or in the lesion, the stylet is removed and the 21- or 22-gauge aspirating needle is then placed through the introducer needle into the lesion. A 10-ml syringe is then attached to the thin needle, and, using a series of up and down and rotatory motions, an aspirate is obtained. The specimen should be immediately placed on glass slides and fixed with a number of available quick stains. If a core biopsy is used, the tissue can be rinsed into either formalin or saline. If the cytologist thinks the original pass with the aspirating needle is nondiagnostic or negative, additional samples may be taken, as well as core samples, using the coaxial technique. If inflammatory changes are present or there is a suspicion of active infection, specimens should also be sent to the bacteriology laboratory.

Postprocedure management

We consider "positional" precautions to be the best postprocedure management option. Patients are removed from the CT table and immediately placed with the puncture side dependent. For example, if the needle

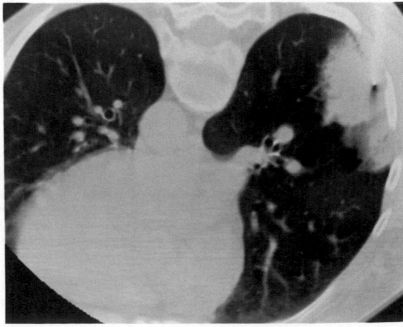

Fig. 19-4 Right lower lobe mass. The patient was placed in the prone position, and the most direct vertical path was used.

has been introduced through the back with the patient in prone position, he or she is immediately turned into the supine position. The patient is then transferred to a holding area where blood pressure and oxygen saturation (with a pulse oximeter) are monitored by the nursing staff. If the patient is asymptomatic he or she is kept quiet on a stretcher, and a radiograph is obtained 1 hour later to determine if a pneumothorax is present. If no pneumothorax is noted another film is obtained at 3 hours, and the patient can be discharged. If a small pneumothorax is present, it is followed for an additional 2 hours, and if there is no change in size the patient can also be discharged. However, symptomatic or enlarging pneumothoraces will require treatment.

The vast majority of TNBs are performed on outpatients. The patient should be instructed to come to the hospital with someone and be prepared to spend the evening of the biopsy in someone's company. Detailed instructions of signs and symptoms of pneumothorax are provided to the patients on discharge with instructions to return to the nearest hospital if such symptoms do occur. However, discharge when there is no pneumothorax or a small, stable pneumothorax is considered to be extremely safe because 98% to 100% of all pneumothoraces requiring chest tube drainage are detected within 1 hour of biopsy.

Complications

The most common complications of TNB (Box 19-3) are pneumothorax and hemoptysis. The incidence of pneumothorax has variously been reported to occur between 0% and 60%, with most institutions reporting approximately a 20% to 30% rate. Risk factors for the development of pneumothorax include the size and depth of the lesion, the presence of emphysema and COPD, the

use of multiple pleural punctures, and the transgression of a fissure. The percentage of biopsies requiring treatment (i.e., chest tube drainage) is much lower and ranges again from about 5% to 15%.

Small pneumothoraces can be managed conservatively as described previously with monitoring of vital signs and follow-up radiographs to confirm stability. Large or symptomatic pneumothoraces require placement of a chest tube. Adequate treatment can usually be accomplished with small-bore percutaneously inserted catheters. Such catheters may be attached to suction or to a Heimlich valve. There is controversy whether such patients with small-bore chest catheters can be managed on an inpatient or outpatient basis. We prefer to admit all patients who require chest tubes. Many do have continuing air leaks that require suction. Most chest tubes, however, can be removed within 24 to 48 hours.

Hemoptysis occurs in 1% to 10% of cases. A large degree of hemoptysis or significant hemorrhage is unusual if no bleeding diathesis exists. The incidence of hemorrhage increases with the size and gauge of the needle used (Fig. 19-5). Hemorrhage is almost always

---

Box 19-3 Complications of TNB

Pneumothorax (20% to 30%)
Chest tube (5% to 15%)
Hemoptysis (1% to 10%)
Seeding of biopsy track
Air embolism

TNB, transthoracic needle biopsy.

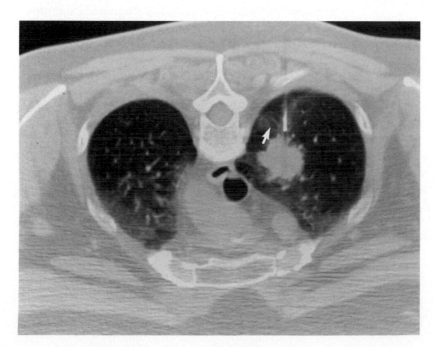

Fig. 19-5 Hemorrhage at biopsy site. There is a small area of ground-glass opacification around the needle *(arrow)* posterior to the mass. This represents a small area of bleeding. The patient did not experience hemoptysis.

self-limiting. In cases with more severe hemorrhage careful monitoring is required and the patient with hemoptysis should be reassured and placed biopsy-side down to prevent transbronchial aspiration of blood.

Malignant seeding of the biopsy track is a very rare complication. The use of an introducer needle with a coaxial technique provides protection from seeding. Most cases of seeding have been reported in malignant pleural tumors such as mesothelioma.

Systemic arterial air embolism is a rare but potentially fatal complication. It may produce myocardial infarction or stroke and occasionally death. The mechanism is presumed to be air entry via a pulmonary vein to the left atrium and systemic circulation. Precipitating factors may include coughing and positive pressure ventilation. We usually place saline in the introducer needle after the stylet is removed and before the aspirating needle is introduced into the lesion. This may prevent the sudden sucking of air through the needle and possibly lessen the danger of air embolism.

Diagnostic value

Transthoracic needle biopsy is extremely accurate in the diagnosis of cancer. Needle aspiration technique alone with excellent cytopathology has provided accurate diagnoses of over 90% of lung cancers in most large series. However, despite the high sensitivity for the diagnosis of intrathoracic malignancy, TNB is somewhat more limited in differentiating among different cell types of lung cancer. Several studies have shown approximately 80% accuracy in the typing of thoracic malignancies preoperatively. Generally the accuracy is less in the diagnosis of thoracic malignancies that are not carcinomas. The diagnosis of lymphoma usually requires larger core needle specimens to allow for the use of typing of lymphoma with immunoperoxidase staining.

A negative biopsy for malignancy should not be considered diagnostic. Thirty percent of nonspecific negative biopsies are eventually proven to represent malignancy. It is extremely important therefore to establish a precise benign diagnosis in lesions that prove by biopsy to be nonmalignant. The ability of TNB to accurately diagnose benign disease has been cited as a major limitation of the technique. This limitation is primarily attributable to the aspiration technique with small gauge needles. Active infections can be diagnosed using aspiration alone with a combination of cytologic analysis and appropriate stains or smears and cultures of aspirated material. However, the diagnosis of other benign nonactive infections such as well-established granulomas, hamartomas, lipoid pneumonia, and such has been disappointingly low—in the range of 10% to 40% in most series. However, the ability to obtain a specific benign diagnosis is greatly improved with the use of core needle biopsies. Such needles can provide histologic specimens

in over 80% of cases and can aid in the diagnosis of such lesions. The advent of small gauge spring-loaded automatic cutting needles has allowed for both reliable and safe retrieval of core tissue specimens from the lung, mediastinum, hila, and pleura. Small 20-gauge core needles can be introduced through an ultrathin 19-gauge introducing needle, permitting the use of the coaxial technique.

As has been mentioned previously, TNB may not be cost effective in adults with a high pretest likelihood of lung cancer who are candidates for curative surgical resection. However, there are several clinical situations in which needle biopsy may be extremely useful. It will establish the diagnosis in patients who are not operative candidates, and it may be useful in certain patient populations, for example, when the prevalence of granulomatous disease is very high—such as in river valleys in the United States where most solitary pulmonary nodules are due to histoplasmosis. In a recent as yet unpublished report from our institution, we have found that TNB had a major impact on clinical decision making in approximately 50% of the cases in which it was performed and resulted in marked cost savings compared with alternative diagnostic techniques, which included video-assisted thoracoscopic biopsy and thoracotomy.

TRANSTHORACIC HILAR AND MEDIASTINAL BIOPSY

Indications and Results

Most hilar lesions are biopsied via bronchoscopy. However, TNB may be useful in those cases in which bronchoscopy is negative, and the hilar mass is extrinsic to the airway. Most mediastinal masses proceed directly to surgery without a preoperative diagnosis. Exceptions, however, occur in the staging of lung cancer and also when lymphoma is suspected. TNB has a high sensitivity and specificity for the diagnosis of metastatic carcinoma to the hilum and mediastinum. Sensitivities over 90% have been reported. TNB has advantages over mediastinoscopy for nodal evaluation. It is faster, better tolerated, can be performed without general anesthesia, and also is less costly. Other alternative procedures include transbronchial (Wang needle) aspiration. This technique is useful when enlarged nodes are immediately adjacent to the trachea or are in the subcarinal location.

Fine needle aspiration biopsy has a lower diagnostic accuracy for lymphoma than for carcinoma. Sensitivity for fine needle aspiration has been reported in the range of 42% to 82%. However, the use of core biopsies has increased the yield, and patients can often be treated on the results of core needle biopsy alone.

In summary, the technique of TNB of the mediastinum is most useful for: (1) staging lung carcinoma where it is a less expensive and minimally invasive alternative to mediastinoscopy; and (2) for the diagnosis of lymphoma when advances in immunohistochemistry are combined with core biopsy techniques.

Technique

An anterior parasternal approach is preferred for most anterior mediastinal masses, while a posterior paravertebral approach is used for posterior mediastinal masses. Often a direct mediastinal approach can be used in which a passing through the lung and pleura is avoided. This lessens the likelihood of pneumothorax because a transpulmonary approach often requires puncturing the pleural space in two locations. The pleural or extrapleural approach to the mediastinum can be enhanced by widening the tract with injections of saline or air.

The hilum is usually approached through the lung obliquely (Fig. 19-6). It is important to administer contrast prior to the biopsy to determine the exact location of the major pulmonary arteries and veins.

Complications

Serious complications from transthoracic biopsy of the mediastinum are rare. Occasional mediastinal bleeding occurs, but this is usually self limited. However, at least one death due to pericardial tamponade has been reported. The incidence of hemoptysis and pneumothorax is similar to that for biopsy of lung lesions when the pulmonary parenchyma and pleura are traversed.

OTHER INTERVENTIONAL PROCEDURES IN THE THORAX

There are a spectrum of additional interventional procedures that radiologists may perform in the thorax. Many are related to pleural disease and processes. These include ultrasound-guided thoracenteses, drainage of empyemas or noninfected pleural collections, drainage of lung and mediastinal abscesses, and pleural sclerosis. Treatment of pneumothorax has already been discussed.

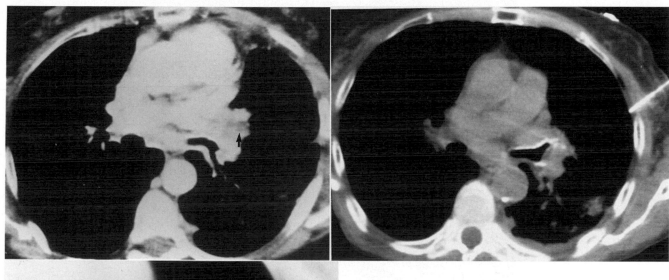

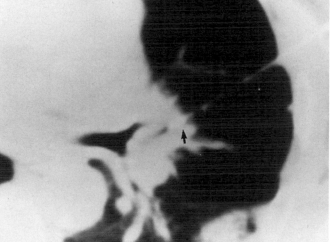

Fig. 19-6   TNB of left hilar mass. **A,** A preliminary scan with contrast reveals a nonopacified lesion in the left hilum *(arrow)*. **B,** An oblique anterior approach was used. **C,** Needle has entered the lesion *(arrow)* avoiding the pulmonary vessels. Biopsy positive for small cell carcinoma. A bronchoscopy showed extrinsic bronchial compression but no endobronchial lesion that could be biopsied.

Diagnosis and Treatment of Thoracic Fluid Collections

Thoracentesis

Most large pleural fluid collections can be tapped for diagnostic purposes by the attending clinician without the need for imaging guidance. Radiologic guidance increases the likelihood of obtaining pleural fluid and decreases the risk of pneumothorax. Ultrasound guidance is most useful when there are small amounts of fluid or when the fluid is loculated. Aspirated fluid can be sent for the usual diagnostic studies including gram stain, microbacteriologic culture, cytology, and chemistry evaluations, as well as pH levels.

Small 5 to 9 French (Fr) catheters may be inserted under ultrasound guidance along the guiding localizing needle to permit therapeutic thoracentesis when the fluid is serous and noninfected. Ultrasound is the guid-

ance procedure of choice for most thoracenteses; CT is reserved for loculated collections.

Empyema

If diagnostic aspiration reveals infection by gram stain or culture, drainage is indicated. Large free-flowing empyemas can be drained under ultrasound guidance. CT is usually reserved for loculated collections (Fig. 19-7). Radiologically guided catheters are usually used after large-bore thoracostomy tubes that have been introduced without imaging guidance have proved ineffective.

A needle is usually placed for localization, and then, using a Seldinger or trocar technique, a catheter is introduced. Such a technique is useful when collections are multiloculated or multiple collections are present. Routinely 12-Fr catheters are used, but larger catheters approaching the size of surgical chest tubes may be uti-

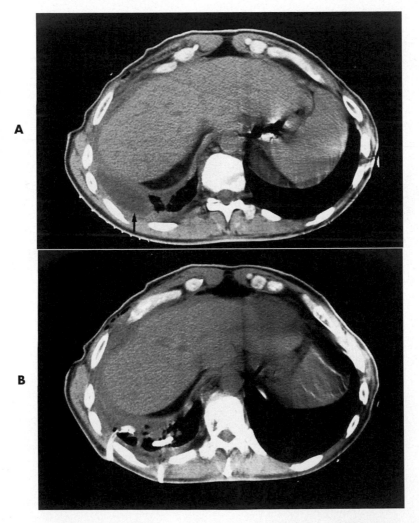

Fig. 19-7 CT-guided empyema drainage. **A,** Preliminary CT shows a small loculated fluid collection posteriorly *(arrow).* **B,** Successful drainage has been achieved with a radiologically placed catheter.

lized. Most catheters contain several holes for better drainage. Empyema drainage is effective in 80% to 90% of patients and complications occur in fewer than 10% of cases.

Mediastinal abscesses

Many mediastinal abscesses will be drained surgically. However, radiologically guided percutaneous techniques used for drainage are particularly useful in extremely ill patients. These are performed under CT guidance and either an anterior or posterior approach can be used. The pathway chosen to enter the collection should not traverse the pleura or the lung but only mediastinal structures.

Lung abscesses

Most lung abscesses are treated effectively with antibiotics, and they drain spontaneously via the bronchial tree. However, occasionally lung abscesses will fail to heal—particularly if there is bronchial obstruction, for example, secondary to a primary lung carcinoma. Drainage of lung abscesses can also be successfully treated with percutaneous catheter drainage. The access route should be through the contiguous abnormal pleura so that the normal lung is not punctured.

Sclerotherapy

Sclerotherapy of the pleural cavity can be performed for recurrent malignant effusion. Although a number of different agents such as bleomycin and tetracycline have been used, talc pleurodesis is now preferred. Several sessions may be necessary for successful treatment, and the lung must be well expanded in order for the treatment to be effective.

SUGGESTED READINGS

Austin JH, Cohen MB: Value of having a cytopathologist present during percutaneous fine-needle aspiration biopsy of lung: Report of 55 cancer patients and metaanalysis of the literature, *AJR* 160:175-177, 1993.

Cameron EWJ, Witton ID: Percutaneous drainage in the treatment of *Klebsiella pneumoniae* lung abscess, *Thorax* 32:673-676, 1977.

Casola G, vanSonnenberg E, Keightley A, Ho M, Withers C, Lee AS: Pneumothorax: Radiologic treatment with small catheters, *Radiology* 166:89-91, 1988.

Haramati LB: CT-guided automated needle biopsy of the chest, *AJR* 165:53-55, 1995.

Khouri NF, Stitik FP, Erozan YS, et al: Transthoracic needle aspiration biopsy of benign and malignant lung lesions, *AJR* 144:281-288, 1985.

Klein JS, Salomon G, Stewart EA: Transthoracic needle biopsy with a coaxially placed 20-gauge automated cutting needle: Results in 122 patients, *Radiology* 198:715-720, 1996.

Lee SI, Shepard JO, Boiselle PM, Trotman-Dickenson B, McLoud TC. Role of transthoracic needle biopsy in patient treatment decisions (abstract), *Radiology* 201(suppl):269, 1996.

Moore EH, Shepard JO, McLoud TC, et al: Positional precautions in needle aspiration lung biopsy, *Radiology* 175:733-735, 1990.

Morrissey B, Adams H, Gibbs AR, Crane MD: Percutaneous needle biopsy of the mediastinum: Review of 94 procedures, *Thorax* 48:632-637, 1993.

Naidich DP, Sussman R, Kutcher WL, Aranda CP, Garay SM, Ettenger NA: Solitary pulmonary nodules: CT-bronchoscopic correlation, *Chest* 93:595-598, 1988.

Pappa VI, Hussain HK, Reznek RH, et al: Role of image-guided core-needle biopsy in the management of patients with lymphoma, *J Clin Oncology* 14:2427-2430, 1996.

Parker SH, Hopper KD, Yakes WF, et al: Imaging-directed percutaneous biopsies with a biopsy gun, *Radiology* 171:663-669, 1989.

Protopapas Z, Westcott JL: Transthoracic needle biopsy of mediastinal lymph nodes for staging lung and other cancers, *Radiology* 199:489-496, 1996.

Schenk DA, Bower JH, Bryan CL, et al: Transbronchial needle aspiration staging of bronchogenic carcinoma, *Am Rev Respir Dis* 134:146-148, 1986.

Schenk DA, Bryan CL, Bower JH, Myers DL: Transbronchial needle aspiration in the diagnosis of bronchogenic carcinoma, *Chest* 92:83-85, 1987.

Seyfer AE, Walsh DS, Graeber GM, et al: Chest wall implantation of lung cancer after thin-needle aspiration biopsy, *Ann Thorac Surg* 48:284-286, 1989.

Sider L, Davis TM Jr: Hilar masses: Evaluation with CT-guided biopsy after negative bronchoscopic examination, *Radiology* 164:107-109, 1987.

Silverman SG, Mueller PR, Saini S, Hahn PF, Simeone JF, Forman BH, Steiner E, Ferrucci JT Jr: Thoracic empyema: Management with image-guided catheter drainage, *Radiology* 169:5-9, 1988.

vanSonnenberg E, D'Agostino H, Casola G, Wittich GR, Varney RR, Harker C: Lung abscess: CT-guided drainage, *Radiology* 178:347-351, 1991.

vanSonnenberg E, Nakamoto SK, Mueller PR, Casola G, Neff CC, Friedman PJ, Ferrucci JT Jr, Simeone JF: CT- and ultrasound-guided catheter drainage of empyema after chest-tube failure, *Radiology* 151:349-353, 1984.

Wang KP, Brower R, Haponik EF, Siegelman S: Flexible transbronchial needle aspiration for staging of bronchogenic carcinoma, *Chest* 84:571-576, 1983.

Weisbrod GL: Percutaneous fine-needle aspiration biopsy of the mediastinum, *Clin Chest Med* 8:27-41, 1987.

Weisbrod GL: Transthoracic percutaneous fine-needle aspiration biopsy in the chest and mediastinum, *Semin Interven Radiol* 8:1-14, 1991.

Westcott JL: Direct percutaneous needle aspiration of localized pulmonary lesions: Results in 422 patients, *Radiology* 137:31-35, 1980.

Westcott JL: Percutaneous needle aspiration of hilar and mediastinal masses, *Radiology* 141:323-329, 1981.

Wholey MH, Machek JS, Rhinehart ER, et al: Automated, percutaneous biopsy device, *Radiology* 174:567-568, 1990.

Zafar N, Moinuddin S: Mediastinal needle biopsy: A 15 year experience with 139 cases, *Cancer* 76:1065-1068, 1995.

Index